Hartman's Nursing Assistant Care
Long-Term Care and Home Care

Susan Alvare Hedman
Jetta Fuzy, RN, MS
and Suzanne A. Rymer, MSTE, RN, LSW

THIRD EDITION

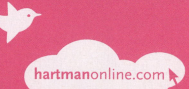

hartmanonline.com

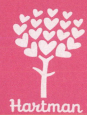

Hartman

Credits

Managing Editor
Susan Alvare Hedman

Designer
Kirsten Browne

Cover Illustrator
Iveta Vaicule

Production
Bill Brooks

Photography
Matt Pence
Pat Berrett
Art Clifton
Dick Ruddy

Proofreaders
Joanna Owusu
Emily Dings
Sarah Garrigan

Sales/Marketing
Deborah Rinker
Kendra Robertson
Erika Walker
Belinda Midyette
Carol Castillo

Customer Service
Fran Desmond
Thomas Noble
Angela Storey
Eliza Martin
Col Foley

Warehouse Coordinator
Chris Midyette

Copyright Information

© 2018 by Hartman Publishing, Inc.
1313 Iron Avenue SW
Albuquerque, New Mexico 87102
(505) 291-1274
web: hartmanonline.com
email: orders@hartmanonline.com
Twitter: @HartmanPub

ISBN 978-1-60425-070-1
ISBN 978-1-60425-073-2 (Hardcover)

PRINTED IN CANADA

Notice to Readers

Though the guidelines and procedures contained in this text are based on consultations with healthcare professionals, they should not be considered absolute recommendations. The instructor and readers should follow employer, local, state, and federal guidelines concerning healthcare practices. These guidelines change, and it is the reader's responsibility to be aware of these changes and of the policies and procedures of her or his healthcare facility.

The publisher, authors, editors, and reviewers cannot accept any responsibility for errors or omissions or for any consequences from application of the information in this book and make no warranty, express or implied, with respect to the contents of the book. The publisher does not warrant or guarantee any of the products described herein or perform any analysis in connection with any of the product information contained herein.

Gender Usage

This textbook uses the pronouns *he*, *his*, *she*, and *her* interchangeably to denote healthcare team members and residents and clients.

Special Thanks

A heartfelt thank you goes to our insightful and wonderful reviewers, listed in alphabetical order:

Sylette DeBois, DNP, MSN-Ed, RN
Kennesaw, GA

Laura R. Hoffmeister, RN, BSN, MA
Wausau, WI

Katherine Howard, MS, RN-BC, CNE
Edison, NJ

Charles A. Illian, RN, BSN
Orlando, FL

Elaine Amo Kafle, PhD, MS, RN
San Jose, CA

Gloria Nunn, PhD, RN
Suwanee, GA

We are very appreciative of the many sources who shared their informative photos with us:

- Briggs Corporation

- Detecto

- Dreamstime

- Exergen Corporation

- Harrisburg Area Community College

- Hollister Incorporated

- Invacare Corporation

- Laerdal Medical

- Dr. Jere Mammino

- Medline Industries

- The Medcom Group, Ltd.

- Motion Control, Inc.

- National Pressure Ulcer Advisory Panel

- North Coast Medical, Inc.

- Nova Medical Products

- RG Medical Diagnostics of Wixom, MI

- Sage Products LLC

- Standard Textile

- Teleflex

- Vancare, Inc.

- Welch Allyn

iv

Contents

Procedures

xii

Using a Hartman Textbook

Understanding how this book is organized and what its special features are will help you make the most of this resource!

We have assigned each chapter its own colored tab. Each colored tab contains the chapter number and title, and is located on the side of every page.

1. List examples of legal and ethical behavior

Everything in this book, the student workbook, and the instructor's teaching material is organized around learning objectives. A learning objective is a very specific piece of knowledge or a very specific skill. After reading the text, if you can do what the learning objective says, you know you have mastered the material.

bloodborne pathogens

Bold key terms are located throughout the text, followed by their definitions. They are also listed in the glossary at the back of this book.

Making an occupied bed

All care procedures are highlighted by the same black bar for easy recognition.

Guidelines: Handwashing

Guidelines and Observing and Reporting lists are colored green for easy reference.

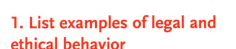

Residents' Rights
Food Choices
...ght to make...

Blue Residents' Rights boxes teach important information about how to support and promote legal rights and person-centered care.

Chapter Review

Chapter-ending questions test your knowledge of the information found in the chapter. If you have trouble answering a question, you can return to the text and reread the material.

Beginning and ending steps in care procedures

For most care procedures, these steps should be performed. Understanding why they are important will help you remember to perform each step every time care is provided.

Beginning Steps

Identify yourself by name. Identify the resident by name.	A resident's room is his home. Residents have a right to privacy. Before any procedure, knock and wait for permission to enter the resident's room. Upon entering his room, identify yourself and state your title. Residents have the right to know who is providing their care. Identify and greet the resident. This shows courtesy and respect. It also establishes correct identification. This prevents care from being performed on the wrong person.
Wash your hands.	Handwashing provides for infection prevention. Nothing fights infection in facilities like performing consistent, proper hand hygiene. Handwashing may need to be done more than once during a procedure. Practice Standard Precautions with every resident.
Explain procedure to resident. Speak clearly, slowly, and directly. Maintain face-to-face contact whenever possible.	Residents have a legal right to know exactly what care you will provide. This promotes understanding, cooperation, and independence. Residents are able to do more for themselves if they know what needs to happen.
Provide for the resident's privacy with a curtain, screen, or door.	Doing this maintains residents' rights to privacy and dignity. Providing for privacy in a facility is not simply a courtesy; it is a legal right.
Adjust the bed to a safe level, usually waist high. Lock the bed wheels.	Locking the bed wheels is an important safety measure. It ensures that the bed will not move as you are performing care. Raising the bed helps you to remember to use proper body mechanics. This helps prevent injury to you and to residents.

Ending Steps

Make resident comfortable.

Make sure the sheets are wrinkle-free and lie flat under the resident's body. This helps prevent pressure injuries. Replace bedding and pillows. Check that the resident's body is in proper alignment. This promotes comfort and health after you leave the room.

Return bed to lowest position. Remove privacy measures.

Lowering the bed provides for the resident's safety. Remove extra privacy measures added during the procedure. This includes anything you may have draped over and around the resident, as well as privacy screens.

Place call light within resident's reach.

A call light allows the resident to communicate with staff as necessary. It must always be left within the resident's reach. You must respond to call lights promptly.

Wash your hands.

Handwashing is the most important thing you can do to prevent the spread of infection.

Report any changes in the resident to the nurse. Document procedure using facility guidelines.

You will often be the person who spends the most time with a resident, so you are in the best position to note any changes in a resident's condition. Every time you provide care, observe the resident's physical and mental capabilities, as well as the condition of his or her body. For example, a change in a resident's ability to dress himself may signal a greater problem. After you have finished giving care, document the care using facility guidelines. Do not record care before it is given. If you do not document the care you gave, legally it did not happen.

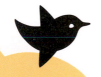

In addition to the beginning and ending steps listed above, remember to follow infection prevention guidelines. Even if a procedure in this book does not tell you to wear gloves or other PPE, there may be times when it is appropriate.

For example, the procedure for giving a back rub does not include gloves. Gloves are usually not required for a back rub. However, if the resident has open sores on his back, gloves are necessary.

1

Understanding Healthcare Settings

1. Discuss the structure of the healthcare system and describe ways it is changing

Health care is a growing field. The healthcare system refers to the different kinds of providers, facilities, and payers involved in delivering medical care. **Providers** are people or organizations that provide health care, including doctors, nurses, clinics, and agencies. **Facilities** are places where care is delivered or administered, including hospitals, long-term care facilities, and treatment centers (such as for cancer). **Payers** are people or organizations paying for healthcare services. These include insurance companies, government programs like Medicare and Medicaid, and individual patients or clients. Together, these people, places, and organizations make up the healthcare system.

This textbook will focus on two types of care: long-term care and home health care. **Long-term care (LTC)** is given in long-term care facilities for people who need 24-hour skilled care. **Skilled care** is medically necessary care given by a skilled nurse or therapist; it is available 24 hours a day. It is ordered by a doctor and involves a treatment plan. This type of care is given to people who need a high level of care for ongoing conditions. The term *nursing homes* was once widely used to refer to these facilities. Now they are often known as *long-term care facilities, skilled nursing facilities, rehabilitation centers,* or *extended care facilities.*

People who live in long-term care facilities may be disabled. They are often elderly, but younger adults sometimes require long-term care, too. They may arrive from hospitals or other healthcare settings. Their **length of stay** (the number of days a person stays in a healthcare facility) may be short, such as a few days or months, or longer than six months. Some of these people will have a **terminal illness**, which means that the illness will eventually cause death. Other people may recover and return to their homes or to other care facilities or situations.

Most people who live in long-term care facilities have **chronic** conditions. This means the conditions last a long period of time, even a lifetime. Chronic conditions include physical disabilities, heart disease, and dementia. (Chapter 18 has more information about these disorders and diseases.) People who live in these facilities are usually referred to as residents because the facility is where they reside or live. These places are their homes for the duration of their stay (Fig. 1-1).

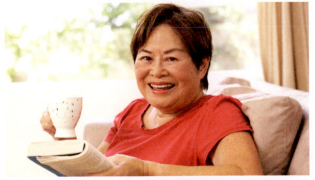

Fig. 1-1. People who live in long-term care facilities are called residents because the facility is where they reside for the duration of their stay.

Home health care, or home care, is provided in a person's home (Fig. 1-2). This type of care is also generally given to people who are older and are chronically ill but who are able to and wish to remain at home. Home health care may also be needed when a person is weak after a recent hospital stay. Skilled assistance or monitoring may be required. People who receive home health care are usually referred to as *clients*.

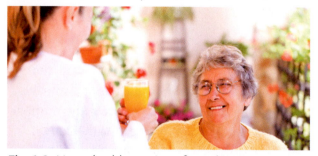

Fig. 1-2. Home health care is performed in a person's home. People receiving home care are generally referred to as clients.

In some ways, working as a home health aide is similar to working as a nursing assistant. Almost all care described in this textbook applies to both nursing assistants and home health aides. Most of the basic medical procedures and many of the personal care procedures are the same. Home health aides may also clean, shop for groceries, do laundry, and cook. (Information about home health care may be found in Chapters 24 through 30 of this textbook.)

Home health aides may have more contact with the client's family than nursing assistants do. They also will work more independently, although a supervisor monitors their work. The advantage of home care is that clients do not have to leave home. They may have lived there for many years, and staying at home can be comforting.

People who need long-term care or home health care will have different **diagnoses**, or medical conditions determined by a doctor. The stages of illnesses or diseases affect how sick people are and how much care they will need. The jobs of nursing assistants and home health aides will also vary. This is due to each person's different symptoms, abilities, and needs.

Other healthcare settings include the following:

Assisted living facilities are residences for people who need some help with daily care, such as showering, meals, and dressing. Help with medications may also be given. People who live in these facilities do not need 24-hour skilled care. Assisted living facilities allow for more independent living in a homelike environment. A resident can live in a single room or an apartment; however, some residents have roommates. An assisted living facility may be attached to a long-term care facility, or it may stand alone. Some assisted living facilities have *memory care* units for people who have mild dementia. These people are unable to live alone but are still fairly independent. **Dementia** is defined as the serious loss of mental abilities, such as thinking, remembering, reasoning, and communicating. There is more information about dementia in Chapter 19.

Adult day services are for people who need some assistance and supervision during certain hours, but who do not live in the facility where care is provided. Generally, adult day services are for people who need some help but are not seriously ill or disabled. Adult day services can also provide a break for spouses, family members, and friends.

Acute care is 24-hour skilled care given in hospitals and ambulatory surgical centers for people who require short-term, immediate care for illnesses or injuries (Fig. 1-3). People are also admitted for short stays for surgery.

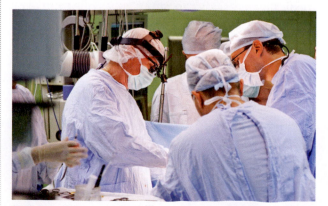

Fig. 1-3. Acute care is performed in hospitals for illnesses or injuries that require immediate care.

Subacute care is care given in hospitals or long-term care facilities. It is used for people who need less care than for an acute (sudden onset, short-term) illness, but more care than for a chronic (long-term) illness. Treatment usually ends when the condition has stabilized or after the predetermined time period for treatment has been completed. The cost is usually less than for acute care but more than for long-term care. Subacute care is covered in Chapter 22.

Outpatient care is usually given to people who have had treatments, procedures, or surgeries and need short-term skilled care. They do not require an overnight stay in a hospital or other care facility.

Rehabilitation is care given by specialists. Physical, occupational, and speech therapists help restore or improve function after an illness or injury. Information about rehabilitation and related care is located in Chapter 21.

Hospice care is given in facilities or homes for people who have approximately six months or less to live. Hospice workers give physical and emotional care and comfort until a person dies, while also supporting families during this process. There is more information about hospice care in Chapter 23.

Often payers control the amount and types of healthcare services people receive. The kind of care a person receives and where he receives it may depend, in part, on who is paying for it.

In 2010, the Patient Protection and Affordable Care Act (PPACA) was signed into law by President Barack Obama. This law is commonly referred to as the Affordable Care Act. Its goals include increasing the quality of health insurance, expanding insurance coverage (both public and private), and reducing healthcare costs. The Affordable Care Act has been controversial and, like any law, it may be changed by elected officials.

Public health insurance programs include Medicare and Medicaid, the Children's Health Insurance Program (CHIP), military health benefits from TRICARE and the Veterans Health Administration, and the Indian Health Service.

Private health insurance plans may be purchased by a person's employer, and costs are paid for by the employer or the employee, or shared by both. An individual may also purchase private health insurance directly. Coverage of medical services varies from plan to plan.

The healthcare system is constantly changing, and with these changes come new costs. New technologies and medications are being created, and better ways of caring for people in a wide variety of healthcare settings are being developed. Better health care helps people live longer, which leads to a larger elderly population that may need additional health care. New discoveries and expensive equipment have also increased healthcare costs (Fig. 1-4).

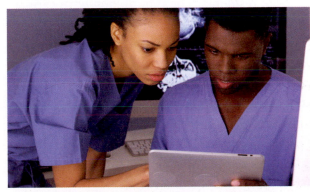

Fig. 1-4. *Technology makes it possible to offer better health care, but equipment can be expensive.*

Many health insurance plans employ cost-control strategies called **managed care. Health maintenance organizations (HMOs)** and **preferred provider organizations (PPOs)** are examples of managed care. Managed care seeks to control costs by limiting plan members' choice of healthcare providers and facilities. There is an increasing emphasis within managed care on promoting wellness as a means of reducing the need for healthcare services (and, as a result, reducing costs).

In the past, the goal of health care was simply to make sick people well. Today things are more complicated. Cost control is a consideration, as is the coordination of the many types of care a person might receive. While in many cases a person who is seriously ill will still be admitted to a hospital, hospital stays are often shorter now due to cost-control measures. After release from the hospital, many people need continuing care. This care may be provided in a long-term care facility, a rehabilitation hospital, or by a home health agency, depending on the needs of the patient or client.

2. Describe a typical long-term care facility

Long-term care facilities are businesses that provide skilled nursing care 24 hours a day. These facilities may offer assisted living housing, dementia care, or subacute care. Some facilities offer specialized care, while others care for all types of residents. The typical long-term care facility offers personal care for all residents and focused care for residents with special needs. Personal care includes bathing; skin, nail and hair care; mouth care; and assistance with walking, eating and drinking, dressing, transferring, and elimination. All of these daily personal care tasks are called **activities of daily living**, or **ADLs**. Other common services offered at these facilities include the following:

- Physical, occupational, and speech therapy

- Wound care

- Care of different types of tubes, including **catheters** (thin tubes inserted into the body to drain fluids or inject fluids)

- Nutrition therapy

- Management of chronic diseases, such as Alzheimer's disease, acquired immune deficiency syndrome (AIDS), diabetes, chronic obstructive pulmonary disease (COPD), cancer, and congestive heart failure (CHF)

When specialized care is offered at long-term care facilities, the employees must have special training. Residents with similar needs may be placed in units together. Nonprofit companies or for-profit companies can own long-term care facilities.

3. Describe residents who live in long-term care facilities

There are some general statements that can be made about residents in long-term care facilities. While it is helpful to understand the entire population, it is more important for nursing assistants to understand each individual for whom they will care. Residents' care should be based on their specific needs, illnesses, and preferences.

According to a survey conducted in 2013–2014 by the National Center for Health Statistics (cdc.gov/nchs), 84.9 percent of long-term care residents in the United States are over age 65. Almost 67 percent of residents are female. More than 76 percent are white and non-Hispanic (Fig. 1-5). About one-third of residents come from a private residence; over 50 percent come from a hospital or other facility.

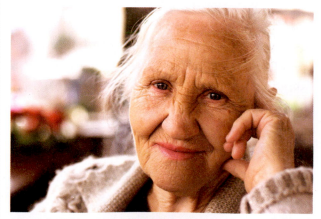

Fig. 1-5. *White, non-Hispanic women make up a high percentage of residents in long-term care facilities.*

The length of stay of over two-thirds of residents in long-term care is six months or longer. These residents need enough help with their activities of daily living to require 24-hour care. Often, they do not have caregivers available to give sufficient care for them to live in the community. The group with the longest average stay are people who are developmentally disabled. They are often younger than 65. More information about developmental disabilities may be found in Chapter 8.

The other third of residents stay for less than six months. This group generally falls into two categories. The first category is made up of residents admitted for terminal care. Due to their disease or condition, they will probably die in the facility. The second category is made up of residents admitted for rehabilitation or temporary illness. They will usually recover and return to the community. Care of these residents may be very different than care provided for permanent residents.

Dementia and other mental disorders are major causes of admissions to care facilities. Various studies place the number of residents with dementia in long-term care facilities as high as 90 percent. Many residents are admitted with other disorders as well. However, the disorders themselves are often not the main reason for admission. It is most often the lack of ability to care for oneself and the lack of a support system that leads people into a facility. A support system is vital in allowing the elderly to live outside a facility.

Some residents have very little outside support from family or friends. This is one reason it is essential to care for the whole person and his or her individual needs instead of only the illness or disease. Residents have many needs besides bathing, eating, drinking, and elimination. These needs will go unmet if staff do not work to meet them.

4. Explain policies and procedures

All facilities have manuals outlining their policies and procedures. A **policy** is a course of action that should be taken every time a certain situation occurs. For example, a very basic policy is that healthcare information must remain confidential. A **procedure** is a method, or way, of doing something. For example, a facility will have a procedure for reporting information about residents. The procedure explains what

form to complete, when and how often to fill it out, and to whom it is given. New employees will be told where to find a list of policies and procedures that all staff are expected to follow. Common policies at long-term care facilities include the following:

- All resident information must remain confidential. This is not only a facility rule, it is also the law. More information about confidentiality, including the Health Insurance Portability and Accountability Act (HIPAA), can be found in Chapter 3.

- The plan of care must always be followed. Nursing assistants should perform tasks assigned by the care plan. Tasks that are not listed in the care plan or approved by the nurse should not be performed.

- Nursing assistants should not do tasks that are not included in the job description.

- Nursing assistants must report important events or changes in residents to a nurse.

- Nursing assistants should not discuss personal problems with residents or their families.

- Nursing assistants should not take money or gifts from residents or their families (Fig. 1-6).

- Nursing assistants must be on time for work and must be dependable.

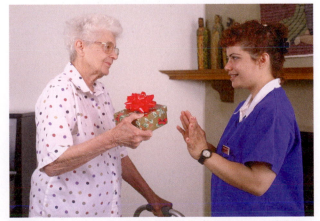

Fig. 1-6. *Nursing assistants should not accept money or gifts because it is unprofessional and may lead to conflict.*

Employers will have policies and procedures for every resident care situation. These have been developed to give quality care and protect resident safety. Procedures may seem long and complicated, but each step is important. It is essential that nursing assistants become familiar with and always follow policies and procedures.

5. Describe the long-term care survey process

Inspections are performed to help ensure that long-term care facilities (and home health agencies) follow state and federal regulations. Inspections are done periodically by the state agency that licenses facilities. These inspections are called surveys. They may be done more often if a facility has been cited for problems. To **cite** means to find a problem through a survey. Inspections may be done less often if the facility has a good record. Inspection teams include a variety of trained healthcare professionals.

Surveyors study how well staff care for residents. They focus on how residents' nutritional, physical, social, emotional, and spiritual needs are being met. They interview residents and their families and observe the staff's interactions with residents and the care given. They review resident charts and observe meals. Surveys are one reason the documentation done by nursing assistants is so important.

Surveyors use tags that identify specific federal regulations (F-Tags) to note any problems. When surveyors are in a facility, staff should try not to be nervous. They should give the same quality care they give every day, and answer any questions to the best of their abilities. If an employee does not know the answer to a surveyor's question, she should be honest and never guess. She should tell the surveyor that she does not know the answer but will find out as quickly as possible. Then she should follow up with the surveyor after she has the answer.

The **Joint Commission** is an independent, not-for-profit organization that evaluates and accredits healthcare organizations. Its standards focus on improving the quality and safety of care given to patients, clients, and residents. For an organization to receive accreditation from the Joint Commission, it must undergo a comprehensive survey process at least every three years. The survey process includes carefully checking performance in specific areas, such as patient rights, treatment, and infection prevention.

The Joint Commission's surveys are not associated with state inspections. Healthcare organizations are not required to participate in the Joint Commission's survey process; they may do so on a voluntary basis. Types of healthcare facilities that are accredited by the Joint Commission include hospitals, long-term care facilities, rehabilitation centers, hospice services, home health care agencies, laboratories, and other organizations.

6. Explain Medicare and Medicaid

The **Centers for Medicare & Medicaid Services (CMS)** is a federal agency within the United States Department of Health and Human Services. CMS runs two national healthcare programs: Medicare and Medicaid. They both help pay for health care and health insurance for millions of Americans. CMS has many other responsibilities as well.

Medicare (medicare.gov) is a federal health insurance program that was established in 1965 for people aged 65 or older. It also covers people of any age with permanent kidney failure or certain disabilities. Medicare has four parts. Part A (hospital insurance) helps pay for care in a hospital or skilled nursing facility or for care from a home health agency or hospice. Part B (medical insurance) helps pay for doctor services and other medical services and equipment. Part C (Medicare Advantage Plans) allows private health insurance companies to provide Medicare benefits. Part D (prescription drug coverage) helps pay for medications prescribed for treatment. Medicare will only pay for care it determines to be medically necessary.

Medicaid (medicaid.gov) is a medical assistance program for people who have a low income, as well as for people with disabilities. It is funded by both the federal government and each state. Eligibility is determined by income and special circumstances. People must qualify for this program.

Medicare and Medicaid pay long-term care facilities a fixed amount for services. This is based on the resident's needs upon admission and throughout his stay at the facility.

Home Care Focus

For home care, Medicare pays for intermittent, not continuous, services provided by a certified home health agency. The agency must meet specific guidelines established by Medicare. To qualify for home health care, Medicare recipients generally must be homebound, and their doctors must determine that they need home health care. Medicare will pay the full cost of most covered home healthcare services. However, Medicare will not pay for 24-hour-a-day home health care. Home health care plays an important role when skilled care is needed on a part-time basis.

---

7. Discuss the terms *culture change* and *person-centered care*

Many long-term care facilities promote meaningful environments with individualized approaches to care. **Culture change** is a term given to the process of transforming services for elders so that they are based on the values and practices of the person receiving care. Culture change involves respecting both elders and those working with them. Core values are promoting choice, dignity, respect, self-determination, and purposeful living. To honor culture change, healthcare settings may need to change their organization, practices, physical environments, and relationships.

Person-centered care (also known as *person-directed care*) emphasizes the individuality of the person who needs care, and recognizes and develops his or her capabilities. Person-centered care revolves around the resident and promotes his or her individual preferences, choices, dignity, and interests. Each person's background, culture, language, beliefs, and traditions are respected (Fig. 1-7). Improving each resident's quality of life is an important goal. Giving person-centered care will be an ongoing focus throughout this textbook.

The Pioneer Network (pioneernetwork.net) and Eden Alternative (edenalt.org) have more information.

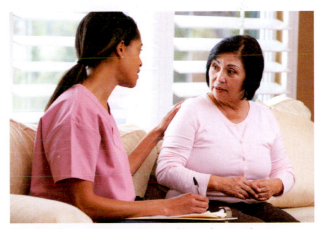

Fig. 1-7. *Person-centered care places the emphasis on the person needing care and his or her individuality and capabilities.*

Chapter Review

1. What is long-term care?

2. What is home health care?

3. List one fact about each of the following healthcare settings: assisted living facilities, adult day services, acute care, subacute care, outpatient care, rehabilitation, and hospice care.

4. List five services commonly offered at long-term care facilities.

5. Who makes up the majority of residents in long-term care—men or women?

6. What are two general categories of residents who stay in a care facility for less than six months?

7. List five common policies at long-term care facilities.

8. When surveyors visit a facility, what do they study and observe?

9. Whom does Medicare insurance cover?

10. Define *person-centered care*.

2

The Nursing Assistant and the Care Team

1. Identify the members of the care team and describe how the care team works together to provide care

Residents will have different needs and problems. Healthcare professionals with a wide range of education and experience will help care for them. This group is known as the *care team*. Members of the care team include the following:

Nursing Assistant (NA) or Certified Nursing Assistant (CNA): The nursing assistant (NA) performs assigned tasks, such as measuring vital signs, and provides or assists with personal care, such as bathing residents and helping with elimination needs. Nursing assistants spend more time with residents than other members of the care team. That is why they act as the "eyes and ears" of the team. Observing and reporting changes in the resident's condition or abilities is a very important role of the NA (Fig. 2-1). Nursing assistants must have at least 75 hours of training, and in many states, training exceeds 100 hours.

Registered Nurse (RN): In a long-term care facility, a registered nurse coordinates, manages, and provides skilled nursing care. This includes administering special treatments and giving medication as prescribed by a physician. A registered nurse also assigns tasks and supervises daily care of residents by nursing assistants. A registered nurse is a licensed professional who has graduated from a two- to four-year nursing program. RNs have diplomas or college degrees and

have passed a national licensure examination. Registered nurses may have additional academic degrees or education in specialty areas.

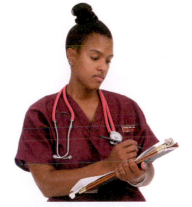

Fig. 2-1. *Observing carefully and reporting accurately are some of the most important duties nursing assistants perform.*

Licensed Practical Nurse (LPN) or Licensed Vocational Nurse (LVN): A licensed practical nurse or licensed vocational nurse administers medications and gives treatments. A licensed practical nurse or vocational nurse is a licensed professional who has completed one to two years of education and has passed a national licensure examination.

Physician or Doctor (MD [medical doctor] or DO [doctor of osteopathy]): A doctor diagnoses disease or disability and prescribes treatment (Fig. 2-2). Doctors have graduated from four-year medical schools, which they attended after receiving bachelor's degrees. Many doctors also attend specialized training programs after medical school.

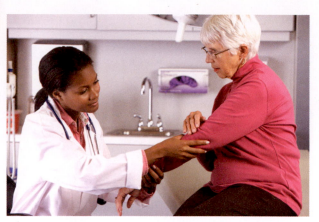

Fig. 2-2. A doctor makes a diagnosis and prescribes treatment.

Physical Therapist (PT or DPT): A physical therapist evaluates a person and develops a treatment plan to increase movement, improve circulation, promote healing, reduce pain, prevent disability, and regain or maintain mobility (Fig. 2-3). A PT administers therapy in the form of heat, cold, massage, ultrasound, electrical stimulation, and exercise to muscles, bones, and joints. A physical therapist has graduated from a three-year doctoral degree program (doctor of physical therapy, or DPT) after receiving an undergraduate degree. PTs have to pass a national licensure examination before they can practice.

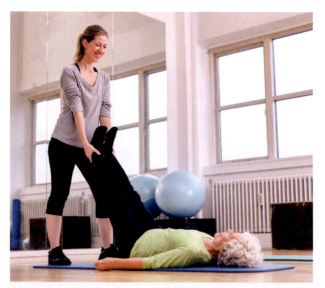

Fig. 2-3. A physical therapist helps exercise muscles, bones, and joints to improve strength or restore abilities.

Occupational Therapist (OT): An occupational therapist helps residents learn to adapt to disabil-

ities. An OT may help train residents to perform **activities of daily living (ADLs)**, such as bathing, dressing, and eating. This often involves the use of special equipment called **assistive** or **adaptive devices** (Fig. 2-4). (Chapter 21 has more information.) The OT evaluates the resident's needs and develops a treatment program. Occupational therapists have earned a master's degree and must pass a national licensure examination before they can practice.

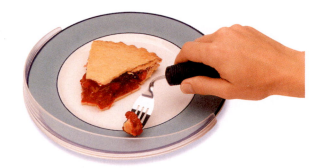

Fig. 2-4. An occupational therapist will help residents learn to use adaptive devices, such as this special fork and plate. (PHOTO COURTESY OF NORTH COAST MEDICAL, INC., 800-821-9319, WWW.NCMEDICAL.COM)

Speech-Language Pathologist (SLP): A speech-language pathologist, or speech therapist, identifies communication disorders, addresses factors involved in recovery, and develops a plan of care to meet recovery goals. An SLP teaches exercises to help the resident improve or overcome speech problems. An SLP also evaluates a person's ability to swallow food and drink. Speech-language pathologists have earned a master's degree in speech-language pathology and are licensed or certified to work.

Registered Dietitian (RD or RDN): A registered dietitian assesses a resident's nutritional status and develops a treatment plan to improve health and manage illness. A registered dietitian creates diets to meet residents' special needs and may also supervise the preparation of food and educate people about nutrition. Registered dietitians have completed a bachelor's degree and may also have completed postgraduate work. Most states require that registered dietitians be licensed or certified.

Medical Social Worker (MSW): A medical social worker determines residents' needs and helps get them support services, such as counseling and financial assistance. He may help residents obtain clothing and personal items if the family is not involved or does not visit often. A medical social worker may book appointments and transportation. Medical social workers have usually earned a master's degree in social work.

Activities Director: The activities director plans activities for residents to help them socialize and stay physically and mentally active. These activities are meant to improve and maintain residents' well-being and to prevent further complications from illness or disability. Games, performances, and arts and crafts are some types of activities that the activities director may plan or lead. An activities director has usually earned a bachelor's degree; however, he or she may have an associate's degree or qualifying work experience. An activities director may be called a *recreational therapist* or *recreation worker*, depending upon education and experience.

Resident and Resident's Family: The resident is an important member of the care team. Providing person-centered care means placing the resident's well-being first, and giving her the right to make decisions and choices about her own care. The resident helps plan care and the resident's family may also be involved in these decisions. The care team revolves around the resident and her condition, goals, priorities, treatment, and progress. Without the resident, there is no care team.

Information on home health aides as members of the care team is located in Chapter 24.

2. Explain the nursing assistant's role

A nursing assistant (NA) performs assigned nursing tasks, such as measuring a resident's temperature. A nursing assistant also provides personal care, such as bathing residents, helping

them eat and drink, and helping with hair care. Promoting independence and self-care are other very important tasks that a nursing assistant does. Common nursing assistant duties include the following:

- Bathing residents
- Assisting with grooming tasks
- Helping residents with elimination needs
- Assisting with range of motion exercises and ambulation (walking)
- Transferring residents from bed to chair or wheelchair
- Measuring vital signs (temperature, pulse rate, respiratory rate, blood pressure, and pain level)
- Assisting with meals (Fig. 2-5)
- Helping residents dress and undress
- Giving backrubs
- Helping with mouth care
- Making and changing beds
- Keeping residents' living areas neat and clean
- Caring for supplies and equipment

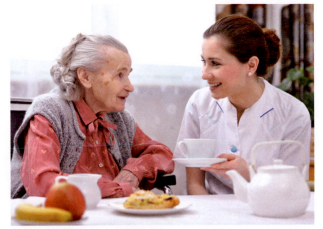

Fig. 2-5. *Helping residents eat and drink is an important part of a nursing assistant's job.*

Nursing assistants are not allowed to insert or remove tubes, give tube feedings, or change sterile dressings.

Some states allow nursing assistants to give medications if they have completed an additional, specialized course for medications and meet the requirements of the individual facility.

Nursing assistants spend more time with residents than other care team members. Observing changes in a resident's condition and reporting them is a very important duty of the NA. Residents' care can be revised or updated as conditions change. Another duty of the nursing assistant is noting important information about the resident; this is called **charting**, or documenting.

Nursing assistants are part of a team of health professionals. The team includes doctors, nurses, social workers, therapists, dietitians, and specialists. The resident and resident's family are part of the team. Everyone, including the resident, works closely together to meet goals. Goals include helping residents recover from illnesses and being able to do as much as possible for themselves.

Nursing assistants can have many different titles. *Nurse aide, certified nurse aide, patient care technician,* and *certified nursing assistant* are some examples. The title given varies by state requirements. This textbook will use the term *nursing assistant.*

Residents' Rights

Responsibility for Residents

All residents are the responsibility of each nursing assistant. A nursing assistant will receive assignments to perform tasks, care, and other duties for specific residents. If an NA sees a resident who needs help, even if the resident is not on his assignment sheet, the NA should provide the needed care.

3. Explain professionalism and list examples of professional behavior

Professional means having to do with work or a job. **Personal** refers to life outside a job, such as family, friends, and home life. **Professionalism** is behaving properly when on the job. It includes dressing appropriately and speaking well. It also includes being on time, completing tasks, and

reporting to the nurse. For a nursing assistant, professionalism means following the care plan, making careful observations, and reporting accurately. Following policies and procedures is an important part of professionalism. Residents, coworkers, and supervisors respect employees who behave professionally. Professionalism helps people keep their jobs and may also help them earn promotions and raises.

A professional relationship with residents includes the following:

- Providing person-centered care

- Keeping a positive attitude

- Doing only the assigned tasks that are in the care plan and that the NA is trained to do

- Keeping all residents' information confidential

- Always being polite and cheerful (Fig. 2-6)

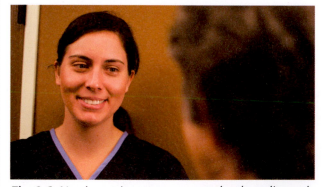

Fig. 2-6. *Nursing assistants are expected to be polite and cheerful in all circumstances.*

- Not discussing personal problems

- Not using personal phones in residents' rooms or in any resident care area

- Not using profanity, even if a resident does

- Listening to the resident

- Calling a resident *Mr., Mrs., Ms.,* or *Miss,* and his or her last name, or by the name he or she prefers; terms such as *sweetie, honey, dearie,* etc. are disrespectful and should not be used

- Never giving or accepting gifts

- Always explaining care before providing it
- Following practices, such as handwashing, to protect oneself and residents

A professional relationship with an employer includes the following:

- Completing tasks efficiently
- Always following policies and procedures
- Documenting and reporting carefully and correctly
- Reporting problems with residents or tasks
- Reporting anything that keeps a nursing assistant from completing duties
- Asking questions when the nursing assistant does not know or understand something
- Taking directions or feedback without becoming upset
- Being clean and neatly dressed and groomed
- Always being on time
- Communicating with the employer if the nursing assistant cannot report for work
- Following the chain of command
- Participating in education programs
- Being a positive role model for the facility

Nursing assistants must be:

Compassionate: Being **compassionate** means being caring, concerned, considerate, empathetic, and understanding. Demonstrating **empathy** means identifying with the feelings of others. People who are compassionate understand other people's problems. They care about them. Compassionate people are also sympathetic. Showing **sympathy** means sharing in the feelings and difficulties of others.

Honest: An honest person tells the truth and can be trusted. Residents need to feel that they can trust the people who care for them. The care team depends on honesty in planning care. Employers count on truthful records of the care provided and the observations made.

Tactful: Being **tactful** means showing sensitivity and having a sense of what is appropriate when dealing with others. It is the ability to speak and act without offending others.

Conscientious: People who are **conscientious** try to do their best. They are guided by a sense of right and wrong. They are alert, observant, accurate, and responsible. Giving conscientious care means making accurate observations and reports, following the care plan, and taking responsibility for one's actions (Fig. 2-7). For example, accurately measuring vital signs, such as temperature or pulse, is important. Other members of the care team will make treatment decisions based on the documented measurements. Without conscientious care, a resident's health and well-being are in danger.

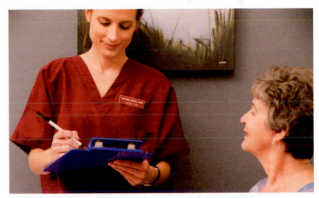

Fig. 2-7. *Nursing assistants must be conscientious about documenting observations and procedures.*

Dependable: Nursing assistants must be able to make and keep commitments. They must report to work on time. They must skillfully do assigned tasks, avoid absences, and help their peers when needed.

Patient: People who are patient do not lose their tempers easily. They do not act irritated or complain when things are hard. Residents are often elderly and may be sick or in pain. They may take a long time to do things. They may become upset. Nursing assistants must be patient. They must not rush residents or act annoyed.

Respectful: Being respectful means valuing other people's individuality, including their age, religion, culture, feelings, practices, and beliefs.

People who are respectful treat others politely and kindly. They care about other people's self-esteem and do not gossip about them.

Unprejudiced: Nursing assistants work with people from many different backgrounds. They must give each resident the same quality care regardless of age, gender, sexual orientation, religion, race, ethnicity, or condition.

Tolerant: Being tolerant means respecting others' beliefs and practices and not judging them. Nursing assistants may not like or agree with things that residents or their families do or have done. However, their job is to care for each resident as assigned, not to judge him or her. NAs should put aside their opinions and see each resident as an individual who needs their care.

4. Describe proper personal grooming habits

Regular grooming makes people feel good about themselves, and it makes a positive impression on others. The nursing assistant's grooming habits affect how confident residents feel about the care given. Professional nursing assistants have the following personal grooming habits:

- Bathing or showering daily and using deodorant (do not use perfume, cologne, aftershave, or scented body creams or lotions, as residents may not like scents or may have illnesses that are worsened by scents)

- Brushing teeth frequently and using mouthwash when necessary

- Keeping hair clean and neatly brushed or combed and tying long hair back in a bun or ponytail

- Keeping facial hair short, clean, and neat

- Dressing neatly in a uniform that has been washed and ironed

- Not wearing clothes that are too tight or too baggy, torn or stained, or too revealing (short skirts, low-cut blouses, see-through fabrics)

- Not wearing large jewelry (the main exception to this rule is a simple, waterproof watch that may be used to measure vital signs and record events)

- Wearing an identification badge as required by the facility

- Not having visible tattoos and body piercings (except for pierced ears)

- Wearing comfortable, clean, high-quality, closed-toe shoes (Fig. 2-8)

- Keeping fingernails short, smooth, and clean

- Not wearing artificial nails (acrylic, gel, sculptured, or wraps) because they harbor bacteria

- Wearing little or no makeup

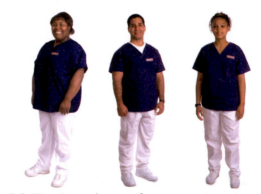

Fig. 2-8. *Wearing a clean uniform, a watch, and an identification badge, as well as keeping long hair tied back and wearing clean, closed-toe shoes, are all parts of proper grooming.*

Nursing assistants should follow any specific rules a facility has regarding their appearance.

5. Explain the chain of command and scope of practice

A nursing assistant carries out instructions given to her by a nurse. The nurse is acting on the instructions of a physician or other member of the care team. This is called the **chain of command**. It describes the line of authority and helps to make sure that residents get proper health care. The chain of command also protects employees and employers from liability. **Liabil-**

ity is a legal term that means someone can be held responsible for harming someone else. For example, imagine that a task a nursing assistant performs for a resident harms that resident. However, the task was in the care plan and was done according to policy and procedure. In this case, the NA may not be liable, or responsible, for hurting the resident. However, if the NA does something that is not in the care plan that harms a resident, she could be held responsible. That is why it is important for team members to follow instructions in the care plan and for the facility to have a chain of command (Fig. 2-9).

Nursing assistants must understand what they can and cannot do. This is important so that they do not harm residents or involve themselves or their employers in lawsuits. Some states certify that nursing assistants are qualified to work. However, nursing assistants are not licensed healthcare providers. Everything they do in their job is assigned to them by a licensed healthcare professional. That is why these professionals will show great interest in what nursing assistants do and how they do it.

Every state grants the right to practice various jobs in health care through licensure. Examples include a license to practice nursing, medicine, or physical therapy. Each member of the care team works under his or her scope of practice. A **scope of practice** defines the tasks that healthcare providers are legally allowed to do as permitted by state or federal law.

Laws and regulations about what nursing assistants can and cannot do vary from state to state. However, some procedures are not performed by nursing assistants under any circumstances. Tasks that are outside the scope of practice for a nursing assistant include the following:

* NAs do not honor a request to do something outside the scope of practice, not listed in the care plan, or not on the assignment sheet. In this situation, an NA should explain that he cannot do the task requested.

The request should then be reported to a nurse. This is true even if a nurse or doctor asks the NA to perform the task. The NA should refuse to perform the task and explain why. Refusing to do something that the NA cannot legally do is the NA's right and responsibility.

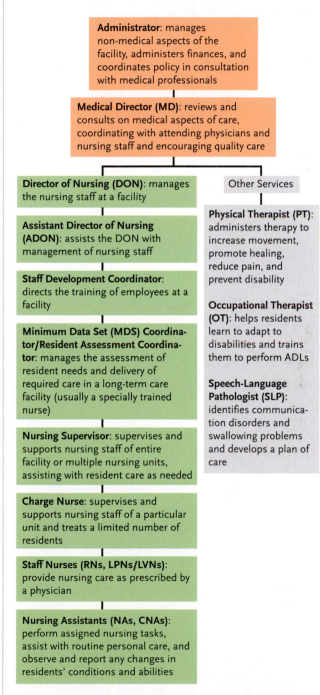

Fig. 2-9. The chain of command describes the line of authority in a facility and helps ensure that the resident receives proper care.

- NAs do not perform procedures that require sterile technique. For example, changing a sterile dressing on a deep, open wound requires sterile technique.

- NAs do not diagnose illnesses or prescribe treatments or medications.

- NAs do not tell the resident or the family the diagnosis or the medical treatment plan. This is the responsibility of the doctor or nurse.

Nursing assistants are also not allowed to administer medications unless their state permits it and they have completed additional training for medications.

An instructor or an employer may provide a list of other tasks outside the nursing assistant's scope of practice. In some cases, an NA may have received training to do a particular task but her employer does not want her to perform it. It is important that NAs know which tasks these are and not perform them. Many of these specialized tasks require more training. NAs must learn how to refuse a task for which they have not been trained or which is outside their scope of practice.

6. Discuss the resident care plan and explain its purpose

The resident's care plan is individualized for each resident. It is developed to help achieve the goals of care. The care plan lists the tasks that team members, including nursing assistants, must perform (Fig. 2-10). It states how often these tasks should be performed and how they should be carried out.

The care plan is a guide to help the resident reach and maintain the best possible level of health. It must be followed very carefully. **Activities not listed on the care plan should not be performed.**

Centers for Medicare and Medicaid Services (CMS) requires that facilities do comprehensive,

person-centered care planning for each resident. Care planning should involve input from the resident and/or the family, as well as from health professionals. When the resident is involved in care planning, he is more likely to participate in and continue treatment. In addition, the resident has a legal right to participate in his own care. Person-centered care places special emphasis on the importance of the resident's input.

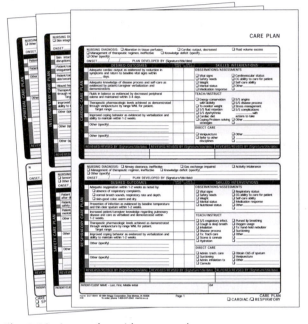

Fig. 2-10. *A sample resident care plan.* (REPRINTED WITH PERMISSION OF BRIGGS CORPORATION, 800-247-2343, BRIGGSCORP.COM)

When planning care, professionals will assess the resident's physical, financial, social, and psychological needs. The resident's history, preferences, and goals are also assessed. The care team helping to plan care includes a doctor, nurse, nursing assistant, nutrition services staff, a social worker, and the resident, as well as other team members. Many factors are considered when formulating a care plan. These include the following:

- The resident's goals, priorities, or expectations

- The resident's health and physical condition

- The resident's diagnosis and treatment

Multiple care plans may be necessary for some residents. In these situations, the nurse will coordinate the resident's overall care. There will be one care plan for the nursing assistant to follow. There will be separate care plans for other providers, such as the physical therapist.

Care plans must be reviewed regularly and updated as the resident's condition or needs change. It is essential that nursing assistants make observations and report them to the nurse. Sometimes even simple observations are very important. The information that NAs collect, such as vital signs, and the changes that they observe are important in determining how care plans may need to change. Because nursing assistants spend so much time with residents, they have a lot of valuable information that will help in care planning. Nursing assistants may be asked to attend care planning meetings. If they attend these meetings, it is important that they share their observations of residents. Nursing assistants who are not sure what is important to share can speak to a nurse before the meeting to find out.

7. Describe the nursing process

To communicate with other care team members and to help plan and evaluate the resident's care needs, nurses use the nursing process (Fig. 2-11). The process has five steps:

- **Assessment**: getting information from many sources, including medical history, physical assessment, and environment, and reviewing this information; the purpose is to identify actual or potential problems

- **Diagnosis**: identifying health problems after looking at all the resident's needs

- **Planning**: setting goals and creating a care plan in accordance with the resident's preferences to meet the resident's needs

- **Implementation**: putting the care plan into action; giving care

- **Evaluation**: a careful examination to see if the goals were met or progress was achieved

The nursing process constantly changes as new information is collected. Clear communication between all team members and the resident is vital to ensure success of the process. The nursing assistant's accurate observations and reports are an important part of planning and evaluating care.

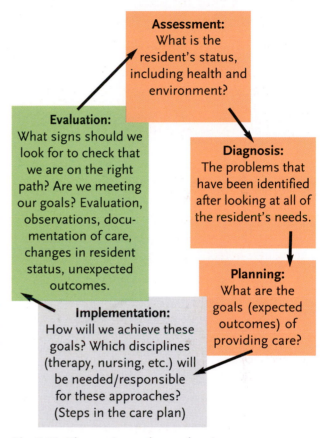

Assessment: What is the resident's status, including health and environment?

Evaluation: What signs should we look for to check that we are on the right path? Are we meeting our goals? Evaluation, observations, documentation of care, changes in resident status, unexpected outcomes.

Diagnosis: The problems that have been identified after looking at all of the resident's needs.

Planning: What are the goals (expected outcomes) of providing care?

Implementation: How will we achieve these goals? Which disciplines (therapy, nursing, etc.) will be needed/responsible for these approaches? (Steps in the care plan)

Fig. 2-11. The nursing and care planning process.

8. Describe *The Five Rights of Delegation*

When planning care, nurses decide which tasks to delegate to others, including nursing assistants. **Delegation** means transferring responsibility to a person for a specific task. Nursing assistants do not delegate tasks; they have tasks delegated to them. Licensed nurses are accountable for care, including all delegated tasks. The National Council of State Boards of Nursing (NCSBN, ncsbn.org) has identified *The Five Rights of Delegation*. This can be used as a mental checklist to help nurses in the decision-making process.

The Five Rights of Delegation are the *Right Task, Right Circumstance, Right Person, Right Direction/ Communication,* and *Right Supervision/Evaluation.* Before delegating tasks, nurses consider these questions:

- Is there a match between the resident's needs and the nursing assistant's skills, abilities, and experience?

- What is the level of resident stability?

- Is the nursing assistant the right person to do the job?

- Can the nurse give appropriate direction and communication?

- Is the nurse available to give the supervision, support, and help that the nursing assistant needs?

There are questions nursing assistants may want to consider before accepting a task:

- Do I have all the information I need to do this job? Are there questions I should ask?

- Do I believe that I can do this task? Do I have the necessary skills?

- Do I have the needed supplies, equipment, and other support?

- Do I know who my supervisor is and how to reach him/her?

- Do we both understand who is doing what?

A nursing assistant should never be afraid to ask for help. She should always ask if she needs any more information or is unsure about something. If an NA feels that she does not have the skills for a task or that the task is not within her scope of practice, she should talk to the nurse.

9. Demonstrate how to manage time and assignments

Nursing assistants must manage their time well when taking care of residents. There are many tasks that must be done during their shifts. Managing time properly helps NAs complete these tasks. Many of the following ideas for managing time on the job can be used to manage personal time as well:

Plan ahead. Planning is the single best way to manage time better. Sometimes it is hard to find time to plan, but it is important that a person takes the time to sit down and list everything that has to be done. NAs must take time to check to see if they have all the supplies needed for a procedure. Often just making the list and taking the time to recheck will help a caregiver feel better and help him focus.

The nurse creates the nursing assistant's work assignments based on the needs of residents and availability of staff. The assignments allow staff to work as a team. The NA's responsibilities in completing assignments include the following:

- Helping others when needed

- Never ignoring a resident who needs help

- Answering all call lights even when not assigned to a particular resident

- Notifying the nurse if he cannot complete an assignment

Prioritize. Identify the most important tasks to get done and do these first.

Make a schedule. Write out the hours of the day and fill in what needs to be done and when. This allows for a realistic schedule.

Combine activities. Nursing assistants can visit with residents while providing care, which combines two important tasks. Work more efficiently whenever possible.

Get help. It is a simple reality that it is not possible for a nursing assistant to do everything. Sometimes NAs will need help to ensure a resident's safety, and they should not be afraid to ask for help.

Chapter Review

1. Describe what each of these care team members does: nursing assistant, registered nurse, physician, physical therapist, occupational therapist, speech-language pathologist, registered dietitian, medical social worker, activities director, and resident.

2. List six examples of duties that nursing assistants perform.

3. List two duties that nursing assistants do not usually perform.

4. By what name should a nursing assistant call a resident?

5. List seven examples of professional behavior with an employer.

6. List eight personal qualities that are important for nursing assistants to have.

7. Why should nursing assistants avoid wearing artificial nails?

8. Why would wearing comfortable shoes be important to nursing assistants?

9. Give one reason why the chain of command is important.

10. List three tasks that are said to be outside the scope of practice of a nursing assistant.

11. Why are observing and reporting even simple observations about a resident important?

12. What are three factors considered when forming a care plan?

13. List five steps in the nursing process.

14. List *The Five Rights of Delegation.*

15. What should a nursing assistant do if he feels he does not have the skills necessary to perform a task?

16. List five steps in managing time and assignments.

3
Legal and Ethical Issues

1. Define the terms *law* and *ethics* and list examples of legal and ethical behavior

Ethics and laws guide behavior. **Ethics** are the knowledge of right and wrong. An ethical person has a sense of duty and responsibility toward others. He tries to do what is right. If ethics tell people what they *should* do, **laws** tell them what they *must* do. Laws are usually based on ethics. Governments establish laws to help people live peacefully together and to ensure order and safety. When someone breaks the law, he may be punished by having to pay a fine or spend time in prison.

Ethics and laws are extremely important in health care (Fig. 3-1). They protect people receiving care and guide people giving care. Nursing assistants, home health aides, and other healthcare providers should be guided by a code of ethics. They must know the laws that apply to their jobs.

Guidelines: Legal and Ethical Behavior

G Be honest at all times. Stealing or lying about the care you provided are examples of dishonesty. Communicate honestly with all team members.

G Protect residents' privacy. Do not discuss their cases except with other members of the care team. Keeping resident information confidential is one of the Residents' Rights,

which are covered later in this chapter. All team members must keep resident information confidential.

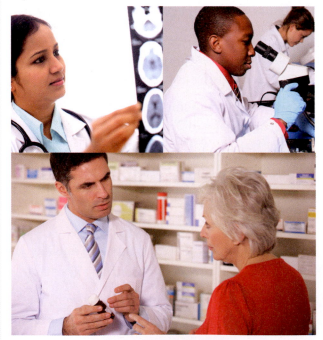

Fig. 3-1. *All healthcare providers must behave ethically and follow the law.*

G Keep staff information confidential. You should not share information about your coworkers at home or anywhere else.

G Report abuse or suspected abuse of residents. Help residents report abuse if they wish to make a complaint of abuse. This is covered later in this chapter.

G Follow the care plan and your assignments. Report any mistakes you make promptly. This helps prevent any further problems.

Reporting mistakes promotes the safety and well-being of all residents.

G Do not perform any task outside your scope of practice.

G Report all resident observations and incidents to the nurse.

G Document accurately and promptly.

G Follow rules about safety and infection prevention. Chapters 5 and 6 contain information about these rules.

G Do not accept gifts or tips.

G Do not get personally or sexually involved with residents or their family members or friends.

Many organizations and companies have created a code of ethics for their members or employees to follow. These vary, but generally they focus on promoting proper conduct and high standards of practice. If a facility has its own code of ethics, all staff members will be given a copy and expected to follow it.

Crimes in Healthcare Settings

Most of the crimes that occur in the community can also occur in healthcare settings. Theft is frequently reported. Physical abuse, including hitting, punching, shoving, rough handling, and many other types of abuse can occur. Violations of Residents' Rights are reported and can be prosecuted as crimes. It is important for nursing assistants to know what to observe and how to report any illegal activity. Being vigilant can help prevent crimes and promote legal and ethical behavior in the workplace.

2. Explain the Omnibus Budget Reconciliation Act (OBRA)

The **Omnibus Budget Reconciliation Act (OBRA)** was passed in 1987. It has been updated several times since. OBRA was passed in response to reports of poor care and abuse in long-term care facilities. Congress decided to set minimum standards of care, which included standardized training of nursing assistants.

OBRA requires that the Nurse Aide Training and Competency Evaluation Program (NATCEP) sets minimum standards for nursing assistant training. Nursing assistants must complete at least 75 hours of training that covers topics like communication, preventing infections, safety and emergency procedures, and how to promote residents' independence and legal rights. Training must also include basic nursing skills, such as how to measure vital signs, as well as performing personal care skills and how to observe and report changes in residents' conditions. In addition, nursing assistants must know how to respond to mental health and social services needs, rehabilitative skills, and how to care for residents who are cognitively impaired. In many states, training requirements exceed the minimum set by the federal government.

OBRA requires that nursing assistants must pass a competency evaluation (testing program) before they can be employed. The exam consists of both written and demonstrated nursing skills. Nursing assistants must also attend regular in-service education classes (minimum of 12 hours per year) to keep their skills updated.

OBRA also requires that states keep a current list of nursing assistants in a state registry. In addition, OBRA identifies standards that instructors must meet in order to train nursing assistants. OBRA sets guidelines for minimum staff requirements and specifies services that long-term care facilities must provide.

The resident assessment requirements are another important part of OBRA. OBRA requires that complete assessments be done on every resident. The assessment forms are the same for every facility. The **Minimum Data Set (MDS)** is a resident assessment system that was developed in 1990 and is revised periodically (Fig. 3-2). The MDS is a detailed form with guidelines for assessing residents. It also lists what to do if resident problems are identified. The manual

Resident _____ Identifier _____ Date _____

MINIMUM DATA SET (MDS) - Version 3.0
RESIDENT ASSESSMENT AND CARE SCREENING
Nursing Home Comprehensive (NC) Item Set

CAA's = ▮   QM's = ⬤   PPS = 💲

Code "-" if information unavailable or unknown

Section A	**Identification Information**

A0050. Type of Record

Enter Code ☐
1. **Add new record** → Continue to A0100, Facility Provider Numbers
2. **Modify existing record** → Continue to A0100, Facility Provider Numbers
3. **Inactivate existing record** → **Skip to X0150**, Type of Provider

A0100. Facility Provider Numbers

A. **National Provider Identifier (NPI):**
B. **CMS Certification Number (CCN):**
C. **State Provider Number:**

A0200. Type of Provider

Enter Code ☐
Type of provider
1. **Nursing home (SNF/NF)**
2. **Swing Bed**

A0310. Type of Assessment `CAA`

Enter Code ☐☐
A. **Federal OBRA Reason for Assessment**
💲 01. **Admission** assessment (required by **day 14**) `11`
💲 02. **Quarterly** review assessment
💲 03. **Annual** assessment `1,8`
💲 04. **Significant change in status** assessment `1,8`
💲 05. **Significant correction** to **prior comprehensive** assessment `1,8`
💲 06. **Significant correction** to **prior quarterly** assessment
💲 99. **None of the above**

Enter Code ☐☐
B. **PPS Assessment**
PPS Scheduled Assessments for a Medicare Part A Stay
💲 01. **5-day** scheduled assessment
💲 02. **14-day** scheduled assessment
💲 03. **30-day** scheduled assessment
💲 04. **60-day** scheduled assessment
💲 05. **90-day** scheduled assessment
💲 06. **Readmission/return** assessment
PPS Unscheduled Assessments for a Medicare Part A Stay
💲 07. **Unscheduled assessment used for PPS** (OMRA, significant or clinical change, or significant correction assessment)
Not PPS Assessment
💲 99. **None of the above**

A0310 continued on next page

QUALITY MEASURES (QM)

SHORT STAY QUALITY MEASURES:
- 76 (#0676) Residents who self report moderate to severe pain
- 78 (#0678) Residents with pressure ulcers that are new or worsened
- 80 (#0680) Residents who were assessed and appropriately given the seasonal Influenza Vaccine
- 80A (#0680A) Residents who received the seasonal Influenza Vaccine
- 80B (#0680B) Residents who were offered and declined the seasonal Influenza Vaccine
- 80C (#0680C) Residents who did not receive, due to medical contraindication, the seasonal Influenza Vaccine
- 82 (#0682) Residents accessed and appropriately given the Pneumococcal Vaccine
- 82A (#0682A) Residents who received the Pneumococcal Vaccine
- 82B (#0682B) Residents who were offered and declined the Pneumococcal Vaccine
- 82C (#0682C) Residents who did not receive, due to medical contraindication, the Pneumococcal Vaccine

LONG STAY QUALITY MEASURES
- 74 (#0674) Residents experiencing one or more falls with major injury
- 77 (#0677) Residents who self-report moderate to severe pain
- 79 (#0679) High-risk residents with pressure ulcers
- 81 (#0681) Residents assessed and appropriately given the seasonal Influenza Vaccine
- 81A (#0681A) Residents who received the seasonal Influenza Vaccine
- 81B (#0681B) Residents who were offered and declined the seasonal Influenza Vaccine
- 81C (0681C) Residents who did not receive, due to medical contraindication, the seasonal Influenza Vaccine
- 83 (#0683) Residents assessed and appropriately given the Pneumococcal Vaccine
- 83A (#0683A) Residents who received the Pneumococcal Vaccine
- 83B (#0683B) Residents who were offered and declined the Pneumococcal Vaccine

- 83C (#0683C) Residents who did not receive, due to medical contraindication, the Pneumococcal Vaccine
- 84 (#0684) Residents with a Urinary Tract Infection
- 85 (#0685) Low Risk residents who lose control of their bowel or bladder
- 86 (#0686) Residents who have/had a catheter inserted and left in their bladder
- 87 (#0687) Residents who were physically restrained
- 88 (#0688) Residents whose need for help with activities of daily living has increased
- 89 (#0689) Residents who lose too much weight
- 90 (#0690) Residents who have depressive symptoms
- 300 (#300) Prevalence of Falls
- 400 (#400) Prevalence of psychoactive medication use, in the absence of psychotic or related conditions
- 500 (#500) Prevalence of anxiety/hypnotic use
- 600 (#600) Prevalence of behavior symptoms affecting others

⬤ Indicates responses that may impact QM items identified by a number in a solid blue oval   ⭕ Indicates responses that may impact covariate for the QM identified by a number in an outline blue oval

CARE AREA ASSESSMENT LEGEND
1 Delirium	5 ADL Function/Rehabilitation Potential	7 Psychosocial Well-Being
2 Cognitive Loss/Dementia	6 Urinary Incontinence & Indwelling Catheter	8 Mood State
3 Visual Function		9 Behavioral Symptoms
4 Communication		10 Activities

11 Falls · 12 Nutritional Status · 13 Feeding Tubes · 14 Dehydration/Fluid Maintenance · 15 Dental Care · 16 Pressure Ulcer · 17 Psychotropic Drug Use · 18 Physical Restraints · 19 Pain · 20 Return to Community Referral

Form 1851P-12R 5/12   2012 BRIGGS, Des Moines, IA 50306 (800) 247-2343 www.BriggsCorp.com
BRIGGS Healthcare®
MDS 3.0 Nursing Home Comprehensive (NC) Version 1.10.4 Effective 04/01/2012   1 of 40

Fig. 3-2. *A sample MDS form.* (REPRINTED WITH PERMISSION OF THE BRIGGS CORPORATION, 800-247-2343, WWW.BRIGGSCORP.COM)

provides examples and definitions for nurses to help them complete the assessments accurately.

Nurses must complete the MDS for each resident within 14 days of admission to the care facility and again each year. In addition, the MDS for each resident must be reviewed every three months. A new MDS must be done when there is any major change in the resident's condition.

OBRA made major changes in the survey process (Chapter 1). The results from surveys are available to the public and posted in the facility.

OBRA also identifies important rights for residents in long-term care facilities. The next learning objective has information about these rights.

3. Explain Residents' Rights and discuss why they are important

Residents' Rights specify how residents must be treated while living in a facility. They provide an ethical code of conduct for healthcare workers. Facility staff give residents a list of these rights and review each right with them. In 2016, Centers for Medicare and Medicaid Services (CMS) finalized a rule to improve the care and safety of residents in long-term care facilities. It was the first comprehensive update since 1991. It includes strengthening the rights of residents who live in long-term care facilities. Nursing assistants must be familiar with these legal rights.

Residents' Rights include the following:

Quality of life: Residents have the right to the best care available. Dignity, choice, and independence are important parts of quality of life. The facility must give equal access to quality care regardless of a resident's condition, diagnosis, or payment source.

Services and activities to maintain a high level of wellness: Residents must receive the correct care. Healthcare professionals at facilities are required to develop a care plan for residents, and their care should keep them as healthy as possible. A baseline care plan for residents must be developed within 48 hours of admission, which includes instructions for providing person-centered care. Residents' health should not decline as a direct result of the care given at the facility.

The right to be fully informed about rights and services: Residents must be told what services are available and what the fee is for each service. They must be informed of charges both orally and in writing. Residents must be given a written copy of their legal rights, along with the facility's rules and regulations. Legal rights must be explained in a language that each resident can understand. Residents must be given contact information for state agencies related to monitoring the quality of care, such as those that employ ombudsmen. When requested, survey results must be shared with residents. Residents have the right to be notified about any change of room or roommate. They have the right to communicate with someone who speaks their language. They have the right to assistance for any sensory impairment, such as vision loss.

The right to participate in their own care: Residents have the right to participate in planning their treatment, care, and discharge. Residents have the right to see and sign their care plans after all significant changes. Residents have the right to be informed of risks and benefits of care and treatment, including treatment options and alternatives, and to choose the options they prefer. They have the right to request, refuse, and/or discontinue treatment and care. They can refuse restraints and refuse to participate in experimental research.

Residents have the right to be told of changes in their condition. They have the right to review their medical record. They have the right to choose and change their care providers at any time.

Informed consent is a concept that is part of participating in one's own care. A person has the legal and ethical right to direct what happens to his or her body. Doctors also have an ethical duty to involve the person in his or her health care. **Informed consent** is the process by which a person, with the help of a doctor, makes informed decisions about his or her health care.

The right to make independent choices: Residents can make choices about their doctors, care, and treatments. They can make personal decisions, such as what to wear and how to spend their time. They can join in community activities, both inside and outside the care facility. They have a right to participate in resident or family groups, such as a Resident Council.

A Resident Council is a group of residents who meet regularly to discuss issues related to the long-term care facility. This council gives residents a voice in facility operations. Topics of discussion may include facility policies, decisions regarding activities, concerns, and problems. The Resident Council offers residents a chance to provide suggestions on improving the quality of care. Council executives are elected by residents. Family members are invited to attend meetings with or on behalf of residents. A designated staff member is required to participate in resident and family groups. The staff member must be approved by council members.

The right to privacy and confidentiality: Residents have the right to speak privately with anyone, the right to privacy during care, and the right to confidentiality regarding every aspect of their lives (Fig. 3-3). Their medical and personal information cannot be shared with anyone but the care team.

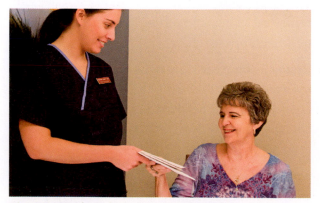

Fig. 3-3. *Residents have the right to privacy, which includes private communication with anyone; they have the right to send and receive mail that is unopened.*

The right to dignity, respect, and freedom: Residents must be respected and treated with dignity by caregivers. Residents must not be abused, mistreated, or neglected in any way.

The right to security of possessions: Residents' personal possessions must be safe at all times. Facilities must make an effort to protect residents' property from loss or theft. Possessions cannot be taken or used by anyone without a resident's permission. Residents have the right to manage their own finances or choose someone else to do it for them. Residents can request that the facility handle their money. If the care facility handles residents' financial affairs, residents must have access to their accounts and financial records, and they must receive quarterly statements, among other things. Residents have the right to not be charged for any care that is covered by Medicaid or Medicare.

Rights during transfers and discharges: Residents have the right to be informed of and to consent to any location changes. Residents have the right to stay in a facility unless a transfer or discharge is needed. Residents can be moved from the facility due to safety reasons (their safety or others' safety), if their health has improved or worsened, or if payment for care has not been received for a determined period of time.

The facility must develop an effective discharge plan for residents that involves each resident's goals and preferences. This plan must be regularly reviewed and updated as appropriate. If the resident is planning to stay at the facility long-term, discharge planning still needs to occur, keeping the resident's preferences in mind.

The right to complain: Residents have the right to make complaints and voice grievances without fear for their safety or care. Facilities must work quickly to address their concerns.

The right to visits: Residents have the right to visits from doctors, family members (including spouses and domestic partners), friends, ombudsmen, clergy members, legal representatives, or any other person. Visits cannot be restricted, limited, or denied on the basis of race, color, national origin, religion, sex, gender identity, sexual orientation, or disability.

Rights with regard to social services: The facility must provide residents with access to social services, including counseling, assistance in solving problems with others (mediation), and help contacting legal and financial professionals.

There are blue boxes throughout this textbook that explain how to promote Residents' Rights and how to reinforce person-centered care.

The Americans with Disabilities Act (ADA)

The Americans with Disabilities Act (ADA, dol.gov/general/topic/disability/ada) became a federal law in 1990. It was passed to help people with disabilities gain skills, do jobs they want to do, and take part in desired activities. The ADA prohibits discrimination because of a disability. The law requires that employers, schools, and businesses offer equal opportunities to individuals with disabilities to use the services in society and improve their quality of life.

People with disabilities must be able to get into and around in buildings and use the bathrooms, drinking fountains, and other areas. The law requires new buildings to be accessible and older buildings to be updated when they are renovated.

Americans with disabilities have the right to education, employment, and all the services offered to the public. Schools, colleges, and many employers are not allowed to discriminate and must make reasonable accommodations, or changes, to make their services available. Examples of accommodations are providing a large screen for a computer or allowing a service dog. Providers of health care, social services, transportation, restaurants, hotels, and recreation are also not allowed to discriminate against people with disabilities. They must provide equal opportunities, which may include making some changes to their services.

4. Discuss abuse and neglect and explain how to report abuse and neglect

Elder abuse and neglect is a growing problem. The National Council on Aging (NCOA, ncoa.org) cites a study by the National Center on Elder Abuse (NCEA, ncea.aoa.gov) that estimates approximately one in ten Americans aged 60 and older has experienced some form of elder abuse. In addition, NCOA states that estimates range as high as five million elderly people are abused each year. As the elderly population grows, this problem may become worse.

Elderly people may be abused intentionally or unintentionally, through ignorance, inexperience, or inability to care for them. People who abuse elders may mistreat them physically, psychologically, sexually, verbally, financially, and/or materially. They may deprive them of their rights, or they may neglect them by failing to provide food, clothing, shelter, or medical care. Some older adults may also become self-abusive or neglect their own needs.

Neglect is the failure to provide needed care that results in physical, mental, or emotional harm to a person. Neglect can be divided into two categories: active neglect and passive neglect. **Active neglect** is the purposeful failure to provide needed care, resulting in harm to a person. Examples of active neglect are leaving a bedridden resident alone for a long time or denying the resident food, dentures, or eyeglasses. **Passive neglect** is the unintentional failure to provide needed care, resulting in physical, mental, or emotional harm to a person. The caregiver may not know how to properly care for the resident, or may not understand the resident's needs.

Negligence means actions, or the failure to act or provide the proper care for a resident, resulting in unintended injury. An example of negligence is an NA forgetting to lock a resident's wheelchair before transferring her. The resident then falls and is injured. **Malpractice** occurs when a person is injured due to professional misconduct through negligence, carelessness, or lack of skill.

Abuse is purposeful mistreatment that causes physical, mental, or emotional pain or injury to someone. There are many forms of abuse, including the following:

Physical abuse is any treatment, intentional or unintentional, that causes harm to a person's body. This includes slapping, bruising, cutting, burning, physically restraining, pushing, shoving, or even rough handling.

Psychological abuse is emotional harm caused by threatening, scaring, humiliating, intimidating, isolating, or insulting a person, or treating him or her as a child.

Verbal abuse is the use of spoken or written words, pictures, or gestures that threaten, embarrass, or insult a person.

Assault is a threat to harm a person, resulting in the person feeling fearful that he or she will be harmed. Telling a resident that she will be slapped if she does not stop yelling is an example of assault.

Battery is the intentional touching of a person without his or her consent. An example is an NA hitting or pushing a resident, which is also considered physical abuse. Forcing a resident to eat a meal is another example of battery.

Sexual abuse is the forcing of a person to perform or participate in sexual acts against his or her will. This includes unwanted touching and exposing oneself to a person. It also includes sharing pornographic material.

Financial abuse is the improper or illegal use of a person's money, possessions, property, or other assets.

Domestic violence is abuse by spouses, intimate partners, or family members. It can be physical, sexual, or emotional. The victim can be a man or woman of any age or a child.

Workplace violence is abuse of staff by other staff members, residents, or visitors. It can be verbal, physical, or sexual. This includes improper touching and discussion about sexual subjects.

False imprisonment is unlawful restraint that affects a person's freedom of movement. Both the threat of being physically restrained and actually being physically restrained are types of false imprisonment. Not allowing a resident to leave the facility is also considered false imprisonment.

Involuntary seclusion is the separation of a person from others against the person's will. An example is an NA confining a resident to his room.

Sexual harassment is any unwelcome sexual advance or behavior that creates an intimidating, hostile, or offensive working environment. Requests for sexual favors, unwanted touching, and other acts of a sexual nature are examples of sexual harassment.

Substance abuse is the repeated use of legal or illegal drugs, cigarettes, or alcohol in a way that harms oneself or others. For the NA, substance abuse can lead to unsafe practices that result in negligence, malpractice, neglect, and abuse. It can also lead to the loss of the NA's job. Chapter 20 contains more information about substance abuse.

Nursing assistants must never abuse residents in any way. They must also try to protect residents from others who abuse them. If a nursing assistant ever sees or suspects that another caregiver, family member, or resident is abusing a resident, she must report this immediately to the nurse in charge. **Reporting abuse or suspected abuse is not optional—it is the law.**

Observing and Reporting: Abuse and Neglect

The following injuries are considered suspicious and should be reported:

O/R Poisoning or traumatic injury

O/R Teeth marks

O/R Belt buckle or strap marks

O/R Bruises, contusions, and welts

O/R Scars

O/R Fractures, dislocation

O/R Burns of unusual shape and in unusual locations, cigarette burns

O/R Scalding burns

o/R Scratches or puncture wounds

o/R Scalp tenderness or patches of missing hair

o/R Swelling in the face, broken teeth, nasal discharge

o/R Bruises, bleeding, or discharge from the vaginal area

The following signs could indicate abuse:

o/R Yelling obscenities

o/R Fear, apprehension, fear of being alone

o/R Poor self-control

o/R Constant pain

o/R Threatening to hurt others

o/R Withdrawal or apathy (Fig. 3-4)

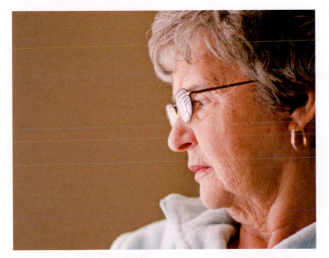

Fig. 3-4. *Withdrawing from others is an important change to report.*

o/R Alcohol or drug abuse

o/R Agitation or anxiety, signs of stress

o/R Low self-esteem

o/R Mood changes, confusion, disorientation

o/R Private conversations are not allowed, or the family member/caregiver is present during all conversations

o/R Reports of questionable care by the resident or her family

The following signs could indicate neglect:

o/R Pressure injuries

o/R Unclean body

o/R Body lice

o/R Unanswered call lights

o/R Soiled bedding or incontinence briefs not being changed

o/R Poorly fitting clothing

o/R Unmet needs relating to hearing aids, eyeglasses, etc.

o/R Weight loss, poor appetite

o/R Uneaten food

o/R Dehydration

o/R Fresh water or beverages not being offered regularly

Residents' Rights

Vulnerable Adults

Some states have Vulnerable Adults Acts or Adult Protective Services (APS) laws. These laws are created by each state and are not the same throughout the country. There are states that do not have any such laws. In general, these Vulnerable Adults Acts or Adult Protective Services laws protect individuals who, because of a physical or mental impairment, need help from other people for their care. The residents of long-term care and assisted living facilities, as well as other care facilities, fit into this category.

It is important that NAs know the laws in their state. However, even if a state does not have a specific law like the ones above, residents of long-term care facilities are covered by the federal laws relating to Residents' Rights, which also forbid abuse and neglect and require reporting if these acts do occur.

Nursing assistants are in an excellent position to observe and report abuse or neglect. NAs have an ethical and legal responsibility to observe for signs of abuse and to report suspected cases to the proper person. Nursing assistants are considered mandated reporters. **Mandated reporters** are people who are legally required to report suspected or observed abuse or neglect because they have regular contact with vulnerable populations, such as the elderly in care facilities. In some facilities, training on how to observe and report abuse is required as part of the orientation process after an employee is hired.

Nursing assistants must follow the chain of command when reporting abuse. If action is not taken, the NA should keep reporting up the chain of command until action is taken. If no appropriate action is taken at the facility, she can call the state abuse hotline or contact the proper state agency. Abuse can be reported anonymously. If a life-or-death situation is witnessed, the NA should remove the resident to a safe place if possible. The NA should get help immediately or have someone go for help. The resident should not be left alone.

If abuse is suspected or observed, the NA should give the nurse as much information as possible. If residents want to make a complaint of abuse, NAs must assist them in every way. This includes telling them about the process and their rights. Nursing assistants must never retaliate against (punish) residents complaining of abuse. If an NA sees someone being cruel or abusive to a resident who made a complaint, she must report it. All care team members are responsible for residents' safety and should take this responsibility seriously.

Residents' Rights

Elder Justice Act

The Elder Justice Act was passed as part of the Affordable Care Act in March of 2010. It is the first federal law designed specifically to combat elder abuse. Under the Elder Justice Act, the federal Department of Health and Human Services has established an Elder Justice Coordinating Council and an Advisory Board on Elder Abuse, Neglect, and Exploitation. These groups are intended to coordinate educational resources, support, and grant funding to aid efforts to stop elder abuse.

5. List examples of behavior supporting and promoting Residents' Rights

Nursing assistants can help protect residents' legal rights by following these guidelines:

Guidelines: Protecting Residents' Rights

G   Never abuse a resident physically, psychologically, verbally, or sexually. Watch for and immediately report any signs of abuse or neglect to the charge nurse.

G   Call the resident by the name he or she prefers.

G   Involve residents in planning. Allow residents to make as many choices as possible about when, where, and how care is performed.

G   Always explain a procedure to a resident before performing it.

G   Do not unnecessarily expose a resident while giving care.

G   Respect a resident's refusal of care. Residents have a legal right to refuse treatment and care. However, report the refusal to the nurse immediately.

G   Tell the nurse if a resident has questions, concerns, or complaints about treatment or the goals of care.

G   Be truthful when documenting care.

G   Do not talk or gossip about residents. Keep all resident information confidential.

G   Knock and ask for permission before entering a resident's room. (Fig. 3-5).

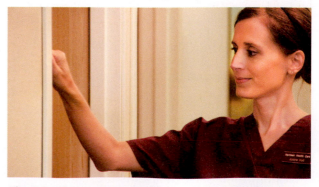

Fig. 3-5. *Always respect residents' privacy. Knock before entering their rooms, even if the door is open.*

G   Do not accept gifts or money from residents.

G   Do not open a resident's mail or look through his belongings.

G Respect residents' personal possessions. Handle them gently and carefully. Keep personal items labeled and stored according to facility policy.

G Report observations about a resident's condition or care.

G Help resolve disputes by reporting them to the nurse.

Residents' Rights

Voting

People retain their legal right to vote when they are living in a care facility. They may request and receive absentee ballots. Sometimes they will be driven to polling places to cast their vote by family, friends, or a facility employee. If an NA is asked to assist a resident with voting, he should ask the resident how she wants the NA to help. For example, a resident may want the NA to read the ballot aloud and/or mark the ballot for her. The NA should understand how to complete the ballot if asked to assist. He can ask the nurse for help if needed. The NA should not discuss his opinions with the resident, even if asked. He should try not to influence the resident in any way or discuss how the resident voted with anyone.

6. Describe what happens when a complaint of abuse is made against a nursing assistant

When a report of abuse against a nursing assistant is made, the NA is usually suspended immediately, pending investigation. The facility's staff will launch an investigation according to the facility's policies and procedures. If staff believe that abuse has occurred, a report must be made to the relevant state agency.

The nursing assistant will be notified of any complaint made about him or her to the state agency. The nursing assistant can request a hearing. The state agency will investigate the claims and, if the findings show that abuse did occur, this is noted in the state's nurse aide registry. There may be additional legal penalties as well, such as revocation of the nursing assistant's certification. The registry is accessible to others (many are available

online), and employers check this registry before hiring nursing assistants.

7. Explain how disputes may be resolved and identify the ombudsman's role

In long-term care facilities in the United States, an **ombudsman** is assigned by law as the legal advocate for residents (ltcombudsman.org). The Older Americans Act (OAA) is a federal law that requires all states to have an ombudsman program. An ombudsman visits facilities and listens to residents. He or she decides what action to take if there are problems. Ombudsmen can help resolve conflicts and settle disputes concerning residents' health, safety, welfare, and rights. The ombudsman will gather information and try to resolve the problem on the resident's behalf and may suggest ways to solve the problem. Ombudsmen provide an ongoing presence in long-term care facilities. They monitor care and conditions. Ombudsmen typically do the following tasks:

- Advocate for Residents' Rights and quality care

- Educate consumers and care providers

- Investigate and resolve complaints

- Appear in court and/or legal hearings

- Work with investigators from the police, adult protective services, and health departments to resolve complaints (Fig. 3-6)

- Give information to the public

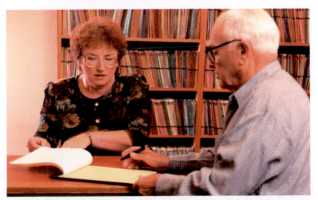

Fig. 3-6. *An ombudsman is a legal advocate for residents. He or she visits the facility and listens to residents, and may work with other agencies to resolve complaints.*

Each state has a department that performs surveys and is responsible for enforcing laws and rules at long-term care facilities. Generally, this is the responsibility of the state's department of health. Complaints may be made directly to the state agency. Each agency has policies and procedures that are used to follow up on complaints.

8. Explain HIPAA and list ways to protect residents' privacy

To respect **confidentiality** means to keep private things private. Nursing assistants will learn confidential (private) information about residents. They may learn about a resident's state of health, finances, and personal relationships. Ethically and legally, they must protect this information. This means that nursing assistants should not share information about residents with anyone other than the care team.

Congress passed the Health Insurance Portability and Accountability Act (HIPAA, hhs.gov/hipaa) in 1996. It has been further defined and revised since then. One reason this law was passed was to help keep health information private and secure. All healthcare organizations must take special steps to protect health information. They and their employees can be fined and/or imprisoned if they do not follow special rules to protect patient privacy.

Under this law, a person's health information must be kept private. **Protected health information (PHI)** is information that can be used to identify a person and relates to the patient's physical or mental condition, any health care that the person has had, and payment for that health care. Examples of PHI include a person's name, address, telephone number, social security number, email address, and medical record number. Only people who must have information to provide care or to process records should know a person's private health information. They must make sure they protect the information so that it does not become known or used by anyone else. It must be kept confidential.

The Health Information Technology for Economic and Clinical Health (HITECH) Act became law at the end of 2009. It was enacted as a part of the American Recovery and Reinvestment Act of 2009. HITECH was created to expand the protection and security of consumers' electronic health records (EHR). HITECH increases civil and criminal penalties for sharing or accessing PHI and expands the ability to enforce these penalties. HITECH also offers incentives to providers and organizations to adopt the use of EHR.

HIPAA applies to all healthcare providers, including doctors, nurses, nursing assistants, and any other members of the care team. NAs cannot give out any information about a resident to anyone who is not directly involved in the resident's care unless the resident gives official consent or unless the law requires it. For example, if a neighbor asks an NA how a resident is doing, she should reply, "I'm sorry, but I cannot share that information. It's confidential." That is the correct response to anyone who does not have a legal reason to know about the resident.

Guidelines: Protecting Privacy

G Make sure you are in a private area when you are listening to or reading your messages.

G Know with whom you are speaking on the phone. If you are not sure, get a name and number to call back after you find out it is all right to share information with this person.

G Do not talk about residents in public (Fig. 3-7). Public areas include elevators, grocery stores, lounges, waiting rooms, parking garages, schools, restaurants, etc.

G Use confidential rooms when reporting to other care team members.

G If you see a resident's family member or a former resident in public, be careful with your greeting. He or she may not want others to know about the family member or that he or she has been a resident.

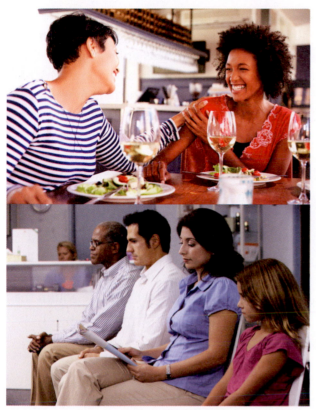

Fig. 3-7. *Do not discuss residents in public places, such as restaurants and waiting rooms.*

G Do not bring family or friends to the facility to meet residents.

G Make sure nobody can see private and protected health or personal information on your computer screen while you are working. Log out and/or exit the browser when you are finished with any computer work.

G Do not give confidential information in emails; you do not know who has access to your messages.

G Do not share resident information, photos, or videos on any social networking site, such as Facebook, Instagram, Pinterest, or Twitter.

G Make sure fax numbers are correct before faxing healthcare information. Use a cover sheet with a confidentiality statement.

G Do not leave documents where others may see them.

G Store, file, or shred documents according to your facility's policy. If you find documents with a resident's information, give them to the nurse.

All healthcare workers must comply with HIPAA regulations, no matter where they are or what they are doing. There are serious penalties for violating these regulations, including the following:

• Fines ranging from $100 to $1.5 million

• Prison sentences of up to ten years

Maintaining confidentiality is a legal and ethical obligation. It is part of respecting residents and their rights. Discussing a resident's care or personal affairs with anyone other than members of the care team violates the law.

9. Explain the Patient Self-Determination Act (PSDA) and discuss advance directives and related medical orders

The Patient Self-Determination Act (PSDA) is a federal law passed in 1990 as an amendment to OBRA. The PSDA requires all healthcare agencies that receive Medicare and Medicaid funds to give adults, during admission or enrollment, information about their rights related to advance directives. **Advance directives** are legal documents that allow people to decide what kind of medical care they wish to have in the event they are unable to make those decisions themselves. An advance directive can also designate someone else to make medical decisions for a person if that person becomes ill or disabled.

Living wills and durable powers of attorney for health care are examples of advance directives. A **living will** outlines the medical care a person wants, or does not want, in case he or she becomes unable to make those decisions. It is called a *living will* because it takes effect while the person is still alive. It may also be called a *directive to physicians, health care declaration,* or *medical directive.* A living will is not the same thing as a will. A will is a legal declaration of how a person wishes his or her possessions to be distributed after death.

A **durable power of attorney for health care** (sometimes called a *health care proxy*) is a signed, dated, and witnessed legal document that appoints someone else to make the medical decisions for a person in the event he or she becomes unable to do so. This can include instructions about medical treatment that the person does not want.

These different types of advance directives may be used together, or a person may only use one type or none at all. Having an advance directive is not legally required. However, it is a good way to make sure a person's wishes regarding medical care are known. An advance directive can be changed or canceled at any time, either in writing or verbally, or both.

According to the Patient Self-Determination Act, rights relating to advance directives that must be given upon admission include the following:

- The right to participate in and direct healthcare decisions

- The right to accept or refuse treatment

- The right to prepare an advance directive

- Information on the facility's policies that govern these rights

The PSDA requires documentation of patient information and ongoing community education on advance directives. The act prohibits discriminating against a patient who does not have an advance directive.

A **do-not-resuscitate (DNR)** order is another tool that helps medical providers honor a person's wishes about health care. A DNR order is a medical order that instructs medical professionals not to perform cardiopulmonary resuscitation (CPR) in the event of cardiac or respiratory arrest. CPR refers to medical procedures used when the heart and lungs have stopped working. A DNR order

means that medical personnel will not attempt emergency CPR if the heartbeat or breathing stops.

Another type of medical order for end-of-life planning is **Physician Orders for Life-Sustaining Treatment (POLST)**. This order specifies treatments to be used when a person is very ill. These treatments are what the person wants to receive, not what he wishes to avoid. Decisions made are based on conversations between the patient and his healthcare providers. The patient discusses his beliefs and goals and is informed of his diagnosis, prognosis, and options, along with the benefits and drawbacks of the treatment options. The decisions made are turned into actionable medical orders. The form is readily accessible to medical personnel and aims to honor preferences whenever possible within the healthcare system.

Advance Directives

Laws related to advance directives vary from state to state. Here are a few resources for locating the proper forms for a particular state:

- The National Hospice and Palliative Care Organization (NHPCO) is a nonprofit organization that represents hospice and palliative care programs in the United States. NHPCO works to improve care for people who are dying and their loved ones. More information can be located on their website, caringinfo.org, or by calling 800-658-8898.

- The U.S. Living Will Registry is a privately held organization that electronically stores advance directives, organ donor information, and emergency contact information and makes them available to healthcare providers across the country 24 hours a day. More information can be found on their website, uslivingwillregistry.com, or by calling 800-LIV-WILL (800-548-9455).

Chapter Review

1. What is the difference between ethics and laws?

2. List eight examples of legal and ethical behavior for a nursing assistant.

3. According to the Omnibus Budget Reconciliation Act's (OBRA) requirements, how many hours of training must nursing assistants complete at a minimum?

4. How soon must a Minimum Data Set (MDS) be completed on new residents after admission?

5. What is the purpose of Residents' Rights?

6. If a nursing assistant sees abuse or suspects that a resident is being abused, what is her responsibility?

7. What are mandated reporters?

8. List five possible signs of abuse that should be reported by the nursing assistant. List five possible signs of neglect that should be reported by the nursing assistant.

9. If a resident wants to make a complaint of abuse, what is the nursing assistant's responsibility?

10. Pick three of the examples of behavior promoting Residents' Rights in Learning Objective 5. Describe how each example supports or promotes specific Residents' Rights.

11. What happens if a nursing assistant is accused of abusing a resident?

12. What is the role of an ombudsman?

13. What is one important reason that HIPAA was passed?

14. List five examples of a person's protected health information (PHI).

15. With whom is a nursing assistant allowed to share information about a resident?

16. To which members of the healthcare team is HIPAA applicable?

17. Define *advance directives* and briefly describe two examples.

18. List three rights relating to advance directives that the Patient Self-Determination Act (PSDA) requires be given to a resident at the time of admission.

4

Communication and Cultural Diversity

1. Define *communication*

Communication is the process of exchanging information with others. It is a process of sending and receiving messages. People communicate by using signs and symbols, such as words, drawings, and pictures. They also communicate through their behavior.

The simplest form of communication is a three-step process that takes place between two people (Fig. 4-1). In the first step, the sender (the person who communicates first) sends a message. In the second step, the receiver receives the message. Receiver and sender constantly switch roles as they communicate. The third step involves providing feedback. The receiver repeats the message or responds to it in some way. This lets the sender know that the message was received and understood. Feedback is especially important when working with the elderly. Nursing assistants must take time to make sure residents understand messages.

All three steps must occur before the communication process is complete. During a conversation, this process is repeated over and over.

Effective communication is a critical part of a nursing assistant's job. Nursing assistants must communicate with supervisors, the care team, residents, and family members. A resident's health depends on how well an NA communicates observations and concerns to the nurse. The NA will also need to communicate clearly and respectfully in stressful or confusing situa-

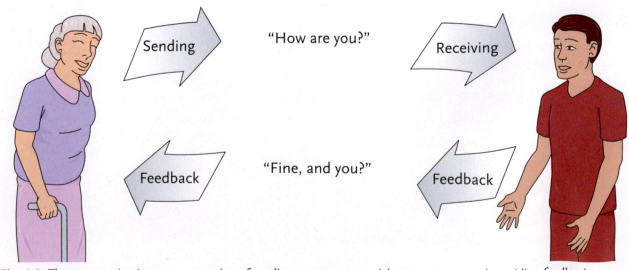

Sending   "How are you?"   Receiving

Feedback   "Fine, and you?"   Feedback

Fig. 4-1. *The communication process consists of sending a message, receiving a message, and providing feedback.*

tions. Some family members may need help in communicating clearly with each other or with the care team.

2. Explain verbal and nonverbal communication

Communication is either verbal or nonverbal. **Verbal communication** involves the use of words, spoken or written. Oral reports are an example of verbal communication. When communicating verbally, it is important to use words that have the same meaning to both the sender and the receiver. Misunderstandings may occur if each person interprets the same words differently. For example, if a nursing assistant asks a resident to "turn on the light" when she needs help, the resident may not understand that the NA meant for her to push the call button.

Nonverbal communication is communicating without using words. An example of nonverbal communication is a person shrugging his shoulders. Nonverbal communication also includes how a person says something. For example, an NA says cheerfully, "I'll be right there, Mrs. Gonzales." This communicates that the NA is ready and willing to help. But saying the same phrase in a different tone or emphasizing different words can communicate frustration and annoyance: *"I'll be right there, Mrs. Gonzales!"*

Body language is another form of nonverbal communication. Movements, facial expressions, and posture can express different attitudes or emotions. Just as with speaking, body language sends messages. Other people receive and interpret them. For example, slouching in a chair and sitting erect send two different messages (Fig. 4-2). Slouching says that a person is bored, tired, or hostile. Sitting up straight says that the person is interested and respectful. Other examples of positive nonverbal communication include smiling, nodding one's head, and looking at the person who is speaking.

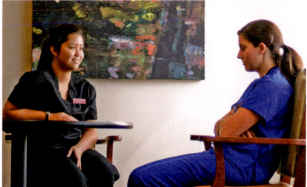

Fig. 4-2. Body language sends messages just as words do. Which of these people seems more interested in their conversation—the person on the right who is looking down with her arms crossed or the person on the left who is sitting up straight and smiling?

Sometimes people send one message verbally and a very different message nonverbally. Nonverbal communication often illustrates how someone is feeling. This message may be quite different from what he is saying. For example, a resident who says "I'm feeling fine today," but does not want to get out of bed and winces in pain, is sending two very different messages. Paying attention to nonverbal communication helps nursing assistants give better care. In this example, the NA should communicate to the nurse that the resident is staying in bed and appears to be wincing in pain, despite what he says.

Nursing assistants must also be aware of their own verbal and nonverbal messages. If an NA says "It's nice to see you today, Mr. Lee," but does not smile or look him in the eye, Mr. Lee may feel that the NA is not really happy to see him.

When communication is confusing, the NA should try to clarify it by asking for an explanation. The NA can say "Mrs. Jones, you've just told me something that I don't understand. Would you explain it to me?" Or she can state what she has observed and ask if the observation is correct. For example, "Mrs. Jones, I see that you're smiling, but I hear by the sound of your voice that you may be sad. Are you sad?" Taking time to clarify communication can help avoid misunderstandings.

3. Describe ways different cultures communicate

The term **cultural diversity** refers to different groups of people with varied backgrounds and experiences living together in the world. Positive responses to cultural diversity include acceptance and knowledge, not **bias**, or prejudice. A **culture** is a system of learned beliefs and behaviors that is practiced by a group of people. Each culture may have different knowledge, behaviors, beliefs, values, attitudes, religions, and customs.

Nonverbal communication may depend on personality or cultural background. Some people are more animated when they speak. They use a lot of gestures and facial expressions. Other people speak quietly or calmly, regardless of their moods. Depending on their cultural background, people may make motions with their hands when they talk. They may stand close to the person with whom they are speaking or touch the person.

People from some cultural groups stand further apart when talking than people from other groups. When one person moves closer, the other person may view it as a threat.

The use of touch and eye contact also varies with cultural background and personality (Fig. 4-3). For some people, touching is welcome. It expresses caring and warmth. For others, it seems intrusive, threatening, or even harassing. In the United States, it is common to talk about "looking someone straight in the eye" or speaking "eye to eye." Eye contact is often viewed as a sign of honesty. However, in some cultures, looking someone in the eye may seem overly bold or disrespectful.

It is important for nursing assistants to be sensitive to each resident's needs. This is key to providing professional, person-centered care. Learning each resident's behavior and preferences can be a challenge, but it is an important part of communication. It is especially vital in a multicultural society (a society made up of many cultures), such as the United States. Being aware

of all the messages sent and received and listening and observing carefully will help an NA better understand residents' needs and feelings.

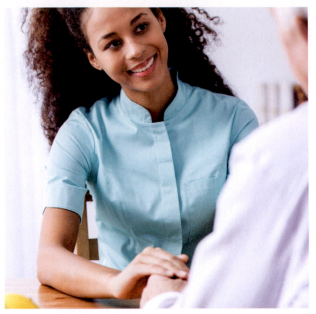

Fig. 4-3. How a person perceives touch may depend on his cultural background.

4. Identify barriers to communication

Communication can be blocked or disrupted in many ways (Fig. 4-4). The following are some communication barriers and ways for a nursing assistant to avoid them:

Resident does not hear NA, does not hear correctly, or does not understand. The NA should stand directly facing the resident. He should speak slowly and clearly. He should not shout, whisper, or mumble. The NA should speak in a low voice, using a pleasant tone. If the resident

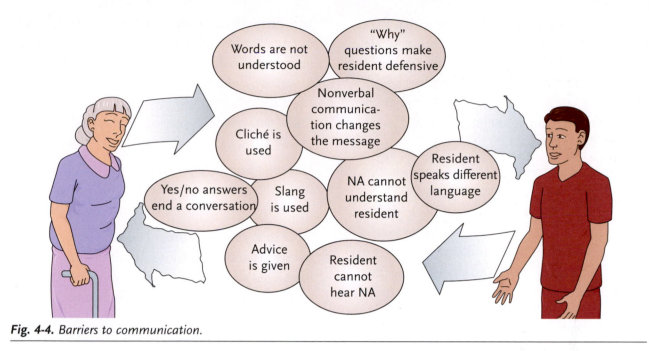

Fig. 4-4. Barriers to communication.

wears a hearing aid, the NA should check to ensure that it is on and is working properly.

Resident is difficult to understand. The NA should be patient and take time to listen. He can ask the resident to repeat or explain the message, and then state the message in his own words to make sure he has understood.

NA, resident, or others use words that are not understood. An NA should not use medical terminology with residents or their families. He should speak in simple, everyday words and ask what a word means if he is not sure.

NA uses slang or profanity. The NA should avoid using slang words and expressions. They are unprofessional and may not be understood. He should not use profanity, even if the resident does.

NA uses clichés. Clichés are phrases that are used over and over again and do not really mean anything. For example, "Everything will be fine" is a cliché. Instead of using a cliché, the NA should listen to what the resident is really saying and respond with a meaningful message. For example, if a resident is afraid of having a bath, the NA can say "I understand that it seems scary to you. What can I do to make you feel more at ease?" instead of saying "Oh, it'll be over before you know it."

NA responds with "Why?" The NA should avoid asking "Why?" when a resident makes a statement. "Why" questions make people feel defensive. For example, a resident may say she does not want to go for a walk today. If the NA asks "Why not," he may receive an angry response. Instead, he can ask "Are you too tired to take a walk? Is there something else you want to do?" The resident may then be willing to discuss the issue.

NA gives advice. The NA should not offer his opinion or give advice. Giving medical advice is not within an NA's scope of practice. It could be dangerous.

NA asks questions that only require yes/no answers. The NA should ask open-ended questions that need more than a "yes" or "no" answer. Yes and no answers end conversation. For example, if an NA wants to know what a resident likes to eat, he should not ask "Do you like vegetables?" Instead, he should ask "Which vegetables do you like best?"

Resident speaks a different language. If a resident speaks a different language than the NA does, the NA should speak slowly and clearly. He should keep his messages short and simple. He should be alert for words the resident understands and also be alert for signs that the resident is only pretending to understand. He may need to use pictures or gestures to communicate. The NA can ask the resident's family, friends, or other staff members who speak the resident's language for help. He should be patient and calm.

NA or resident uses nonverbal communication. Nonverbal communication can change a message. The NA should be aware of his body language and gestures. He can look for nonverbal messages from residents and clarify them. For example, "Mr. Feldman, you say you're feeling fine but you seem to be in pain. Is that true? What can I do to help?"

5. List ways to make communication accurate and explain how to develop effective interpersonal relationships

In addition to avoiding the barriers above, using the following techniques will help NAs send and receive clear, complete messages.

Be a good listener. The NA should allow the other person to express her ideas completely. He should concentrate on what the resident is saying and not interrupt. The NA should not finish the resident's sentences even if he knows what she is going to say. When the resident is finished, the NA should restate the message in his own words to make sure he has understood.

Provide feedback. Active listening means focusing on the person sending the message and giving feedback. Feedback might be an acknowledgment, a question, or repeating the sender's message. The NA should offer general but leading responses, such as "Oh?" or "Go on," or "Hmm." By doing this, he is actively listening, providing feedback, and encouraging the sender to expand the message.

Bring up topics of concern. If the NA knows of a topic that might concern a resident, he can raise the issue in a general, nonthreatening way. This

lets the resident decide whether or not to discuss it. For example, if the NA observes that a resident is unusually quiet, he could say, "Mrs. Jones, you seem so quiet today." Or he may notice a certain emotion. He might say, "Mrs. Jones, you seemed upset earlier. Would you like to talk about it?"

Let some pauses happen. Using silence for a few moments at a time encourages the resident to gather her thoughts and compose messages.

Tune in to other cultures. The NA should learn the words and expressions of a resident's culture. This shows respect and interest and promotes person-centered care. It will help the NA understand the resident more fully. He should be careful about using new words and terms, though, because some may have a different meaning than what he thinks. The focus should be on understanding words and expressions when others use them. The NA should not be judgmental; he should accept people who are different from him.

Accept a resident's religion or lack of religion. Religious differences also affect communication. Religion can be very important in people's lives, particularly when they are ill or dying. Other people are not religious and may feel strongly about that. The NA should respect residents' religious beliefs, practices, or lack of beliefs, especially if they are different from his own. He should not question residents' beliefs or discuss his beliefs with them.

Understand the importance of touch. Softly patting residents' hands or shoulders or holding their hands may communicate caring. Some people's backgrounds may make them less comfortable being touched. The NA should ask permission before touching residents and should be sensitive to their feelings. NAs must touch residents in order to do their jobs. However, they should recognize that some residents feel more comfortable when there is little physical contact. The NA should learn about his residents and adjust care to their needs.

Ask for more. When residents report symptoms, events, or feelings, the NA should have them repeat what they have said and ask them for more information.

Make sure communication aids are clean and in proper working order (Fig. 4-5). These include hearing aids, eyeglasses, dentures, and wrist or hand braces. The NA should inform the nurse if they do not work properly or are dirty or damaged.

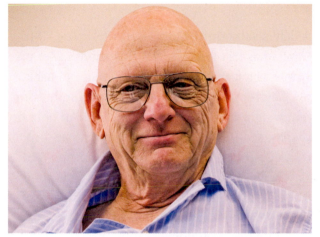

Fig. 4-5. Eyeglasses must fit well, be clean, and be in good condition. A nurse should be informed if communication aids are not working properly.

Proper Communication

When communicating with residents, the nursing assistant should remember to do the following:

- Always greet the resident by his or her preferred name.

- Identify herself.

- Focus on the topic to be discussed.

- Face the resident while speaking and avoid talking into space.

- Talk with the resident while giving care. The NA should not have personal conversations with other staff members while providing care.

- Listen and respond when the resident speaks.

- Praise the resident and smile often.

- Encourage the resident to interact with her and others.

- Be courteous.

- Tell the resident when she is leaving the room.

Residents' Rights

Names

Nursing assistants should call residents by the names that they prefer. Residents should not be referred to by their first names unless they have asked the NA to do so. Terms such as *sweetie, honey, dearie,* or *Gramps* are disrespectful and should not be used.

Developing good relationships with residents, their family members, and the care team will help NAs provide excellent care. Although an NA should not try to become friends with residents, she should try to develop warm professional relationships with them that are based on trust. In addition to the strategies already discussed, these suggestions can promote effective communication and lead to good relationships:

Avoid changing the subject when a resident is discussing something. This is true even if the subject makes the NA feel uncomfortable or helpless. For example, a resident might say "I'm having so much pain today." The NA should not try to avoid the topic by asking the resident if he wants to watch television. This makes the resident feel that the NA is not interested in him or what he is talking about.

Do not ignore a resident's request. Ignoring a request is considered negligent behavior. The NA should honor the request if she can or explain why the request cannot be fulfilled. These requests should always be reported to the nurse.

Do not talk down to an elderly or disabled resident. An NA should talk to residents and their families as she would talk to any person. She can make adjustments if someone has a visual or hearing impairment. Guidelines for residents who have a visual or hearing impairment are found later in the chapter.

Sit or stand near the resident who has started the conversation. Sitting or standing near the resident shows that the NA finds what she is saying important and worth listening to (Fig. 4-6).

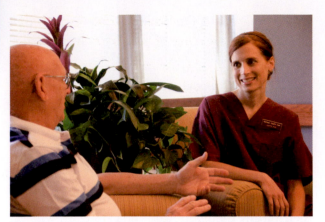

Fig. 4-6. Nursing assistants should sit near residents and look at them while they talk to show that they are interested in the conversation.

Lean forward in the chair when a resident is speaking. Leaning forward communicates interest. The NA should pay attention to her nonverbal communication. If she folds her arms in front of her body, she sends the negative message that she wishes to distance herself from the speaker.

Talk directly to the resident. The NA should not talk to other staff members, the resident's family members, or anyone else while helping residents. She should not gossip about other staff members or residents.

Approach the resident. Even if the NA is in another area of the room, she should approach the resident. This tells the resident she is interested in what the resident has to say.

Be empathetic. The NA should try to understand and identify with what the resident is going through. This is called empathy. She can ask herself how she would feel if she were confined to bed or needed help to go to the bathroom. The NA should not tell residents she knows how they feel, because she does not know exactly how they feel. She can say things like, "I can imagine this must be difficult for you."

Have time for residents' family and friends. The NA should not discuss a resident's care with friends or family members, but she can listen if they want to talk. The NA should be respectful and pleasant and give privacy for visits. She

should not interfere with private family business. Families are great sources of information for residents' personal preferences, history, diet, habits, and routines. The NA should ask them questions. If any abusive behavior toward a resident is observed during a visit, it must be reported immediately to the nurse.

6. Explain the difference between facts and opinions

A fact is something that is definitely true. "Mr. Garcia has lost four pounds this month," for example, is a fact. This fact has evidence to back it up: weighing Mr. Garcia and comparing his current weight to his weight last month. An opinion is something someone believes to be true, but is not definitely true or cannot be proven. "Mr. Garcia looks thinner" is an opinion. This statement might be true, but it cannot be backed up with evidence. It is important to be able to separate facts from opinions.

Using facts instead of opinions is a more professional and effective way to communicate. When communicating with the care team, distinguishing between facts and opinions is important. For example, "Mr. Morgan is acting like he had a stroke" is an opinion and could very well be wrong. Instead, the facts should be reported: "Mr. Morgan has lost strength on his right side, and his speech is slurred." When reporting opinions, the NA can introduce them with "I think." Then it is clear that she is offering her opinion and not a fact she has observed.

7. Explain objective and subjective information and describe how to observe and report accurately

When making any kind of report, the right kind of information must be collected before documenting it. Facts, not opinions, are most useful to the nurse and the care team. Two kinds of factual information are needed in reporting. **Objective information** is based on what a person sees, hears, touches, or smells. Objective information is collected by using the senses. It is also called signs. **Subjective information** is something a person cannot or did not observe, but is based on something that the resident reported, and it may or may not be true. It is also called symptoms.

An example of objective information is "Mr. McClain is holding his head and rubbing his temples." A subjective report of the same situation might be "Mr. McClain says he has a headache." The nurse and the care team need factual information in order to make decisions about care and treatment. Both objective and subjective reports are valuable.

In any report, what is observed (signs) and what the resident reports (symptoms) need to be clearly noted. "Ms. Scott reports pain in left shoulder" is an example of clear reporting. Nursing assistants are not expected to make diagnoses based on signs and symptoms they observe. This is beyond their scope of practice. Their observations, however, can alert the care team to possible problems.

In order to report accurately, an NA must observe residents accurately. To observe accurately, as many senses as possible should be used to gather information (Fig. 4-7).

Sight. The NA should look for changes in the resident's appearance. These include rashes, redness, paleness, swelling, discharge, weakness, sunken eyes, and posture or gait (walking) changes.

Hearing. The NA should listen to what the resident says about his condition, family, or needs. Is the resident speaking clearly and making sense? Does he show emotions, such as anger, frustration, or sadness? Is his breathing normal? Does he wheeze, gasp, or cough? Is the area calm and quiet enough for him to rest as needed?

Touch. Does the resident's skin feel hot or cool, moist or dry? Is the pulse rate normal?

Smell. Are there any odors coming from the resident's body? Odors could suggest poor bathing, infections, or incontinence. **Incontinence** is the

inability to control the bladder or bowels. Breath odor could suggest use of alcohol or tobacco, indigestion, or poor mouth care.

Using all of the senses will allow an NA to make the most complete report of a resident's situation.

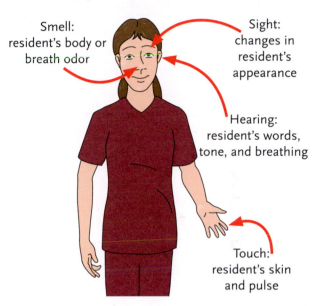

Smell: resident's body or breath odor

Sight: changes in resident's appearance

Hearing: resident's words, tone, and breathing

Touch: resident's skin and pulse

Fig. 4-7. Reporting observations accurately requires using more than one sense.

8. Explain how to communicate with other team members

Nursing assistants will communicate regularly with care team members, residents, and residents' families and friends. NAs should communicate freely with the charge nurse regarding residents. They should keep the nurse informed of all important issues during their shift and share information with other staff members as needed. A nursing assistant may need to share a resident's personal information with another nursing assistant to help her give care to a resident. However, the activities staff may have no need to know that same information. NAs should refer any doctor's questions to the nurse.

It is important to always respect residents' privacy. When giving information to other members of the care team, NAs should be sure that other residents or staff cannot overhear. They should be cautious when communicating with residents and their families and friends. NAs should not share new information about residents' conditions or new diagnoses. That is the nurse's or doctor's responsibility. When in doubt, NAs can ask the nurse what they can say. A resident may not want information shared with family members and that is his legal right.

The chain of command should be used to voice any complaints that NAs may have. The charge nurse should be approached first. If a complaint is not resolved, NAs can continue reporting up the chain of command. If an NA feels that her charge nurse has abused a resident, she must communicate this to the nurse's supervisor.

9. Describe basic medical terminology and abbreviations

Throughout a nursing assistant's training, he will learn medical terms for specific conditions. For example, the medical term for a runny nose is *nasal discharge*; skin that is blue or gray is called **cyanotic**. Medical terms are often made up of roots, prefixes, and suffixes. A root is a part of a word that contains its basic meaning or definition. The prefix is the word part that precedes the root to help form a new word. The suffix is the word part added to the end of a root that helps form a new word. Prefixes and suffixes are called *affixes* because they are attached, or affixed, to a root. Here are some examples:

- The root *derm* or *derma* means skin. The suffix *itis* means inflammation. Dermatitis is an inflammation of the skin.

- The prefix *brady* means slow. The root *cardia* means heart. Bradycardia is slow heartbeat or pulse.

- The suffix *pathy* means disease. The root *neuro* means of the nerve or nervous system. Neuropathy is a nerve disease or disease of the nervous system.

When speaking with residents and their families, NAs should use simple, nonmedical terms. Medical terms should not be used because they

may not be understood. But when speaking with the care team, using medical terminology will help give more complete information.

Abbreviations are another way to communicate more efficiently with care team members. For example, the abbreviation *prn* means *as necessary*. *BP* means *blood pressure*. Nursing assistants should learn the standard medical abbreviations their facility uses. They can use them to report information briefly and accurately. They may also need to know these abbreviations to read assignments or care plans. A brief list of abbreviations follows, and more are located at the end of this textbook and in the instructor's guide. There may be other terms in use at a facility, so it is important for NAs to follow facility policy.

Common Abbreviations	
ā	before
abd	abdomen
ac, AC	before meals
ad lib	as desired
ADLs	activities of daily living
amb	ambulate, ambulatory
AP	apical pulse
b.i.d., bid	two times a day
BM	bowel movement
BP, B/P	blood pressure
c̄	with
C	Celsius degree
c/o	complains of
CHF	congestive heart failure
CPR	cardiopulmonary resuscitation
DNR	do not resuscitate
dx, DX	diagnosis
F	Fahrenheit degree
FBS	fasting blood sugar

ft	foot
FWB	full weight-bearing
GI	gastrointestinal
H_2O	water
h, hr, hr.	hour
hs, HS	hours of sleep
inc	incontinent
I&O	intake and output
NKDA	no known drug allergies
NPO	nothing by mouth
NWB	non-weight-bearing
O_2	oxygen
OOB	out of bed
$\bar{p}$	after
pc, p.c.	after meals
PO	by mouth
prn, PRN	as necessary
PWB	partial-weight-bearing
$\bar{q}$	every
ROM	range of motion
$\bar{s}$	without
SOB	shortness of breath
stat, STAT	at once, immediately
t.i.d., tid	three times a day
TPR	temperature, pulse, respiration
v.s., VS	vital signs
w/c, W/C	wheelchair

10. Explain how to give and receive an accurate report of a resident's status

Nursing assistants must make brief and accurate oral and written reports to residents and staff. Careful observations are used to make these reports and are very important to the health and well-being of all residents. Signs and symptoms that should be reported will be discussed throughout this textbook. Some observations will need to be reported immediately to the nurse. Deciding what to report immediately involves critical thinking. Anything that endangers residents should be reported immediately, including the following:

- Falls
- Chest pain
- Severe headache
- Difficulty breathing
- Abnormal pulse, respiration, or blood pressure
- Change in mental status
- Sudden weakness or loss of mobility
- High fever
- Loss of consciousness
- Change in level of consciousness
- Bleeding
- Swelling of body part
- Change in resident's condition
- Bruises, abrasions, or other signs of possible abuse (Chapter 3)

Nursing assistants use oral reports to discuss experiences with residents and observations of residents' conditions. Facts, not opinions, should be used for oral reports. It is a good idea for NAs to write notes so that important details are not forgotten (Fig. 4-8). When needing to give an oral report, unless the situation is urgent, the NA should approach the nurse and wait for the nurse to complete the task she is currently doing. Once the nurse has acknowledged the NA, she can briefly state the message and deliver the written summary as well if there is one. Waiting until the nurse is done helps reduce the risk of error. Following an oral report, NAs must document when, why, about what, and to whom an oral report was given. Documentation should always occur after the report was given, not before.

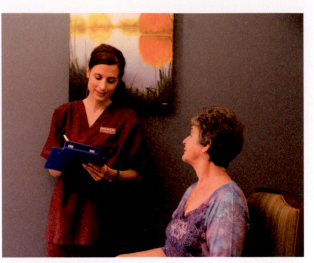

Fig. 4-8. *Taking notes helps nursing assistants remember facts and report accurately.*

Sometimes the nurse or another member of the care team will give an NA a brief oral report on one of her residents. The NA should listen carefully and take notes. She should ask about anything she does not understand. At the end of the report, the NA can restate what she has been told to make sure she understands.

When making reports about residents, NAs must remember that all resident information is confidential. Information should only be shared with members of the care team.

11. Explain documentation and describe related terms and forms

Nursing assistants spend more time with residents than other members of the care team. They may observe things about residents that nurses or doctors have not noticed. NAs do not make diagnoses or decide on treatment. However, they have valuable information about residents that will help in care planning. Documenting accurately is the key to care planning. A thorough record shows an NA's observations to others. It helps the NA to remember details about each resident.

Because nursing assistants see many residents during the day, they cannot remember everything that each resident did or said, or every observation they made. Documentation gives an up-to-date record of each resident's care. NAs must learn to document accurately. They must always take the time to observe and record carefully. Because documentation is so important, it should be recorded immediately and not be put off until later.

A medical chart is a legal document. What is included in the chart is considered in court to be what actually happened. If an NA gave a resident a bath and took her temperature, but never documented these things, the NA could not necessarily prove that he actually performed the care. In general, if something does not appear in a resident's chart, it did not legally happen. Failing to document care could cause very serious legal problems for nursing assistants and their employers. It could also harm residents. It is important for NAs to remember that if it was not documented, it was not done.

Information found in a medical chart includes the following:

• Admission sheet (protected health information about the person, such as name, address, social security number, date of birth, and email address, among other items)

• Medical history (illnesses, immunizations, medications, previous surgeries, and family and social histories)

• Doctor's orders (instructions given to other members of the care team)

• Progress notes (updates from all care team members detailing changes or new information about the person's condition)

• Test results (blood tests, lab results, and other tests)

• Graphic sheet (vital signs, intake and output, and bladder and bowel elimination)

• Nurse's notes (the person's reported symptoms and actions taken to address them)

• Flow sheets (check-off sheets for documenting care; may also be called an ADL [activities of daily living] sheet) (Fig. 4-9)

Communication and Cultural Diversity

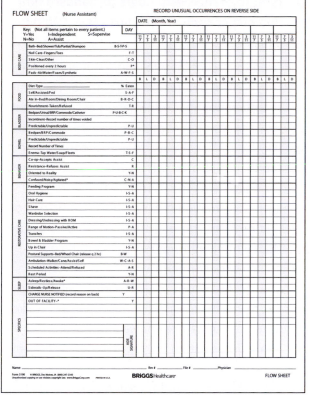

Fig. 4-9. *Some facilities use an ADL flow sheet for documenting care.* (REPRINTED WITH PERMISSION OF BRIGGS CORPORATION, 800-247-2343, WWW.BRIGGSCORP.COM)

There are legal aspects to careful documentation that are important to remember:

- It is the only way to guarantee clear and complete communication among all the members of the care team.

- Documentation is a legal record of every part of a resident's treatment. Medical charts can be used in court as legal evidence.

- Documentation helps protect nursing assistants and their employers from liability by proving what they did when caring for residents.

- Documentation gives an up-to-date record of the status and care of each resident.

Guidelines: Careful Documentation

G Document care immediately after it is given. This makes details easier to remember. Always wait to document until after care has been completed. Do not record any care before it has been done.

G Think about what you want to say before documenting. Be as brief and as clear as possible.

G Use facts, not opinions.

G Use black ink when documenting by hand. Write as neatly as you can.

G If you make a mistake, draw one line through it, and write the correct information. Put your initials and the date (Fig. 4-10). Do not erase what you have written. Do not use correction fluid. Documentation done on a computer is time-stamped; it can only be changed by entering another notation.

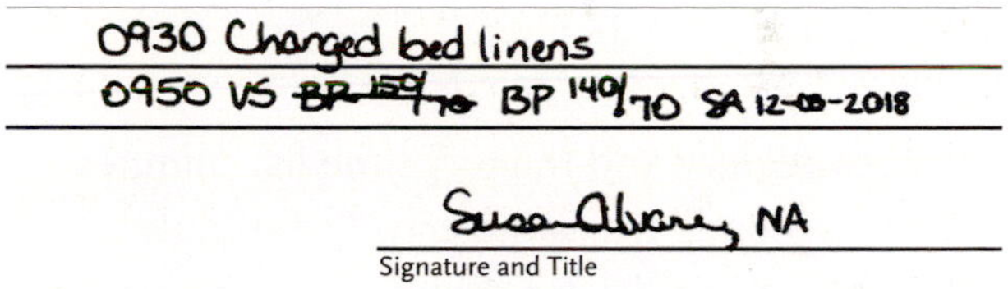

0930 Changed bed linens
0950 VS ~~BP 159/70~~ BP 140/70 SA 12-03-2018

Susan Abvary, NA
Signature and Title

Fig. 4-10. *One example of how to correct a mistake.*

G Sign your full name and title (for example, Sara Martinez, CNA) and write the correct date.

G Document as specified in the care plan.

G Documentation may be done by code. For example, when documenting activities of daily living on a flow sheet, you may need to choose a code to explain what the resident was able to do. Zero may be classified as independent, 1 as needs supervision, 2 as needs limited assistance, 3 as needs extensive assistance, and 4 as total dependence. You will be trained to use the proper procedures for documentation at your facility.

G Documentation may need to be done using the 24-hour clock, or military time (Fig. 4-11). Regular time uses the numbers 1 to 12 to show each of the 24 hours in a day. In military time, the hours are numbered from 00 to 23. Midnight is expressed as 0000 (or 2400), 1:00 a.m. is 0100, 1:00 p.m. is 1300, and so on.

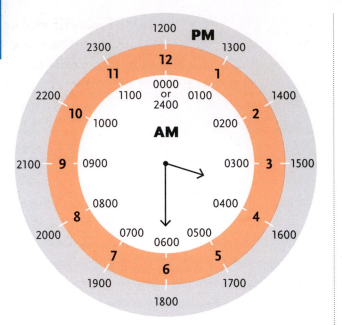

Fig. 4-11. *Illustration showing the divisions in the 24-hour clock.*

Both regular and military time list minutes and seconds the same way. The minutes and seconds do not change when converting from regular to military time. The abbreviations a.m. and p.m. are used in regular time to show what time of day it is. However, these are not used in military time, since specific numbers show each hour of the day. For example, to change 4:22 p.m. to military time, add 4 + 12. The minutes do not change. The time is expressed as 1622 hours.

To change the hours between 1:00 p.m. to 11:59 p.m. to military time, add 12 to the regular time. For example, to change 3:00 p.m. to military time, add 3 + 12. The time is expressed as 1500 (fifteen hundred) hours.

Midnight is the only time that differs. Midnight can be written as 0000, and it can also be written as 2400. This follows the rule of adding 12 to the regular time. Follow your facility's policy on how to express midnight.

To change from military time to regular time, subtract 12. The minutes do not change. For example, to change 2200 hours to standard time, subtract 12 from 22. The answer is 10:00

p.m. To change 1610 hours to standard time, subtract 12 from 16. The answer is 4:10 p.m.

G   At some facilities, computers or tablets are used to document information. A computer may remain in a resident's room for care team members to input information each time they visit the room. A computer may be in the hallway for staff members to use. A computer or tablet may also be carried from room to room for documentation. Computers record and store information that can be retrieved when it is needed. This is faster and more accurate than writing information by hand. If your facility uses computers for documentation, you will be trained to use them. HIPAA privacy guidelines apply to computer use. Make sure nobody can see private and protected health information on your computer screen. Confidential information should not be shared with anyone except the care team.

12. Describe incident reporting and recording

An **incident** is an accident, problem, or unexpected event during the course of care. It is something that is not part of the normal routine. A mistake in care, such as feeding a resident from the wrong meal tray, is an incident. A resident fall or injury is another type of incident. Accusations made by residents against staff, as well as employee injuries, are other types of incidents.

State and federal guidelines require that incidents be recorded in an incident report (Fig. 4-12). An incident report (also called an occurrence, accident, accident/incident, or event report) is a report that documents the incident and the response to it. The report is a factual, objective account of what happened. The information in an incident report is confidential and is intended for internal use to help prevent future incidents. Incident reports should be filed when any of the following occur:

INCIDENT/ACCIDENT REPORT

PERSON INVOLVED	(Last name)	(First name)	(Middle initial)					
				Adult ☐	Child ☐	Male ☐	Female ☐	Age_____

Date of incident/accident	Time of incident/accident	A.M. ☐ P.M. ☐	Exact location of incident/accident
			Resident's room ☐ (No._____) Hallway ☐ Bathroom ☐ Other ☐ Specify _____

RESIDENT ☐
List diagnosis if contributed to incident/accident:

Resident's condition before incident/accident

Normal ☐   Confused ☐   Disoriented ☐   Sedated ☐ (Drug_____ Dose_____ Time_____)   Other ☐ (Specify)_____

Were bed rails ordered? Yes ☐ No ☐	Were bed rails present? Yes ☐ No ☐	If Yes, Up ☐ Down ☐	Was height of bed adjustable? Yes ☐ No ☐	If Yes, Up ☐ Down ☐

Was a restraint in use?   Yes ☐   No ☐

Physical restraint ☐   Type_____   Chemical restraint ☐   Specify_____

EMPLOYEE ☐	Department	Job title	Length of time in this position

VISITOR ☐ **OTHER** ☐	Home address	Home phone
	Occupation	Reason for presence at this facility

Equipment involved ☐ Property involved ☐ Describe	Was person authorized to be at location of incident/accident? Yes ☐ No ☐

Describe exactly what happened; why it happened; what the causes were. If an injury, state part of body injured. If property or equipment damaged, describe damage.

_____

_____

Indicate on diagram location of injury:

Temp. _____   Pulse _____   Resp. _____

B.P. _____

TYPE OF INJURY

1. Laceration ☐
2. Hematoma ☐
3. Abrasion ☐
4. Burn ☐
5. Swelling ☐
6. None apparent ☐
7. Other (specify below) ☐

LEVEL OF CONSCIOUSNESS

_____

_____

Name of physician notified	Time of notification _____ A.M./P.M.	Time of response _____ A.M./P.M.
Name and relationship of family member/resident representative notified	Time of notification _____ A.M./P.M.	Time of response _____ A.M./P.M.

Was person involved seen by a physician? Yes ☐ No ☐ If Yes, physician's name	Where	Date	Time A.M. ☐ P.M. ☐
Was first aid administered? Yes ☐ No ☐ If Yes, type of care provided and by whom	Where	Date	Time A.M. ☐ P.M. ☐
Was person involved taken to a hospital? Yes ☐ No ☐ If Yes, hospital name	By whom	Date	Time A.M. ☐ P.M. ☐

Name, title (if applicable), address & phone no. of witness(es)	Additional comments and/or steps taken to prevent recurrence:

SIGNATURE / TITLE / DATE	SIGNATURE / TITLE / DATE
Person preparing report	Medical Director
Director of Nursing	Administrator

Form 3322/2R   Rev. 11/00   © 1991 BRIGGS, Des Moines, IA (800) 247-2343
Unauthorized copying or use violates copyright law. www.BriggsCorp.com   PRINTED IN U.S.A.

BRiGGS Healthcare®

INCIDENT/ACCIDENT REPORT

Fig. 4-12. *A sample incident report.* (REPRINTED WITH PERMISSION OF BRIGGS CORPORATION, 800-247-2343, WWW.BRIGGSCORP.COM)

- A resident falls (all falls must be reported, even if the resident says he or she is fine)

- A nursing assistant or a resident breaks or damages something

- A nursing assistant makes a mistake in care

- A resident or a family member makes a request that is outside the nursing assistant's scope of practice

- A resident or a family member makes sexual advances or remarks

- Anything happens that makes a nursing assistant feel uncomfortable, threatened, or unsafe

- A nursing assistant gets injured on the job

- A nursing assistant is exposed to blood or body fluids

Reporting and documenting incidents is done to protect everyone involved. This includes the resident, the employer, and the nursing assistant. When documenting incidents, NAs should complete the report as soon as possible and give it to the charge nurse. This is important so that they do not forget any details.

If a resident falls, and the NA did not see it, she should not write, "Mr. G fell." Instead, she should write "Found Mr. G on the floor" or "Mr. G states that he fell." Nursing assistants should write brief and accurate descriptions of the events as they happened without placing blame or liability within the report.

Guidelines: Incident Reporting

G Tell what happened. State the time and the mental and physical condition of the person.

G Describe the person's reaction to the incident.

G State the facts; do not give opinions.

G Do not write anything in the incident report on the medical record.

G Describe the action taken to give care.

Sentinel Event

A **sentinel event** is an unexpected occurrence that results in serious physical or psychological injury or death. Events are called sentinel because they signal the need for an immediate investigation and response. An example of this type of event is a medication error that results in a resident's death. A sentinel event is required to be reported to the proper agency.

13. Demonstrate effective communication on the telephone

Nursing assistants may be asked to make a call or answer the telephone at their facility. A home health aide working in the home may need to answer the phone for clients or call a supervisor.

Guidelines: Telephone Communication

When making a call, follow these steps:

G Always identify yourself before asking to speak to someone. Never ask, "Who is this?" when someone answers your call.

G After you have identified yourself, ask for the person with whom you need to speak.

G If the person you are calling is available, identify yourself again. State why you are calling. Planning your call before you pick up the phone will help you be as efficient as possible.

G If the person is not available, ask if you can leave a message. Always leave a brief message, even if it is only to say you called. The message shows that you were trying to reach someone.

G Leave a brief and clear message. Do not give more information than necessary. A basic message includes your name, your facility's name, the phone number where you can be reached, and a brief description of the reason for your call.

G Thank the person who takes the message for you. Always be polite over the telephone, as you would be in person.

When answering calls, follow these steps:

G Always identify your facility's name, your name, and your position. Be friendly and professional.

G If you need to find the person the caller wishes to speak with, place the caller on hold after asking if it is OK to do so.

G If the caller has to leave a message, write it down and repeat it to make sure you have the correct message. Ask for proper spellings of names. Do not ask for more information than the person needs to return the call: a name, short message, and phone number is enough. Do not give out any information about staff or residents.

G Thank the person for calling and say goodbye.

14. Explain the resident call system

Long-term care facilities are required to have a call system—often called *call lights*—so that residents can call for help whenever they need it. They are in resident rooms and bathrooms. Some have strings for residents to pull and others have buttons to be pushed (Fig. 4-13). The signal is usually both a light outside the room and a sound that can be heard in the nurses' station. This is the primary way a resident can call for help. Nursing assistants should always respond immediately when they see the light or hear the sound. They should respond in a courteous and respectful manner. If the resident needs something that is outside of the NA's scope of practice or not part of the NA's responsibilities, she should let the resident know what she will do to address the issue. Then the NA should direct the request to the correct person. Once that has been done, she should follow up and let the resident know how long he can expect to wait.

It is important for the nursing assistant to check each time before leaving a room to make sure that the call light is within reach of the resident's unaffected/stronger hand and that the resident knows how to use it.

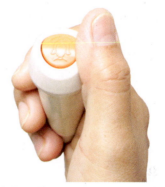

Fig. 4-13. *Call lights allow residents to signal staff when needed. This is one type of call light that requires a button to be pushed. There are other types of call systems available for residents who are not able to push buttons. Nursing assistants must always respond to call lights promptly.*

15. List guidelines for communicating with residents with special needs

Due to illness or impairments, some residents need special techniques to aid communication. An **impairment** is a loss of function or ability; it can be a partial or complete loss. Special techniques for different conditions are listed below. Information about communicating with residents who have dementia, such as Alzheimer's disease, is in Chapter 19. Guidelines for communicating with residents who have a mental illness are in Chapter 20.

Hearing Impairment

There are many different kinds of hearing loss. A person may be born with a hearing impairment or it may happen gradually. Deafness is a partial or complete loss of hearing. It can occur as the result of heredity, disease, or injury. In the elderly, aging commonly causes loss of hearing, as well as impaired vision, smell, and taste. If a person has a gradual hearing loss, he may not be conscious of it. Signs of hearing loss include the following:

- Speaking loudly

- Leaning forward when someone is speaking

- Cupping the ear to hear better

- Responding inappropriately

- Asking the speaker to repeat what has been said

- Speaking in a monotone

- Avoiding social gatherings or acting irritable in the presence of people who are having a conversation

- Suspecting others of talking about them or of deliberately speaking softly

People who have hearing impairment may use a hearing aid, read lips, or use sign language. People with impaired hearing also closely observe the facial expressions and body language of others to add to their knowledge of what is being said.

Guidelines: Hearing Impairment

G If the person has a hearing aid, make sure he or she is wearing it and that it is turned on.

G Many different types of hearing aids exist. Follow the manufacturer's directions for cleaning and handling the hearing aid. In general, the hearing aid needs to be cleaned daily. Wipe it with a special cleaning solution and a soft cloth. Do not put the hearing aid in water. Handle it carefully; do not drop it. Always keep it in the same safe place, such as its case, when it is not being worn. Turn it off when it is not in use. Remove it before bathing, showering, or shampooing hair. Some hearing aids have rechargeable batteries. Some need to be recharged nightly. Follow instructions in the care plan.

G Reduce or remove background noise, such as televisions, radios, and loud speech. Close doors if needed.

G Get the resident's attention before speaking. Do not startle residents by approaching from behind. Walk in front of them or touch them lightly on the arm to let them know you are near.

G Speak clearly, slowly, and in good lighting. Directly face the person (Fig. 4-14). The light should be on your face, not on the resident's. Ask if she can hear what you are saying.

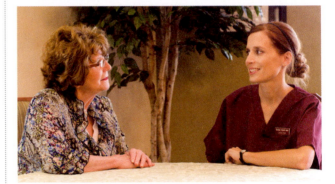

Fig. 4-14. *Speak face-to-face in good light.*

G Do not shout or mouth the words in an exaggerated way.

G Keep the pitch of your voice low.

G Residents may read lips, so do not chew gum or eat while speaking. Keep your hands away from your face while talking.

G If the resident hears better out of one ear, try to speak and stand on that side.

G Use short sentences and simple words. Avoid sudden topic changes.

G Repeat what you have said using different words when needed. Some people who are hearing impaired want you to repeat exactly what was said because they miss only a few words.

G Use picture cards or a notepad as needed.

G Residents who are hearing impaired may hear less when they are tired or ill. This is true of everyone. Be patient and empathetic. Avoid long, tiring conversations.

G Some residents who are hearing-impaired have speech problems and may be difficult to understand. Do not pretend you understand if you do not. Ask the resident to repeat what was said. Observe the lips, facial expressions, and body language. Then tell the resident what you think you heard. You can also request that the resident write down words.

G Hearing decline can be a normal aspect of aging. Be understanding and supportive.

Vision Impairment

Vision impairment can affect people of all ages. It can exist at birth or develop gradually. It can occur in one eye or in both. It can also be the result of injury, illness, or aging.

Some vision impairment causes people to wear corrective lenses, such as contact lenses or eyeglasses. **Farsightedness** (hyperopia) is the ability to see objects in the distance better than objects nearby. It develops in most people as they age. **Nearsightedness** (myopia) is the ability to see things near but not far. It may occur in younger persons. Some people need to wear eyeglasses all the time. Others only need them to read or for activities that require seeing distant objects, such as driving. Surgery can also be performed to correct these eye problems. Chapter 18 has more information about vision impairment.

Guidelines: Vision Impairment

G Encourage the use of eyeglasses or contact lenses (contacts) if worn.

G If the resident has eyeglasses, make sure they are clean. Clean glass lenses with water and a soft tissue. Clean plastic lenses with cleaning fluid and/or a lens cloth. Make sure that eyeglasses are in good condition and fit correctly. Report to the nurse if they do not.

G Contact lenses are made of many types of plastic. Some can be worn and disposed of daily; others are worn for longer periods. If the resident is able, it is best to leave contact lens care to him or her.

G Knock on the door and identify yourself immediately when you enter the room. Do not touch the resident until you have said your name. Explain why you are there and what you would like to do. Let the resident know when you are leaving the room.

G Make sure there is proper lighting in the room. Face the resident when speaking.

G When you enter a new room with the resident, orient him to where things are. Describe the things you see around you. Try not to use words such as "see," "look," and "watch."

G Always tell the resident what you are doing while caring for him. Give specific directions, such as "on your right" or "in front of you." Talk directly to the resident whom you are assisting. Do not talk to other residents or staff members.

G Use the face of an imaginary clock as a guide to explain the position of objects that are in front of the resident. For example, "There is a sofa at 7 o'clock" (Fig. 4-15).

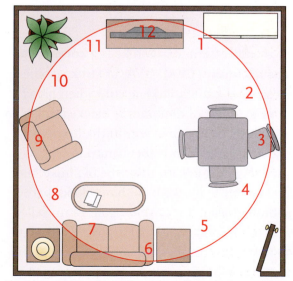

Fig. 4-15. *Use the face of an imaginary clock to explain the position of objects.*

G   Do not move personal items, furniture, or other objects. Put everything back where you found it.

G   Tell the resident where the call light is.

G   Leave doors completely open or completely closed, never partly open.

G   If the resident needs guidance in getting around, walk slightly ahead. Let the resident touch or grasp your arm lightly. This allows you to guide the resident and warn him of steps, etc. Walk at the resident's pace, not yours.

G   Give assistance with cutting food and opening containers as needed.

G   Use large clocks, clocks that chime, and radios to help keep track of time.

G   Large-print books, audiobooks, digital books, and Braille books are available. Learning to read Braille, however, takes a long time and requires training.

G   If the resident has a guide dog, do not play with, distract, or feed it.

G   Encourage the use of the other senses, such as hearing, touch, and smell. Encourage the resident to feel and touch things, such as clothing, furniture, or items in the room.

CVA or Stroke

The medical term for a stroke is a **cerebrovascular accident (CVA)**. CVA, or stroke (sometimes called *brain attack*), occurs when blood supply to a part of the brain is blocked or a blood vessel leaks or ruptures within the brain. An ischemic stroke is the most common type of stroke (Fig. 4-16). With this type of stroke, the blood supply is blocked. Without blood, part of the brain does not receive oxygen. Brain cells begin to die, and additional damage can occur due to leaking blood, clots, and swelling of the tissues. Swelling can also cause pressure on other areas of the brain.

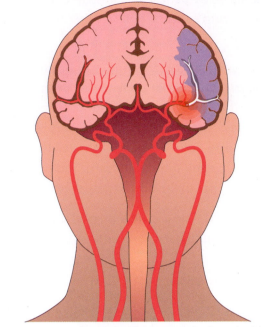

Fig. 4-16. *An ischemic stroke is caused when the blood supply to the brain is blocked.*

Strokes can be mild or severe. After a stroke, a resident may experience any of the following:

- Paralysis on one side of the body, called **hemiplegia**

- Weakness on one side of the body, called **hemiparesis**

- Tendency to ignore one side of the body, called *one-sided neglect*

- Loss of ability to tell where affected body parts are

- Trouble communicating thoughts through speech or writing, called **expressive aphasia**

- Difficulty understanding spoken or written words, called **receptive aphasia**

- Inappropriate or unprovoked emotional responses, including laughing, crying, and anger, called **emotional lability**

- Loss of sensations such as temperature or touch

- Loss of bowel or bladder control

- Cognitive impairments, such as poor judgment, memory loss, loss of problem-solving abilities, and confusion

- Difficulty swallowing, called **dysphagia**

Depending on the severity of the stroke and speech loss or confusion, these guidelines may be helpful:

Guidelines: Communication and Stroke

G   Keep questions and directions simple. Give directions one step at a time.

G   Phrase questions so they can be answered with a "yes" or "no." For example, when helping a resident with eating, ask "Would you like to start with a drink of milk?"

G   Agree on signals, such as shaking or nodding the head or raising a hand or finger to indicate "yes" or "no."

G   Give residents time to respond. Listen attentively.

G   Use a pencil and paper if the resident is able to write. A thick handle or tape wrapped around the pencil may help the resident hold it more easily.

G   Never call the weaker side the "bad side," or talk about the "bad" leg or arm. Use the term *weaker* or *involved* to refer to the side with paralysis or weakness.

G   Keep the call signal within reach of residents. They can let you know when you are needed.

G   Use both verbal and nonverbal communication to express your positive attitude. Let the resident know you have confidence in his or her abilities through smiles, touches, and gestures. Gestures and pointing can also help give information or allow the resident to communicate with you.

G   Use communication boards or special cards to make communication easier (Fig. 4-17).

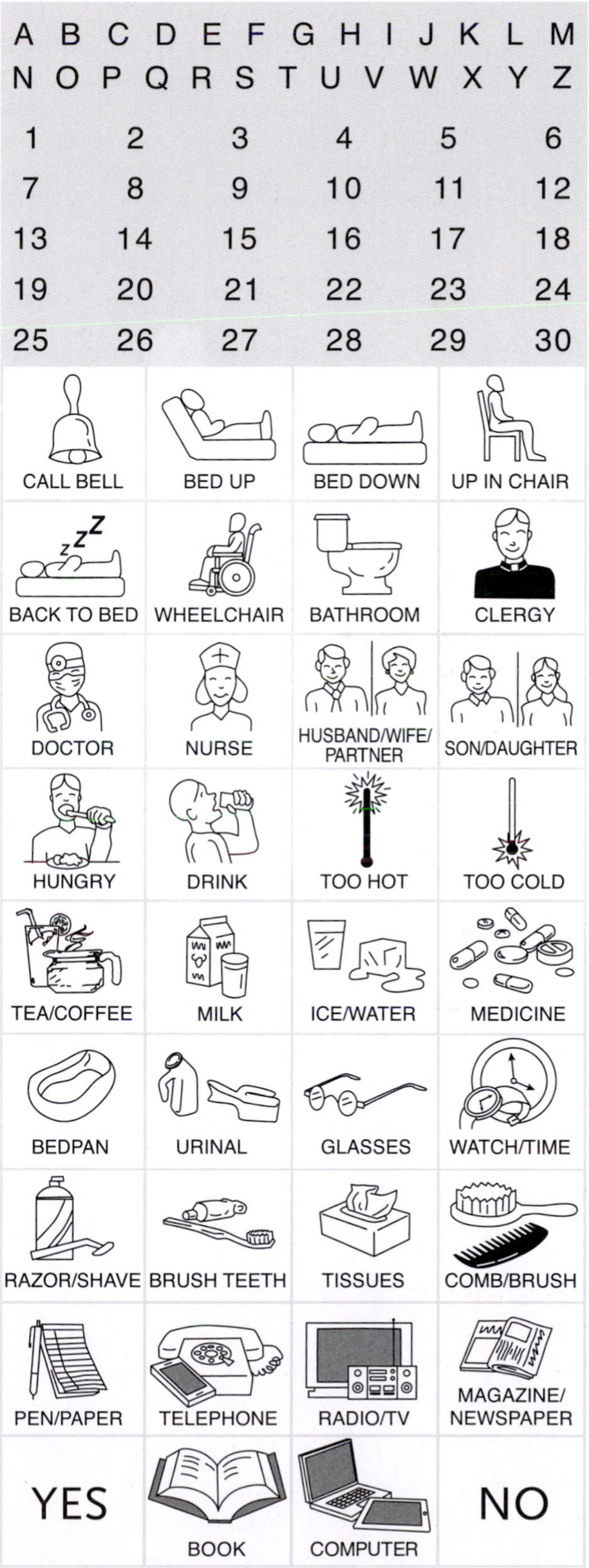

Fig. 4-17. A sample communication board.

More information about strokes and related care may be found in Chapter 18.

Combative Behavior

Residents may display **combative**, meaning violent or hostile, behavior. Such behavior may include hitting, pushing, kicking, or verbal attacks. This behavior may be the result of disease affecting the brain. It may be an expression of frustration, or it may just be part of someone's personality. In general, combative behavior is not a reaction to the caregiver and should not be taken personally.

Nursing assistants should always report and document combative behavior. Even if an NA does not find the behavior upsetting, the care team needs to be aware of it.

Guidelines: Combative Behavior

G Block physical blows or step out of the way, but never hit back (Fig. 4-18). No matter how much a resident hurts you, or how angry or afraid you are, never hit or threaten a resident.

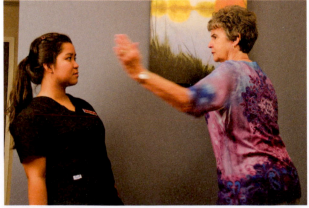

Fig. 4-18. *When dealing with combative residents, step out of the way, but never hit back.*

G Allow the resident time to calm down before the next interaction.

G Ensure the resident is safe and give him or her space. When possible, stand at least an arm's length away.

G Remain calm. Lower the tone of your voice.

G Be flexible and patient.

G Stay neutral. Do not respond to verbal attacks. Do not argue or accuse the resident of wrongdoing. If you must respond, say something like "I understand that you're angry and frustrated. How can I make things better?"

G Do not use gestures that could frighten or startle the resident. Try to keep your hands open and in front of you.

G Be reassuring and supportive.

G Consider what provoked the resident. Sometimes something as simple as a change in caregiver or routine can be very upsetting to a resident. Get help to take the resident to a quieter place if needed.

G Report inappropriate behavior to the nurse.

Anger

Anger is a natural emotion that has many causes, such as disease, fear, pain, loneliness, and loss of independence. Anger may also just be a part of someone's personality. Some people get angry more easily than others.

People express anger in different ways. Some may shout, yell, threaten, throw things, or pace. Others express their anger by withdrawing, being silent, or sulking. Angry behavior should always be reported to the nurse.

Guidelines: Angry Behavior

G Stay calm. Do not argue or respond to verbal attacks.

G Empathize with the resident. Try to understand what he or she is feeling.

G Try to find out what caused the resident's anger. Using silence may help the resident explain. Listen attentively as the resident speaks.

G Treat the resident with dignity and respect. Explain what you are going to do and when you will do it.

G Answer call lights promptly.

G Stay at a safe distance if the resident becomes combative.

Assertive vs. Aggressive Behavior

A person is behaving assertively when he expresses thoughts, feelings, and beliefs in a direct and honest way. Being assertive involves respect for one's own needs and feelings and for those of other people. It is not the same as being aggressive, combative, or angry.

A person is behaving aggressively when he expresses thoughts, feelings, and beliefs in ways that humiliate, disgrace, or overpower the other person. Little or no respect is shown for the needs or feelings of others. Nursing assistants should report aggressive behavior when they witness it.

Inappropriate Behavior

Inappropriate behavior from a resident includes trying to establish a personal, rather than a professional, relationship with a nursing assistant. Examples include asking personal questions, requesting visits on personal time, asking for or doing favors, giving tips or gifts, and lending or borrowing money.

Inappropriate behavior includes making sexual advances and comments. Sexual advances include any sexual words, comments, or behavior that makes the person to whom the advances are directed feel uncomfortable.

Inappropriate behavior may include residents removing their clothes or touching themselves in public. Illness, dementia, confusion, and medication may cause this behavior.

Confused residents may have problems that mimic inappropriate sexual behavior. They may have an uncomfortable rash, clothes that are too tight, too hot, or too scratchy, or they may need to go to the bathroom. Nursing assistants need to observe for these problems.

Guidelines: Inappropriate Behavior

G If you think a light approach will work, say something like "I'm sorry, but I'm not allowed to do that."

G Address the behavior directly, saying something like "That makes me uncomfortable." If the resident persists, call the nurse immediately.

G Respond to personal questions by saying "I really can't talk about my personal life on the job." If the resident is sharing thoughts or feelings that make you uncomfortable, say "That's not something I can help you with. If you'd like to speak with a social worker or someone else, I can let the nurse know."

G Firmly refuse gifts, tips, and favors. Say "I really can't accept that. It's against the facility's rules."

G If you encounter a resident in any embarrassing situation, remain professional. Do not overreact, as that may actually reinforce the behavior. Try to distract the resident. If that does not help, take the resident to a private area, and notify the nurse.

G Always report inappropriate behavior to the nurse, even if you think it was harmless.

Chapter Review

1. Briefly describe three steps in the communication process.

2. Define *nonverbal communication* and give one example that is not listed in the textbook.

3. What does the word *culture* mean?

4. What is one positive response to cultural diversity?

5. Why should "why" questions be avoided when talking with residents?

6. If a resident speaks a different language than the nursing assistant does, what can the nursing assistant do?

7. What is one way to provide feedback while listening?

8. What can silence or pauses help a resident do?

9. What is one reason that a nursing assistant should not ignore a resident's request?

10. Why should a nursing assistant sit near a resident who has started a conversation with her?

11. For each statement, decide whether it is a fact or an opinion. Write *F* for fact and *O* for opinion.

    ___ Mrs. Kim does not eat enough.

    ___ Mr. Moore looked terrible today.

    ___ Mr. Gaston had a fever of 100.7° F.

    ___ Ms. Martino needs to make some friends.

    ___ Mr. Klein has not had a visitor since last Tuesday.

    ___ The doctor says Mrs. Storey has to walk once a day.

12. What is objective information? What is subjective information?

13. With whom should NAs use medical terminology—care team members or residents and their families?

14. When making an oral report, should the nursing assistant use facts or opinions?

15. When should care be documented—before or after it is done?

16. Convert 8:43 p.m. to military time.

17. Convert 1400 hours to regular time.

18. When should an incident report be completed?

19. Give an example of a proper greeting when answering the phone.

20. Give two reasons why computers may be used in a facility.

21. What is the purpose of the resident call light or call system?

22. When a resident has a hearing impairment, on whose face should the light be shining while communicating—the resident's or the nursing assistant's?

23. How can a nursing assistant explain the position of objects in front of a resident who is visually impaired?

24. How should questions be phrased to a resident who has had a stroke?

25. How should a nursing assistant refer to the weaker side of a resident who has had a stroke?

26. What should a nursing assistant always do after a resident behaves inappropriately?

5

Infection Prevention and Control

1. Define *infection prevention* and discuss types of infections

Infection prevention is the set of methods practiced in healthcare facilities to prevent and control the spread of disease. Preventing the spread of infection is very important and is the responsibility of all care team members. Nursing assistants must know and follow their facility's policies relating to infection prevention; these policies help protect staff members, residents, visitors, and others from disease.

A **microorganism** (MO) is a living thing that is so small that it is only visible under a microscope. A **microbe** is another name for a microorganism. Microorganisms are always present in the environment (Fig. 5-1). **Infections** occur when harmful microorganisms, called **pathogens**, invade the body and multiply.

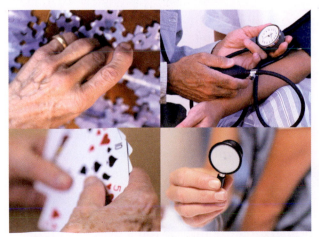

Fig. 5-1. *Microorganisms are always present in the environment. They are on almost everything a person touches.*

There are two main types of infections: localized and systemic. A **localized infection** is an infection that is limited to a specific location in the body. It has local symptoms, which means the symptoms are near the site of infection. For example, if a wound becomes infected, the area around it may become red, swollen, warm, and painful. A **systemic infection** affects the entire body. This type of infection travels through the bloodstream and is spread throughout the body. It causes general symptoms, such as fever, chills, or mental confusion.

A type of infection that can be localized or systemic is a **healthcare-associated infection (HAI)**. A healthcare-associated infection is an infection acquired in a healthcare setting during the delivery of medical care. Healthcare settings include hospitals, long-term care facilities, and outpatient surgery centers, among others.

Nursing assistants need to be able to recognize signs and symptoms of infections so that they can report them to the nurse promptly.

Observing and Reporting: Infections

Signs and symptoms of a localized infection include the following:

O/R Pain

O/R Redness

O/R Swelling

O/R Pus

O/R Drainage (fluid from a wound or cavity)

O/R Heat

Signs and symptoms of a systemic infection include the following:

O/R Fever

O/R Body aches

O/R Chills

O/R Nausea

O/R Vomiting

O/R Weakness

O/R Headache

O/R Mental confusion

O/R Drop in person's normal blood pressure

2. Describe the chain of infection

To understand how to prevent disease, it is helpful to first understand how it is spread. The **chain of infection** is a way of describing how disease is transmitted from one human being to another (Fig. 5-2). Definitions and examples of each of the six links in the chain of infection follow.

Chain Link 1: The **causative agent** is a pathogenic microorganism that causes disease. Microorganisms are small living bodies that cannot be seen without a microscope. They are everywhere—on skin, in food, in the air, and in water. Causative agents include bacteria, viruses, fungi, and parasites.

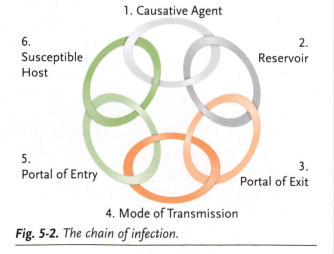

Fig. 5-2. The chain of infection.

Normal flora are the microorganisms that live in and on the body and normally do not cause harm to a healthy person, as long as the flora remain in that particular area. When they enter a different part of the body, they may cause an infection.

Chain Link 2: A **reservoir** is where the pathogen lives and multiplies. A reservoir can be a human, animal, plant, soil, or substance. Warm, dark, and moist places are the ideal environments for microorganisms to live, grow, and multiply. Some microorganisms need oxygen to survive, while others do not. Examples of reservoirs include the lungs, blood, and the large intestine.

Chain Link 3: The **portal of exit** is any body opening on an infected person that allows pathogens to leave (Fig. 5-3). These include the nose, mouth, eyes, or a cut in the skin.

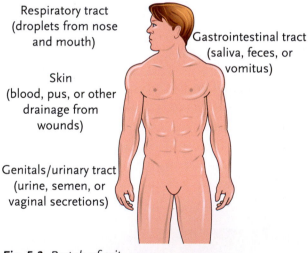

Fig. 5-3. Portals of exit.

Chain Link 4: The **mode of transmission** describes how the pathogen travels. Transmission can occur through the air or through direct or indirect contact. **Direct contact** happens by touching the infected person or his secretions. **Indirect contact** results from touching an object contaminated by the infected person, such as a needle, dressing, tissue, or bed linen. The primary route of disease transmission within the healthcare setting is via the hands of healthcare workers.

Chain Link 5: The **portal of entry** is any body opening on an uninfected person that allows pathogens to enter (Fig. 5-4). These include the nose, mouth, eyes, and other mucous membranes, cuts in the skin, and cracked skin. **Mucous membranes** are the membranes that line body cavities that open to the outside of the body. These include the linings of the mouth, nose, eyes, rectum, and genitals.

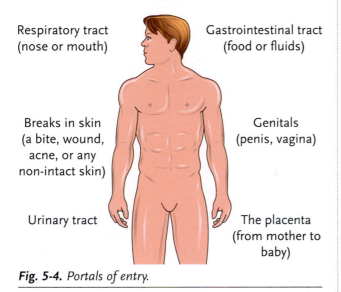

Respiratory tract (nose or mouth)

Gastrointestinal tract (food or fluids)

Breaks in skin (a bite, wound, acne, or any non-intact skin)

Genitals (penis, vagina)

Urinary tract

The placenta (from mother to baby)

Fig. 5-4. Portals of entry.

Chain Link 6: A **susceptible host** is an uninfected person who could become ill. Examples include all healthcare workers and anyone in their care who is not already infected with that particular disease.

If one of the links in the chain of infection is broken, then the spread of infection is stopped. Infection prevention practices help stop pathogens from traveling (Link 4) and from getting on a person's hands, nose, eyes, mouth, skin, etc. (Link 5). Immunizations (Link 6) reduce a person's chances of getting sick from diseases such as hepatitis B and influenza.

Transmission (passage or transfer) of most **infectious** diseases can be blocked by using proper infection prevention practices, such as handwashing. Handwashing is the most important way to stop the spread of infection. All caregivers should wash their hands often.

Handwashing is a part of medical asepsis. **Medical asepsis** refers to measures used to reduce and prevent the spread of pathogens. Medical asepsis is used in all healthcare settings. **Surgical asepsis**, also known as sterile technique, makes an object or area completely free of all microorganisms (not just pathogens). Surgical asepsis is used for many types of procedures, such as changing catheters.

3. Explain why the elderly are at a higher risk for infection

The elderly are at a higher risk for infection. This is due, in part, to weakened immune systems as a result of aging. Weakened immune systems can also result from chronic illnesses. Other physical changes of aging, such as decreased circulation and slow wound healing, may also contribute to infections in the elderly.

Older adults are at risk for **malnutrition** and dehydration. A person who is malnourished is not getting the proper nutrition. **Dehydration** is a condition that occurs when there is an inadequate amount of fluid in the body. These conditions can result from difficulty chewing and/or swallowing, lack of appetite and thirst, illnesses, weakness, and medication. Both malnutrition and dehydration are serious conditions (Chapter 15 has more information). When the body is not getting the nutrients and fluid it needs, the risk of infection greatly increases. Also, the elderly may have limited mobility, which is another risk factor for serious problems, such as pressure injuries, skin infections, and pneumonia.

The elderly are hospitalized more often than younger people. This makes them more likely to get healthcare-associated infections. Difficulty swallowing and incontinence increase the risk of respiratory and urinary tract infections. Feeding tubes, oxygen tubes, and other types of tubing, such as catheters (Chapter 16), also increase the risk of infection.

Infection is more dangerous for the elderly because even a simple cold can turn into a life-threatening illness such as pneumonia. It also may take longer for older people to recover from an infection or illness. This is why preventing infection is so important. Nursing assistants play an important role in preventing infection.

4. Explain Standard Precautions

State and federal government agencies have guidelines and laws concerning infection prevention. The **Occupational Safety and Health Administration (OSHA)** (osha.gov) is a federal government agency that makes rules to protect workers from hazards on the job. The **Centers for Disease Control and Prevention (CDC)** (cdc.gov) is a federal government agency that issues guidelines to protect and improve the health of individuals and communities. Through education, the CDC aims to prevent and control disease, injury, and disability, as well as to promote public health.

In 1996, the CDC created a new infection prevention system to reduce the risk of contracting infectious diseases in healthcare settings. Some additions and changes were made to this system in 2007. There are two levels of precautions within the CDC's infection prevention system: Standard Precautions and Transmission-Based Precautions.

Following **Standard Precautions** means treating blood, body fluids, nonintact skin (like abrasions, pimples, or open sores), and mucous membranes as if they were infected. Body fluids include tears, saliva, sputum (mucus coughed up), urine, feces, semen, vaginal secretions, pus or other wound drainage, and vomit. They do not include sweat.

Standard Precautions must be used with every resident; this promotes safety. A nursing assistant cannot tell by looking at residents or even by reading their medical charts whether residents have a contagious disease such as tuberculosis,

hepatitis, or influenza. Many diseases can be spread even before the infected person shows signs or has been diagnosed.

Standard Precautions and Transmission-Based Precautions (Learning Objective 9) are ways to stop the spread of infection by interrupting the mode of transmission. In other words, these guidelines do not stop an infected person from giving off pathogens. However, by following these guidelines, nursing assistants help prevent those pathogens from infecting them or those in their care.

- Standard Precautions must be practiced with every single person in a nursing assistant's care.

- Transmission-Based Precautions vary based on how an infection is transmitted. When indicated, these precautions are used **in addition** to Standard Precautions. More information about these precautions is located later in the chapter.

Guidelines: Standard Precautions

G **Wash your hands** before putting on gloves. Wash your hands immediately after removing your gloves. Be careful not to touch clean objects with your used gloves.

G **Wear gloves** if you may come into contact with any of the following: blood; body fluids or secretions; broken or open skin, such as abrasions, acne, cuts, stitches, or staples; or mucous membranes. Such contacts occur during mouth care; toilet assistance; perineal care; helping with a bedpan or urinal; ostomy care; cleaning up spills; cleaning basins, urinals, bedpans, and other containers that have held body fluids; and disposing of wastes.

G **Remove gloves** immediately when finished with a procedure and wash your hands.

G **Immediately wash all skin surfaces that have been contaminated** with blood and body fluids.

G   **Wear a disposable gown** that is resistant to body fluids if you may come into contact with blood or body fluids or when splashing or spraying of blood or body fluids is likely. If a resident has a contagious illness, wear a gown even if it is not likely you will come into contact with blood or body fluids.

G   **Wear a mask and protective goggles and/or a face shield** if you may come into contact with blood or body fluids or when splashing or spraying of blood or body fluids is likely (for example, when emptying a bedpan).

G   **Wear gloves and use caution when handling razor blades, needles, and other sharps.** Avoid nicks and cuts when shaving residents. Place sharps carefully in a biohazard container for sharps. **Sharps** are needles or other sharp objects. Biohazard containers used for sharps are puncture-resistant, leakproof containers. They are clearly labeled and warn of the danger of the contents inside (Figs. 5-5 and 5-6). They must be closable and kept in an upright position to keep items inside from spilling out. They should not be filled past the line indicating that the container is full. There are also biohazard bags that are used for biomedical waste that is not sharp, such as soiled dressings, contaminated tubing, and other items. OSHA recommends that biomedical/biohazard waste be disposed of at the *point of origin*, or where the waste occurs.

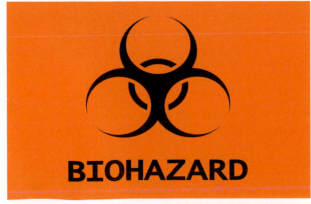

Fig. 5-5. *This label indicates that the material is potentially infectious.*

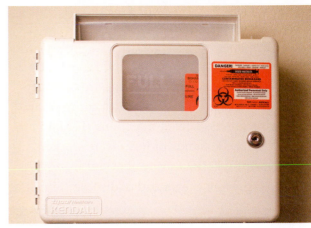

Fig. 5-6. *One type of container for sharps.*

G   **Never attempt to recap needles or sharps after use.** You might stick yourself. Dispose of them in a biohazard container for sharps.

G   **Carefully bag all contaminated supplies.** Depending on policy, you may need to double bag some items. This means putting the contaminated bag into another bag. Dispose of contaminated items according to policy.

G   **Clearly label body fluids that are being saved for a specimen** with the resident's name, date of birth, room number, date, and a biohazard label. Keep them in a container with a lid. Put in a biohazard specimen bag for transportation if required.

G   **Dispose of contaminated wastes according to your facility's policy.** Waste containing blood or body fluids is considered biohazardous waste. Liquid waste can usually be disposed through the regular sewer system as long as there is no splashing, spraying, or aerosolizing of the waste as it is being disposed. Appropriate personal protective equipment needs to be worn, followed by proper removal and handwashing. Follow instructions.

Standard Precautions should always be practiced on all residents, regardless of their infection status. This greatly reduces the risk of transmitting infection. There is more information about Standard Precautions in the next several learning objectives.

5. Explain hand hygiene and identify when to wash hands

Nursing assistants use their hands constantly while they work. Microorganisms are on everything they touch. The single most common way for healthcare-associated infections (HAIs) to be spread is via the hands of healthcare workers. Handwashing is the most important thing NAs can do to prevent the spread of disease (Fig. 5-7).

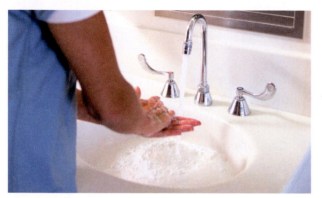

Fig. 5-7. *All people working in health care must wash their hands often. Handwashing is the most effective way to prevent the spread of disease.*

The CDC has defined **hand hygiene** as washing hands with either plain or antiseptic soap and water or using alcohol-based hand rubs. Alcohol-based hand rubs (often referred to as *hand sanitizer*) include gels, rinses, and foams that do not require the use of water.

Alcohol-based hand rubs have proven effective in reducing bacteria on the skin. However, they are not a substitute for frequent, proper handwashing. When hands are visibly soiled, they should be washed using plain or antimicrobial soap and water. An **antimicrobial** agent destroys, resists, or prevents the development of pathogens. Hand rubs can be used in addition to handwashing any time hands are not visibly soiled. When using a hand rub, the hands must be rubbed together until the product has completely dried. Hand lotion can help prevent dry, cracked skin.

Nursing assistants should avoid wearing rings or bracelets while working because they may increase the risk of contamination. (Smooth,

plain bands may be acceptable at some facilities.) Fingernails should be short, smooth, and clean. Artificial (acrylic, gel, or wraps) nails should not be worn because they harbor bacteria and increase the risk of contamination even if hands are washed often. Nursing assistants should wash their hands at these times:

- When first arriving at work
- Whenever hands are visibly soiled
- Before, between, and after all contact with residents
- Before putting on gloves and after removing gloves
- After contact with any body fluids, mucous membranes, nonintact skin, or wound dressings
- After handling contaminated items
- After contact with any object in the resident's room (care environment)
- Before and after touching meal trays and/or handling food
- Before and after assisting residents with meals
- Before getting clean linen
- Before and after using the toilet
- After touching garbage or trash
- After picking up anything from the floor
- After blowing the nose, wiping the nose, or coughing or sneezing into the hands
- Before and after eating
- After smoking
- After touching areas on the body, such as the mouth, face, eyes, hair, ears, or nose
- Before and after applying makeup
- After any contact with pets and after contact with pet care items
- Before leaving the facility

Washing hands (hand hygiene)

Equipment: soap, paper towels

1. Turn on water at sink. Keep your clothes dry because moisture breeds bacteria. Do not let your clothing touch the outside portion of the sink or counter.

2. Wet hands and wrists thoroughly (Fig. 5-8).

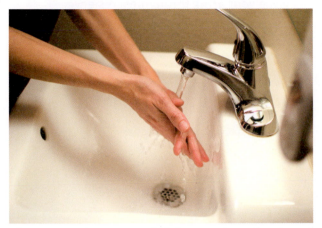

Fig. 5-8. *Keeping arms angled downward, wet hands and wrists thoroughly.*

3. Apply soap to your hands.

4. Keep your hands lower than your elbows and your fingertips down. Rub hands together and fingers between each other to create a lather. Lather all surfaces of wrists, fingers, and hands, using friction for at least 20 seconds. Friction helps clean (Fig. 5-9).

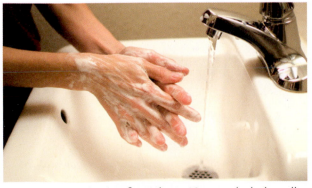

Fig. 5-9. *Using friction for at least 20 seconds, lather all surfaces of wrists, fingers, and hands.*

5. Clean your fingernails by rubbing them in the palm of your other hand.

6. Keep your hands lower than your elbows and your fingertips down. Being careful not to touch the sink, rinse thoroughly under running water. Rinse all surfaces of your hands and wrists. Run water down from wrists to fingertips (Fig. 5-10). Do not run water over unwashed arms down to clean hands.

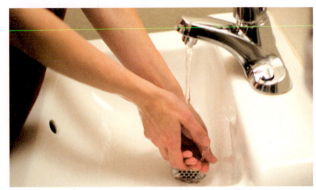

Fig. 5-10. *Rinse wrists and hands thoroughly without touching the sink. Let water run down from wrists to fingertips.*

7. Use a clean, dry paper towel to dry all surfaces of your hands, wrists, and fingers. Do not wipe towel on unwashed forearms and then wipe clean hands. Dispose of paper towel into waste container without touching the container. If your hands touch the sink or wastebasket, start over.

8. Use a clean, dry paper towel to turn off the faucet (Fig. 5-11). Dispose of paper towel into waste container. Do not contaminate your hands by touching the surface of the sink or faucet.

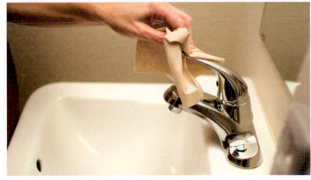

Fig. 5-11. *Use a clean, dry paper towel to turn off the faucet, so that you do not contaminate your hands.*

6. Discuss the use of personal protective equipment (PPE) in facilities

Personal protective equipment (PPE) is equipment that helps protect employees from serious workplace injuries or illnesses resulting from contact with workplace hazards. In long-term care facilities, PPE helps protect nursing assistants from contact with potentially infectious material. Employers are responsible for providing nursing assistants with the appropriate PPE to wear.

Personal protective equipment includes gowns, masks, goggles, face shields, and gloves. Gowns protect the skin and/or clothing. Masks protect the mouth and nose. Goggles protect the eyes. Face shields protect the entire face—the eyes, nose, and mouth. Gloves protect the hands. Gloves are used most often by all caregivers.

Nursing assistants must wear personal protective equipment if there is a chance of coming into contact with body fluids, mucous membranes, or open wounds. They must wear, or **don**, gowns, masks, goggles, and face shields when splashing or spraying of body fluids or blood could occur. Hand hygiene should be performed before donning PPE and after removing and discarding PPE.

Gowns

Clean, non-sterile gowns protect exposed skin. They also prevent the soiling of clothing. Gowns should fully cover the torso. They should fit comfortably over the body, and have long sleeves that fit snugly at the wrists.

OSHA requires fluid-resistant gowns if fluid penetration is likely. If a gown becomes wet or soiled during care, it should be discarded and a new gown should be donned. When finished with a procedure, the NA should remove, or **doff**, the gown as soon as possible and wash her hands.

1. Wash your hands.

2. Open the gown. Hold it out in front of you and allow gown to open/unfold (Fig. 5-12). Do not shake the gown or touch it to the floor. Facing the back opening of the gown, place your arms through each sleeve.

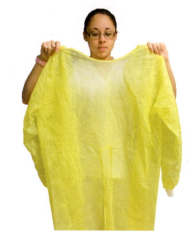

Fig. 5-12. *Let the gown unfold without shaking it.*

3. Fasten the neck opening.

4. Reaching behind you, pull the gown until it completely covers your clothing. Secure the gown at your waist (Fig. 5-13).

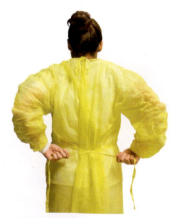

Fig. 5-13. *Reaching behind you, secure the gown at the waist.*

5. Put on your gloves after putting on the gown. The cuffs of the gloves should overlap the cuffs of the gown (Fig. 5-14).

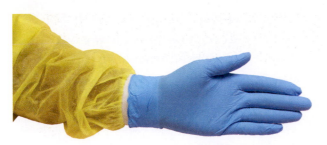

Fig. 5-14. *The cuffs of the gloves should overlap the cuffs of the gown.*

6. When removing a gown, first remove and discard gloves properly (see procedure later in the chapter). Then unfasten the gown at the neck and waist. Remove the gown without touching the outside of the gown. Roll the dirty side in, while holding the gown away from your body. Dispose of the gown properly and wash your hands.

Masks and Goggles

Masks can prevent inhalation of microorganisms through the nose or mouth. Masks should be worn when caring for residents with respiratory illnesses. They should also be worn when it is likely that contact with blood or body fluids may occur. Sometimes special masks (respirators) are required for certain diseases, such as tuberculosis (TB). Masks should fully cover the nose and mouth and prevent fluid penetration. Masks should fit snugly over the nose and mouth.

Masks can only be worn once before they need to be discarded. Masks that become wet or soiled must be changed immediately without touching the outside of the soiled mask. Nursing assistants must always change their masks when moving between residents; the same mask should not be worn from one resident to another.

Goggles are worn with a mask and are used whenever it is likely that blood or body fluids may be splashed or sprayed into the eye area or into the eyes. Eyeglasses alone do not provide proper eye protection. Goggles should fit snugly over and around the eyes or eyeglasses.

Putting on (donning) mask and goggles

1. Wash your hands.

2. Pick up the mask by the top strings or the elastic strap. Do not touch the mask where it touches your face.

3. Pull the elastic strap over your head, or if the mask has strings, tie top strings first, then bottom strings. Do not wear a mask hanging from only the bottom ties or straps.

4. Pinch the metal strip at the top of the mask (if part of the mask) tightly around your nose so that it feels snug (Fig. 5-15). Fit the mask snugly around your face and below the chin.

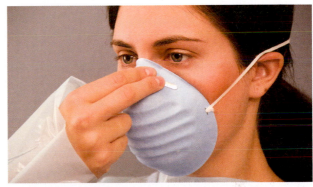

Fig. 5-15. *Adjust the metal strip until the mask fits snugly around your nose.*

5. Put on the goggles over your eyes or eyeglasses. Use the headband or earpieces to secure them to your head. Make sure they are on snugly.

6. Put on gloves after putting on the mask and goggles.

Face Shields

Face shields may be worn when blood or body fluids may be splashed or sprayed into the eyes or eye area. A face shield can be substituted for a mask or goggles, or it can be worn with a mask. The face shield should cover the forehead, go below the chin, and wrap around the sides of the face. The headband can secure it to the head.

Gloves

Non-sterile gloves are used for basic care. They are available in different sizes, and may be made of nitrile, vinyl, or latex. However, due to allergy issues, some facilities have banned the use of latex gloves. In addition, in 2017 the Food and Drug Administration (FDA, fda.gov) banned the use of all powdered patient examination gloves. This is due to the powder posing numerous risks to patients and workers.

Gloves should fit the hands comfortably and should not be too loose or too tight. Facilities have specific policies and procedures on when to wear gloves. Nursing assistants must learn and follow these rules. Gloves must always be worn for the following tasks:

- Anytime the caregiver might come into contact with blood or any body fluid, open wounds, or mucous membranes

- When performing or helping with mouth care or care of any mucous membrane

- When performing or helping with **perineal care** (care of the genitals and anal area)

- When performing personal care on **non-intact skin**—skin that is broken by abrasions, cuts, rashes, acne, pimples, lesions, surgical incisions, or boils

- When the caregiver has open sores or cuts on her hands

- When shaving a resident

- When disposing of soiled bed linens, gowns, dressings, and pads

- When touching a surface or equipment that is either visibly contaminated or may be contaminated

Disposable gloves can be worn only once; they cannot be washed or reused. Gloves should be changed immediately if they become wet, worn, soiled, or torn. Gloves should also be changed before contact with mucous membranes or bro-ken skin. After removing gloves, the NA should wash his hands before donning new gloves. Non-intact areas on the hands should be covered with bandages or gauze before putting on gloves.

Putting on (donning) gloves

1. Wash your hands.

2. If you are right-handed, slide one glove on your left hand (reverse if left-handed).

3. Using your gloved hand, slide the other hand into the second glove.

4. Interlace your fingers to smooth out folds and create a comfortable fit.

5. Carefully look for tears, holes, or discolored spots. Replace the glove if needed.

6. Adjust gloves until they are pulled up over your wrist and fit correctly. If wearing a gown, pull the cuff of the gloves over the sleeves of the gown (Fig. 5-16).

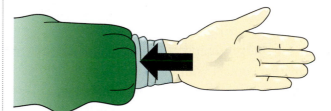

Fig. 5-16. *Adjust gloves until they are pulled up over the sleeves of the gown.*

Gloves should be removed, or doffed, promptly after use, and the NA should wash his hands directly after removing gloves. He should be careful not to contaminate his skin or clothing when removing gloves. Gloves are worn to protect the skin from becoming contaminated. After giving care, gloves are contaminated. If an NA opens a door with the gloved hand, the doorknob becomes contaminated. Later, anyone who opens the door with an ungloved hand will be touching a contaminated surface. Before touching surfaces or leaving residents' rooms, the NA must remove gloves and wash his hands. Afterward, new gloves can be donned if necessary.

Removing (doffing) gloves

1. Touch only the outside of one glove. With one gloved hand, grasp the other glove at the palm and pull the glove off (Fig. 5-17).

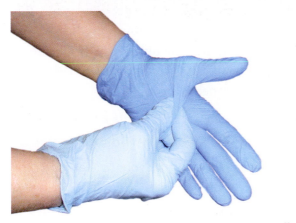

Fig. 5-17. *Grasp the glove at the palm and pull it off.*

2. With the fingertips of your gloved hand, hold the glove you just removed. With your ungloved hand, slip two fingers underneath the cuff of the remaining glove at the wrist. Do not touch any part of the outside of the glove (Fig. 5-18).

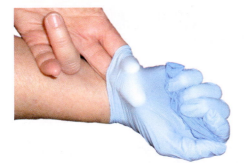

Fig. 5-18. *Reach inside glove at wrist, without touching any part of the outside of glove.*

3. Pull down, turning this glove inside out and over the first glove as you remove it.

4. You should now be holding one glove from its clean inner side and the other glove should be inside it.

5. Drop both gloves into the proper container without contaminating yourself.

6. Wash your hands.

The nursing assistant's employer will provide personal protective equipment as needed. PPE will be readily available and accessible in a variety of sizes. It is the NA's responsibility to know where it is kept and how to use it (Fig. 5-19). A specific order must be followed when donning and doffing PPE.

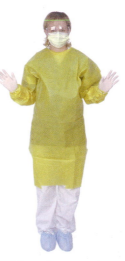

Fig. 5-19. *Using PPE is an important way to reduce the spread of infection.*

Donning a full set of PPE

1. Wash your hands.

2. Open the gown. Hold it out in front of you and allow the gown to open/unfold. Do not shake the gown to touch it to the floor. Facing the back opening of the gown, place your arms through each sleeve.

3. Fasten the neck opening.

4. Reaching behind you, pull the gown until it completely covers your clothing. Secure the gown at your waist.

5. Pick up the mask by the top strings or the elastic strap. Do not touch the mask where it touches your face.

6. Pull the elastic strap over your head, or if the mask has strings, tie top strings first, then bottom strings. Do not wear a mask hanging from only the bottom ties or straps.

7. Pinch the metal strip at the top of the mask (if part of the mask) tightly around your nose so that it feels snug. Fit the mask snugly around your face and below the chin.

8. Put on the goggles over your eyes or eyeglasses. Use the headband or earpieces to secure them to your head. Make sure they fit snugly.

9. If you are right-handed, slide one glove on your left hand (reverse if left-handed).

10. Using your gloved hand, slide the other hand into the second glove.

11. Interlace your fingers to smooth out folds and create a comfortable fit.

12. Carefully look for tears, holes, or discolored spots. Replace the glove if needed.

13. Pull the cuff of the gloves over the sleeves of the gown.

___

All personal protective equipment, except a respirator (if worn), must be removed before exiting the resident's room. A respirator is removed after leaving the room and closing the door.

Doffing a full set of PPE

1. Touch only the outside of one glove. With one gloved hand, grasp the other glove at the palm and pull the glove off.

2. With the fingertips of your gloved hand, hold the glove you just removed. With your ungloved hand, slip two fingers underneath the cuff of the remaining glove at the wrist. Do not touch any part of the outside of the glove.

3. Pull down, turning this glove inside out and over the first glove as you remove it.

4. You should now be holding one glove from its clean inner side and the other glove should be inside it.

5. Drop both gloves into the proper container without contaminating yourself.

6. Grasp headband or earpieces of goggles with your ungloved hands.

7. Lift the goggles away from your face.

8. Put the goggles in the proper container.

9. Unfasten the gown at the neck and waist. Remove the gown without touching the outside of the gown. Roll the dirty side in, while holding the gown away from your body. Dispose of gown properly.

10. If the mask has strings, untie the bottom strings first, then the top strings.

11. Remove the mask from your face and discard in the proper container.

12. Wash your hands. Washing hands is always the final step after removing and disposing of PPE.

___

OSHA and PPE

OSHA states that it is the employer's responsibility to instruct the staff on how to properly don PPE, how to wear PPE effectively, and how to safely doff PPE. This instruction needs to be given before the employee is in a situation where PPE is indicated, and as an annual review.

7. List guidelines for handling equipment and linen

In health care, an object is called **clean** if it has not been contaminated with pathogens. An object that is **dirty** has been contaminated with pathogens. Measures like disinfection and sterilization decrease the spread of pathogens that could cause disease.

Disinfection is a process that kills pathogens but does not destroy all pathogens. It reduces the pathogen count to a level that is considered not infectious. Disinfection is carried out with pasteurization or chemical germicides. Examples of items that are usually disinfected are reusable oxygen tanks, wall-mounted blood pressure cuffs, and any reusable resident care equipment.

Sterilization is a cleaning measure that destroys all microorganisms, including pathogens. This includes those that form spores. Spore-forming microorganisms are a special group of organisms that produce a protective covering that is difficult to penetrate. Sterilization is part of surgical asepsis and is accomplished through the use of special machines and devices. An autoclave is a machine that sterilizes objects by using hot steam under pressure. Liquid or gas chemicals and dry heat are other ways to sterilize objects. Items that need to be sterilized are ones that go directly into the bloodstream or into other normally sterile areas of the body (for example, surgical instruments).

Facilities have special rooms or areas for clean and dirty items, such as equipment, linen, and supplies. There are separate rooms for supplies that are considered clean and for supplies that are considered dirty or contaminated (Fig. 5-20). Nursing assistants will be told where these rooms are located and what types of equipment and supplies are found in each room. NAs should wash their hands before entering clean rooms and before leaving dirty rooms. This helps prevent the spread of pathogens.

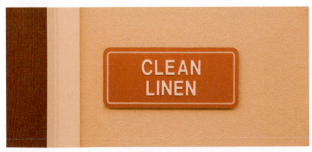

Fig. 5-20. There are separate rooms in facilities for clean and dirty equipment, linen, and supplies.

Guidelines: Handling Equipment, Linen, and Clothing

G   Handle all equipment in a way that prevents

- Skin/mucous membrane contact

- Contamination of your clothing

- Transfer of disease to other residents or areas

G   Do not use reusable equipment again until it has been properly cleaned and reprocessed.

G   Dispose of all single-use, or disposable, equipment properly. **Disposable** means it is discarded after one use. Disposable razors and disposable thermometers are examples of disposable equipment.

G   Clean and disinfect

- All environmental surfaces

- Beds, bedrails, and all bedside equipment

- All frequently touched surfaces (such as doorknobs, call lights, and handles on dressers and tables)

G   Handle, transport, and process soiled linens and clothing in a way that prevents

- Skin and mucous membrane exposure

- Contamination of clothing (hold linen and clothing away from your uniform)

- Transfer of disease to other residents and areas (do not shake linen or clothes; fold or roll linen so that the dirtiest area is inside; do not put soiled linen on floor)

G   Bag soiled linen at the point of origin.

G   Sort soiled linen away from resident care areas.

G   Place wet linen in leakproof bags.

More information about cleaning equipment and supplies is located in Chapter 12.

8. Explain how to handle spills

Spills, especially those involving blood or body fluids, can pose a serious risk of infection, as well as put residents and staff at risk for falls. The housekeeping department may be responsible for cleaning spills. If nursing assistants must clean spills, here are general guidelines to follow:

Guidelines: Cleaning Spills Involving Blood, Body Fluids, or Glass

G   Notify the proper department about the spill immediately if it is not your responsibility to clean the spill.

G   If you need to clean the spill, don gloves immediately. You may need to use special heavy-duty gloves, depending on the spill.

G   First, absorb the spill with whatever product is used by the facility. It may be an absorbing powder.

G   Scoop up the absorbed spill, and dispose of it in a designated container.

G   Apply the proper disinfectant to the spill area and allow it to stand wet for a minimum of 10 minutes (follow directions on the label).

G   Clean up spills immediately with the proper cleaning solution.

G   Do not pick up any pieces of broken glass, no matter how large, with your hands. Use a dustpan and broom or other tools.

G   Waste containing broken glass, blood, or body fluids should be properly bagged. Waste containing blood or body fluids may need to be placed in a special biohazard waste bag. Follow facility policy.

Cleaning Spills

Many facilities use special cleanup kits for spills. Nursing assistants should follow directions when using these kits. The CDC states that it is important to absorb and remove the fluid first. Disinfectant should not be placed directly on the spilled fluid. The spilled fluid may neutralize the disinfectant upon contact.

9. Explain Transmission-Based Precautions

The CDC set forth a second level of precautions beyond Standard Precautions. These guidelines are used for persons who are infected or may be infected with certain infectious diseases. These precautions are called **Transmission-Based**

Precautions. When ordered, these precautions are used in addition to Standard Precautions. These precautions will always be listed in the resident's care plan and on the nursing assistant's assignment sheet. Following these precautions promotes the nursing assistant's safety, as well as the safety of others.

There are three categories of Transmission-Based Precautions: Airborne Precautions, Droplet Precautions, and Contact Precautions. The category used depends on what type of pathogen or disease the person has or may have and how it spreads. They may also be used in combination for diseases that have multiple routes of transmission. Conditions that require Transmission-Based Precautions in addition to Standard Precautions include the following:

• **Multidrug-resistant organisms (MDROs)** (microorganisms, mostly bacteria, that are resistant to one or more antimicrobial agents that are commonly used for treatment), such as methicillin-resistant *Staphylococcus aureus* (MRSA) and vancomycin-resistant *enterococcus* (VRE) *

• *Clostridium difficile (C. diff or C. difficile)* *

• Scabies (a skin disease that causes itching)

• Lice

• Influenza (during an outbreak)

* There is more information about these infections later in the chapter.

Airborne Precautions

Airborne Precautions prevent the spread of pathogens that can be transmitted through the air after being expelled (Fig. 5-21). The pathogens are able to remain floating in the air for some time. They are carried by moisture, by air currents, and by dust. Tuberculosis is an example of an airborne disease. Precautions include wearing special masks, such as N95 or HEPA masks, to avoid being infected. More information on tuberculosis may be found later in this chapter.

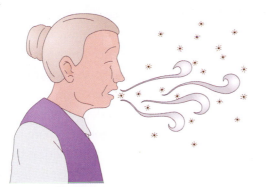

Fig. 5-21. *Airborne Precautions are used for diseases that can be transmitted through the air.*

Droplet Precautions

Droplet Precautions are used for diseases that are spread by droplets in the air. Droplets normally do not travel more than six feet. Talking, coughing, sneezing, laughing, singing, or suctioning can spread droplets (Fig. 5-22). An example of a droplet disease is influenza.

Droplet Precautions include wearing a face mask when providing care and restricting visits from uninfected people. In addition, nursing assistants should cover their noses and mouths with a tissue when they sneeze or cough and ask others to do the same. Used tissues should be disposed of in the nearest waste container. Used tissues should not be placed in a pocket for later use. If a tissue is not available, NAs should cough or sneeze into their upper sleeve or elbow, not their hands. They should wash their hands immediately afterward. Residents should wear masks when being moved from room to room.

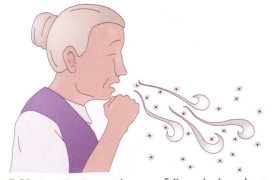

Fig. 5-22. *Droplet Precautions are followed when the disease-causing microorganism does not remain in the air.*

Respiratory Hygiene/Cough Etiquette

The CDC has set forth special infection prevention measures to prevent the transmission of all respiratory infections in healthcare settings. They are a part of Standard Precautions and include the following:

1. Post visual alerts at the entrances of care facilities instructing that all patients and visitors inform staff of symptoms of respiratory infections and practice respiratory hygiene/cough etiquette.

2. All individuals with signs and symptoms of a respiratory infection must do the following:

- Cover their noses/mouths with a tissue when coughing or sneezing.

- Dispose of used tissues in the nearest no-touch waste container after use.

- Perform hand hygiene (washing hands with soap and water, using an alcohol-based hand rub or an antiseptic handwash) after contact with respiratory secretions and contaminated objects.

Healthcare facilities must make these items available to staff, patients, and visitors:

- Tissues and no-touch receptacles for used tissue disposal

- Conveniently located hand rub dispensers and handwashing supplies in areas where sinks are located

3. During times of increased respiratory infections, offer masks to anyone who is coughing, and encourage coughing people to sit at least three feet away from others in waiting areas.

4. Advise healthcare personnel to observe Droplet Precautions, in addition to Standard Precautions, when examining a patient with symptoms of a respiratory infection, particularly if fever is present.

Contact Precautions

Contact Precautions are used when the resident is at risk of spreading an infection by direct contact with a person or object. The infection can be spread by touching a contaminated area on the client's body or her blood or body fluids (Fig. 5-23). It may also be spread by touching contaminated items, linen, equipment, or supplies. Conjunctivitis (pink eye) and *Clostridium difficile*

(*C. diff*) infection are examples of situations that require Contact Precautions. *Clostridium difficile* is discussed later in the chapter.

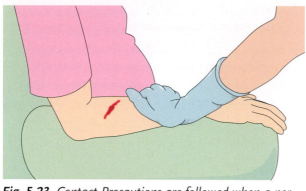

Fig. 5-23. *Contact Precautions are followed when a person is at risk of transmitting a microorganism by touching an object or person.*

Contact Precautions include wearing gloves and a gown and resident isolation. To **isolate** means to keep something separate, or by itself. Contact Precautions require washing hands with antimicrobial soap and not touching infected surfaces with ungloved hands or uninfected surfaces with contaminated gloves.

Staff often refer to residents who need Transmission-Based Precautions as being "in isolation." A sign should be on the door indicating *Contact Precautions* and alerting people to see the nurse before entering the room. Other guidelines for NAs to follow include the following:

Guidelines: Isolation

G When they are indicated, Transmission-Based Precautions are always used **in addition** to Standard Precautions.

G Nurses will set up the isolation unit. Some facilities have a special room where isolation supplies are kept. Some facilities keep supplies within the room itself, while other facilities set up an isolation cart outside the room. Isolation supplies consist of gloves, masks, gowns or aprons, and, if indicated, goggles, face shields, respirator masks, or other forms of specialized personal protective equipment (PPE).

G You will be told the proper PPE to wear for care of each resident in isolation. Make sure to put on PPE properly and remove it safely. Remove PPE and place it in the appropriate container before exiting a resident's room. PPE cannot be worn outside the resident's room. Perform hand hygiene following the removal of PPE and again after exiting the resident's room. In addition to handwashing areas within the resident's room, there may be an alcohol-based hand rub dispenser mounted on the wall inside the room as you exit the door.

G Do not share equipment between residents. Use disposable supplies that can be discarded after use whenever possible. Use dedicated (only for use by one resident) equipment when disposable is not an option. For example, a resident in isolation has her own (dedicated) blood pressure cuff and stethoscope. Disposable thermometers are used to take her temperature. When using disposable supplies, discard them in the resident's room before leaving. Be careful not to contaminate reusable equipment by setting it on furniture or counters in the resident's room. When the resident is discharged or no longer needs the additional precautions, properly dispose of dedicated equipment if required. If the dedicated equipment is to be used for other residents, it should be cleaned and disinfected after use.

G Wear the proper PPE, if indicated, when serving food and drink to residents in isolation. Do not leave uneaten food uncovered in the resident's room. When the meal is completed, remove the meal tray and take it to the designated area, or put it back on the food cart. When the food carts are returned to the kitchen, all soiled trays will be handled with gloves by the dietary staff, and the tray and dinnerware will be cleaned and sanitized.

G Follow Standard Precautions when dealing with body waste removal. Wear gloves when touching or handling waste. Wear gowns and goggles when indicated. The waste must be disposed of in such a manner as to minimize splashing and spraying.

G If required to take a specimen from a resident in isolation, wear the proper PPE. Collect the specimen and place it in the appropriate container without the outside of the container coming into contact with the specimen. Properly remove your PPE and dispose of it in the room. Perform hand hygiene before leaving the room and take the specimen to the nurse.

G Residents need to feel that their circumstances and feelings are appreciated and understood by members of the care team without criticism or judgment. Listen to what residents are telling you and allow time to talk with residents about concerns. Reassure residents. Explain why these steps are being taken. Relay any requests outside your scope of practice to the nurse.

Residents' Rights

Isolation

Residents' basic needs remain the same while in isolation. Basic human needs do not change, even though physical conditions may change. Do not avoid a resident in isolation. Do not rush through care tasks or make the resident feel that he or she should be avoided. Being professional, caring, and competent may help lessen a resident's worries or concerns and feelings about being isolated. If an NA has questions about the care he is providing, he should talk to the charge nurse.

10. Define *bloodborne pathogens* and describe two major bloodborne diseases

Bloodborne pathogens are microorganisms found in human blood that can cause infection and disease in humans. They may also be found in body fluids, draining wounds, and mucous membranes. These pathogens are transmitted by infected blood entering the bloodstream, or if infected semen or vaginal secretions contact mucous membranes. Having sexual contact with someone carrying the disease can also transmit a bloodborne disease. Sexual contact includes sexual intercourse (vaginal and anal), contact of the mouth with the genitals or anus, and contact of the hands with the genital area. Sharing infected drug needles is another way to spread bloodborne diseases. Infected pregnant women may transmit bloodborne diseases to their babies in the womb or at birth.

In health care, contact with infected blood or body fluids is the most common way to be infected with a bloodborne disease. Infections can be spread through contact with contaminated blood or body fluids, needles or other sharp objects, or contaminated supplies or equipment. Standard Precautions, handwashing, isolation, and using PPE are all methods of preventing transmission of bloodborne diseases. Employers are required by law to help prevent exposure to bloodborne pathogens. Following Standard Precautions and other procedures helps protect caregivers from bloodborne diseases.

Bloodborne diseases cannot be spread by casual contact. Nursing assistants can safely touch, hug, and spend time talking with residents who have a bloodborne disease (Fig. 5-24). These residents need the same thoughtful, personal attention given to all residents. NAs need to follow Standard Precautions, but should never isolate residents emotionally because they have a bloodborne disease.

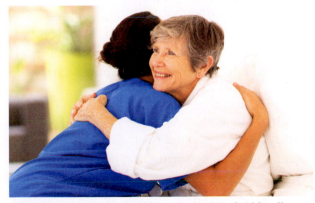

Fig. 5-24. Hugs and touches cannot spread a bloodborne disease.

Two major bloodborne diseases in the United States are acquired immune deficiency syndrome (AIDS) and the viral hepatitis family. **HIV** stands for human immunodeficiency virus, and it is the virus that can cause AIDS. Over time, HIV weakens the immune system so that the body cannot effectively fight infections. The final stage of HIV infection is AIDS. People with AIDS lose all ability to fight infection and can die from illnesses that a healthy immune system could handle. Chapter 18 contains more information about HIV and AIDS.

Hepatitis is inflammation of the liver caused by certain viruses and other factors, such as alcohol abuse, some medications, and trauma. Liver function can be permanently damaged by hepatitis. Several different viruses can cause hepatitis. The most common types of hepatitis are A, B, and C. Hepatitis B and C are bloodborne diseases that can cause death. Many more people have hepatitis B (HBV) than HIV. In the United States today, the risk of getting hepatitis is greater than the risk of acquiring HIV.

The virus causing hepatitis A (HAV) is a result of fecal-oral contamination, which means through food or water contaminated by stool from an infected person.

Hepatitis B (HBV) is a bloodborne disease. It is spread through sexual contact, by sharing infected needles, and from a mother to her baby during delivery. It can be spread through improperly sterilized needles used for tattoos and piercings and through grooming supplies, such as razors, nail clippers, and toothbrushes. It is also spread by exposure at work from accidental contact with infected needles or other sharps or from splashing blood.

The hepatitis B virus can survive outside the body for at least seven days and can still cause infection in others during that time. HBV may cause few symptoms or may become a severe infection. HBV can cause short-term illness that leads to the following:

- Loss of appetite

- Diarrhea and vomiting

- Fatigue

- **Jaundice** (a condition in which the skin, whites of the eyes, and mucous membranes appear yellow)

- Pain in muscles, joints, and stomach

It can also cause long-term illness that leads to

- Liver damage (cirrhosis)

- Liver cancer

- Death

HBV is a serious threat to healthcare workers. Employers must offer nursing assistants a free vaccine to protect them from hepatitis B. The hepatitis B vaccine is usually given as a series of three shots. Prevention is the best option for dealing with this disease, and employees should take the vaccine when it is offered.

Hepatitis C (HCV) is also transmitted through blood or body fluids. Hepatitis C can lead to cirrhosis and liver cancer; it can even cause death. There is no vaccine for hepatitis C.

Less common types of hepatitis in the United States are hepatitis D (HDV) and hepatitis E (HEV). Hepatitis D is transmitted by blood. It is only found in people who carry the hepatitis B virus. Hepatitis E (HEV) is transmitted by the fecal-oral route, usually through contaminated water. Although HEV is rare in the United States, it is more common in many other parts of the world. There is no vaccine for hepatitis D and hepatitis E.

11. Explain OSHA's Bloodborne Pathogens Standard

OSHA has set standards for special procedures that must be followed in healthcare facilities. One of these is the **Bloodborne Pathogens Standard**. This law requires that healthcare facilities protect employees from bloodborne health hazards. By law, employers must follow these rules to reduce or eliminate the risk of exposure to infectious diseases. The standard also guides employers and employees through the steps to follow if exposed to infectious material. Significant exposures include the following:

* Exposure by injection; a needle stick

* Mucous membrane contact

* A cut from an object containing a potentially infectious body fluid (includes human bites)

* Having nonintact skin (OSHA includes acne in this category)

Guidelines employers must follow include the following:

* Employers must have a written **exposure control plan** designed to eliminate or reduce employee exposure to infectious material. This plan identifies, step by step, what to do if an employee is exposed to infectious material (for example, if an NA is stuck by a needle). This includes medical treatment and plans to prevent any similar exposures. It also includes specific work practices that must be followed. This plan must be accessible to all employees, and they must receive training on the plan.

* Employers must give all employees, visitors, and residents proper personal protective equipment (PPE) to wear when needed at no cost. Employers must make sure PPE is available in the appropriate sizes and is readily accessible.

* Employers must make biohazard containers available for disposal of sharps and other infectious waste. These containers must be puncture-resistant, labeled or color-coded, and leakproof.

* Employers must provide a free hepatitis B vaccine to all employees after hire.

* Warning labels must be affixed to waste containers and refrigerators and freezers that contain blood or any other potentially infectious material.

* Employers must keep a log of injuries from contaminated sharps. The information recorded must protect the confidentiality of the injured employee. Employers are also required to select safer needle devices and to involve employees in choosing these devices.

* Employers must provide in-service training on bloodborne pathogens and updates on any new safety standards at the time of hire and annually to all employees.

When an employee is exposed to blood or other potentially infectious material, an incident report or a special exposure report form must be completed. Tests and follow-up care may be needed. The employer will take steps to prevent the employee from becoming sick. Steps will also be taken to help keep similar incidents from occurring again. Nursing assistants must report any potential exposures immediately. Doing this helps protect their health and that of others. OSHA's website has more information at osha.gov.

12. Define *tuberculosis* and list infection prevention guidelines

Tuberculosis, or **TB**, is a highly contagious disease caused by a bacterium, *Mycobacterium tuberculosis*, that is carried on mucous droplets suspended in the air. The bacteria usually affect the lungs, which is known as pulmonary tuberculosis. TB is an airborne disease. People can be exposed to TB when they spend time with a person who is infected with TB. When the infected person talks, coughs, breathes, sings, laughs, or sneezes, he may spread the disease. Tuberculosis causes coughing, trouble breathing, fever, weight loss, and fatigue (Fig. 5-25). Usually it can be cured by taking all prescribed medication. However, if left untreated, TB may cause death.

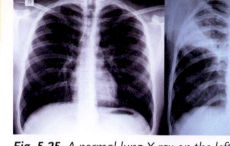

Fig. 5-25. A normal lung X-ray on the left, and an X-ray of a lung with tuberculosis on the right.

There are two types of tuberculosis: **latent TB infection (LTBI)** and **TB disease**. Someone with latent TB infection carries the disease but does not show symptoms and cannot infect others. A person with TB disease shows symptoms of the disease and can spread TB to others. Latent TB infection can progress to TB disease. These are some signs and symptoms of TB:

- Fatigue
- Loss of appetite
- Weight loss
- Slight fever and chills
- Night sweats
- Prolonged coughing
- Coughing up blood
- Chest pain
- Shortness of breath
- Trouble breathing

Tuberculosis is more likely to be spread in areas with poor ventilation or in small, confined spaces. People are more likely to get TB disease if their immune systems are weakened by illness, malnutrition, cancer, HIV/AIDS, alcoholism, or drug abuse.

Multidrug-resistant TB (MDR-TB) is a form of tuberculosis that is caused by an organism that is resistant to medication that is used to treat TB. **Resistant** means that drugs no longer work to kill the specific bacteria. It may develop when a person infected with TB does not take all of

his prescribed medication. When the full course of medication is not taken, bacteria remain in the body and are less likely to be killed by the medication. The disease becomes more difficult to cure. Other reasons for drug resistance are that the TB medication is used incorrectly or the medication is ineffective due to poor quality or poor storage conditions.

Employees are generally required to be tested for tuberculosis before they can begin working, and then they may be tested again annually. Nursing assistants must follow their facility's policy.

Guidelines: Tuberculosis

G Follow Standard Precautions and Airborne Precautions.

G Wear personal protective equipment as instructed during care. Special masks (respirators), such as N95 or high efficiency particulate air (HEPA) masks, may be needed. These masks help prevent a person from inhaling droplets. You must be fitted for these special masks and will be trained how to use them.

G Use special care when handling sputum or phlegm. **Phlegm** is thick mucus from the respiratory passage.

G Residents with TB will be placed in an airborne infection isolation room (AIIR). These rooms have a controlled flow of air. All of the air inside the room will be exhausted directly to the outside, or all air will first be recirculated through a special HEPA filter before returning to circulation. The room will be marked with a sign identifying it as a special respiratory isolation room. Keep doors to these rooms closed except when entering or exiting the room. When entering this room, do not open or close the door quickly. This pulls contaminated room air into the hallway.

G Follow isolation procedures for airborne diseases if directed.

G Help the resident remember to take all medication prescribed. Failure to take all medication is a major factor in the spread of TB.

13. Discuss MRSA, VRE, and *C. Difficile*

Multidrug-resistant organisms (MDROs) are microorganisms, mostly bacteria, that are resistant to one or more antimicrobial agents that are commonly used for treatment. There has been an increase in MDROs, and this is a serious problem. Two common types of MDROs are methicillin-resistant *Staphylococcus aureus*, commonly referred to as MRSA, and vancomycin-resistant *enterococcus, called VRE*.

Staphylococcus aureus is a common type of bacteria that can cause infection. Methicillin is a powerful antibiotic often used in healthcare facilities. **MRSA** is an antibiotic-resistant infection to methicillin. This type of MRSA is also known as HA-MRSA, which stands for hospital-associated MRSA.

Community-associated methicillin-resistant *Staphylococcus aureus* (CA-MRSA) is a type of MRSA infection that occurs in people who have not recently been admitted to healthcare facilities and who have no past diagnosis of MRSA. Often CA-MRSA manifests as skin infections, such as boils or pimples. This type of infection is becoming more common.

MRSA is almost always spread by direct physical contact with infected people. This means if a person has MRSA on his skin, especially on his hands, and touches another person, he may spread MRSA. Spread also occurs through indirect contact by touching equipment or supplies (for example, towels, sheets, wound dressings, or clothes) contaminated by a person with MRSA.

Symptoms of MRSA infection include drainage, fever, chills, and redness. Nursing assistants can help prevent the spread of MRSA by practicing proper hygiene. Handwashing, using soap and warm water, is the single most important measure to control the spread of MRSA. NAs must always follow Standard Precautions, along with Transmission-Based Precautions as ordered. Cuts and abrasions should be kept clean and covered with a proper dressing (e.g., bandage) until healed. Contact with other people's wounds or material that is contaminated from wounds should be avoided.

Enterococci are bacteria that live in the digestive and genital tracts. Although they normally do not cause problems in healthy people, they can sometimes cause infection. Vancomycin is a powerful antibiotic used to treat infections caused by *enterococci*. If the *enterococci* become resistant to vancomycin, then it is called vancomycin-resistant *enterococcus*, or **VRE**.

VRE is spread through direct and indirect contact. Symptoms of VRE infection include fever, fatigue, chills, and drainage. VRE infections are often difficult to treat and may require the use of several medications. VRE infections can cause life-threatening infections in those with compromised immune systems—the very young, the very old, and the very ill.

Preventing VRE is much easier than trying to treat it. Proper hand hygiene can help prevent the spread of VRE. Nursing assistants should wash their hands often and wear PPE as directed. NAs must always follow Standard Precautions, along with Transmission-Based Precautions as ordered. Items may need to be disinfected and that information should be listed in the care plan.

Clostridium difficile infection is commonly known as **C. diff** or **C. difficile.** It is a spore-forming bacterium which can be part of the normal intestinal flora. When the normal intestinal flora is altered, *C. difficile* can flourish in the intestinal tract and can cause infection. It produces a toxin that causes watery diarrhea. Enemas, nasogastric tube insertion, and GI tract surgery increase a person's risk of developing the infection. The elderly are at a higher risk of getting *C. difficile* infection. The overuse of antibiotics may alter the normal intestinal flora and increase the risk of developing *C. difficile*. It can also cause colitis, a more serious intestinal condition.

When released in the environment, *C. difficile* can form a spore that makes it difficult to kill. These spores can be carried on the hands of people who have direct contact with infected residents or with environmental surfaces (floors, bedpans, toilets, etc.) contaminated with *C. difficile*. Touching an object contaminated with *C. difficile* can transmit *C. difficile*. Alcohol-based hand sanitizer is not considered effective on *C. difficile*. Soap and water must be used each time hand hygiene is performed.

Symptoms of *C. difficile* include frequent, foul-smelling, watery stools. Other symptoms are fever, diarrhea that contains blood and mucus, nausea, lack of appetite, and abdominal cramps. Proper handwashing with soap and water is vital in preventing the spread of the infection. Handling contaminated wastes properly can help prevent the spread of the infection. Cleaning surfaces with an appropriate disinfectant, such as a bleach solution, can also reduce transmission. Limiting the use of antibiotics helps lower the risk of developing *C. difficile* infection.

14. List employer and employee responsibilities for infection prevention

Several state and federal government agencies have guidelines and laws concerning infection prevention. OSHA requires employers to provide for the safety of their employees through rules and suggested guidelines. The CDC issues guidelines for healthcare workers to follow on the job. Some states have additional requirements. Facilities consider these rules very carefully when writing their policies and procedures. It is important that nursing assistants learn these policies and procedures and follow them. They exist to protect all staff members and residents. Employers and employees both have key roles in infection prevention.

The employer's responsibilities for infection prevention include the following:

- Establish infection prevention procedures and an exposure control plan to protect workers

- Provide continuing in-service education on infection prevention, including education on bloodborne and airborne pathogens and updates on any new safety standards

- Have written procedures to follow should an exposure occur, including medical treatment and plans to prevent similar exposures

- Provide personal protective equipment (PPE) for employees to use, and teach them when and how to properly use it

- Provide free hepatitis B vaccinations for all employees

The employee's responsibilities for infection prevention include the following:

- Follow Standard Precautions

- Follow all facility policies and procedures

- Follow resident care plans and assignments

- Use provided personal protective equipment as indicated or as appropriate

- Take advantage of the free hepatitis B vaccination

- Immediately report any exposure to infection, blood, or body fluids

- Participate in annual education programs covering the prevention of infection

Chapter Review

1. What does infection prevention mean?

2. Which link in the chain of infection is broken by wearing gloves, and why?

3. Why are elderly people at a higher risk for infection?

4. Under Standard Precautions, what substances are considered body fluids?

5. On whom should Standard Precautions be practiced?

6. What is the single most important thing a nursing assistant can do to prevent the spread of disease?

7. What is hand hygiene?

8. For how long should a nursing assistant use friction when washing her hands?

9. How many times can disposable gloves be worn?

10. In what order should personal protective equipment be put on and removed?

11. Define *sterilization*. Define *disinfection*.

12. How should soiled linen be carried?

13. When blood or body fluids are spilled, what should an NA do first, before starting to clean the spill?

14. What are Transmission-Based Precautions?

15. If an NA needs to sneeze and does not have a tissue, into what area of the body should she sneeze?

16. How are bloodborne diseases transmitted? What is the most common way to be infected with a bloodborne disease in a healthcare setting?

17. What does HIV do to a person's immune system?

18. What is hepatitis?

19. How is hepatitis B (HBV) contracted?

20. Describe an exposure control plan.

21. In which people is tuberculosis more likely to develop?

22. What are multidrug-resistant organisms (MDROs)?

23. What is one of the best ways to prevent the spread of MRSA and VRE?

24. What are two ways that an NA can help prevent the spread of *C. difficile*?

25. What is an employer required to do with regard to the hepatitis B vaccination?

6

Safety and Body Mechanics

1. Identify the persons at greatest risk for accidents and describe accident prevention guidelines

All staff members, including nursing assistants, are responsible for safety in a facility. Elderly people have more safety concerns due to issues like dementia, confusion, illness, disability, and diminished senses. Walking aids, such as crutches, walkers, canes, and boots for foot or leg injuries put people at risk for falling. Residents who take medications that cause dizziness and light-headedness are likely to have accidents.

The senses of sight, hearing, touch, smell, and taste relay information about surroundings and help keep people safe. As people grow older, however, they suffer sensory losses. The senses of vision, hearing, taste, and smell decrease. Sensitivity to heat and cold decreases. And in addition to normal aging changes, diseases can cause diminished senses. Diseases of the circulatory and integumentary (skin) systems and paralysis can reduce the skin's ability to feel. **Paralysis** is the loss of ability to move all or part of the body. It often includes loss of feeling in the affected area. Strokes and brain or spinal injuries affect sensation and awareness of surroundings. A loss of sensation can lead to burns or other accidents. Drowsiness due to illness, lack of sleep, medications, or even feeling depressed can also cause a lack of awareness. Being in pain may reduce awareness. Individuals who are less aware may not know the positions of their body parts. Re-

flexes slow, making it more difficult to react in time to avoid accidents such as falls. Visual or hearing problems can also cause falls. Residents with vision problems may not see hazards, such as an object or water on the floor. Those who cannot hear well may not understand directions.

There are many factors that put residents at risk for serious injury. This is why it is very important to try to prevent accidents *before* they occur. Prevention is the key to safety. As nursing assistants work, they should observe for safety hazards and report unsafe conditions to the supervisor promptly.

Falls

A fall is any sudden, uncontrollable descent from a higher to a lower level, with or without injury resulting. Falls make up the majority of accidents that occur in long-term care facilities. They can be caused by an unsafe environment, loss of abilities, diseases, and medications. Problems resulting from falls range from minor bruises to fractures and life-threatening injuries. A **fracture** is a broken bone. Falls are particularly common among the elderly. Older people are often more seriously injured by falls because their bones are more fragile. Hip fractures are one of the most common types of fractures from falls. Hip fractures can lead to severe health problems and cause the greatest number of deaths. NAs should be especially alert to the risk of falls. All falls must be reported to the supervisor. An incident report must be completed, even if the resident says he or she is fine.

These factors increase the risk of falls:

- Clutter
- Throw rugs
- Exposed electrical cords
- Slippery or wet floors
- Uneven floors or stairs
- Poor lighting
- Call lights that are out of reach or not promptly answered

Personal conditions that increase the risk of falls include medications, loss of vision, gait (walking) or balance problems, weakness, paralysis, and disorientation. **Disorientation** means confusion about person, place, or time.

Guidelines: Preventing Falls

G Clear all walkways of clutter, trash, throw rugs, and cords.

G Use rugs or mats with a nonslip backing.

G Have residents wear nonskid, sturdy shoes. Make sure shoelaces are tied.

G Residents should not wear clothing that is too long or drags on the floor.

G Keep personal items that are used often close to residents, including call lights (Fig. 6-1).

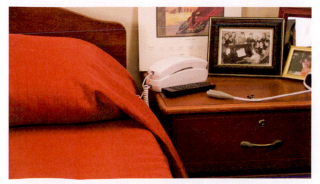

Fig. 6-1. Keep call lights within reach of residents so they can use them when needed. Respond to call lights promptly.

G Answer call lights right away.

G Immediately clean up spills on the floor.

G Report loose handrails immediately.

G Mark uneven flooring or stairs with tape of a contrasting color to indicate a hazard.

G Improve lighting where needed.

G Lock wheels and move footrests out of the way before helping residents into or out of wheelchairs (Fig. 6-2).

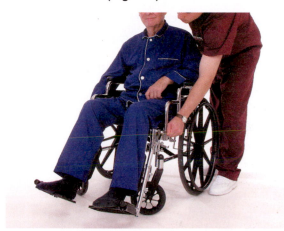

Fig. 6-2. Always lock a wheelchair and then remove the footrests before transferring a resident into or out of it.

G Lock bed wheels before helping a resident into and out of bed or when giving care (Fig. 6-3).

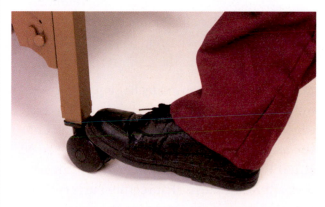

Fig. 6-3. Always lock the bed wheels before helping a resident into or out of bed and before giving care.

G Before giving care, there are many times that you will need to raise beds to make your job easier and safer. After completing care, return beds to their lowest positions.

G   Get help when moving a resident; do not assume you can do it alone. When in doubt, ask for help. Keep residents' walking aids, such as canes or walkers, within their reach.

G   Offer help with elimination regularly. Respond to requests for help immediately. Think about how you would feel if you had to wait for help to go to the bathroom.

G   Leave furniture in the same place as you found it.

G   Know which residents are at risk for falls and pay attention so that you can give help often.

G   If a resident starts to fall, be in a good position to help support her. Never try to catch a falling resident. Use your body to slide her to the floor. If you try to reverse a fall, you may hurt yourself and/or the resident.

G   Whenever a resident falls, it must be reported to the nurse. Always complete an incident report, even if the resident says he or she feels fine.

Burns/Scalds

Burns can be caused by dry heat (e.g., a hot iron, stove, other electrical appliances), wet heat (e.g., hot water or other liquids, steam), or chemicals (e.g., lye, acids). Small children, older adults, or people with loss of sensation (such as from paralysis or diabetes) are at the greatest risk for burns.

Scalds are burns caused by hot liquids. It takes five seconds or less for a serious burn to occur when the temperature of a liquid is 140°F. Coffee, tea, and other hot drinks are usually served at 160°F to 180°F. These temperatures can cause almost instant burns that require surgery. Preventing burns is very important.

Guidelines: Preventing Burns and Scalds

G   Always check water temperature with a water thermometer or on the inside of your wrist before using.

G   Immediately report frayed electrical cords or appliances that look unsafe. Do not use these appliances. Remove them from the room.

G   Let residents know that you are about to pour or set down a hot liquid.

G   Pour hot drinks away from residents. Keep hot drinks and liquids away from edges of tables. Put lids on them.

G   Make sure residents are sitting down before serving them hot drinks.

G   If plate warmers or other equipment that produces heat are used, monitor them carefully.

Resident Identification

Residents must always be identified before giving care or serving food. Failure to identify residents can cause serious problems, even death. Facilities have different methods of identification. Some have pictures to identify residents. Others have signs outside residents' doors (Fig. 6-4). Nursing assistants must identify each resident before beginning any procedure or giving any care. They should identify residents before placing meal trays or helping with feeding. The diet card should be checked against the resident's identification to make sure they match. The resident should be called by name and asked to state his or her name if able.

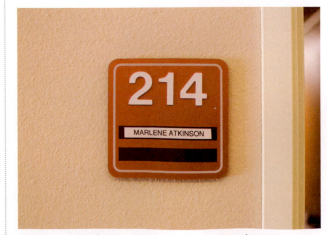

Fig. 6-4. A resident's name may be displayed outside the room to identify who is living in that room. Before giving any care, nursing assistants must always identify residents.

Choking

Choking can occur when eating, drinking, or swallowing medication. Babies and young children who put objects in their mouths are at great risk for choking. People who are weak, ill, or unconscious may choke on their own saliva. A person's tongue can also become swollen and obstruct the airway. To guard against choking, residents should eat in as upright a position as possible (Fig. 6-5). Residents with swallowing problems may have special diets with liquids thickened to the consistency of honey or syrup. Thickened liquids are easier to swallow. More information about helping with feeding and thickened liquids is located in Chapter 15.

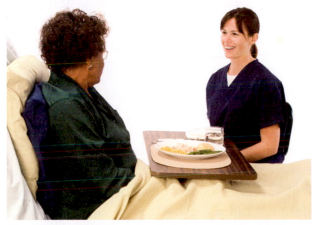

Fig. 6-5. *Residents must be sitting upright when eating, whether in a bed or a chair.*

Poisoning

There are many harmful substances in facilities that should not be swallowed. These include cleaning products, paints, medicines, toiletries, and glues. These products should be locked away from confused residents or those with limited vision. Cleaning products should not be left in residents' rooms. Residents with dementia may hide food and let it spoil in closets, drawers, or other places. Nursing assistants should investigate any odors they notice. The number for the Poison Control Center should be posted near all telephones.

Cuts/Abrasions

Cuts or abrasions typically occur in the bathroom at a facility or in the kitchen or bathroom when at home. An **abrasion** is an injury that rubs off the surface of the skin. Sharp objects, such as scissors, nail clippers, and razors, should be put away after use. Nursing assistants should take care when transferring residents into and out of beds, chairs, and wheelchairs. When moving residents in wheelchairs, NAs should push the wheelchair forward. Wheelchairs should not be pulled from behind. When using elevators, wheelchairs should be turned around before entering, so that residents are facing forward.

Nursing assistants should also follow these additional guidelines for working safely in facilities:

- Do not run in halls, on stairs, or in the dining room.
- Keep paths clear and free of clutter.
- Wipe up spilled liquids right away.
- Discard trash properly.
- Follow instructions. Ask about anything you do not understand.
- Report injuries immediately.

Promoting safety is part of nursing assistants' responsibilities. Reporting hazards immediately makes workplaces safer for everyone.

Residents' Rights

Safety

The Omnibus Budget Reconciliation Act (OBRA) requires that residents in long-term care facilities have the right to a safe environment. Nursing assistants should observe the environment carefully to identify safety hazards. If any safety hazard exists, such as a frayed electrical cord on a resident's radio, it should be reported immediately. Residents have the right to have personal items and to have these items treated with respect. However, if a resident's possession is a potential safety hazard, it should be reported to the nurse. The safety of all residents and staff members is most important.

2. List safety guidelines for oxygen use

Oxygen therapy is the administration of oxygen to increase the supply of oxygen to the lungs. This increases the availability of oxygen to the body tissues. Oxygen therapy is used to treat breathing difficulties and is prescribed by a doctor. Nursing assistants never stop, adjust, or administer oxygen.

Oxygen can be delivered in various ways. It may be piped into a resident's room through a central system. It may come in large tanks or in small, portable tanks. It may be produced by an oxygen concentrator. An oxygen concentrator is a box-like device that changes air in the room into air with more oxygen. Chapter 14 has more information about oxygen therapy.

Oxygen is a very dangerous fire hazard because it makes other things burn (supports combustion). **Combustion** means the process of burning. Working around oxygen requires special safety precautions.

Guidelines: Working Safely around Oxygen

G   Post *No Smoking* and *Oxygen in Use* signs. Never allow smoking where oxygen is used or stored.

G   Remove all fire hazards from the room or area. Fire hazards include electrical equipment, such as electric razors and hair dryers. Other fire hazards are cigarettes, matches, and flammable liquids. **Flammable** means easily ignited and capable of burning quickly. Examples of flammable liquids are alcohol and nail polish remover. Read the labels on liquids if you are unsure. If they say *flammable*, remove them from the area. Notify the nurse if a resident does not want a fire hazard removed.

G   Do not burn candles, light matches, or use lighters around oxygen. Any type of open flame that is present around oxygen is a dangerous fire hazard.

G   Do not use an extension cord with an oxygen concentrator.

G   Do not place electrical cords or oxygen tubing under rugs or furniture.

G   Avoid using fabrics such as nylon and wool that can cause static electricity discharges.

G   Oxygen can be irritating to the nose and mouth. The strap of the nasal cannula or face mask can also cause irritation around the ears. Check the nasal area and behind the ears for signs of irritation. Report and document any irritation you observe.

G   Do not use any petroleum-based products, such as Vaseline or Chapstick, on the resident or on any part of the cannula or mask. Oil-based lubricants can be a fire hazard.

G   Learn how to turn oxygen off in case of fire. Never adjust the oxygen setting or dose.

3. Explain the Safety Data Sheet (SDS)

The Occupational Safety and Health Administration (OSHA, osha.gov) requires that all hazardous chemicals have a Safety Data Sheet (SDS) (formerly called *Material Safety Data Sheet*, or *MSDS*). This sheet details the chemical ingredients, chemical dangers, and safe handling, storage, and disposal procedures for the product. Information about emergency response actions to be taken are also included. Some facilities use a toll-free number to access SDS information. These sheets must be accessible in work areas for all employees. Important information about the SDS includes the following:

• Employers must have an SDS for every chemical used.

• Employers must provide easy access to the SDS.

• Staff members must know where these sheets are kept and how to read them. They should ask for help if they do not know how to do this.

The list of hazardous chemicals that must have an SDS will be updated as new chemicals are purchased.

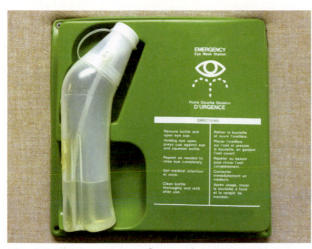

Fig. 6-6. *This is one type of eyewash station.*

4. Define the term *restraint* and give reasons why restraints were used

A **restraint** is a physical or chemical way to restrict voluntary movement or behavior. A *physical restraint* is any method, device, material, or equipment that restricts a person's freedom of movement. Types of physical restraints include vest restraints, belt restraints, wrist/ankle restraints, and mitt restraints. *Chemical restraints* are medications used to control a person's mood or behavior.

An *enabler* is equipment or a device that promotes a resident's safety, comfort, independence, and mobility. Wheelchairs, geriatric chairs, cushions and pillows, and certain types of assistive devices, such as special utensils, are examples of enablers. However, if a person cannot remove an enabler independently, it may be considered a restraint. Raised side rails on beds and geriatric chairs with tray tables attached may

be considered enablers or physical restraints, depending upon their intended use and the resident's condition or abilities (Figs. 6-7 and 6-8).

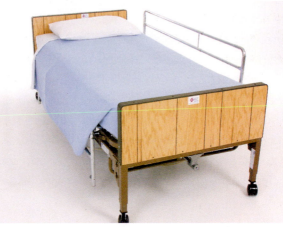

Fig. 6-7. *Raised side rails may be considered restraints, depending on their intended use and on the resident's abilities.*

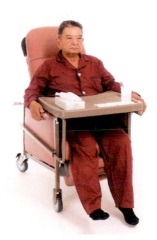

Fig. 6-8. *If a resident cannot remove an attached or locked tray table, a geriatric chair may be considered a restraint.*

In the past, restraints were commonly used to prevent confused people from wandering, to prevent falls, to keep people from injuring themselves or others, or to prevent people from pulling out tubing needed for treatment. Restraints were often overused by caregivers, and residents were injured. This led to new laws restricting the use of restraints.

Today, long-term care facilities are prohibited from using restraints unless they are medically necessary. They are only used as a last resort and only after less restrictive measures have been tried. If a restraint is needed, a doctor must order it. Very specific guidelines apply to carrying out a restraint order, including frequent monitoring of the resident. This is important because residents have been severely injured and have died due to improper restraint use and lack of monitoring. Nursing assistants cannot use physical restraints unless a doctor has ordered it in the care plan and they have been trained in the restraint's use. It is against the law for staff to apply a restraint for convenience or to discipline a resident. Nursing assistants can check with their supervisor for policies regarding restraints.

5. List physical and psychological problems associated with restraints

There are many serious problems associated with restraint use, including the following:

- Pressure injuries
- Pneumonia
- Risk of suffocation (**suffocation** is the stoppage of breathing from a lack of oxygen or excess of carbon dioxide in the body that may result in unconsciousness or death)
- Reduced blood circulation
- Stress on the heart
- Incontinence
- Constipation
- Muscle **atrophy** (weakening or wasting away of the muscle)
- Loss of bone mass
- Poor appetite and malnutrition
- Depression and/or withdrawal
- Sleep disorders
- Loss of dignity
- Loss of independence
- Stress and anxiety
- Increased agitation (anxiety, restlessness)

- Loss of self-esteem
- Severe injury
- Death

Nursing assistants must never use restraints unless their supervisor has told them to do so and they have been instructed in the proper use of the restraint. They must follow the care plan. The care plan will include instructions on frequent monitoring and repositioning.

6. Discuss restraint alternatives

Restraint usage has significantly decreased in facilities. State and federal agencies encourage facilities to take steps to create restraint-free environments. **Restraint-free care** means that restraints are not kept or used for any reason. Creative ideas that help avoid the need for restraints are being used instead. **Restraint alternatives** are measures used in place of a restraint or that reduce the need for a restraint. Many scientific studies have shown that restraints are not needed. People tend to respond better to the use of creative ways to reduce tension and behaviors such as pulling at tubes, wandering, and boredom. Examples of restraint alternatives include the following:

- Make sure call lights are within reach, and respond to call lights promptly.
- Improve safety measures to prevent accidents and falls. Improve lighting.
- Ambulate the resident when he is restless. The doctor or nurse may add exercise into the care plan.
- Provide activities for those who wander at night.
- Encourage activities and independence. Escort the resident to social activities. Increase visits and social interaction.
- Give frequent help with toileting. Help with cleaning immediately after an episode of incontinence.

- Offer food or drink. Offer reading materials.

- Distract or redirect interest. Give the resident a repetitive task.

- Decrease the noise level. Listen to soothing music. Offer back massages or use relaxation techniques.

- Reduce pain levels through medication. The resident should be monitored closely and complaints of pain should be reported immediately.

- Provide familiar caregivers, and increase the number of caregivers with family and volunteers.

- Use a team approach to meeting the resident's needs. Offer training to teach gentle approaches to difficult people.

There are also several types of pads, belts, special chairs, and alarms that can be used instead of restraints. If a resident is ordered to have an alarm on his bed or chair, the nursing assistant should make sure it is there and is turned on.

7. Describe guidelines for what must be done if a restraint is ordered

OBRA sets specific rules for restraint use. Restraints are used only after everything else has been ruled out and can only be applied with a doctor's order.

Guidelines: Restraints

G Know your state's laws and facility rules regarding applying restraints. Check to make sure there is a doctor's order for restraint use and that it is in the care plan before applying one. Make sure that you have been trained on how to apply the restraint.

G Follow the manufacturer's instructions when applying restraints.

G Check to make sure that the restraint is not too tight. You should be able to place your hand in a flat position between the resident and the restraint. This helps to ensure that the device fits properly and is comfortable.

G Make sure that the breasts or skin are not caught in the restraint.

G Place the call light within the resident's reach. Answer call lights immediately.

G Document restraint use according to facility policy.

A restrained resident must be monitored constantly; the resident must be checked at least every 15 minutes. At a minimum, every two hours the restraint must be released and the resident must be given proper care:

G Offer help with elimination. Check for episodes of incontinence, and provide skin care.

G Offer fluids and food.

G Measure vital signs.

G Check the skin for signs of irritation. Report any red, purple, blue, gray, or pale skin or any discolored areas to the nurse immediately.

G Check for swelling of the body part and report any swelling to the nurse immediately.

G Reposition the resident.

G Ambulate the resident if he is able.

If any problems occur with the restraint, especially injury, notify the nurse and complete an incident report as soon as possible.

8. Explain the principles of body mechanics

Back strain or injury can be a serious problem for nursing assistants. In fact, an increasing injury rate is one reason why many long-term care facilities have *lift-free* or *zero-lift* policies. These policies set strict guidelines on the use of lifts and transfers of residents in order to reduce injuries. Using proper body mechanics is an important step in preventing back strain and injury.

Body mechanics is the way the parts of the body work together when a person moves. Using proper body mechanics helps save energy and prevent injury. Nursing assistants can keep themselves and their residents safer if they understand the basic principles of body mechanics.

Alignment: Alignment is based on the word *line*. When a person stands up straight, a vertical line could be drawn through the center of his body and his center of gravity (Fig. 6-9). When the line is straight, the body is in alignment. Whether standing, sitting, or lying down, the body should be in alignment and should have good posture. This means that the two sides of the body are mirror images of each other, with body parts lined up naturally. **Posture** is the way a person holds and positions his body. A person can maintain correct body alignment when lifting or carrying an object by keeping the object close to his body. His feet and body should be pointed in the direction he is moving. He should avoid twisting at the waist.

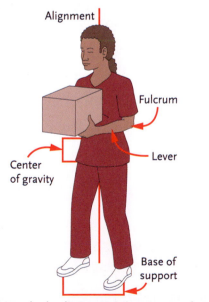

Alignment

Fulcrum

Center
of gravity

Lever

Base of
support

Fig. 6-9. Proper body alignment is important when standing and sitting.

Base of support: The base of support is the foundation that supports an object. The feet are the body's base of support. The wider the support, the more stable a person is. Standing with legs shoulder-width apart allows for a greater base of support. This is more stable than standing with the feet together.

Fulcrum and lever: A **lever** moves an object by resting on a base of support, called a *fulcrum*. For example, on a seesaw, the flat board a person sits on is the lever. The triangular base that the board rests on is the fulcrum. When two children sit on opposite sides of the seesaw, they easily move each other up and down. This is because the fulcrum and lever of the seesaw are doing the work.

Thinking of the body as a set of fulcrums and levers can be helpful when trying to find smart ways to lift without working as hard. For example, an arm is a lever and the elbow is the fulcrum. When a person lifts something, he can rest it against his forearm. This will shorten the lever and make the item easier to lift than it would be if he were holding it in his hands.

Center of gravity: The center of gravity in the body is the point where the most weight is concentrated (Fig. 6-10). This point will depend on the position of the body. When a person stands, weight is centered in the pelvis. A low center of gravity gives a more stable base of support. Bending the knees when lifting an object lowers the pelvis and, therefore, lowers a person's center of gravity. This gives more stability and makes the person less likely to fall or strain the working muscles.

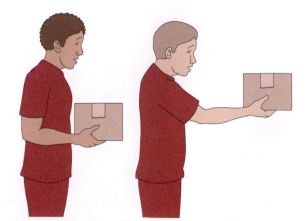

Fig. 6-10. Holding things close to the body moves weight toward the center of gravity. In this illustration, who is more likely to strain his back muscles?

9. Apply principles of body mechanics to daily activities

By applying the principles of body mechanics to daily activities, injury can be avoided and less energy used. Procedures for properly transferring, positioning, and ambulating residents are located throughout this textbook. These procedures include instructions for maintaining proper body mechanics. In addition, the following guidelines are helpful:

Guidelines: Using Proper Body Mechanics

G Assess the situation first. Clear the path and remove any obstacles.

G Use both arms and hands to lift, push, or carry objects.

G When lifting a heavy object from the floor, spread your feet shoulder-width apart. Bend your knees. Use the strong, large muscles in your thighs, upper arms, and shoulders to lift the object. Raise your body and the object together (Fig. 6-11).

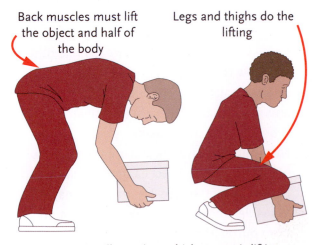

Back muscles must lift the object and half of the body

Legs and thighs do the lifting

Fig. 6-11. In this illustration, which person is lifting correctly?

G Hold objects close to you when you are lifting or carrying them. This keeps the object closer to your center of gravity and base of support.

G Push or slide objects rather than lifting them.

G Avoid bending and reaching as much as possible. Move or position furniture so that you do not have to bend or reach.

G If you are making an adjustable bed, adjust the height to a safe working level, usually waist high. If you are making a regular bed, lean or kneel to support yourself at working level. Avoid bending at the waist.

G When a task requires bending, use a good stance. Bend your knees to lower yourself (squat), rather than bending from the waist. This uses the big muscles in your legs and hips rather than the smaller muscles in your back.

G Do not twist when you are lifting or moving an object. Instead, turn your whole body. Pivot your feet instead of twisting at the waist. Your feet should point toward what you are lifting or moving.

G Get help from coworkers when possible for lifting or helping residents.

G Talk to residents before moving them. Let them know what you will do so they can help if possible. Agree on a signal, such as counting to three. Lift or move on three so that everyone moves together.

G To help a resident sit up, stand up, or walk, place your feet shoulder-width apart. Place one foot in front of the other and bend your knees. Your upper body should stay upright and in alignment. Do this whenever you have to support a resident's weight.

G Never try to catch a falling resident. If the resident falls, assist her to the floor (Fig. 6-12). If you try to reverse a fall in progress, you could injure yourself and/or the resident.

G Report to the nurse any task you feel that you cannot safely do. Never try to lift an object or a resident that you feel you cannot handle.

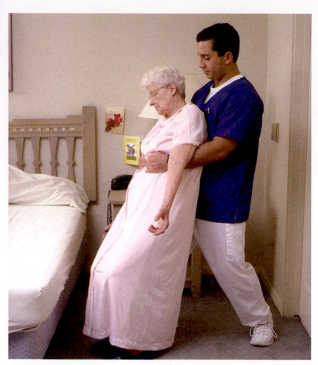

Fig. 6-12. Maintaining a wide base of support and low center of gravity will enable you to help a falling resident.

10. Identify major causes of fire and list fire safety guidelines

In order for a fire to occur, three elements must be present: heat, fuel, and oxygen. A fire can be prevented or extinguished by removing any one of these elements.

Nursing assistants must be able to recognize and report any fire hazards they observe. There are many potential fire hazards in facilities and in the home, including the following:

- Smoking

- Frayed or exposed electrical wires

- Damaged electrical equipment

- Oxygen use

- Flammable liquids or rags with oils on them

- Overloaded electrical sockets

In addition, in the home, any of the following can be a fire hazard:

- Wood stoves and kerosene, gas, or electric heaters that appear old, damaged, or faulty

- Unvented heaters used in small, enclosed areas or sleeping areas

- Space heaters used near fabrics such as draperies, bedspreads, or towels, or used to dry clothing or towels

- Flammable materials such as gasoline, kerosene, or paint thinner stored near stoves, heaters, furnaces, hot water heaters, or other appliances

- Matches or lighters left within reach of children or incapacitated adults

- Careless cooking

All facilities have a fire safety plan, and all workers need to know this plan. Guidelines regarding fires and evacuations will be explained to all employees. Evacuation routes are posted in facilities. Nursing assistants should read and review them often and should attend fire and disaster in-service trainings when they are offered. These in-services will explain what NAs must do in an emergency. A fast, calm, and confident response by the staff saves lives.

Guidelines: Reducing Fire Hazards and Responding to Fires

G Some facilities are nonsmoking, while others allow residents to smoke. If residents smoke, make sure they are in the proper area for smoking. Be sure that cigarettes are extinguished. Empty ashtrays often. Before emptying ashtrays, make sure there are no hot ashes or hot matches in the ashtray. Burn-resistant aprons for smokers may be available. These aprons help protect a person from burns from hot ashes and lit cigarettes if they are dropped. If residents wear these aprons when smoking, make sure buckles and snaps are properly fastened and that the apron covers their torso and lap. Never leave any smoker unattended.

G Residents may use electronic cigarettes (e-cigarettes, e-cigs). E-cigarettes do not contain tobacco. They contain liquid nicotine that is heated and turned into a vapor that the person inhales and exhales. Matches or lighters are not needed to light this type of cigarette; they use a battery to turn the liquid nicotine into vapor. Fires involving e-cigarettes have been reported due to the battery overcharging or overheating or when using a non-approved power source to recharge the battery. To reduce the risk of fire, e-cigarettes should only be charged using the appliance supplied by the manufacturer. Batteries may need to be turned off manually after residents are finished using e-cigarettes. Batteries may need to be removed from chargers after they are fully charged. Follow instructions given with regard to these devices.

G Report frayed or damaged electrical cords immediately. Report electrical equipment in need of repair immediately.

G Fire alarms and exit doors should not be blocked. If they are, report this to the nurse.

G Every facility will have multiple fire extinguishers (Fig. 6-13). Learn where they are located. The PASS acronym will help you understand how to use an extinguisher:

- **P**ull the pin.
- **A**im at the base of the fire when spraying.
- **S**queeze the handle.
- **S**weep back and forth at the base of the fire.

G In case of fire, the RACE acronym is a good rule to follow:

- **R**emove anyone in danger if you are not in danger.
- **A**ctivate alarm or call 911.
- **C**ontain the fire if possible by closing all doors and windows.
- **E**xtinguish the fire, or the fire department will extinguish it. Evacuate the area if instructed to do so.

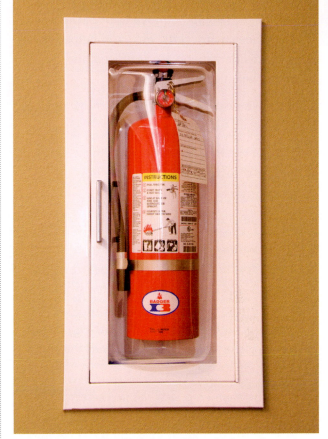

Fig. 6-13. Know the locations of your facility's fire extinguishers and how to use them.

Follow these guidelines for helping residents exit the building safely:

G Know the facility's fire evacuation plan.

G Stay calm. Do not panic.

G Follow the directions of the fire department.

G Know which residents need one-on-one help or assistive devices. Immobile residents can be moved in several ways. If they have a wheelchair, help them into it. You can also use other wheeled transporters, such as carts, bath chairs, stretchers, or beds. A blanket can be used as a stretcher or even pulled across the floor with someone on it.

G Residents who can walk will also need assistance getting out of the building. Those who are hearing impaired may not hear the warnings and instructions. Staff will need to tell them directly what to do while guiding them to the nearest safe exit. People with visual problems should be moved out of the way of the wheelchairs, carts, etc., and helped to the exit. Residents who are confused and disoriented will also need guidance.

G Remove anything blocking a window or door that could be used as a fire exit.

G Do not get into an elevator during a fire unless directed to do so by the fire department.

G Stay low in a room to escape a fire.

G If the door of the room you are in is closed, check for heat coming from it before opening it. If the door or doorknob feels hot, stay in the room if there is no safe exit. Plug the doorway (use wet towels or clothing) to prevent smoke from entering. Stay in the room until help arrives.

G Use the *stop, drop, and roll* fire safety technique to extinguish a fire on clothing or hair. Stop running or stay still. Drop to the ground, lying down if possible. Roll on the ground to try to extinguish the flames.

G Use a damp covering over the mouth and nose to reduce smoke inhalation.

G After leaving the building, move away from it.

Chapter Review

1. List five reasons that elderly people have more safety concerns than other people do.

2. What type of accident occurs most frequently in long-term care facilities?

3. What should the nursing assistant do before helping a resident into or out of a wheelchair?

4. What should nursing assistants always do before giving care or serving meal trays?

5. In what position should residents eat to avoid choking?

6. What are three guidelines for working safely around oxygen?

7. What important information does the Safety Data Sheet (SDS) provide about chemicals?

8. When can a restraint be used?

9. List ten problems associated with restraint use.

10. What are restraint alternatives?

11. What is body mechanics?

12. What is the name for the point in the body where the most weight is concentrated?

13. When lifting a heavy object from the floor, how should the feet be placed? How should the knees be positioned?

14. When a task requires bending, which of the following demonstrates proper body mechanics: bending the knees or bending from the waist?

15. Is it better to push an object or to lift an object?

16. What three elements are needed for a fire to occur?

17. Define the *PASS* and *RACE* acronyms.

18. If a fire has started, what should the nursing assistant do before opening a closed door?

7

Emergency Care and Disaster Preparation

1. Demonstrate how to recognize and respond to medical emergencies

Medical emergencies may be the result of accidents or sudden illnesses. This chapter discusses how to respond appropriately to medical emergencies. Heart attacks, strokes, diabetic emergencies, choking, automobile accidents, and gunshot wounds are all medical emergencies. Falls, burns, and cuts can also be emergencies. In an emergency situation, it is important for responders to remain calm, act quickly, and communicate clearly. The following steps illustrate the correct response to emergencies:

Assess the situation. The responder should try to determine what has happened. She must make sure she is not in danger and notice the time.

Assess the victim. The responder should ask the injured or ill person what has happened. If the person is unable to respond, he may be unconscious. Being **conscious** means being mentally alert and having awareness of surroundings, sensations, and thoughts. Tapping the person and asking if he is all right helps to determine if a person is conscious. The responder should speak loudly and use the person's name if she knows it. If there is no response, she should assume the person is unconscious and that an emergency situation exists. She should call for help right away or send someone else to call.

If a person is conscious and able to speak, then he is breathing and has a pulse. The responder should talk with the person about what happened. She should get his permission to touch him. (Anyone who is unable to give consent for treatment, such as a child with no parent near or an unconscious or seriously injured person, may be treated with *implied consent*. This means that if the person were able or the parent were present, they would have given consent.) The person should be checked for the following:

- Severe bleeding
- Changes in consciousness
- Irregular breathing
- Unusual color or feel to the skin
- Swollen places on the body
- Medical alert tags
- Pain

If any of these conditions exists, professional medical help may be needed. When a nursing assistant is responding to an emergency, she should always get help and call the nurse before doing anything else. If an injured or ill person is conscious, he may be frightened. Whoever responds to the emergency should listen to the person and tell him what actions are being taken to help him. A calm and confident response will help reassure him that he is being taken care of.

After the emergency is over, the NA will need to document the emergency and complete an incident report. It is important to include as many details as possible and report only facts. For example, if the NA thinks a resident had a heart attack, she should only document the signs and symptoms she observed and the actions she took. Knowing the kind of information to document will help the NA remember the important facts during the emergency. For instance, it is especially important to remember the time at which a resident became unconscious.

Reporting Emergencies

If a resident needs emergency help, the nurse may ask a nursing assistant to call emergency services. The NA should know the procedure for dialing an outside line. Emergency medical services can be reached by dialing 911. The NA should be prepared to give the following information when calling emergency services:

- The phone number and address of the emergency, including exact directions or landmarks, and the location within the building if necessary

- The person's condition, including any known medical background

- The NA's name and position

- Details of any first aid being given

The dispatcher may need other information or may want to give other instructions. The NA should not hang up the phone until the dispatcher hangs up or tells her to hang up.

A home health aide working in a home should remember this: if in doubt about calling for help, she should call! If the HHA is alone, she should make the call herself. If she is not alone, she can shout for help and have someone else make the call. After calling 911, the supervisor should be notified about what is happening and that 911 or emergency services has been called. The supervisor can notify the family or friends who need to know this information. If in a home, the HHA should unlock the front door so emergency personnel can get in when they arrive.

2. Demonstrate knowledge of first aid procedures

Emergency situations can happen to anyone at any time. **First aid** is emergency care given immediately to an injured person by the first people to respond to an emergency. **Cardiopulmonary resuscitation (CPR)** refers to medical procedures used when a person's heart or lungs have stopped working. CPR is used until medical help arrives.

Quick action is necessary. CPR must be started immediately to help prevent or lessen brain damage. Brain damage can occur within four to six minutes after the heart stops beating and breathing stops. The person can die within ten minutes.

Employers often arrange for nursing assistants to be trained in CPR. If not, the American Heart Association (heart.org) and Red Cross (redcross.org) have more information about training. CPR is an important skill to learn.

Nursing assistants need to know their facility's policies on initiating CPR. Some facilities do not allow nursing assistants to begin CPR without direction of the nurse. This is due, in part, to residents' advance directives. Some people have made the decision that they do not want CPR. The nurse should be notified immediately if an emergency occurs.

Residents' Rights

CPR

Nursing assistants can protect the privacy of residents who need CPR by pulling the privacy curtain around the bed and closing the door. Anyone who is not directly involved in giving care should leave the room. NAs should remain calm and be professional. They should remember that a resident may be able to hear what is being said. Some residents have do-not-resuscitate (DNR) orders in place, which means that no CPR may be given. This is a legal order; the resident's decision for a DNR order and other advance directives must be honored. NAs should not judge these very personal decisions.

Choking

When something is blocking the tube through which air enters the lungs, the person has an **obstructed airway**. When people are choking, they usually put their hands to their throats (Fig. 7-1). Nursing assistants may encounter residents who are choking or seem to be choking. As long as the resident can speak, breathe, or cough, the NA should only encourage her to cough as forcefully as possible to get the object out. The NA should stay with the resident at all times, until she stops choking or can no longer speak, breathe, or cough.

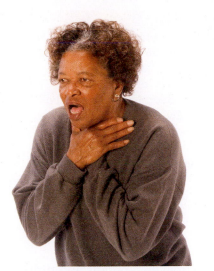

Fig. 7-1. People who are choking usually put their hands to their throats.

If a resident can no longer speak, breathe, or cough, the NA should call for help immediately by using the call light or emergency cord. The choking victim should not be left alone. **Abdominal thrusts** are a method of attempting to remove an object from the airway of someone who is choking. These thrusts work to remove the blockage upward, out of the throat.

The NA should make sure the resident needs help before starting to give abdominal thrusts. The resident must show signs of a severely obstructed airway. These signs include poor air exchange, an increase in trouble breathing, silent coughing, blue-tinged skin (cyanosis), and an inability to speak, breathe, or cough. The NA should ask, "Are you choking? I know what to do. Can I help you?" If the resident nods her head yes, she has a severe airway obstruction and needs immediate help. The NA should begin giving abdominal thrusts. This procedure should never be performed on a person who is not choking. Abdominal thrusts risk injury to the ribs or internal organs.

Performing abdominal thrusts for the conscious person

1. Stand behind the person and bring your arms under her arms. Wrap your arms around the person's waist.

2. Make a fist with one hand. Place the thumb side of the fist against the person's abdomen, above the navel but below the breastbone (Fig. 7-2).

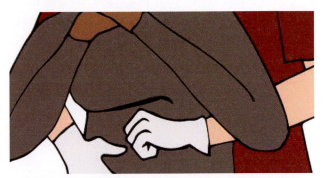

Fig. 7-2. Place the flat, thumb side of your fist against the person's abdomen, above the navel but below the breastbone.

3. Grasp the fist with your other hand. Pull both hands toward you and up, quickly and forcefully.

4. Repeat until the object is pushed out or the person loses consciousness.

5. Report and document the incident properly.

If the resident becomes unconscious while choking, she should be helped to the floor gently so she is lying on her back on a hard surface with her face up. The NA should begin CPR for an unconscious person if trained and allowed to do so. The NA should make sure help is on the way. The resident may have a completely blocked airway and needs professional medical help immediately. The NA should stay with the victim until help arrives.

Home health aides working in the home need to know how to clear an obstructed airway in an infant. The infant will need to receive back blows and chest thrusts after the responder makes sure the airway is obstructed.

Clearing an obstructed airway in a conscious infant

1. Lay the infant face down on your forearm; if you are sitting, rest the arm holding the in-

fant's torso on your lap or thigh. Support her jaw and head with your hand. Keep her head lower than the rest of her body.

2. Using the heel of your free hand, deliver up to five back blows. Back blows are performed by striking the infant between the shoulder blades (Fig. 7-3).

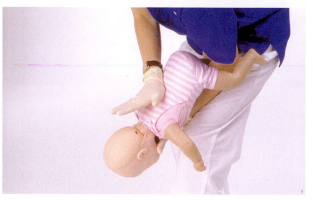

Fig. 7-3. Keeping the infant's head below the rest of her body, deliver back blows.

3. If the obstruction is not expelled with back blows, turn the infant onto her back while supporting the head. Deliver up to five chest thrusts by placing two or three fingers in the center of the breastbone (Fig. 7-4).

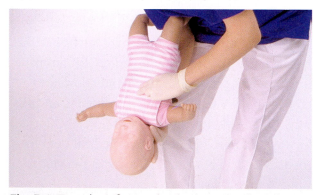

Fig. 7-4. Turn the infant on her back to give chest thrusts if the obstruction is not expelled with back blows.

4. Repeat alternating five back blows and five chest thrusts until the object is pushed out or the infant loses consciousness.

5. Call 911 immediately if the infant loses consciousness. Follow any instructions you are given. Report and document the incident properly.

Emergency Codes

Facilities often use codes to inform staff of emergencies while preventing panic and stress among residents and visitors. These codes are frequently described by color. For example, *Code Red* usually means fire. *Code Blue* usually means cardiac arrest. However, the meanings of these codes vary from facility to facility. It is important for nursing assistants to know the codes for their facility. NAs should not panic when codes are announced; they should respond calmly and professionally.

Shock

Shock occurs when organs and tissues in the body do not receive an adequate blood supply. Bleeding, heart attack, severe infection, and falling blood pressure can lead to shock. Shock can become worse when the person is extremely frightened or in severe pain.

Shock is a dangerous, life-threatening situation. Signs of shock include pale or bluish skin, staring, increased pulse and respiration rates, low blood pressure, and extreme thirst. A nursing assistant should always call for help if she suspects a resident is experiencing shock.

Responding to shock

1. Notify the nurse immediately. Victims of shock should always receive medical care as soon as possible.

2. If you need to control bleeding, put on gloves first. This procedure is described later in the chapter.

3. Have the person lie down on her back. If the person is bleeding from the mouth or vomiting, place her on her side. Elevate the legs about eight to 12 inches unless the person has a head, neck, back, spinal, or abdominal injury; breathing difficulties; or fractures (Fig. 7-5). Elevating the legs allows blood to flow back to the brain (and other vital areas). Never elevate a body part if the person has a broken bone or if it causes pain.

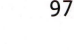

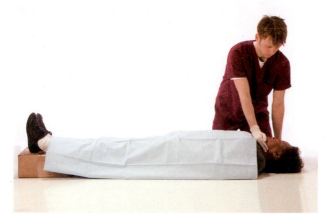

Fig. 7-5. If a person is in shock, elevate the legs, unless she has head, neck, back, spinal, or abdominal injuries; breathing difficulties; or fractures.

4. Check pulse and respirations if possible (see Chapter 14). Begin CPR if breathing and pulse are absent and if you are trained and allowed to do so.

5. Keep the person as calm and comfortable as possible.

6. Maintain normal body temperature. If the weather is cold, place a blanket around the person. If the weather is hot, provide shade.

7. Do not give the person liquids or food.

8. Report and document the incident properly.

Myocardial Infarction or Heart Attack

Myocardial infarction (MI), or heart attack, occurs when the heart muscle itself does not receive enough oxygen because blood vessels are blocked (Chapter 18 contains more information). A myocardial infarction is an emergency that can result in serious heart damage or death. The following are signs and symptoms of MI:

- Sudden, severe pain, pressure, or squeezing in the chest, usually on the left side or in the center, behind the breastbone

- Pain or discomfort in other areas of the body, such as one or both arms, the back, neck, jaw, or stomach

- Indigestion or heartburn

- Nausea and vomiting

- **Dyspnea** or difficulty breathing

- Dizziness

- Pale or bluish (cyanotic) skin color, indicating lack of oxygen

- Perspiration

- Cold and clammy skin

- Weak and irregular pulse rate

- Low blood pressure

- Anxiety and a sense of doom

- Denial of a heart problem

The pain of a heart attack is commonly described as a crushing, pressing, squeezing, stabbing, piercing pain, or, "like someone is sitting on my chest." The pain may go down the inside of the left arm. A person may also feel it in the neck and/or in the jaw. The pain usually does not go away.

As with men, women may experience chest pain or discomfort. Women, though, can have heart attacks without chest pressure. Women are more likely to have shortness of breath, nausea, light-headedness, stomach pain, sweating, fatigue, and back, neck, or jaw pain. Some women's symptoms seem more flu-like, and women are more likely to deny that they are having a heart attack. A nursing assistant must take immediate action if a resident experiences any of these symptoms.

Responding to a myocardial infarction

1. Notify the nurse immediately. If working in the home, call 911 immediately and call your supervisor.

2. Place the person in a comfortable position. Encourage him to rest and reassure him that you will not leave him alone.

3. Loosen clothing around the person's neck (Fig. 7-6).

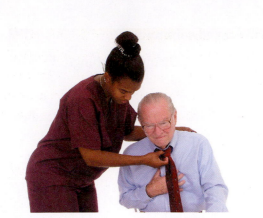

Fig. 7-6. Loosen clothing around the person's neck if you suspect he is having an MI.

4. Do not give the person liquids or food.

5. Monitor the person's breathing and pulse. If the person stops breathing or has no pulse, begin CPR if trained and allowed to do so.

6. Stay with the person until help arrives.

7. Report and document the incident properly.

Some states allow nursing assistants to offer heart medication, such as nitroglycerin, to a resident having a heart attack. If allowed to do this, NAs can only offer the medication; they cannot place it in the resident's mouth.

Bleeding

Severe bleeding can cause death quickly and must be controlled.

Controlling bleeding

1. Notify the nurse immediately.

2. Put on gloves. Take the time to do this. If the resident is able, he can hold his bare hand over the wound until you can put on gloves.

3. Hold a thick sterile pad, clean cloth, or clean towel against the wound.

4. Press down hard directly on the bleeding wound until help arrives. Do not decrease pressure (Fig. 7-7). Put additional pads or cloths over the first pad if blood seeps through. Do not remove the first pad.

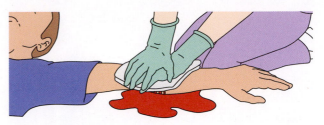

Fig. 7-7. Press down hard directly on the bleeding wound; do not decrease pressure.

5. If you can, raise the wound above the level of the heart to slow the bleeding. Prop up the limb if the wound is on an arm, leg, hand, or foot and there are no broken bones. Use towels or other absorbent material.

6. When bleeding is under control, secure the dressing to keep it in place. Check for symptoms of shock (pale skin, staring, increased pulse and respiration rates, low blood pressure, and extreme thirst). Stay with the person until help arrives.

7. Remove and discard gloves and wash hands thoroughly when finished.

8. Report and document the incident properly.

Poisoning

Facilities contain many harmful substances that should not be swallowed. Signs and symptoms of poisoning vary widely, depending on the substance that the person ingested. However, poisoning may be suspected when a resident vomits, has heavy, difficult breathing, is very drowsy, is confused, or has burns or red areas around the mouth. If an NA suspects poisoning, he should notify the nurse immediately. The NA may be asked to don gloves and look for a container that will help determine what the resident has taken or eaten.

Burns

Care of a burn depends on its depth, size, and location. There are three types of burns: first-degree (superficial), second-degree (partial-thickness), and third-degree (full-thickness) (Fig. 7-8). First-degree burns involve just the outer layer of skin. The skin becomes red, painful, and swollen, but no blisters appear. Second-degree burns extend from the outer layer of skin to the next deeper layer of skin. The skin is red, painful, and swollen, and blisters appear. Third-degree burns involve all three layers of the skin and may extend to the bone. The skin is shiny and appears hard. It may be white in color.

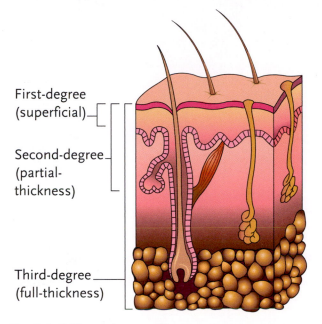

First-degree (superficial)

Second-degree (partial-thickness)

Third-degree (full-thickness)

Fig. 7-8. *Different degrees of burns.*

Burns in the Home

When working in a home, the home health aide should call for emergency help in any of the following situations:

- An infant or child, or an elderly, ill, or weak person has been burned, unless the burn is very minor

- The burn occurs on the head, neck, hands, feet, face, or genitals, or burns cover more than one body part

- The person who has been burned is having trouble breathing

- The burn was caused by chemicals, electricity, or an explosion

Treating burns

To treat a minor burn:

1. Notify the nurse immediately. Put on gloves.

2. Use cool, clean water to decrease the skin temperature and prevent further injury (Fig. 7-9). Do not use ice or ice water, as ice may cause further skin damage. Dampen a clean cloth with cool water and place it over the burn.

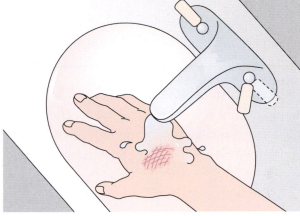

Fig. 7-9. *Use cool, clean water, not ice, on burned skin.*

3. Once the pain has eased, you may cover the area with a dry, clean dressing or nonadhesive sterile bandage.

4. Remove and discard gloves. Wash your hands.

5. Never use any kind of ointment, salve, or grease on a burn.

For more serious burns:

1. Remove the person from the source of the burn. If clothing has caught fire, have the person stop, drop, and roll, or smother the fire with a blanket or towel to put out flames. Protect yourself from the source of the burn.

2. Notify the nurse immediately. Put on gloves.

3. Check for breathing, pulse, and severe bleeding. If the person is not breathing and has no pulse, begin CPR if trained and allowed to do so.

4. Do not use any type of ointment, water, salve, or grease on the burn.

5. Do not try to pull away any clothing from burned areas. Cover the burn with sterile

gauze or a clean sheet. Apply the gauze or sheet lightly. Take care not to rub the burned area.

6.   Monitor vital signs and wait for emergency medical help.

7.   Remove and discard gloves. Wash your hands.

8.   Report and document the incident properly.

Chemical burns require special care. The NA should call for help immediately. The chemical must be washed away thoroughly. A shower or a hose may be needed when the burns cover a large area.

Fainting

Fainting, called **syncope**, occurs as a result of decreased blood flow to the brain, causing a loss of consciousness. Fainting may be the result of hunger, hypoglycemia (low blood glucose), dehydration, fear, pain, fatigue, standing for a long time, poor ventilation, certain medications, pregnancy, or overheating. Fainting may sometimes be caused by orthostatic hypotension, which is also called postural hypotension. **Orthostatic hypotension** is a sudden drop in blood pressure that occurs when a person stands or sits up. Signs and symptoms of fainting include dizziness, lightheadedness, nausea, perspiration, pale skin, weak pulse, shallow respirations, and blackness in the visual field.

Responding to fainting

1.   Notify the nurse immediately.

2.   Have the person lie down or sit down before fainting occurs.

3.   If the person is in a sitting position, have him bend forward (Fig. 7-10). He can place his head between his knees if he is able. If the person is lying flat on his back, elevate his legs about 12 inches.

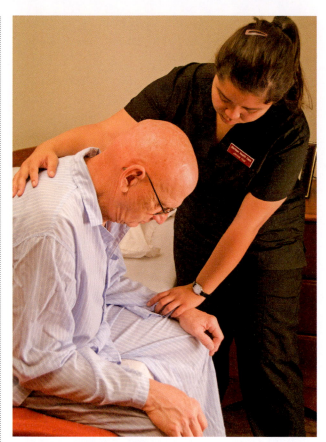

Fig. 7-10. *Have the person bend forward if he is sitting.*

4.   Loosen any tight clothing.

5.   Have the person stay in position for at least five minutes after symptoms disappear.

6.   Help the person get up slowly. Continue to observe him for symptoms of fainting. Stay with him until he feels better. If you need help but cannot leave him, use the call light.

7.   If a person does faint, lower him to the floor or other flat surface. Position him on his back. If he has no head, neck, back, spinal, or abdominal injuries, elevate his legs eight to 12 inches. If unsure about injuries, leave him flat on his back. Loosen any tight clothing. Check to make sure the person is breathing. He should recover quickly, but keep him lying down for several minutes. Report the incident to the nurse immediately. Fainting may be a sign of a more serious medical condition.

8.   Report and document the incident properly.

Nosebleed

A nosebleed can occur suddenly when the air is dry, when injury has occurred, or when a person has taken certain medications. The medical term for a nosebleed is **epistaxis**.

1. Notify the nurse immediately.

2. Elevate the head of the bed, or tell the person to remain in a sitting position, leaning forward slightly. Offer tissues or a clean cloth to catch the blood. Do not touch blood or bloody clothes, tissues, or cloths without gloves.

3. Put on gloves. Apply firm pressure on both sides of the nose, on the soft part, up near the bridge. Squeeze the sides with your thumb and forefinger (Fig. 7-11). Have the resident do this until you are able to put on gloves.

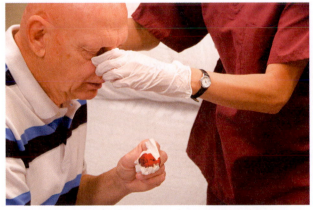

Fig. 7-11. With gloves on, squeeze near the bridge of the nose on both sides, using your thumb and forefinger.

4. Apply pressure until the bleeding stops.

5. Use a cool cloth or ice wrapped in a cloth on the bridge of the nose to slow the flow of blood. Never apply ice directly to skin.

6. Remove and discard gloves. Wash your hands.

7. Report and document the incident properly.

Insulin Reaction and Diabetic Ketoacidosis

Insulin reaction and diabetic ketoacidosis are complications of diabetes that can be life-threatening. **Insulin reaction**, or **hypoglycemia**, can result from either too much insulin or too little food. It occurs when insulin is given and the person skips a meal or does not eat all the food required. Even when a regular amount of food is eaten, physical activity may rapidly metabolize the food so that too much insulin is in the body. Vomiting and diarrhea may also lead to insulin reaction in people who have diabetes.

The first signs of insulin reaction include feeling weak or different, nervousness, dizziness, and perspiration. The NA should immediately report these signs to the nurse. These signs signal that the resident needs food in a form that can be rapidly absorbed. A glass of milk, fruit juice, or water with sugar dissolved in it should be consumed right away. A glucose tablet is another quick source of sugar. A fingerstick blood glucose test may need to be done right away (Chapter 18 has more information), and the NA should follow her facility's policies. Signs and symptoms of insulin reaction include the following:

- Hunger
- Headache
- Rapid pulse
- Low blood pressure
- Cold, clammy skin
- Confusion
- Trembling
- Nervousness
- Blurred vision
- Numbness of the lips and tongue
- Unconsciousness

Diabetic ketoacidosis (DKA) is caused by having too little insulin in the body. It can result from undiagnosed diabetes, infection, going without insulin or not taking enough insulin, eating too much, not getting enough exercise, or physical or emotional stress. The signs of the onset of diabetic ketoacidosis include increased hunger, thirst, or urination; abdominal pain; deep or labored breathing; and breath that smells sweet or fruity. The nurse should be notified immediately if a resident has shown signs of diabetic ketoacidosis. Other signs and symptoms include the following:

- Headache
- Weakness
- Rapid, weak pulse
- Low blood pressure
- Dry skin
- Flushed cheeks
- Drowsiness
- Nausea and vomiting
- Shortness of breath or air hunger (person gasping for air and being unable to catch his breath)
- Unconsciousness

More information about diabetes and related care may be found in Chapter 18.

Seizures

Seizures are involuntary, often violent, contractions of muscles. They can involve a small area or the entire body. Seizures are caused by abnormalities in the brain. They can occur in young children who have a high fever. Older children and adults who have a serious illness, fever, head injury, or a seizure disorder such as **epilepsy** may also have seizures.

The main goal during a seizure is to make sure the resident is safe. During a seizure, a person may shake severely and thrust arms and legs uncontrollably. He may clench his jaw, drool, and be unable to swallow. Most seizures last only a short time.

Responding to a seizure

1. Note the time. Put on gloves.

2. Lower the person to the floor. Cradle the head to protect it. If a pillow is nearby, place it under the person's head. Loosen clothing to help with breathing. Try to turn the person to one side to help lower the risk of choking. This may not be possible during a violent seizure.

3. Have someone call the nurse immediately or use the call light. Do not leave a person during a seizure unless you must do so to get medical help.

4. Move furniture away to prevent injury.

5. Do not try to restrain the person or stop the seizure.

6. Do not force anything between the person's teeth. Do not place your hands in the person's mouth for any reason. You could be bitten.

7. Do not give the person liquids or food.

8. When the seizure is over, note the time. Gently turn the person to his left side if you do not suspect head, neck, back, spinal, or abdominal injuries. Turning the person reduces the risk of choking on vomit or saliva. If the person begins to choke, get help immediately. Check for adequate breathing and pulse. Begin CPR if breathing and pulse are absent and if you are allowed and trained to do so. Do not begin CPR during a seizure.

9. Remove and discard gloves. Wash your hands.

10. Report and document the incident properly, including how long the seizure lasted.

CVA or Stroke

Cerebrovascular accident (CVA), or stroke, was first discussed in Chapter 4. A quick response to a suspected stroke is critical. Tests and treatment need to be given within a short time of the stroke's onset (ideally within an hour). Early treatment may be able to reduce the severity of the stroke.

Emergency Care and Disaster Preparation

A **transient ischemic attack (TIA)** is a warning sign of a CVA. It is the result of a temporary lack of oxygen in the brain. Symptoms may last up to 24 hours. They include difficulty speaking, weakness on one side of the body, temporary loss of vision, and numbness or tingling. These symptoms should not be ignored; they should be reported to the nurse immediately. The are also signs that a TIA or CVA is occurring:

- Facial numbness, weakness, or drooping, especially on one side
- Paralysis on one side of the body (hemiplegia)
- Arm numbness or weakness, especially on one side (hemiparesis)
- Slurred speech or inability to speak (expressive aphasia)
- Inability to understand spoken or written words (receptive aphasia)
- Use of inappropriate words
- Severe headache
- Blurred vision
- Ringing in the ears
- Redness in the face
- Noisy breathing
- Elevated blood pressure
- Slow pulse rate
- Nausea or vomiting
- Loss of bowel and bladder control
- Seizures
- Dizziness
- Loss of consciousness

In addition to the symptoms listed above, women may have these symptoms:

- Pain in the face, arms, and legs
- Hiccups
- Weakness
- Chest pain
- Shortness of breath
- Palpitations

F.A.S.T.

The acronym F.A.S.T. can be used as a way to remember the sudden signs that a stroke is occurring.

(F)ace: Is one side of the face drooping? Is it numb? Ask the person to smile. Is the smile uneven?

(A)rms: Is one arm numb or weak? Ask the person to raise both arms. Check to see if one arm drifts downward.

(S)peech: Is the person's speech slurred? Is the person unable to speak? Can the person be understood? Ask the person to repeat a simple sentence and see if the sentence is repeated correctly.

(T)ime: Time is of the utmost importance when responding to a stroke. If the person shows any of the symptoms listed above, report to the nurse immediately.

Websites for the American Stroke Association (strokeassociation.org) and The National Stroke Association (stroke.org) have more information. Chapter 18 in this textbook contains more information about strokes.

Vomiting

Vomiting, or **emesis**, is the act of ejecting stomach contents through the mouth and/or nose. It can be a sign of a serious illness or injury. Some residents, such as those with cancer who are undergoing chemotherapy, may vomit frequently as a result of treatment. Because a nursing assistant may not know when a resident is going to vomit, he may not have time to explain what he will do and assemble supplies ahead of time. The NA should talk to the resident soothingly as he helps him clean up. He should tell the resident what he is doing to help him.

Responding to vomiting

1. Notify the nurse immediately.

2. Put on gloves.

3. Make sure the head is up or turned to one side. Place an emesis basin under the chin. Remove it when vomiting has stopped.

Emergency Care and Disaster Preparation

4. Remove soiled linens or clothes and set aside. Replace with fresh linens or clothes.

5. If the resident's intake and output (I&O) is being monitored (Chapter 15), measure and note the amount of vomitus.

6. Flush vomit down the toilet unless vomit is red, has blood in it, or looks like wet coffee grounds. If these symptoms are observed, show this to the nurse before discarding the vomit. After disposing of vomit, wash and store basin.

7. Remove and discard gloves.

8. Wash your hands.

9. Put on clean gloves.

10. Provide comfort to the resident: wipe face and mouth, position comfortably, and offer a drink of water or oral care (Chapter 13) (Fig. 7-12). Oral care helps get rid of the taste of vomit in the mouth.

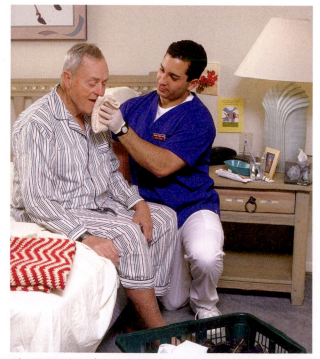

Fig. 7-12. Be calm and comforting when helping a resident who has vomited.

11. Put soiled linen in proper containers.

12. Remove and discard gloves.

13. Wash your hands again.

14. Document time, amount, color, odor, and consistency of vomitus.

Falls

Falls can be minor or severe. All falls should be reported to the nurse immediately, even if the resident says he feels fine. The nursing assistant will need to complete an incident report. In the case of a severe fall, the nurse may ask the NA to call emergency medical services. To help a resident who is falling, the nursing assistant should do the following:

- Widen her stance. Bring the resident's body close to the NA's body to break the fall. The NA should bend her knees and support the resident as she lowers the resident to the floor.

- The nursing assistant should not try to reverse or stop a fall. Doing this can cause more injury.

- The NA should notify the nurse immediately. She should not attempt to get the resident up or move the resident after the fall.

Chapter 6 contains more information about falls and fall prevention.

3. Describe disaster guidelines

Disasters can include fire, flood, earthquake, hurricane, tornado, or severe weather. Man-made dangers, such as acts of terrorism or bomb threats, are also considered disasters. The disasters a person may experience will depend on where he lives. Nursing assistants should know the appropriate action to take when disasters occur. Each facility has a local and area-specific disaster plan, and NAs will be trained on these plans. Annual in-services and disaster drills are often held at facilities. NAs should take advantage of these sessions when offered and pay close attention to instructions.

During natural disasters, a nurse or the administrator will give directions. Nursing assistants should listen carefully to all directions and follow instructions. Facilities may rely on local or state management groups and the American Red Cross to assume overall responsibility for the ill and disabled.

Guidelines: Disasters

The following guidelines apply in any disaster situation:

G   Remain calm.

G   Know the locations of all exits and stairways.

G   Know where the fire alarms and extinguishers are located.

G   Know the appropriate action to take in any situation.

G   Use the internet to stay informed, or keep the radio or television tuned to a local station to get the latest information.

In addition, you will be required to apply specific guidelines for the area in which you work. For example, an NA working where hurricanes are prevalent, such as in Florida, needs to know the guidelines for hurricane preparedness as well as for storms and fires. The following general guidelines are separated by the type of disaster:

Tornadoes

G   Seek shelter inside, ideally in a steel-framed or concrete building.

G   Stay away from windows.

G   Stand in the hallway or in a basement, or take cover under heavy furniture.

G   Do not stay in a mobile home or trailer.

G   Lie as flat as possible.

Lightning

If outdoors, follow these guidelines:

G   Avoid the largest objects, such as trees, and avoid open spaces.

G   Stay out of the water.

G   Seek shelter in buildings.

G   Stay away from metal fences, doors, or other objects.

G   Avoid holding metal objects, such as golf clubs, in your hands.

G   Stay in automobiles.

G   It is safe to perform CPR on lightning victims if you are trained to do so; they carry no electricity.

If indoors, follow these guidelines:

G   Stay inside and away from open doors and windows.

G   Avoid the use of electrical equipment such as hair dryers and televisions.

Floods

G   Fill the bathtub with fresh water.

G   Evacuate if advised to do so.

G   Check the fuel level in automobiles. Make sure there is enough fuel to last through an evacuation if one becomes necessary.

G   Have a portable battery-operated radio, flashlight, and cooking equipment available.

G   Do not drink water or eat food that has been contaminated with floodwater.

G   Do not handle electrical equipment.

G   Do not turn off the gas yourself. Ask the gas company to turn off the gas.

Blackouts

G   Get a flashlight. Take prompt action to keep calm and provide light.

G   Use a backup pack for electrical medical equipment, such as an IV pump. Backup packs do not last more than 24 hours, so contact emergency services when instructed.

Hurricanes

G   Know what category the hurricane is and track the expected path.

G   Know which residents or clients must go to shelters, hospitals, or other facilities, and which need assistance. Be aware of people with special needs. High-risk people include the elderly and those unable to evacuate on their own. High-risk areas include mobile homes or trailers.

G   Call your employer for instructions.

G   Fill the bathtub with fresh water.

G   Board up windows.

G   Evacuate if advised to do so.

G   Check the fuel level in automobiles.

G   Have a portable battery-operated radio, flashlight, and cooking equipment available.

Earthquakes

If indoors, follow these guidelines:

G   Drop to the ground.

G   If possible, get under a sturdy piece of furniture, such as a heavy table, and hold on until the shaking stops.

G   If no table or desk is available, stay crouched down in the inside corner of a building, and cover your face and head with your arms.

G   Stay away from windows, outside walls, and anything that might fall over or fall down.

G   Do not exit a building or house during the shaking.

G   Do not use elevators.

If outdoors, follow these guidelines:

G   Move away from buildings, electric poles and wires, and streetlights. Falling or flying debris is a far greater danger than ground movement.

G   If driving, stop as quickly as is safely possible and stay in the vehicle. Avoid stopping under overpasses or near buildings or wires if possible.

G   If trapped under debris after an earthquake, do not light a match or ignite a lighter, and avoid kicking up dust. Breathe through a handkerchief or clothing and make tapping noises or use a whistle, if available, to get rescuers' attention. Do not shout. Shouting could cause you to inhale dangerous amounts of dust.

In addition to the above, when working in the home, follow these guidelines for disasters:

G   If a disaster is forecast (for example, a tornado or hurricane), be ready. Wear appropriate clothing and shoes. Have family members dressed and ready in case evacuation is necessary.

G   Stay in contact with your supervisor or others if possible. Let someone know where you are, what the conditions are, and where you will go if you must evacuate.

G   Locate disaster supplies. Ideally, a disaster supply kit should meet your needs for at least three days. The kit can be stored in sturdy, easy-to-carry containers such as backpacks, duffel bags, or covered trash containers. It should be assembled before disaster strikes and should include the following:

- A three-day supply of water (one gallon per person, per day) and food that will not spoil

- One change of clothing and footwear per person, and one blanket or sleeping bag per person

- A first aid kit that includes the family's prescription medications

- Emergency tools, including a battery-powered radio, flashlight, and plenty of extra batteries

- An extra set of car keys and a credit card, a debit card, or cash

- Sanitation supplies

- Special items for infant, elderly, or disabled family members

- An extra pair of eyeglasses

- Important family documents in a waterproof container

Chapter Review

1. List two steps to follow when encountering an emergency situation.

2. What kind of information should a nursing assistant be prepared to give when calling emergency services?

3. Why should a nursing assistant not perform CPR if she is not trained to do so?

4. How are abdominal thrusts used to help someone who is choking?

5. If the person becomes unconscious while choking, what should the nursing assistant do?

6. In what position should a person be placed if he is in shock?

7. What symptoms are women more likely to experience than men if they are having a myocardial infarction (heart attack)?

8. What can be done to a wound to slow bleeding?

9. Why should ice not be applied to burns?

10. If a person feels like he is going to faint, in what position should he be placed?

11. Why should a nursing assistant put on gloves if a resident has a nosebleed?

12. What are the first signs that a person is experiencing diabetic ketoacidosis?

13. Why should a nursing assistant not force anything into the mouth of a person who is having a seizure?

14. What is a transient ischemic attack (TIA)?

15. What should a nursing assistant do if a resident starts to fall?

16. What are three things that a nursing assistant should observe for in a resident's vomit?

17. What are four guidelines that apply in any disaster situation?

8

Human Needs and Human Development

1. Identify basic human needs

People have different genes, physical appearances, cultural backgrounds, ages, and social and financial positions. But all human beings have the same basic physical needs:

- Food and water

- Protection and shelter

- Activity

- Sleep and rest

- Comfort, especially freedom from pain

Activities of daily living (ADLs), such as eating, eliminating, bathing, and grooming, are the ways people meet their most basic physical needs. By assisting with ADLs or helping residents learn to perform them independently, nursing assistants help residents meet these needs.

Human beings also have **psychosocial needs**, which involve social interaction, emotions, intellect, and spirituality. Although they are not as easy to define as physical needs, psychosocial needs include the following:

- Love and affection

- Acceptance by others

- Safety and security

- Self-reliance and independence in daily living

- Contact with others (Fig. 8-1)

- Success and self-esteem

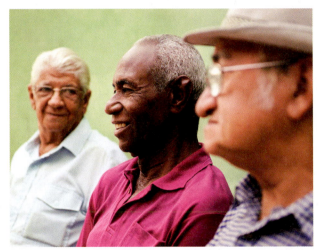

Fig. 8-1. *Interaction with other people is a basic psychosocial need. Nursing assistants can encourage residents to be with friends or relatives. Social contact is important.*

Health and well-being affect how well psychosocial needs are met. Stress and frustration occur when basic needs are not met. This can lead to fear, anxiety, anger, aggression, withdrawal, indifference, and depression. Stress can also cause physical problems that may eventually lead to illness.

Abraham Maslow, a researcher of human behavior, wrote about human physical and psychosocial needs. He arranged these needs by order of importance. He thought that physical needs must be met before psychosocial needs can be met. His theory is called *Maslow's Hierarchy of Needs* (Fig. 8-2).

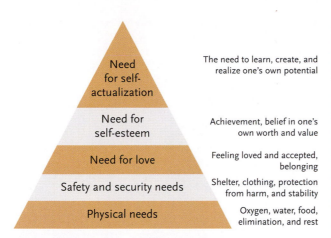

Fig. 8-2. Maslow's Hierarchy of Needs is a model developed by Abraham Maslow to show how physical and psychosocial needs are arranged in order of importance. Maslow believed that physical needs must be met before psychosocial needs can be met.

After meeting physical needs, safety and security needs must be met. Feeling safe means not feeling afraid or unstable. Residents need to feel safe in facilities. Many things can cause a person to feel unsafe. An illness or disability can be frightening and make a person feel fearful and insecure. Losing some independence and needing help from caregivers, such as NAs, may cause some uncertainty or discomfort. Residents need to feel safe with all care team members; they need to know that they and their personal possessions will be protected.

After physical and safety needs are met, the need for love and belonging is important. This level involves feeling accepted, needed, and cared for. Regardless of their condition, residents need to know that their contributions are meaningful.

The need for self-esteem is the next level. This need involves respecting and valuing oneself, which comes from within, as well as from other people. Achievements that make a person feel valued are important. For residents, being able to do a task they were not able to do previously may satisfy this need. Hearing praise from NAs about this new achievement may also help meet this need.

Self-actualization is the highest level. It means that a person tries to be the best person he can

be; he tries to reach his full potential. This may mean different things for each person. The quest to reach this need continues throughout a person's life and may change as a person enters different stages of life.

2. Define *holistic care* and explain its importance in health care

Holistic means considering a whole system, such as a whole person, rather than dividing the system up into parts. **Holistic care** means caring for the whole person—the mind as well as the body (Fig. 8-3). Holistic care takes into account a person's physical, psychological, social, and spiritual needs. This is the approach nursing assistants should use when caring for residents. Caring for a person holistically is part of providing person-centered care. Person-centered care revolves around the resident and promotes his or her individual preferences, choices, dignity, and interests.

A simple example of holistic care is taking time to talk with residents while helping them bathe. The NA is meeting the physical need with the bath and meeting the psychosocial need for interaction with others at the same time. Another way of practicing holistic care is considering psychosocial factors in illness, as well as physical factors. For example, Mr. Hartman looks thin and tired. The cause might be depression rather than an infection. The NA does not need to determine the cause of his condition. However, by talking with him she might learn something that would help the rest of the care team. For example, she might learn that last year at this time his wife died, and he is still coping with that loss. She can and should share this information with the care team and document it.

3. Explain why independence and self-care are important

Any big change in lifestyle, such as moving into a long-term care facility, requires a huge

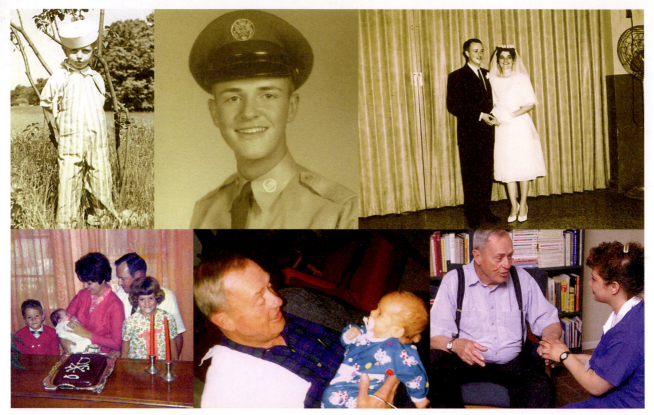

Fig. 8-3. *Residents are people, not just lists of illnesses and disabilities. They have many needs, like any other people. Many have had rich lives with wonderful experiences. Take time to know and care for each resident as a whole person.*

emotional adjustment. Residents may be experiencing fear, loss, and uncertainty, along with a decline in health and independence. Other common reactions to illness are denial, withdrawal, anger, hostility, and depression. All of these feelings may cause residents to behave differently than they have before. Each person adjusts to illness and change in his or her own way and in his or her own time. It is important for nursing assistants to remain supportive and encouraging. NAs should be patient, understanding, and empathetic.

Moving to a care facility represents a tremendous loss of independence for a resident, and loss of independence can be very difficult. Somebody else must now do what residents did for themselves all of their lives. NAs should try to imagine what it would be like to have to call someone to help every time they had to go to the bathroom. The loss of independence is also difficult for residents' friends and family members.

For example, a resident may have been the main provider for his or her family. A resident may have been the person who did all of the cooking for the family. Other losses residents may be experiencing include the following:

- Loss of spouse, family members, or friends due to death

- Loss of workplace and its relationships due to retirement

- Loss of ability to go to favorite places

- Loss of ability to attend services and meetings at faith communities

- Loss of home and personal possessions (Fig. 8-4)

- Loss of health and ability to care for themselves

- Loss of ability to move freely

- Loss of pets

- Lesbian, gay, bisexual, transgender, or queer (LGBTQ) residents may fear the loss of a comfortable and accepting environment.

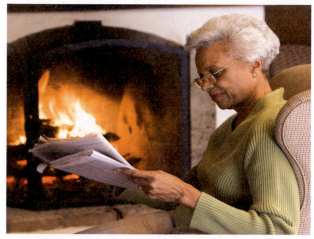

Fig. 8-4. Nursing assistants should understand and be sympathetic to the fact that many residents had to leave familiar places.

Independence often means not having to rely on others for money, daily care, or participation in social activities. Activities of daily living (ADLs) are the personal care tasks a person does every day to care for himself. People may take these activities for granted until they can no longer do them for themselves. ADLs include bathing or showering, dressing, caring for teeth and hair, eliminating, eating and drinking, and moving from place to place. When a person loses independence, the following problems can result:

- Poor self-image

- Anger toward caregivers, others, and self

- Feelings of helplessness, sadness, and hopelessness

- Feelings of being useless

- Increased dependence

- Depression

To prevent these feelings, NAs should encourage residents to do as much as possible for themselves. Even if it seems easier for the NA to do a task for a resident, the resident should be allowed to do it independently. NAs must encourage self-care, regardless of how long it takes

or how poorly residents are able to do it. NAs should be patient (Fig. 8-5).

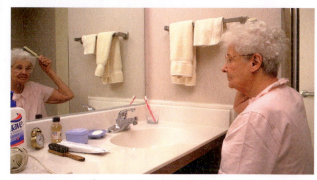

Fig. 8-5. Even if tasks take a long time, residents should be encouraged to do what they can for themselves.

Allowing residents to make choices is another way to promote independence and person-centered care. For example, residents can choose where to sit while they eat. They can choose what they eat and in what order. NAs must respect a resident's right to make choices.

Residents' Rights

Dignity and Independence

Residents are adults; they should not be treated like children. NAs should encourage residents to do self-care without rushing them. Residents have the right to refuse care and to make their own choices. Promoting dignity and independence is part of protecting their legal rights. It is also the proper and ethical way for NAs to work.

4. Describe sexual orientation and gender identity and explain ways to accommodate sexual needs

In addition to the needs discussed earlier, people also have sexual needs. These needs continue throughout their lives (Fig. 8-6). The ability to engage in sexual activity, such as intercourse and masturbation, continues unless a disease or injury occurs to prevent it. **Masturbation** means to touch or rub sexual organs in order to give oneself or another person sexual pleasure.

Residents have the right to choose how they express their sexuality. In all age groups, there is a variety of sexual behavior. This is also true of residents.

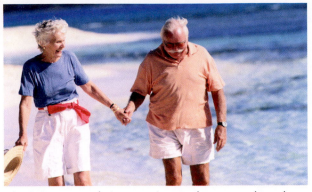

Fig. 8-6. Human beings continue to have sexual needs throughout their lives.

Sexual orientation is a person's physical, emotional, and/or romantic attraction to another person. Sexual orientation plays a big part in human sexuality. **Gender identity** is a deeply felt sense of one's gender. A person may have the gender identity of a man or a woman, or may not fit into either of those two categories. Terms related to sexual orientation and gender identity, listed alphabetically, include the following:

- **Bisexual, Bi**: A person whose physical, emotional, and/or romantic attraction may be for people of the same gender or different gender.

- **Cisgender**: A person whose gender identity matches his or her birth sex (sex assigned at birth due to anatomy).

- **Coming out**: A continual process of revealing one's sexual orientation or gender identity to others.

- **Cross-dresser**: Typically refers to a heterosexual man who sometimes wears clothing and other items associated with women; cross-dressing is not associated with men who permanently wish to change their sex.

- **Gay**: A person whose physical, emotional, and/or romantic attraction is for people of the same sex.

- **Heterosexual**: A person whose physical, emotional, and/or romantic attraction is for people of the opposite sex; also known as *straight*.

- **Lesbian**: A woman whose physical, emotional, and/or romantic attraction is for other women.

- **LGBT**: Acronym for lesbian, gay, bisexual, and transgender.

- **LGBTQ**: Acronym for lesbian, gay, bisexual, transgender, and queer (less commonly, Q can also stand for questioning).

- **Queer**: A term used by some people to describe sexual orientation that is not exclusively heterosexual and who feel terms such as *lesbian* and *gay* are too limiting; once considered a derogatory term, queer may not be accepted by everyone within the LGBT community.

- **Transgender**: A person whose gender identity conflicts with his or her birth sex (sex assigned at birth due to anatomy); transgender identity is not dependent on someone having undergone medical measures like hormones or surgery.

- **Transition**: The process of changing genders, which can include legal procedures, such as changing one's name and/or sex on documents, and medical measures, such as hormone therapy and surgery; it can also include telling others and using new pronouns.

More information may be found at the National Resource Center on LGBT Aging's website (lgbtagingcenter.org) or at GLAAD's website (glaad.org).

Residents' Rights

LGBTQ Residents

The Administration on Aging (AOA, aoa.gov) cites research suggesting that lesbian, gay, bisexual, transgender, and queer (LGBTQ) adults often face discrimination due to their sexual orientation as well as their age (Fig. 8-7). Nursing assistants must treat every resident with respect, no matter what their personal or religious feelings regarding sexuality may be. Part of respecting each resident's sexual orientation is not making the assumption that all residents are heterosexual. NAs must use terms and pronouns residents prefer (using "she," for example, to refer to a resident who is physically male but identifies as female), and must not gossip or break confidentiality regarding residents' sexual behavior, sexual orientation, or gender identity.

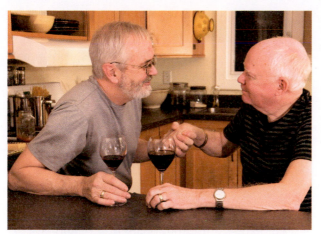

Fig. 8-7. The number of lesbian, gay, bisexual, and transgender older adults continues to increase. It is important to treat all residents with respect.

A common myth is that elderly people no longer have sexual needs or desires. That is not true. Sexual urges do not end due to age or admission to a care facility. Many things can affect a resident's sexual needs. Illness and disability can affect sexual desires, needs, and abilities. Sexual desire may not be lessened by a disability, although the ability to meet sexual needs may be limited. Many people confined to wheelchairs can have sexual and intimate relationships, although adjustments may have to be made. Nursing assistants should not assume they know what impact a disability has had on sexuality.

Sexual needs may also be affected by residents' living environments. A lack of privacy and no available partner are often reasons for a lack of sexual expression in care facilities. NAs should always be sensitive to privacy needs.

Here are some ways that nursing assistants can help meet and respect residents' sexual needs:

Guidelines: Respecting Sexual Needs

G   Always knock or announce yourself before entering residents' rooms. Listen and wait for a response before entering.

G   If you encounter a sexual situation between consenting adult residents, provide privacy and leave the room. Residents are allowed to meet their sexual needs however they choose, such as through sexual relationships or masturbation.

G   Be open and nonjudgmental about residents' sexual attitudes. Respect residents' sexual orientation and gender identity.

G   When possible, ask transgender residents which pronouns they would like you to use and use them. Be patient if a resident takes time to decide which pronouns are best for him or her. The resident may decide a set of pronouns works for a time and then prefer a different set later.

G   Always use a transgender person's chosen name.

G   Honor *Do Not Disturb* signs.

G   Do not view any expression of sexuality by the elderly as disgusting or cute. That attitude is inappropriate and deprives residents of their right to dignity and respect.

Residents' Rights

Sexual Abuse

Residents must be protected from unwanted sexual advances. If an NA sees sexual abuse happening, he should remove the resident from the situation and take the resident to a safe place. The NA should then report to the nurse immediately.

5. Identify ways to help residents meet their spiritual needs

Residents may have spiritual needs, and nursing assistants can help with these needs. **Spiritual** means of, or relating to, the spirit or soul. Helping residents meet their spiritual needs can help them cope with illness or disability. Spirituality is a sensitive area, and NAs should always treat residents and practices with respect.

Residents' beliefs will vary. Some may consider themselves deeply religious, while others may think of themselves as spiritual but not religious. Other residents may not consider themselves spiritual or religious at all. Residents may believe in God or may not believe in God. The important thing for nursing assistants to remember is to respect all residents' beliefs, whatever they are. NAs must never make judgments about residents' spiritual beliefs or try to push their own beliefs on residents.

Guidelines: Respecting Spiritual Needs

G Learn about residents' religions or beliefs. Listen carefully to what residents say.

G Respect residents' decisions to participate in, or refrain from, food-related rituals. Accommodate practices such as dietary restrictions. Never make judgments about them.

G If residents are religious, encourage participation in religious services.

G Respect all religious items.

G Report to the nurse (or social worker) if a resident expresses the desire to see clergy.

G Get to know the priest, rabbi, or minister who visits or calls a resident.

G Allow privacy for clergy visits (Fig. 8-8).

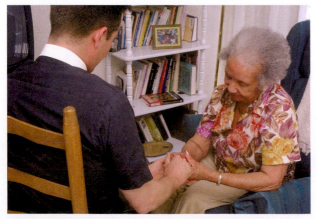

Fig. 8-8. Be open to residents' spiritual needs. Be welcoming and provide privacy when they receive visits from a spiritual leader.

G If asked, read religious materials aloud. If you are uncomfortable doing this, find another staff member who is not.

G If a resident asks you, help find spiritual resources available in the area. Check the internet for churches, synagogues, mosques, and other houses of worship. You can also refer this request to the nurse or social worker.

G You should never do any of the following:

- Try to change someone's religion
- Tell residents their belief or religion is wrong
- Express judgments about a religious group
- Insist residents join in religious activities
- Interfere with religious practices
- Discuss your personal beliefs or opinions, either directly or indirectly

6. Identify ways to accommodate cultural and religious differences

Culture and cultural diversity were first discussed in Chapter 4. A culture is a system of learned beliefs and behaviors that is practiced by a group of people. Cultural diversity refers to different groups of people with varied backgrounds and experiences living together in the world.

Nursing assistants will take care of residents with backgrounds and traditions different from their own. It is important that NAs respect and value each person as an individual. They should respond to differences and new experiences with acceptance, not prejudice.

There are so many different cultures that they cannot all be listed here. One might talk about American culture being different from Japanese culture. But within American culture there are thousands of different groups with their own cultures: Japanese-Americans, African-Americans, and Native Americans are just a few. Even people from a particular region, state, or city can be said to have a different culture (Fig. 8-9). The culture of the South is not the same as the culture of New York City.

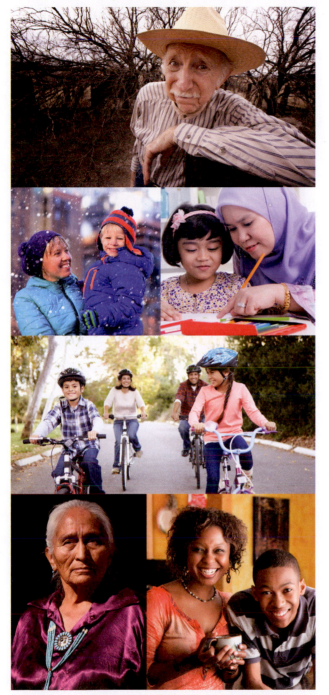

Fig. 8-9. *There are many different cultures in the United States.*

Cultural background affects how friendly people are to strangers. It can affect how close they want others to stand to them when talking. It can affect how they feel about NAs performing care for them or discussing their health with them. For example, a care team member asks a resident when he last had a bowel movement. One resident may freely answer this,

while another may be embarrassed to have this discussion. One resident may be fine with an NA undressing him to help him bathe, while another may be uncomfortable with this. These reactions may also just be a part of a person's personality. Nursing assistants should be sensitive to residents' backgrounds. They may have to adjust their behavior around some residents. Regardless of their backgrounds, all residents must be treated with respect and professionalism. NAs should expect to be treated respectfully as well.

A resident's primary language may be different from the nursing assistant's. If he or she speaks a different language, an interpreter may be necessary. It can be helpful if staff members learn a few common phrases in a resident's native language. Picture cards and flash cards can assist with communication.

Religious differences also influence the way people behave. Religion may be very important in people's lives, particularly when they are ill or dying. Some people belong to a religious group, but do not practice everything that religion teaches. Some people consider themselves spiritual but not religious. Others do not believe in any religion or God, and do not consider themselves spiritual. Nursing assistants must respect the religious beliefs and practices of residents, even if they are different from their own. Common religions, listed alphabetically, follow:

Buddhism: Buddhism started in Asia but has many followers in other parts of the world. Buddhism is based on the teachings of Siddhartha Gautama, called Buddha. Buddhists believe that life is filled with suffering that is caused by desire and that suffering ends when desire ends. Buddhism emphasizes meditation. Proper conduct and wisdom release a person from desire, suffering, and a repeating sequence of births and deaths (**reincarnation**). Nirvana is the highest spiritual plane a person can reach. It is the state of peace and freedom from worry and pain. There are many Buddhist texts. The Tipitaka or

Pali Canon is the standard scripture collection. The Dalai Lama is considered to be the highest spiritual leader.

Christianity: Christians believe Jesus Christ was the son of God and that he died so their sins would be forgiven. Christians may be Catholic or Protestant. There are many subgroups or denominations, such as Baptist, Episcopalian, Evangelical, Lutheran, Methodist, Mormon, Presbyterian, and Roman Catholic. Christians may be baptized and may receive communion as a symbol of Christ's sacrifice. They may attend church on Saturdays or Sundays. Some Christians may try to share their beliefs and convert others to their faith. The Christian Bible is the sacred text and is divided into the Old Testament and the New Testament. Religious leaders may be called priests, ministers, pastors, preachers, or reverends.

Hinduism: Hinduism is the dominant faith of India, but it is practiced in other places as well. According to Hindu beliefs, there are four purposes of life: acting morally and ethically (Dharma), pursuing prosperity (Artha), enjoying life (Kama), and accomplishing enlightenment (Moksha). People move through birth, life, death, and rebirth. How a person moves toward enlightenment is determined by karma. **Karma** is the result of actions in past lives, and actions in this life can determine one's destiny in future lives. Hindus advocate respect for all life, and some Hindus are vegetarians. Hindus who do eat meat almost always refrain from eating beef. Hindus follow the teachings of ancient scriptures like the Vedas and Upanishads, as well as other major scriptures. Holy men are called Sadhus.

Islam: Muslims, or followers of Mohammed, believe that Allah (the Arabic term for God) wants people to follow the teachings of the prophet Mohammed. Many Muslims pray five times a day facing Mecca, the holy city for their religion. Muslims also fast during the month called Ramadan. Muslims worship at mosques and do not drink alcohol or eat pork. There are other dietary restrictions, too. The Qur'an (Koran) is the sacred text of Islam. Islamic religious leaders may be called ayatollah, caliph, imam, mufti, and mullah, among other titles.

Judaism: Judaism is divided into Reform, Conservative, and Orthodox movements. Jewish people believe that God gave them laws through Moses in the form of the Torah (the sacred text), and that these laws should order their lives. Jewish services are held in synagogues or temples on Friday evenings and sometimes on Saturdays. Some Jewish men wear a **yarmulke**, or small skullcap, as a sign of their faith. Some Jewish people observe dietary restrictions. They may not do certain things, such as work or drive, on the Sabbath day (called Shabbat), which lasts from Friday sundown to Saturday sundown. Religious leaders are called rabbis.

Spirituality concerns a person's beliefs about the spirit or the soul. It may center on how a person relates to his community, to nature, or to the divine. It may involve reflection and contemplation and a search for inner peace. It may relate to a person's beliefs about the meaning of life. Spiritual practices can include meditation or prayer, but spirituality does not have to encompass religious beliefs. Many people consider themselves to be spiritual but not religious.

Many Native Americans (American Indians) follow many different spiritual traditions and practices. An emphasis is placed on the personal and the communal, rather than the institutional, and there is a deep connection with nature. There are many varied practices and rituals.

As mentioned earlier, people have varying beliefs in religion, spirituality, and God. Some people may not believe in God or a higher power and identify themselves as agnostic. **Agnostics** believe that they do not know or cannot know if God exists. They do not deny that God might exist, but they feel there is no true knowledge of God's existence.

Atheists are people who believe that there is no God. This is different from what agnostics believe. Atheists actively deny the existence of any deity (higher power). For many atheists, this belief is as strongly held as any religious belief.

Respect for residents' beliefs regarding religion and spirituality is an essential way in which NAs provide person-centered care. NAs should not discuss their own beliefs with residents.

Some specific cultural and religious practices affect a nursing assistant's work. Many religious beliefs include **dietary restrictions**. These are rules about what and when followers can eat and drink. Some examples are listed below:

- Many Buddhists are vegetarians, though some include fish in their diet.

- Some Christians, particularly Roman Catholics, do not eat meat on Fridays during Lent.

- Many Jewish people eat kosher foods, do not eat pork, and do not eat lobster, shrimp, and clams (shellfish). Kosher food is food prepared in accordance with Jewish dietary laws. Kosher and non-kosher foods cannot come into contact with the same plates. Jewish people who observe dietary laws may not eat meat products at the same meal with dairy products.

- Mormons may not drink alcohol, coffee, or tea. They may not use tobacco in any form.

- Muslims do not eat pork and may avoid eating certain birds. They may not drink alcohol. Muslims may have regular periods of fasting. **Fasting** means not eating food or eating very little food.

- Some people are **vegetarians** and do not eat any meat for religious, moral, or health reasons.

- Some people are **vegans** and do not eat any animals or animal products, such as eggs or dairy products. Vegans may also not use or wear any animal products, including leather.

7. Describe the need for activity

Activity is an essential part of a person's life; it improves and maintains physical and mental health. Meaningful activities help promote independence, memory, self-esteem, and quality of life. In addition, physical activity can help manage illnesses, such as diabetes, high blood pressure, or high cholesterol. Regular physical activity can also help by doing the following:

- Lessening the risk of heart disease, colon cancer, diabetes, and obesity

- Relieving symptoms of anxiety and depression

- Improving mood and concentration

- Improving body function

- Lowering the risk of falls

- Improving sleep quality

- Improving the ability to cope with stress

- Increasing energy

- Increasing appetite and promoting better eating habits

Just as activity aids physical and mental health, inactivity and immobility can result in physical and mental problems, such as the following:

- Loss of self-esteem

- Depression

- Anxiety

- Boredom

- Pneumonia

- Urinary tract infection

- Skin breakdown and pressure injuries

- Constipation

- Blood clots

- Dulling of the senses

The Omnibus Budget Reconciliation Act (OBRA) requires that facilities provide an activities program that is designed to meet the interests and the physical, mental, and psychosocial well-being of each resident. The activities are created to help residents socialize and to keep them physically and mentally active. Daily schedules are normally posted with activities for that particular day. Activities include exercise, arts and crafts, board games, newspapers, magazines, music, books, TV and radio, pet therapy, gardening, and group religious events. When activities are scheduled, nursing assistants should help residents with grooming beforehand, as needed and requested. They should assist with any personal care that residents require. NAs may need to help residents with walking and wheelchairs as well.

8. Discuss family roles and their significance in health care

Families play an important part in most people's lives. The concept of family is always changing. Often a family is defined by the level of support and connection people have rather than by biological relationships. There are many different kinds of families (Fig. 8-10):

- Nuclear families (two parents and one or more children)

- Single-parent families (one parent and one or more children)

- Married or committed couples of the same sex or opposite sex, with or without children

- Extended families (parents, children, grandparents, aunts, uncles, cousins, other relatives, and even friends)

- Blended families (divorced or widowed parents who have remarried and have children from previous relationships and/or the current marriage)

Nursing assistants must respect all kinds of families. Residents with no living relatives may have friends or neighbors who function as a family. Whatever kinds of families residents

have, they have an important role to play. Family members help in many ways:

- Helping residents make care decisions

- Communicating with the care team

- Giving support and encouragement

- Connecting the resident to the outside world

- Offering assurance to dying residents that family memories and traditions will be valued and carried on

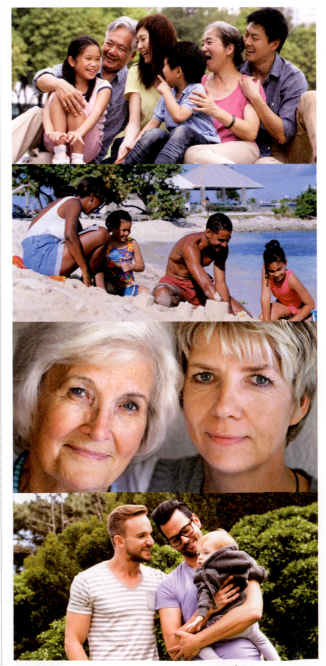

Fig. 8-10. *Families come in all shapes and sizes.*

Families

No matter whether a nursing assistant has the same understanding of family as a resident or not, no resident should ever be denied the right to have the people he loves around him. Families of all descriptions make residents' lives more meaningful. Staff should always make residents' families feel welcome and make it clear that the resident's right to spend time with them is being honored.

Illness or disability requires residents and families to make adjustments. Making these adjustments may be difficult (Fig. 8-11). The family's emotional, spiritual, and financial resources will influence how they adjust. Some personal adjustments include the following:

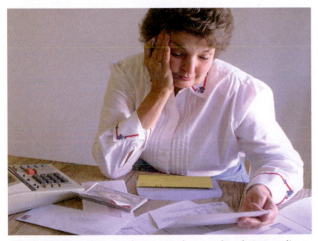

Fig. 8-11. Family members may have a hard time adjusting to the additional responsibilities when a loved one becomes ill or disabled.

- Accepting the illness or disability and its long-term consequences or results

- Finding money needed to pay the expenses of hospitalization or long-term or home care

- Dealing with paperwork involved in insurance, Medicaid, or Medicare benefits

- Taking care of tasks the resident can no longer handle

- Understanding medical information and making difficult care decisions

- Caring for their children while caring for an elderly loved one (called the *sandwich generation*—being "sandwiched" between two generations)

Nursing assistants should be sensitive to the big adjustments residents and their families may be making. NAs can help them by doing their job well. It is important for NAs to be respectful and pleasant to friends and family members and to allow privacy for visits. After any visitor leaves, the NA should observe the effect the visit had on the resident and report any noticeable effects. Some residents have good relationships with their families; others do not. Any abusive behavior from a visitor toward a resident should be reported immediately to the charge nurse.

9. List ways to respond to emotional needs of residents and their families

Residents or family members may come to nursing assistants with problems or needs. Changes in a resident's health status can cause fear, uncertainty, stress, and anger. The nursing assistant's response will depend on many factors, including how comfortable she is with emotions in general, how well she knows the person, and what the need or problem is. The NA should try to empathize, or understand how the person feels. Every person deals with challenges differently, and the NA can consider what response might be best for any given resident. This is part of providing person-centered care. In addition, the NA can use the following ways to respond:

Listen. Often just talking about a problem or concern can make it easier to handle. Sitting quietly and letting someone talk or cry may be the best help a nursing assistant can give (Fig. 8-12). Families often seek out nursing assistants because they are closest to the residents. This is an important responsibility. NAs should show families that they have time for them.

Offer support and encouragement. Saying things like "You have really been under a lot of stress, haven't you?" or "I can imagine that really is scary" can provide a lot of comfort. The NA should avoid using clichés (common phrases that really do not mean anything), like "It'll all work out." Things may not all work out. It is more comforting to the resident if the NA acknowledges how hard the situation is. Feelings should not be simply dismissed with a cliché.

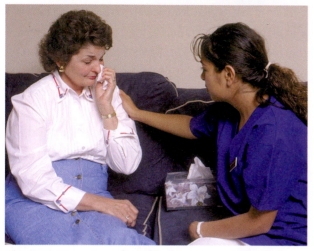

Fig. 8-12. *Sometimes listening to someone is the best way to provide emotional support.*

Refer the problem to a nurse or social worker. When an NA feels that she cannot help the resident, or when someone is asking for help outside her scope of practice, she should get someone else on the care team to handle the situation. She can say something like "Mrs. Pfeiffer, I think my supervisor would be better at getting you the help you need."

10. Describe the stages of human growth and development and identify common disorders for each stage

Throughout their lives, people change physically and psychologically. Physical changes occur in the body. Psychological changes occur in the mind and also in the person's behavior. These changes are called human growth and development.

Everyone will go through the same stages of development during their lives. However, no two people will follow the exact same pattern or rate of development. The age ranges given in this learning objective provide a general idea of devel-

opmental stages, not an exact description. Each resident must be treated as an individual and as a whole person who is growing and developing, rather than someone who is merely ill or disabled.

Infancy (Birth to 12 Months)

Infants grow and develop very quickly. In one year, a baby moves from total dependence to the relative independence of moving around, communicating basic needs, and feeding himself. Physical development in infancy moves from the head down. For example, infants gain control over the muscles of the neck before they are able to control the muscles in their shoulders. Control over muscles in the trunk area, such as the shoulders, develops before control of the arms and legs (Fig. 8-13). This head-to-toe sequence should be respected when caring for infants. For example, newborns must be supported at the shoulders, head, and neck. Babies who cannot sit or crawl should not be encouraged to stand or walk.

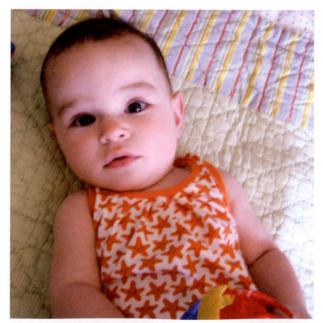

Fig. 8-13. *An infant's physical development moves from the head down.*

Common Disorders: Infancy

CD Babies who are born before 37 weeks gestation (more than three weeks before the due date) are considered **premature**. These babies may weigh from one to six pounds, depending on how early they are born. Often, premature babies will remain in the hospital for some time after birth. At home, premature babies may need special care. This includes medication, heart monitoring, and frequent feedings to ensure weight gain.

CD Babies born at full term but weighing less than five pounds are called low-birth-weight babies. Low-birth-weight babies can have many of the same problems premature babies have. They are cared for in much the same way as premature babies.

CD The term *birth defects* refers to a physical or structural defect that affects an infant from birth. Some birth defects are inherited from parents. Injury or disease during pregnancy causes others. Some of the conditions include cerebral palsy, Down syndrome, and cystic fibrosis.

CD Viral or bacterial infections can cause fever, runny nose, coughing, rash, vomiting, diarrhea, and secondary infections of the sinuses or ears. Viral infections are treated with extra rest, fluids, and sometimes over-the-counter medications for cough and congestion. Bacterial infections can be treated with antibiotics.

CD **Sudden infant death syndrome (SIDS)** is a condition in which babies stop breathing and die for no known reason while asleep. Doctors do not know how to prevent SIDS. However, studies have shown that putting a baby to sleep on his back can reduce the chances of SIDS. Because SIDS is more common among premature or low-birth-weight babies, these infants often wear apnea monitors to alert parents if breathing stops. Another factor that may contribute to SIDS is secondhand smoke. Parents and caregivers should never smoke around infants or children.

Toddler (Ages 1 to 3)

During the toddler years, children gain independence. One part of this independence is new control over their bodies. Toddlers learn to speak, gain coordination of their limbs, and to control their bladders and bowels (Fig. 8-14). Toddlers assert their new independence by exploring. Poisons and other hazards, such as sharp objects, must be locked away. Psychologically, toddlers learn that they are individuals, separate from their parents. Children at this age may try to control their parents. They may try to get what they want by throwing tantrums, whining, or refusing to cooperate. This is a key time for parents to set rules and standards.

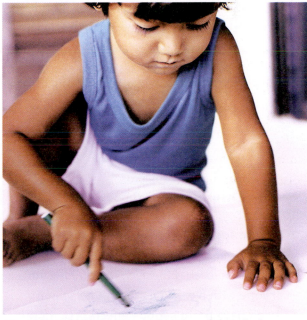

Fig. 8-14. *Toddlers gain coordination of their limbs.*

Preschool (Ages 3 to 6)

Children in their preschool years develop skills that help them become more independent and have social relationships (Fig. 8-15). They develop a vocabulary and language skills. They learn to play in groups. They become more physically coordinated and learn to care for themselves. Preschoolers also develop ways of relating to family members. They begin to learn right from wrong.

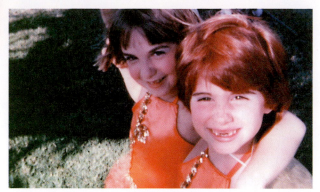

Fig. 8-15. *Children in their preschool years develop social relationships.*

School-Age (Ages 6 to 10)

From ages 6 to about 10 years, children's development is centered on **cognitive** (related to thinking and learning) and social development. As children enter school, they also explore the world around them. They relate to other children through games, peer groups, and classroom activities. In these years, children learn to get along with each other. They also begin to behave in ways common among their gender, and they develop a conscience, morals, and self-esteem.

Common Disorders: Childhood

CD **Chickenpox** is a highly contagious, viral illness. It generally has no serious effects for healthy children. However, in adults or in anyone with a weakened immune system, it can have more serious effects. Taking the varicella-zoster vaccine, commonly called the chickenpox vaccine, can prevent chickenpox.

CD Children, as well as infants, may be susceptible to infections caused by viruses or bacteria. Bacterial infections can be treated with antibiotics. Viral infections are treated with extra rest, fluids, and over-the-counter medications for cough or congestion.

CD **Leukemia** is a form of cancer. It refers to the inability of the body's white blood cells to fight disease. Children with leukemia may be susceptible to infections and other disorders.

Chemotherapy can be used to fight this disease. See Chapter 18 for more information on cancer.

Measles, mumps, rubella, diphtheria, smallpox, whooping cough, and polio are diseases that were once common during childhood. They can all be prevented now with vaccinations.

Abuse and neglect were first discussed in Chapter 3. Child abuse refers to physical, emotional, and sexual mistreatment of children, as well as neglect. Physical abuse includes hitting, kicking, burning, or intentionally causing injury to a child. Psychological abuse includes withholding affection, constantly criticizing, or ridiculing a child. Sexual abuse includes engaging in or allowing another person to engage in a sexual act with a child. Abuse also includes allowing children to use alcohol or drugs, leaving children alone, or exposing them to danger. Child neglect includes not providing adequate food, clothing, or support. Chapters 3 and 27 contain more information.

Preadolescence (Ages 10 to 13)

During the years between 10 and 13, children enjoy a growing sense of self-identity and a strong sense of identity with their peers. They tend to be very social. Friends are generally of the same gender, but relationships with children of the opposite sex may become more complicated as puberty approaches. This is usually a relatively calm period, and preadolescents are often easy to get along with and able to handle more responsibility at home and school. Childhood fears of ghosts or monsters will give way to fears based in the real world, and it is important that preadolescents feel able to trust in the attention and care of parents or other adults.

Girls may reach puberty in the later years of this stage. During puberty, a person develops secondary sex characteristics. In females, secondary sex characteristics include growth of body hair and development of breasts and hips. In males, they include growth of body hair, growth of the testes and penis, broadening of the shoulders, and a lower voice.

Adolescence (Ages 13 to 19)

During adolescence, genders become sexually mature. Boys usually reach puberty during this stage. If girls did not reach puberty during the previous stage, it will start here. Many teenagers have a hard time adapting to the rapid changes that occur in their bodies after puberty. Peer acceptance is important to them. Adolescents may be afraid that they are unattractive or abnormal.

This concern for body image and peer acceptance, combined with changing hormones that influence moods, can cause rapid mood swings. Conflicting pressures develop as they remain dependent on their parents and yet need to express themselves socially and sexually (Fig. 8-16). This can cause conflict and stress.

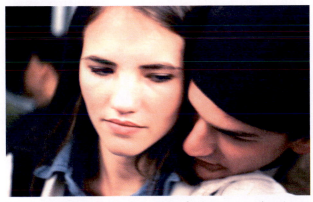

Fig. 8-16. Adolescence is a time of adapting to change.

Common Disorders: Adolescence

CD As their bodies change, adolescents, especially girls, may develop eating disorders. **Anorexia** is an eating disorder in which a person does not eat or exercises excessively to lose weight. A person with **bulimia** binges, eating huge amounts of foods or very fattening foods, and then purges, or eliminates the food by vomiting, using laxatives, or exercising excessively. Eating disorders can

be serious and even life-threatening. These disorders must be treated with therapy and, in some cases, hospitalization.

CD Teenagers can contract sexually transmitted infections (STIs), such as chlamydia, genital herpes, and AIDS, if they are sexually active. If teenagers are sexually active, condoms can reduce, but not eliminate, the risk of STI transmission. Chapter 18 contains more information about STIs.

CD Girls who are sexually active and do not use birth control, or who do not use it properly, can become pregnant. Teenage pregnancy can have terrible consequences for adolescents, their families, and for the babies born to teenage parents. Teenagers should understand that they can avoid pregnancy by using birth control or by practicing abstinence (abstinence means not having sexual contact with anyone). Teenagers who choose to be sexually active should know what birth control methods are available and how to use them. Pregnancy puts a great deal of stress on teenage bodies, which are still developing. In most cases they are not physically ready to bear a child. It is common for teenage mothers to give birth to premature or low-birth-weight babies.

CD Because of the many physical and emotional changes they are experiencing, adolescents may become depressed and even attempt suicide. Parents, teachers, and friends should watch for the signs of depression. These include withdrawal, loss of appetite, weight gain or loss, sleep problems, moodiness, and apathy. Teenagers who are depressed should see a doctor, counselor, therapist, minister, or other trusted adult who can get them the help they need.

CD Adolescents can sustain **trauma**, or severe injury, to the head or spinal cord in car accidents or while playing sports. These injuries can be temporarily or permanently disabling or even fatal.

Young Adulthood (Ages 19 to 40)

Physical growth has usually been completed by this time. Adopting a healthy lifestyle in these years can make life better now and prevent health problems in later adulthood. Psychological and social development continues, however. The developmental tasks of these years include the following:

- Selecting an appropriate education

- Selecting an occupation or career

- Selecting a mate (Fig. 8-17)

- Learning to live with a mate or others

- Raising children

- Developing a satisfying sex life

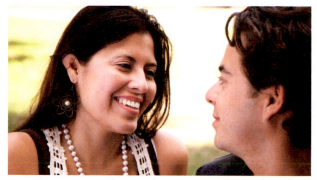

Fig. 8-17. Young adulthood often involves finding mates.

Middle Adulthood (Ages 40 to 65)

In general, people in middle adulthood are more comfortable and stable than they were in previous stages. Many of their major life decisions have already been made. In the early years of middle adulthood people sometimes experience a "midlife crisis." This is a period of unrest centered on a subconscious desire for change and fulfillment of unmet goals.

Physical changes related to aging also occur in middle adulthood. Adults in this age group may notice that they have difficulty maintaining their weight or notice a decrease in strength and energy. Metabolism and other body functions slow down. Wrinkles and gray hair appear. Vision and hearing loss may begin. Women experience **menopause**, the end of menstruation (occurs when a woman has not had a menstrual period for 12 months). This occurs when the ovaries stop secreting hormones. Many diseases and illnesses can develop in these years. These disorders can become chronic and life-threatening.

Late Adulthood (65 years and older)

Persons in late adulthood must adjust to the effects of aging. These changes can include the loss of strength and health, the death of loved ones, retirement, and preparation for their own death. Although the developmental tasks of this age appear to deal entirely with loss, solutions often involve new relationships, friendships, and interests. Common disorders of this age group (arthritis, Alzheimer's disease, cancer, diabetes, and stroke) are covered in Chapters 18 and 19.

11. Distinguish between what is true and what is not true about the aging process

Geriatrics is the study of health, wellness, and disease later in life. It includes the health care of older people and the well-being of their caregivers. **Gerontology** is the study of the aging process in people from midlife through old age. Gerontologists look at the impact of the aging population on society.

Because later adulthood covers an age range of as many as 25 to 35 years, people in this age category can have very different abilities, depending on their health. Some 70-year-old people still enjoy active sports, while others are not active. Many 85-year-old people can still live alone, though others may live with family members or in skilled care facilities.

Ideas and stereotypes about older people are often false. They create prejudices against the elderly that are as unfair as prejudices against racial, ethnic, or religious groups. On television or in movies, older people are often shown as helpless, lonely, disabled, slow, forgetful, dependent, or inactive. However, research indicates that most older people are active and engaged in work, volunteer activities, learning programs, and exercise regimens. Aging is a normal process, not a disease. Most older people live independent lives and do not need assistance (Fig. 8-18). Prejudice toward, stereotyping of, and/or discrimination against older persons or the elderly is called **ageism**.

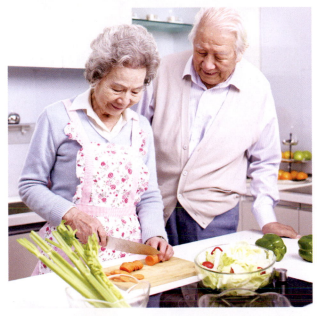

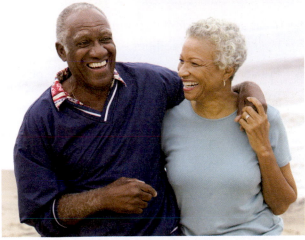

Fig. 8-18. Most older people lead active lives.

Nursing assistants are likely to spend much of their time working with residents who are elderly. They must be able to know what is true about aging and what is not true. Aging causes many physical, psychological, and social changes. However, normal changes of aging do not mean an older person must become depen-

dent, ill, or inactive. Knowing normal changes of aging from signs of illness or disability will allow nursing assistants to better help residents. Normal changes of aging include the following:

- Skin is thinner, drier, more fragile, and less elastic.
- Muscles weaken and lose tone.
- Bones lose density and become more brittle.
- Sensitivity of nerve endings in the skin decreases.
- Responses and reflexes slow.
- Short-term memory loss occurs.
- Senses of vision, hearing, taste, touch, and smell weaken.
- Heart pumps less efficiently.
- Lung strength and lung capacity decrease.
- Oxygen in the blood decreases.
- Urinary elimination is more frequent.
- Appetite decreases.
- Digestion takes longer and is less efficient.
- Levels of hormones decrease.
- Immunity weakens.
- Lifestyle changes occur.

There are also changes that are NOT considered normal changes of aging and should be reported to the nurse. These include the following:

- Signs of depression
- Suicidal thoughts
- Loss of ability to think logically
- Poor nutrition
- Shortness of breath
- Incontinence

This is not a complete list. A nursing assistant's job includes reporting any change, normal or not. More information about normal changes of aging is located in Chapter 9.

12. Explain developmental disabilities and list care guidelines

Developmental disabilities refer to disabilities that are present at birth or emerge during childhood. A developmental disability is a chronic condition that restricts physical and/or mental ability. These disabilities prevent a child from developing at a normal rate. Language, mobility, learning, and the ability to perform self-care may be affected. These disabilities include intellectual disabilities, Down syndrome, cerebral palsy, spina bifida, and autism spectrum disorder.

Intellectual disability: Intellectual disability (formerly called *mental retardation*) is the most common developmental disability. An intellectual disability is neither a disease nor a mental illness. People with an intellectual disability develop at a below-average rate. They have below-average mental functioning. They experience difficulty with learning, communicating, and moving, and may have problems adjusting socially. The ability to care for themselves may be affected. The potential for living independently and for achieving financial independence may be limited.

There are four different degrees of this disability: mild, moderate, severe, and profound. The level of care required can range from relatively independent living with a mild intellectual disability to a need for skilled, 24-hour care for a person who has a profound intellectual disability.

Despite their special needs, residents who have an intellectual disability have the same emotional and physical needs that others have (Fig. 8-19). They experience the same emotions, such as anger, sadness, love, and joy, as others do, but their ability to express their emotions may be limited.

For residents who have an intellectual disability, the main goal of care is to help the person have as normal a life as possible. For a person with an intellectual disability, this means recognizing her individuality, basic human rights, and physical and emotional needs, as well as her special needs.

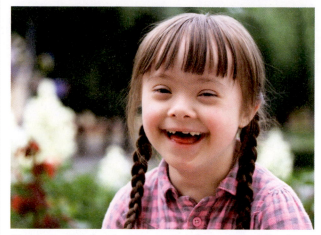

Fig. 8-19. *People who have an intellectual disability have the same emotional and physical needs that others do.*

Some residents and/or their families will use the term *intellectually disabled*, while others may use *developmentally delayed*, *special*, or *challenged*. Nursing assistants should respect the resident's wishes about which term or terms to use.

Guidelines: Intellectual Disability

G Treat adult residents as adults, regardless of their intellectual abilities.

G Praise and encourage often, especially positive behavior.

G Help teach the resident to perform activities of daily living (ADLs) by dividing a task into smaller units.

G Promote independence, but also assist residents with activities and motor functions that are difficult.

G Encourage social interaction.

G Repeat what you say to make sure they understand.

G Be patient.

Down Syndrome: Down syndrome, also called Trisomy 21, is most often caused by an abnormal cell division, resulting in an extra number 21 chromosome (three copies of chromosome

21 instead of the usual two copies). People who are born with Down syndrome experience different degrees of intellectual disability, along with physical symptoms. A person with Down syndrome typically has a small skull, a flattened nose, short fingers, and a wider space between the first two fingers and the first two toes. As with some of the types of intellectual disabilities, a person with Down syndrome can become fairly independent.

Guidelines: Down Syndrome

G   Give the same type of care and instruction that you would for any other person with an intellectual disability.

G   Praise and encourage often, especially positive behavior.

G   Help teach the resident to perform ADLs by dividing a task into smaller units.

Cerebral Palsy: People who have cerebral palsy have suffered brain damage either while in the uterus or during birth. They may have both physical and mental disabilities. Damage to the brain stops the development of the child or causes disorganized or abnormal development. Muscle coordination and nerves are affected. People with cerebral palsy may lack control of the head, have trouble using the arms and hands, and have poor balance or posture. They may be either stiff or limp, and may have impaired speech. Gait and mobility may be affected. Intelligence may also be affected. With or without assistance, a person with cerebral palsy may be able to live independently.

Guidelines: Cerebral Palsy

G   Allow the resident to move slowly. People with cerebral palsy take longer to adjust their body positions. They may repeat movements several times.

G   Keep the resident's body in as normal an alignment as possible.

G   Talk to the resident, even if she cannot speak. Be patient and listen.

G   Use touch as a form of communication.

G   Avoid activities that are tiring or frustrating.

G   Be gentle when handling parts of the body that may be painful (Fig. 8-20).

G   Promote independence and encourage socializing with friends and family.

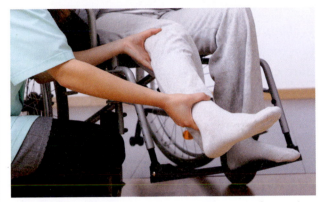

Fig. 8-20. *Be gentle when moving body parts of a resident who has cerebral palsy.*

Spina Bifida: Spina bifida literally means *split spine.* When part of the backbone is not well developed at birth, the spinal cord may bulge out of the person's back. Spina bifida can cause a range of disabilities. Some babies born with spina bifida will be able to walk and will experience no lasting disabilities. Others may be in a wheelchair and/or may have little or no bladder or bowel control. In some cases, complications of spina bifida may cause brain damage.

Guidelines: Spina Bifida

G   If the resident is an adult, provide assistance with range of motion exercises and ADLs. If working in the home, help perform light housecleaning duties.

G   If an infant or child has spina bifida, perform tasks that help the parents manage and stabilize the home.

G   Be a positive role model for the resident and family in learning to deal with the resident's disabilities.

Autism Spectrum Disorder (ASD): Autism spectrum disorder is a developmental disability that causes problems with social skills and communication. It appears in early childhood, usually by age 3. Parents may notice that a child does not engage in pretend play or has problems with communication and social interaction. A diagnosis may be made after comprehensive testing, including physical and neurological examinations, among other screening tests.

Problems with social skills and communication include being withdrawn, unable to communicate using words, and unable to make eye contact. Intense tantrums, repetitive body movements, aggression, a short attention span, and an inability to be empathetic are also problems caused by autism spectrum disorder. Overly focused interests (for example, learning everything about airplanes) are common.

The exact cause of autism spectrum disorder is unknown, but genetics may be a factor. Boys are more likely to have ASD.

Treatment includes many types of therapies, including behavior, speech, and occupational therapies, along with social skills training. Nutrition management can also be beneficial. Having familiar caregivers and keeping a routine may be helpful. Ideally, treatment should be started early and must be tailored to the individual.

13. Identify community resources available to help the elderly and people who are developmentally disabled

Government and private agencies exist in most areas to serve the needs of the elderly. These agencies may have counselors to work with victims of abuse or neglect and other programs to protect senior citizens' rights and contribute to their quality of life. These resources can be located online by searching for terms such as community services, senior citizens, aging, or elder services. Local religious organizations may also have programs for seniors. Here are a few of the many community resources available to help residents meet different needs:

- Eldercare Locator, a public service of the U.S. Administration on Aging (eldercare.gov, 800-677-1116)

- National Association of Agencies on Aging (n4a.org, 202-872-0888)

- National Resource Center on LGBT Aging (lgbtagingcenter.org, 212-741-2247)

- Alzheimer's Association (alz.org, 800-272-3900)

- American Cancer Society (cancer.org, 800-227-2345)

- AIDSinfo, a service of the U.S. Department of Health and Human Services (aidsinfo.nih.gov, 800-448-0440)

- Meals on Wheels Association of America (mealsonwheelsamerica.org, 888-998-6325)

- National Institute of Mental Health (NIMH, nimh.nih.gov, 866-615-6464)

There are many services available to help people who have developmental disabilities, including the following resources:

- American Association on Intellectual and Developmental Disabilities (AAIDD, aaidd.org, 202-387-1968)

- Autism Science Foundation (autismsciencefoundation.org, 914-810-9100)

- National Down Syndrome Congress (ndsccenter.org, 800-232-6372)

- Special Olympics (specialolympics.org, 800-700-8585)

- Spina Bifida Association (spinabifidaassociation.org, 800-621-3141)

- United Cerebral Palsy (ucp.org, 800-872-5827)

If residents ask a nursing assistant for help, the NA should refer them to the nurse or social worker. If no one asks, but the NA thinks help is needed, she should speak to her supervisor.

Chapter Review

1. List six basic human needs.

2. What psychosocial needs do humans have?

3. According to Maslow, which needs must be met first—physical or emotional?

4. Describe what holistic care involves.

5. List six examples of losses that residents may be experiencing.

6. What is one way that a nursing assistant can show respect for residents' sexual identity?

7. If a nursing assistant encounters a sexual situation between two consenting residents, what should she do?

8. List five ways that a nursing assistant can help residents meet their spiritual needs.

9. What should a nursing assistant never do regarding residents' spiritual or religious needs?

10. Pick three religions listed in Learning Objective 6 and briefly describe them. Feel free to add information that is not included in the Learning Objective.

11. If a resident is an atheist, but her nursing assistant believes in God, is it okay for the NA to ask the resident to pray with her?

12. List seven ways that regular physical activity can help a person.

13. List seven ways that inactivity and immobility can cause problems for a person.

14. List four ways that families can help residents.

15. Name three ways nursing assistants can meet the emotional needs of residents and their families.

16. Name at least two common disorders for each stage of human development.

17. What is ageism?

18. In movies, elderly people are often shown as helpless, lonely, disabled, slow, forgetful, dependent, or inactive. What is actually true of most older adults?

19. List ten normal changes of aging.

20. What are developmental disabilities?

21. What is one way to locate community resources for the elderly?

9

The Healthy Human Body

1. Describe body systems and define key anatomical terms

Bodies are organized into body systems. Each system in the body has a condition under which it works best. **Homeostasis** is the name for the condition in which all of the body's systems are balanced and are working together to maintain internal stability. To be in homeostasis, the body's **metabolism**, or physical and chemical processes, must be working at a steady level. When disease or injury occurs, the body's metabolism is disturbed, and homeostasis is lost.

Changes in metabolic processes are called signs (objective information) and symptoms (subjective information). For instance, changes in body temperature could indicate that the body is fighting an infection. Noticing and reporting changes in residents is a very important part of a nursing assistant's job. The changes noted could be signs of significant problems.

Each system in the body has its own unique structure and function. There are also normal, age-related changes for each body system. Knowing normal changes of aging will help nursing assistants be able to recognize any abnormal changes in residents.

The body's systems can be organized in different ways. In this book, the human body is divided into ten systems:

1. Integumentary (skin)
2. Musculoskeletal
3. Nervous
4. Circulatory
5. Respiratory
6. Urinary
7. Gastrointestinal
8. Endocrine
9. Reproductive
10. Immune and Lymphatic

Body systems are made up of **organs**. An organ has a specific function. Organs are made up of **tissues**. Tissues are made up of groups of cells that perform a similar task. For example, in the circulatory system, the heart is one of the organs. It is made up of tissues and cells. **Cells** are the building blocks of the body. Living cells divide, grow, and die, renewing the tissues and organs of the body.

Anatomical Terms of Location

Anatomical terms of location are descriptive terms to help identify positions or directions of the body. Here are some anatomical terms used to describe location in the human body:

- Anterior or ventral: the front of the body or body part

- Posterior or dorsal: the back of the body or body part

- Superior: toward the head

- Inferior: away from the head

- Medial: toward the midline of the body

This chapter discusses the structure and function of each body system, as well as age-related changes and what is important to observe and report about each system. The bulk of information on diseases and disorders of each system and related care will be discussed in Chapter 18. Chapters 16, 17, and 19 also have information about diseases.

2. Describe the integumentary system

The largest organ and system in the body is the skin, a natural protective covering, or **integument**. Skin prevents injury to internal organs, and it protects the body against entry of bacteria. Skin also prevents the loss of too much water, which is essential to life. Skin is made up of layers of tissues. Within these layers are sweat glands, which secrete sweat to help cool the body when needed, and sebaceous glands, which secrete oil (sebum) to keep the skin lubricated. There are also hair follicles, many tiny blood vessels (capillaries), and tiny nerve endings (Fig. 9-1).

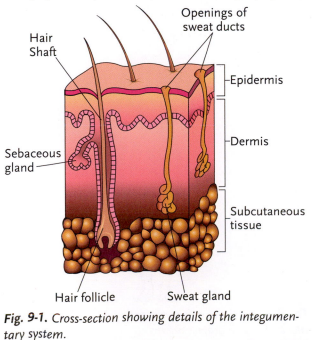

Fig. 9-1. *Cross-section showing details of the integumentary system.*

The skin is also a *sense organ* that feels heat, cold, pain, touch, and pressure. It then tells the brain what it is feeling. Body temperature is regulated in the skin. Blood vessels **dilate**, or widen, when the outside temperature is too high. This brings more blood to the body's surface to cool it off. The same blood vessels **constrict**, or narrow, when the outside temperature is too cold. By restricting the amount of blood reaching the skin, the blood vessels help the body retain heat.

The blood vessels, called capillaries, are located in the dermis, which is the inner layer of skin. The dermis also contains nerves, sweat glands, sebaceous (oil) glands, and hair roots. Sweat glands help control body temperature by secreting sweat. Sweat is made up of mostly water, but it also contains salt and a small amount of waste products. Sweat comes to the body's surface through pores, or tiny openings in the skin. It cools the body as it evaporates. Sebaceous glands in the dermis secrete sebum (oil). Sebum comes to the skin surface through hair follicles, or roots. Sebum keeps the skin and hair lubricated.

No blood vessels and only a few nerve endings are located in the epidermis, which is the outer layer of skin. Thinner than the dermis, the epidermis contains both dead and living cells. The dead cells begin deeper in the epidermis. They are pushed to the surface as other cells divide. They are eventually worn off. The epidermis also contains pigment cells that give skin its color.

Hair grows from roots located in the dermis. It grows through hair follicles that extend through the epidermis to the outside of the body. Hair protects the body from heat and cold. Hair inside the nose and ears keeps out particles and bacteria trying to enter the body.

The functions of the integumentary system are to protect internal organs from injury, protect the body against bacteria, and prevent the loss of too much water. It also responds to heat, cold, pain, touch, and pressure, and it regulates body temperature.

Normal changes of aging include the following:

- Skin is thinner, drier, and more fragile. It is more easily damaged.

- Skin is less elastic.

- Protective fatty tissue is lost, so the person may feel colder.

- Hair thins and may turn gray.

- Wrinkles and brown spots, or "liver spots," appear.

- Nails are harder and more brittle.

- Dry, itchy skin may result from lack of oil from the sebaceous glands.

How the NA Can Help

Older adults perspire less and do not need to bathe as often. Most elderly people generally need a complete bath only twice a week, with sponge baths every day. Using lotions as ordered helps to relieve dry skin. The NA should be gentle; elderly skin may be fragile and can tear easily. Hair also becomes drier and needs to be shampooed less often. Gently brushing dry hair stimulates and distributes the natural oils. Clothing and bed covers can be layered for additional warmth. Bed linens should be kept wrinkle-free. The NA should not cut residents' toenails. Fluid intake should be encouraged.

Observing and Reporting: Integumentary System

During daily care, a resident's skin should be observed for changes that may indicate injury or disease:

O/R Pale, white, reddened, or purple areas

O/R Blisters or bruises

O/R Complaints of tingling, warmth, or burning

O/R Dry or flaking skin

O/R Itching or scratching

O/R Rash or any skin discoloration

O/R Swelling

O/R Cuts, boils, sores, wounds, or abrasions

O/R Fluid or blood draining from the skin

O/R Broken skin

O/R Changes in moistness or dryness

O/R Changes in an injury or wound (size, depth, drainage, color, odor)

O/R Redness or broken skin between toes or around toenails

O/R Scalp or hair changes

O/R Skin that appears different from normal or that has changed

O/R In darker complexions, changes in skin tone, skin temperature, and the feel of the tissue as compared to the skin nearby

3. Describe the musculoskeletal system

Muscles, bones, ligaments, tendons, and cartilage give the body shape and structure. They work together to move the body. The skeleton, or framework, of the human body has 206 bones (Fig. 9-2). In addition to allowing the body to move, **bones** also protect organs. For example, the skull protects the brain and the vertebrae protect the spinal cord. Bones are hard and rigid, but are made up of living cells. Blood vessels supply oxygen and nutrients to the bones, as well as to other tissues of the body.

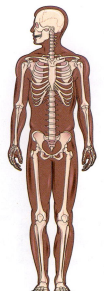

Fig. 9-2. The skeleton is composed of 206 bones that aid movement and protect organs.

Two bones meet at a **joint**. Some joints, such as the ball-and-socket joint, make movement possible in all directions. This joint is a type of synovial joint. In this joint, the round end of one bone fits into the hollow end of the other bone, which allows it to move in all directions. The hip and shoulder joints are examples.

Other joints permit movement in one direction only. The hinge joint is another example of a synovial joint. Like the hinge of a door, a hinge joint permits movement in one direction only. The elbow and knee are hinge joints. They bend in one direction only (Fig. 9-3).

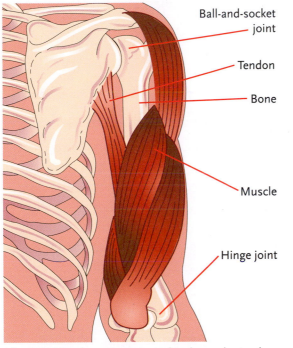

Ball-and-socket joint

Tendon

Bone

Muscle

Hinge joint

Fig. 9-3. Muscles are connected to bones by tendons. Bones meet at different types of joints. The ball and socket joint and the hinge joint are shown here.

Muscles provide movement of body parts to maintain posture and to produce heat. Muscles can be voluntary or involuntary. Voluntary muscles are also called skeletal muscles. They are attached to bones and can be moved when a person wants them to move. Examples of voluntary muscles are the arm and leg muscles, which are consciously controlled. Involuntary muscles cannot be consciously controlled. They automatically regulate the movement of organs and blood vessels. An example of an involuntary muscle is the heart.

Exercise is important for improving and maintaining physical and mental health. Inactivity and immobility can result in a loss of self-esteem, depression, pneumonia, and urinary tract infections. They can also lead to constipation, blood clots, dulling of the senses, and muscle atrophy or contractures. When **atrophy** occurs, the muscle wastes away, decreases in size, and becomes weak. When a **contracture** develops, the muscle or tendon shortens, becomes inflexible, and "freezes" in position. This causes permanent disability of the limb.

Range of motion (ROM) exercises can help prevent these conditions. With these exercises, the joints are extended and flexed in the measured degrees of a circle. Exercise increases circulation of blood, oxygen, and nutrients and improves muscle tone. Chapter 21 has more information on range of motion exercises.

The functions of the musculoskeletal system are to give the body shape and structure, to allow the body to move, to protect body organs, to maintain posture, and to produce heat.

Normal changes of aging include the following:

- Muscles weaken and lose tone.

- Body movement slows.

- Bones lose density. They become more brittle, making them more susceptible to breaks.

- Joints may stiffen and become painful.

- Height is gradually lost.

How the NA Can Help

Falls can cause life-threatening complications, including fractures. The NA can prevent falls by answering call lights immediately. She should keep pathways clear, clean up spills, and not move furniture. Walkers or canes need to be placed where residents can easily reach them. Residents should wear nonskid shoes that are securely fastened. The NA should encourage regular movement and self-care. Residents should perform as many activities of daily living as possible. The NA can help with range of motion exercises as needed.

Observing and Reporting: Musculoskeletal System

Observe and report these signs and symptoms:

%R Changes in ability to perform routine movements and activities

%R Any changes in residents' abilities to perform range of motion exercises

%R Pain during movement

%R Any new or increased swelling of joints

%R White, shiny, red, or warm areas over a joint

%R Bruising

%R Aches and pains reported

4. Describe the nervous system

The nervous system is the control and message center of the body. It controls and coordinates all body functions. The nervous system also senses and interprets information from outside the human body.

The neuron, or nerve cell, is the basic unit of the nervous system. Neurons send messages or sensations from the receptors in different parts of the body, through the spinal cord, to the brain.

The nervous system has two main parts: the **central nervous system (CNS)** and the **peripheral nervous system (PNS)**. The central nervous system is composed of the brain and spinal cord. The peripheral nervous system deals with the periphery, or outer part, of the body via the nerves that extend throughout the body (Fig. 9-4).

The Central Nervous System

The brain is housed within the skull. The spinal cord is housed within the spinal column. The spinal column extends from the brain into the trunk of the body. Both the brain and the spinal cord are covered by a protective membrane made up of three layers. Between two of these layers is the cerebrospinal fluid. This fluid circulates around the brain and spinal cord. It provides a cushion against injuries.

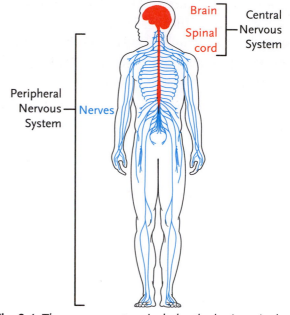

Fig. 9-4. The nervous system includes the brain, spinal cord, and nerves throughout the body.

The brain has three main sections: the cerebrum, the cerebellum, and the brainstem (Fig. 9-5). The largest section of the human brain is the cerebrum. The outside layer of the cerebrum is the cerebral cortex. The cerebral cortex is the part of the brain in which thinking, analysis, association of ideas, judgment, emotions, and memory occur. The cerebral cortex also

- Directs speech and emotions

- Interprets messages from the eyes, ears, nose, tongue, and skin

- Controls voluntary muscle movement

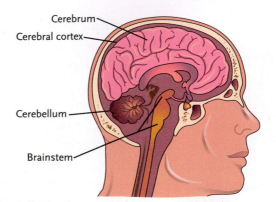

Fig. 9-5. The three main sections of the brain are the cerebrum, cerebellum, and brainstem.

The cerebrum is divided into right and left hemispheres. The right hemisphere controls movement and function in the left side of the body. The left hemisphere controls movement and function in the right side of the body (Fig. 9-6). Any illness or injury to the right hemisphere affects functions on the left side of the body. Illness or injury to the left hemisphere disrupts function on the right side.

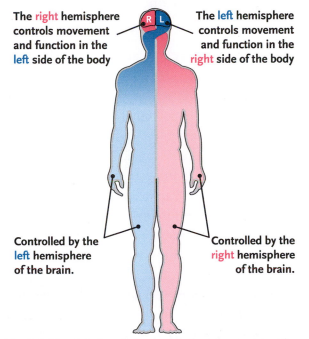

The **right** hemisphere controls movement and function in the **left** side of the body

The **left** hemisphere controls movement and function in the **right** side of the body

Controlled by the **left** hemisphere of the brain.

Controlled by the **right** hemisphere of the brain.

Fig. 9-6. *The right hemisphere controls movement and function in the left side of the body. The left hemisphere controls movement and function in the right side of the body.*

The cerebellum controls balance and regulates the body's voluntary muscles. It produces and coordinates smooth movements. Someone who has a problem in the cerebellum will be uncoordinated and have jerky movements and muscle weakness.

The cerebrum and cerebellum are connected to the spinal cord by the brainstem. The brainstem contains a kind of regulatory center. It controls heart rate, breathing, swallowing, coughing, vomiting, and closing or opening of blood vessels.

The spinal cord is connected to the brain. It is protected by the bones of the spinal column. Nerve pathways run through the spinal cord.

They conduct messages between the brain and the body. Cranial nerves attach to the brain and brainstem. Some of these nerves bring information from the sense organs to the brain. Some control muscles and others are connected to glands or organs, such as the lungs. There are 12 pairs of cranial nerves. Nerves that are attached to the spinal cord and connect the spinal cord to other parts of the body are called spinal nerves. The brain communicates with most of the body through the spinal nerves. There are 31 pairs of spinal nerves.

The functions of the nervous system are to control and coordinate all body functions and to sense, interpret, and respond to changes occurring both inside and outside the human body.

Normal changes of aging include the following:

- Responses and reflexes slow.

- Sensitivity of nerve endings in skin decreases.

- Person may show some memory loss, more often with short-term memory. Long-term memory, or memory of past events, usually remains sharp.

How the NA Can Help

Suggesting residents make lists or write notes about things they want to remember can help with memory loss. Placing a calendar nearby may also help. If residents enjoy reminiscing, the NA can take an interest in their past by asking to see photos or hear stories. The NA should allow time for decision-making and avoid sudden changes in schedule. The NA should allow plenty of time for movement; residents should not be rushed. Reading, thinking, and other mental activities should be encouraged.

Observing and Reporting: Nervous System

Observe and report these signs and symptoms:

O/R Fatigue or pain with movement or exercise

O/R Shaking or trembling

O/R Inability to move one side of body

- °/R Difficulty speaking or slurring of speech
- °/R Numbness or tingling
- °/R Disturbance or changes in vision or hearing
- °/R Dizziness or loss of balance
- °/R Changes in eating patterns and/or fluid intake
- °/R Difficulty swallowing
- °/R Bowel and bladder changes
- °/R Depression or mood changes
- °/R Memory loss or confusion
- °/R Violent behavior
- °/R Any unusual or unexplained change in behavior
- °/R Decreased ability to perform ADLs

The Nervous System: Sense Organs

The eyes, ears, nose, tongue, and skin are the body's major sense organs. They are considered part of the central nervous system because they contain receptors that receive impulses from the environment. They relay these impulses to the nerves.

The eye, which is about an inch in diameter, is located in a bony socket in the skull (Fig. 9-7). The bony socket protects the eye, which is surrounded by muscles that control its movements.

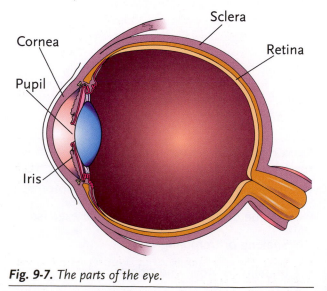

Fig. 9-7. *The parts of the eye.*

The outer part of the eye is called the sclera. The sclera appears white, except in front, where it is called the cornea. The cornea is actually clear, but it appears colored because it lies over the iris, or the colored part of the eye. The pupil, or black circle in the center of the iris, widens or narrows to adjust the amount of light that enters the eye. Inside the back of the eye is the retina. The retina contains cells that respond to light and send a message to the brain, where the picture is interpreted so a person can see.

The ear is a sense organ that provides balance and hearing. It is divided into three parts: the outer, middle, and inner ear (Fig. 9-8). The outer ear is the funnel-shaped outer part, sometimes called the auricle or pinna. It guides sound waves into the auditory canal. This canal is about one inch long and contains many glands that secrete earwax. Earwax and hair in the ear protect the ear from foreign objects. The eardrum, or tympanic membrane, separates the outer ear from the middle ear.

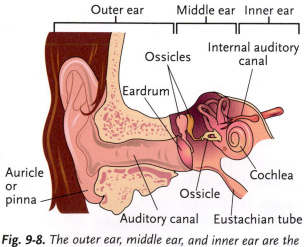

Fig. 9-8. *The outer ear, middle ear, and inner ear are the three main divisions of the ear.*

The middle ear consists of the eustachian tube and three ossicles, small bones that amplify sound. The ossicles transmit sound to the inner ear. The eustachian tube connects the middle ear to the throat. It functions to allow air into the middle ear to equalize pressure on the tympanic membrane. The inner ear contains fluid that carries sound waves from the middle ear to the auditory nerve. The auditory nerve then transmits the impulse to the brain. The inner ear also contains structures that help in maintaining balance.

Normal changes of aging include the following:

- Vision and hearing decrease. Sense of balance may be affected.

- Senses of taste, smell, and touch decrease.

How the NA Can Help

Residents should use their eyeglasses. The NA can help by keeping them clean. Bright colors and proper lighting will also help. Hearing aids should be worn, and they should be kept clean. The NA should face the resident when speaking and speak slowly and clearly. Shouting should be avoided. The loss of senses of taste and smell may lead to decreased appetite. Providing oral care often and offering foods with a variety of tastes and textures may help. The loss of smell may make residents unaware of increased body odor. The NA should help as needed with regular bathing. Due to a decreased sense of touch, residents may not be able to tell if something is too hot for them. The NA should be careful with hot drinks and hot bath water.

Observing and Reporting: Eyes and Ears

Observe and report these signs and symptoms:

O/R Changes in vision or hearing

O/R Dizziness

O/R Complaints of pain in eyes or ears

5. Describe the circulatory system

The circulatory, or cardiovascular, system is made up of the heart, blood vessels, and blood (Fig. 9-9). The heart pumps blood through the blood vessels to the cells. The blood carries food, oxygen, and other substances cells need to function properly. A healthy circulatory system is essential for life. Cells, tissues, and organs need proper circulation to function well. If circulation is reduced, cells do not receive enough oxygen and nutrients. Waste products of cell metabolism are not removed, and organs become diseased.

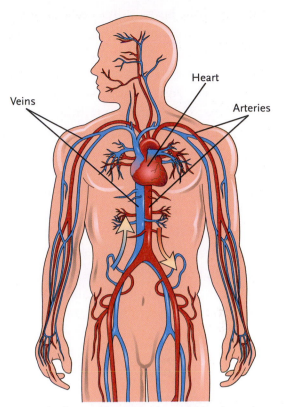

Fig. 9-9. The heart, blood vessels, and blood are the main parts of the circulatory system.

The heart is the pump of the circulatory system (Fig. 9-10). The heart is a muscle. It is located in the middle lower chest, on the left side. The heart muscle is made up of three layers: the pericardium, the myocardium, and the endocardium.

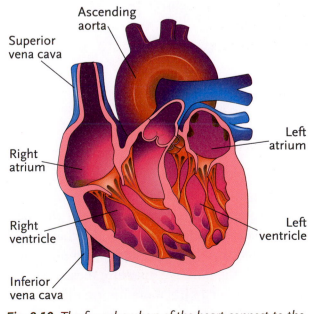

Fig. 9-10. The four chambers of the heart connect to the body's largest blood vessels.

The interior of the heart is divided into four chambers. The two upper chambers are called the left atrium and right atrium. They receive blood. The two lower chambers, or ventricles, pump blood. The right atrium receives blood from the veins. This blood, containing carbon dioxide, then flows into the right ventricle. It is pumped to the blood vessels in the lungs. Carbon dioxide is exchanged for oxygen. The heart's left atrium receives the oxygen-saturated blood. It then flows into the left ventricle. There it is pumped through the arteries to all parts of the body. Two valves, one located between the right atrium and right ventricle and the other between the left atrium and left ventricle, allow the blood to flow in only one direction (Fig. 9-11).

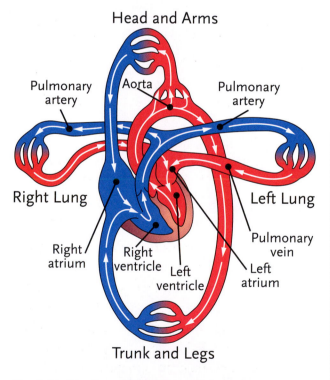

Fig. 9-11. The flow of blood through the heart.

The heart functions in two phases: the contracting phase, or **systole**, when the ventricles pump blood through the blood vessels, and the resting phase, or **diastole**, when the chambers fill with blood. When a person's blood pressure is checked, the numbers measure these two phases. Chapter 14 has more information on how to measure blood pressure.

Three types of blood vessels are found in the body: arteries, capillaries, and veins. Arteries carry oxygen-rich blood away from the heart. The blood is pumped from the left ventricle through the aorta, the largest artery. Blood is then pumped through other arteries that branch off from it. The coronary arteries carry blood to the heart itself.

Capillaries are tiny blood vessels that receive blood from the arteries. Nutrients, oxygen, and other substances in the blood pass from the capillaries to the cells. Waste products, including carbon dioxide, pass from the cells into the capillaries.

Veins carry the blood containing waste products from the capillaries back to the heart. Near the heart, the veins come together to form the two largest veins, the inferior vena cava and the superior vena cava. These empty into the right atrium. The inferior vena cava carries blood from the legs and trunk. The superior vena cava carries blood from the arms, head, and neck.

Blood is made up of blood cells and plasma. There are three different types of blood cells: red blood cells, or erythrocytes; white blood cells, or leukocytes; and platelets, or thrombocytes.

Red blood cells (erythrocytes) carry oxygen from the lungs to all parts of the body. Red blood cells are produced by bone marrow, a substance found inside hollow bones. Iron, found in bone marrow and red blood cells, is essential to blood. It gives it its red color. Red blood cells function for a short time, then die. They are filtered out of the blood by the liver and spleen. Iron in diets allows bodies to produce new red blood cells.

White blood cells (leukocytes) defend the body against foreign substances, such as bacteria and viruses. When the body becomes aware of these invaders, white blood cells rush to the site of infection. They multiply rapidly. The bone marrow, spleen, and thymus gland produce white blood cells.

Platelets (thrombocytes) are also carried by the blood. They cause the blood to clot, preventing excess bleeding. Platelets are also produced by bone marrow.

Plasma is the liquid portion of the blood. It is made up of mostly water and carries many substances, including blood cells, nutrients, and waste products.

The functions of the circulatory system are to supply food, oxygen, and hormones to cells and to supply the body with infection-fighting blood cells. The circulatory system removes waste products from cells and also helps control body temperature.

Normal changes of aging include the following:

- Heart pumps less efficiently.

- Blood flow decreases.

- Blood vessels narrow.

How the NA Can Help

Movement and exercise should be encouraged. Walking, stretching, and even lifting light weights can help maintain strength and promote circulation. Range of motion exercises are important for residents who cannot get out of bed. The NA should allow time to complete activities and try to prevent residents from tiring. Layering clothing helps keep residents warm. Socks, slippers, or shoes help keep the feet warm.

Observing and Reporting: Circulatory System

Observe and report these signs and symptoms:

- O/R Changes in pulse rate

- O/R Weakness, fatigue

- O/R Loss of ability to perform activities of daily living (ADLs)

- O/R Swelling of ankles, feet, fingers, or hands

- O/R Pale or bluish hands, feet, or lips

- O/R Chest pain

- O/R Weight gain

- O/R Shortness of breath, changes in breathing patterns, inability to catch breath

- O/R Severe headache

- O/R Inactivity (which can lead to circulatory problems)

6. Describe the respiratory system

Respiration, the body taking in oxygen and removing carbon dioxide, involves breathing in, **inspiration**, and breathing out, **expiration**. The lungs accomplish this process (Fig. 9-12).

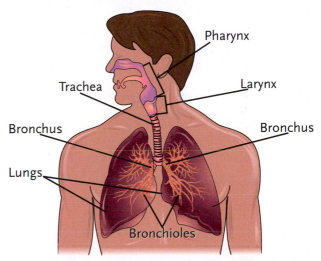

Fig. 9-12. *The respiratory process begins with inspiration through the nose or mouth. The air travels through the trachea and into the lungs via the bronchi, which then branch into bronchioles.*

As the lungs inhale, the air is pulled in through the nose and into the pharynx, a tubular passageway for both food and air. From the pharynx, air passes into the larynx, or voice box. The larynx is located at the beginning of the trachea, or windpipe. The trachea divides into two branches at its lower portion, the right bronchus and the left bronchus, or bronchi. Each bronchus leads into a lung and then subdivides into bronchioles. These smaller airways subdivide further. They end in alveoli: tiny, one-cell sacs that appear in grape-like clusters. Blood is supplied to the alveoli by capillaries. Oxygen and carbon dioxide are exchanged between the alveoli and capillaries.

Oxygen-saturated blood then circulates through the capillaries and venules (small veins) of the lungs into the pulmonary vein and left side of the heart. The carbon dioxide is exhaled through the alveoli into the bronchioles and bronchi of the lungs, the trachea, through the larynx, the pharynx, and out the nose and mouth.

Each lung is covered by the pleura, a membrane with two layers. One is attached to the chest wall. The other is attached to the surface of the lung. The space between the layers is filled with a thin fluid that lubricates the layers, preventing them from rubbing together during breathing.

The functions of the respiratory system are to bring oxygen into the body and to eliminate carbon dioxide produced as the body uses oxygen.

Normal changes of aging include the following:

- Lung strength decreases.
- Lung capacity decreases.
- Oxygen in the blood decreases.
- Voice weakens.

How the NA Can Help

Residents with acute or chronic upper respiratory conditions should not be exposed to cigarette smoke or polluted air. The NA should provide rest periods as needed and encourage exercise and regular movement. The NA should assist with deep breathing exercises as ordered. Residents who have difficulty breathing will usually be more comfortable sitting up rather than lying down.

Observing and Reporting: Respiratory System

Observe and report these signs and symptoms:

O/R Change in respiratory rate

O/R Shallow breathing or breathing through pursed lips

O/R Coughing or wheezing

O/R Nasal congestion or discharge

O/R Sore throat, difficulty swallowing, or swollen tonsils

O/R The need to sit after mild exertion

O/R Pale, bluish, or gray color of the lips, arms, and/or legs

O/R Pain in the chest area

O/R Discolored **sputum**, mucus a person coughs up from the lungs (green, yellow, blood-tinged, or gray)

7. Describe the urinary system

The urinary system is composed of two kidneys, two ureters, one urinary bladder, a single urethra, and a meatus (Figs. 9-13 and 9-14).

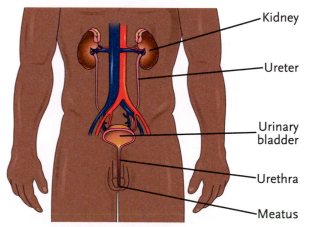

Fig. 9-13. *The urinary system consists of two kidneys and two ureters, the bladder, the urethra, and the meatus. This is an illustration of the male urinary system.*

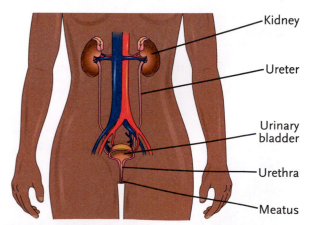

Fig. 9-14. *The female urethra is shorter than the male urethra. This is one reason why the female bladder is more likely to become infected by bacteria.*

The kidneys are located in the upper part of the abdominal cavity on each side of the spine.

These two bean-shaped organs are protected by the muscles of the back and the lower part of the rib cage. When blood flows through the kidneys, waste products and excess water are filtered out. Necessary water and substances are reabsorbed into the bloodstream. Waste and the remaining fluid form urine. The body must maintain a proper balance between water absorbed in the body and waste fluids that are released from the body. Chapter 15 contains information about fluid intake and output.

Each kidney has a ureter, which is attached to the bladder. Urine flows through the ureters to the bladder, a muscular sac in the lower part of the abdomen. Urine flows from the bladder through the urethra. It then passes out of the body through the meatus, the opening at the end of the urethra. In the female, the meatus is located in the genital area just in front of the opening of the vagina. In the male, the meatus is located at the end of the penis.

The urinary system has two important functions. Through urine, the urinary system eliminates waste products created by the cells. The urinary system also maintains the water balance in the body.

Normal changes of aging include the following:

- The ability of kidneys to filter blood decreases.

- Bladder muscle tone weakens.

- Bladder holds less urine, which causes more frequent urination.

- Bladder may not empty completely, causing a greater chance of infection.

How the NA Can Help

The NA should encourage fluids and offer frequent trips to the bathroom. If residents are incontinent, the NA should not show frustration or anger. **Urinary incontinence** is the inability to control the bladder, which leads to an involuntary loss of urine. Residents should be kept clean and dry.

Observing and Reporting: Urinary System

Observe and report these signs and symptoms:

O/R Weight loss or gain

O/R Swelling in the upper or lower extremities

O/R Pain or burning during urination

O/R Changes in urine, such as cloudiness, odor, or color

O/R Changes in frequency and amount of urination

O/R Swelling in the abdominal/bladder area

O/R Complaints that bladder feels full or painful

O/R Urinary incontinence/dribbling

O/R Pain in the kidney or back/flank region

O/R Inadequate fluid intake

O/R Confusion

8. Describe the gastrointestinal system

The gastrointestinal (GI) system, also called the digestive system, is made up of the gastrointestinal tract and the accessory digestive organs (Fig. 9-15). The gastrointestinal tract is a long passageway extending from the mouth to the anus, the opening of the rectum. Food passes from the mouth through the pharynx, esophagus, stomach, small intestine, large intestine, and out of the body as solid waste (*feces* or *stool*). The teeth, tongue, salivary glands, liver, gallbladder, and pancreas are the accessory organs to digestion. They help prepare the food so that it can be absorbed.

Food is first placed in the mouth. The teeth chew it by cutting it, then chopping and grinding it into smaller pieces that can be swallowed. Saliva moistens the food and begins chemical digestion. The tongue helps with chewing and swallowing by pushing the food around between the teeth and then into the pharynx.

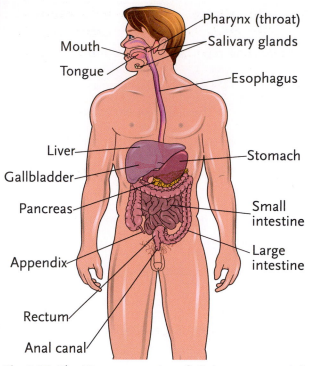

Fig. 9-15. The GI system consists of all the organs needed to digest food and process waste.

Labels:
Mouth
Tongue
Pharynx (throat)
Salivary glands
Esophagus
Liver
Gallbladder
Pancreas
Stomach
Small intestine
Large intestine
Appendix
Rectum
Anal canal

The pharynx is a muscular structure located at the back of the mouth. It extends into the throat. It contracts with swallowing and pushes food into the esophagus. The muscles of the esophagus then move food into the stomach through involuntary contractions called **peristalsis**.

The stomach is a muscular pouch located in the upper left part of the abdominal cavity. It provides physical digestion by stirring and churning the food to break it down into smaller particles. The glands in the stomach lining aid in digestion. They secrete gastric juices that chemically break down food. This process turns food into a semi-liquid substance called chyme. Peristalsis continues in the stomach, pushing the chyme into the small intestine.

The small intestine is about twenty feet long. Here enzymes secreted by the liver and the pancreas finish digesting the chyme. Bile, a green liquid produced by the liver, is stored in the gallbladder and released into the small intestine. Bile helps break down dietary fat. The liver con-

verts fats and sugars into glucose, a sugar that can be carried to cells by the blood. The liver also stores glucose. The pancreas produces insulin, a hormone that works to move **glucose**, or natural sugar, from the blood and into the cells for energy for the body.

The chyme is moved by peristalsis through the small intestine. There villi, tiny projections lining the small intestine, absorb the digested food into the capillaries.

Peristalsis moves the chyme that has not already been digested through the large intestine. In the large intestine, most of the water in the chyme is absorbed. What remains is feces, a semi-solid material of water, solid waste material, bacteria, and mucus. Feces passes by peristalsis through the rectum, the lower end of the colon. It moves out of the body through the anus, the rectal opening.

The gastrointestinal system has the following functions: digestion, absorption, and elimination. **Digestion** is the process of preparing food physically and chemically so that it can be absorbed into the cells. **Absorption** is the transfer of nutrients from the intestines to the cells. **Elimination** is the process of expelling wastes (made up of the waste products of food and fluids) that are not absorbed into the cells.

Normal changes of aging include the following:

- Decreased saliva production affects the ability to chew and swallow.

- Dulled sense of taste may result in poor appetite.

- Absorption of vitamins and minerals decreases.

- Process of digestion takes longer and is less efficient.

- Body waste moves more slowly through the intestines, causing more frequent constipation.

How the NA Can Help

Fluids and nutritious, appealing meals should be encouraged. The NA should allow the resident time to eat and make mealtime enjoyable. Regular oral care should be provided. Dentures must fit properly and should be cleaned regularly. Residents who have trouble chewing and swallowing are at risk of choking. The NA should offer fluids during mealtime. Residents should eat a diet that contains fiber and drink plenty of fluids to help prevent constipation. Residents should be given the opportunity to have a bowel movement around the same time each day.

Observing and Reporting: Gastrointestinal System

Observe and report these signs and symptoms:

- ^O/_R Difficulty swallowing or chewing (including denture problems, tooth pain, or mouth sores)

- ^O/_R **Fecal incontinence** (inability to control the bowels, leading to involuntary passage of stool)

- ^O/_R Weight gain or weight loss

- ^O/_R Loss of appetite

- ^O/_R Abdominal pain and cramping

- ^O/_R Diarrhea

- ^O/_R Nausea and vomiting (especially vomitus that looks like coffee grounds)

- ^O/_R Constipation

- ^O/_R Flatulence

- ^O/_R Hiccups, belching

- ^O/_R Bloody, black, or hard stools

- ^O/_R Heartburn

- ^O/_R Poor nutritional intake

9. Describe the endocrine system

The endocrine system is made up of glands in different areas of the body (Fig. 9-16). **Glands** are organs that produce and secrete chemicals called hormones. **Hormones** are chemical substances created by the body that control numerous body functions. Hormones are carried in the blood to various organs.

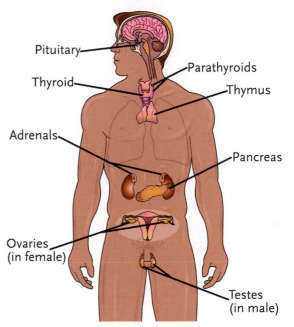

Fig. 9-16. *The endocrine system includes organs that produce hormones that regulate essential body processes.*

The pituitary gland, called the *master gland*, is located behind the eyes at the base of the brain. It secretes key hormones that cause other glands to produce other hormones. The following are some hormones secreted by the pituitary gland:

- Growth hormone, which regulates growth and development

- Antidiuretic hormone (ADH), which controls the balance of fluids in the body

- Oxytocin, which causes the uterus to contract during and after childbirth

The pituitary gland also produces hormones that regulate the thyroid gland and the adrenal glands. The thyroid gland is located in the neck in front of the larynx. It produces thyroid hormone, which regulates metabolism, the burning of food for heat and energy.

The parathyroid glands secrete a hormone that regulates the body's use of calcium. Nerves and muscles require calcium to function smoothly. A deficiency of this hormone can cause severe muscle contractions and spasms. It can be fatal if untreated.

The pancreas, a gland located in the upper mid-section of the abdomen, secretes insulin. Insulin is a hormone that works to move glucose (natural sugar) from the blood and into the cells for energy for the body.

Two adrenal glands are located at the tops of the kidneys. They produce hormones that are essential to life. These hormones are important because they help the body regulate carbohydrate metabolism. They also control the body's reaction to stress and regulate salt and water absorption in the kidneys. Adrenal glands also produce the hormone adrenaline, which regulates muscle power, heart rate, blood pressure, and energy levels during stressful situations or emergencies.

Gonads, or sex glands, produce hormones that regulate the body's ability to reproduce. The testes in the male secrete testosterone. The ovaries in the female secrete estrogen and progesterone.

The functions of the endocrine system are to maintain homeostasis through hormone secretion, influence growth and development, maintain blood sugar levels, and regulate levels of calcium and phosphate in the body. The endocrine system also regulates the body's ability to reproduce and determines how fast cells burn food for energy.

Normal changes of aging include the following:

- Levels of hormones, such as estrogen and progesterone, decrease.
- Insulin production lessens.
- Body is less able to handle stress.

How the NA Can Help

The NA should encourage proper nutrition and try to eliminate or reduce stressors. Stressors are anything that causes stress. Exercise can help reduce stress and should be encouraged. The NA can also help by listening to residents.

Observing and Reporting: Endocrine System

Observe and report these signs and symptoms:

°/R Headache

°/R Weakness

°/R Blurred vision

°/R Dizziness

°/R Irritability

°/R Sweating/excessive perspiration

°/R Change in "normal" behavior

°/R Confusion

°/R Change in mobility

°/R Change in sensation

°/R Numbness or tingling in arms or legs

°/R Weight gain or weight loss

°/R Loss of appetite or increased appetite

°/R Increased thirst

°/R Frequent urination or any change in urine output

°/R Hunger

°/R Dry skin

°/R Skin breakdown

°/R Sweet or fruity breath

°/R Sluggishness or fatigue

°/R Hyperactivity

10. Describe the reproductive system

The reproductive system is made up of the reproductive organs, which are different in men and women. The reproductive system allows human beings to **reproduce**, or create new human life. Reproduction begins when a male's and female's sex cells (sperm and ovum) join. These sex cells are formed in the male and female sex glands. These sex glands are called the gonads.

The Male Reproductive System

In the male, the sex glands or gonads are the testes or testicles. The two oval glands are located outside the body in the scrotum. The scrotum is a sac made of skin and muscle that is suspended between the thighs. The testes produce the male sex cells, called sperm, and testosterone (Fig. 9-17). Testosterone is the male hormone needed for the reproductive organs to function properly. Testosterone also promotes development of male secondary sex characteristics, which include the following:

- Facial hair
- Pubic and underarm hair
- Hair on the chest, legs, and arms
- Deepening of the voice
- Development of muscle mass

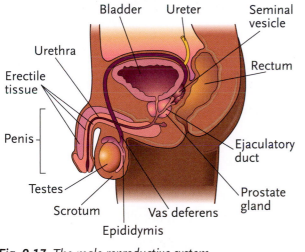

Fig. 9-17. *The male reproductive system.*

Sperm travel from the testes through a coiled tube, the epididymis, and another tube called the vas deferens. Sperm then pass into the seminal vesicle where semen is produced. Semen carries sperm out of the body.

The ducts coming from each seminal vesicle unite to form the ejaculatory ducts. They pass through the prostate gland, where more fluid is added to the semen. In the prostate, the ejaculatory ducts join the urethra, the tube through which both urine and semen pass. The urethra

continues through the penis, the sex organ located outside the body, in front of the scrotum. The penis is composed of erectile tissue that becomes filled with blood during sexual excitement. As the penis fills with blood, it becomes enlarged and erect. It then can enter the vagina, the female reproductive tract, where it releases semen containing sperm.

The Female Reproductive System

In the human female, the gonads are two oval glands called the ovaries. There is one ovary on each side of the uterus (Fig. 9-18). The ovaries make the female sex cells or eggs (ova). They release the female hormones, estrogen and progesterone. Each month, from puberty to menopause, an egg is released from an ovary. This cycle is maintained by estrogen and progesterone. These hormones control development of female secondary sex characteristics, which include the following:

- Increased breast size
- Wider and rounder hips
- Axillary and pubic hair
- A slightly deeper voice

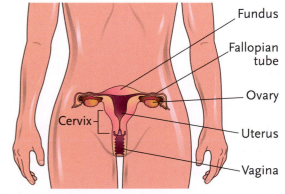

Fig. 9-18. *The female reproductive system.*

Once an egg is released from an ovary, it travels through the fallopian tube to the uterus. The uterus is a hollow, pear-shaped, muscular organ that is located within the pelvis. It lies behind the bladder and in front of the rectum. If sexual intercourse takes place while the egg is in the fallopian tube, the egg may be fertilized by sperm in the fallopian tube. The fertilized egg then travels down into the uterus. It implants in the endometrium, the lining of the uterus. Stimulated by hormones, the endometrium builds up during the menstrual cycle. It has many blood vessels supplying it for the growth and feeding of an embryo. If the egg is not fertilized, the hormones decrease. The blood supply to the endometrium decreases. The endometrium then breaks up in a process called menstruation.

The main section of the uterus is the fundus. This is where the fetus develops after the fertilized egg is implanted. The narrow neck of the uterus extending into the vagina is the cervix. The cervix has an opening through which menstrual fluid can pass and semen can enter the vagina.

The vagina is the muscular canal that opens to the outside of the body. The external vaginal opening is partially closed by the hymen membrane. The vagina is kept moist by secretions from glands in the vaginal walls. The vagina receives the penis during sexual intercourse. It also serves as the birth canal. The baby passes through the cervix, which is made thin by pressure from the baby's head during contractions. Once the cervix opens, the baby can then move out through the vagina.

For males, the function of the reproductive system is to manufacture sperm and the male hormone testosterone. For females, the reproductive system manufactures ova (eggs) and the female hormones estrogen and progesterone. It also provides an environment for the development of a fetus and produces milk for the nourishment of a baby after birth.

Normal changes of aging for males include the following:

- Sperm production decreases.
- Prostate gland enlarges, which can interfere with urination.

Normal changes of aging for females include the following:

- Menstruation ends. Menopause is the end of menstruation; it occurs when a woman has not had a menstrual period for 12 months.
- Decrease in estrogen may lead to a loss of calcium. This can cause brittle bones and, potentially, osteoporosis.
- Vaginal walls become drier and thinner.

How the NA Can Help

Sexual needs and desires continue as people age. The NA should provide privacy when necessary for sexual activity. The NA must respect residents' sexual needs and never judge any sexual behavior. However, any behavior that makes the NA uncomfortable or seems inappropriate should be reported. Inappropriate behavior is not a normal sign of aging and could be a sign of illness.

Observing and Reporting: Reproductive System

Observe and report these signs and symptoms:

- Discomfort or difficulty with urination
- Discharge from the penis or vagina
- Swelling of the genitals
- Blood in urine or stool
- Breast changes, including size, shape, lumps, or discharge from the nipple
- Sores on the genitals
- Redness or rash on the genitals
- Genital itching
- Resident reports erectile dysfunction (ED) (trouble getting or maintaining an erection)
- Resident reports painful intercourse

Residents' Rights

Sexual Expression and Privacy
Residents have the right to sexual freedom and expression. Residents have the right to privacy and to meet their sexual needs.

11. Describe the immune and lymphatic systems

The immune system protects the body from disease-causing bacteria, viruses, and microorganisms in two ways. **Nonspecific immunity** protects the body from disease in general. **Specific immunity** protects against a particular disease that is invading the body at a given time.

Nonspecific Immunity

To protect itself against disease in general, the body has several defenses:

- Anatomic barriers include the skin and the mucous membranes. They provide a physical barrier to keep foreign materials—bacteria, viruses, or microorganisms—from invading the body. Saliva, tears, and mucous secretions also help protect the body by washing away substances.

- Physiologic barriers include body temperature and acidity of certain organs. Most organisms that cause disease cannot survive high temperatures or high acidity. When the body senses foreign organisms, it can raise its temperature (by running a fever) to kill off the invaders. The acidity of organs like the stomach keeps harmful bacteria from growing there.

- Inflammatory response refers to the body's ability to fight infection through inflammation or swelling of an infected area. When inflammation occurs, it indicates that the body has sent extra disease-fighting cells and extra blood to the infected area to fight the infection.

Specific Immunity

To protect itself against specific diseases, the body makes different types of cells that will fight a range of different invaders. Once it has successfully eliminated an invader, the immune system records the invasion in the form of antibodies. Antibodies are carried within cells. They prevent a disease from threatening the body a second time.

Acquired immunity is a kind of specific immunity. The body acquires it either by fighting an infection or by vaccination. For example, a person can acquire immunity to a disease like the measles in two ways:

1. The person gets measles. His body forms antibodies to the disease to make sure he will not get it again; or

2. The person gets a vaccine for the measles. This causes his body to produce the same antibodies to protect him from the disease.

The lymphatic system removes excess fluids and waste products from the body's tissues. It also helps the immune system fight infection. It is closely related to both the immune and the circulatory systems. The lymphatic system consists of lymph vessels and lymph capillaries in which a fluid called lymph circulates (Fig. 9-19). **Lymph** is a clear yellowish fluid that carries disease-fighting cells called lymphocytes.

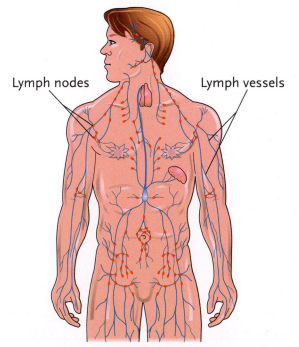

Lymph nodes   Lymph vessels

Fig. 9-19. *Lymph nodes work to fight infection and are located throughout the body.*

When the body is fighting an infection, swelling may occur in the lymph nodes. These are oval-shaped bodies that can be as small as a pinhead or as large as an almond. Located in the neck, groin, and armpits, the lymph nodes filter out germs and waste products carried from the tissues by the lymph fluid. After lymph fluid has been purified in the lymph nodes, it flows into the bloodstream.

Unlike the circulatory system, in which the heart functions as a pump to move the blood, the lymph system has no pump. Lymph fluid is circulated by muscle activity, massage, and breathing. A sore muscle may feel better if it is rubbed. The rubbing action helps the lymph fluid circulate, carrying waste products away from the tired muscle.

The functions of the immune and lymphatic systems are to protect the body against disease-causing bacteria, viruses, and microorganisms and to remove excess fluids and waste products from the body's tissues.

Normal changes of aging include the following:

- Immune system weakens, increasing the risk of all types of infections.

- It may take longer for a person to recover from an illness.

- Number and size of lymph nodes decrease, which results in body being less able to contract a fever to fight infection.

- Response to vaccines decreases.

How the NA Can Help

Factors that weaken the immune system include not getting enough sleep, poor nutrition, chronic illness, and stress. Preventing infection is important. The NA should wash her hands often and keep the resident's environment clean. She can help with personal hygiene as needed. Proper nutrition and fluid intake should be encouraged. A slight temperature increase may indicate that a resident is fighting an infection. The NA should measure vital signs accurately.

Observing and Reporting: Immune and Lymphatic Systems

Observe and report these signs and symptoms:

O/R Recurring infections (such as pneumonia, fevers, and diarrhea)

O/R Swelling of the lymph nodes

O/R Increased fatigue

Chapter Review

1. What is homeostasis?

2. What are three functions of the skin, or integument?

3. How many bones make up the skeleton of the human body?

4. What type of exercises can help prevent contractures and muscle atrophy?

5. What are two functions of the nervous system?

6. What are four functions of the circulatory system?

7. What does respiration mean? What are the two parts involved in respiration?

8. What are two functions of the urinary system?

9. What does digestion mean? What does absorption mean? What does elimination mean?

10. What are glands?

11. What is the function of the reproductive system?

12. What is nonspecific immunity? What is specific immunity?

13. What is the function of the lymphatic system?

10
Positioning, Transfers, and Ambulation

1. Review the principles of body mechanics

This chapter deals with how nursing assistants can safely position and move residents. Using proper body mechanics when assisting with positioning or moving helps prevent injury to both staff and residents. The following guidelines are a brief review of how to use proper body mechanics. Chapter 6 has more information.

Guidelines: Proper Body Mechanics

G   Assess the load. Before lifting, assess the weight of the load. Determine if you can safely move the person or object without help. Know the lift policies at your facility. Never attempt to lift someone you are not sure you can lift.

G   Think ahead, plan, and communicate the move. Check for any objects in your path. Look for any potential risks, such as a wet floor. Make sure the path is clear. Watch for hazards, like high-traffic areas, combative residents, or a loose toilet seat. Decide exactly what you are going to do together. Agree on the verbal cues you will use before attempting to move the resident.

G   Check your base of support and be sure you have firm footing. Use a wide but balanced stance to increase support. Keep this stance when walking. Have enough room to maintain a wide base of support. Make sure you and the resident are wearing nonskid shoes that are securely fastened.

G   Face what you are lifting. Your feet should always face the direction you are moving. This enables you to move your body as a unit and keeps your back straight. Do not twist; twisting at the waist increases the likelihood of injury. Turn and face the area you are moving the object to, then set the object down.

G   Keep your back straight. Keeping your head up and shoulders back will keep the back in the proper position. Taking a deep breath will help you regain correct posture.

G   Begin in a squatting position and lift with your legs. Bend at the hips and knees. Use the strength of your leg muscles to stand and lift the object. You will need to push your buttocks out to do this. Before you stand with the object you are lifting, remember that your legs, not your back, will enable you to lift. You should be able to feel your leg muscles as they work. Lift with the large leg muscles to decrease stress on the back.

G   Tighten your stomach muscles when beginning the lift. This will help to take weight off the spine and maintain alignment.

G   Keep the object close to your body. This decreases stress on your back. Lift objects only to your waist. Carrying them any higher can affect your balance.

G Push when possible rather than lifting. When you lift an object, you must overcome gravity to balance the load. When you push an object, you only need to overcome the friction between the surface and the object. Use your body weight to move the object, rather than your lifting muscles. Stay close to the object. Use both arms and tighten your stomach muscles.

2. Explain positioning and describe how to safely position residents

Residents who spend a lot of time in bed often need help getting into comfortable positions. They also need to change positions periodically to avoid muscle stiffness and skin breakdown. Too much pressure on one area for too long can cause a decrease in circulation, which can lead to pressure injuries and other problems like muscle contractures. (Chapter 13 contains information about pressure injuries and prevention guidelines.)

Positioning means helping residents into positions that promote comfort and health. Bed-bound residents should be repositioned at least every two hours. Residents in wheelchairs or chairs should be repositioned at least every hour. Each time there is a change of position, the nursing assistant should document the position and the time.

Which positions a resident uses depends on the diagnosis, the condition, and the resident's preference. The care plan will give specific positioning instructions. It is important to remember that even residents who are immobile must not remain in the position in which they are placed for long. They should be checked regularly. When positioning residents, nursing assistants must use proper body mechanics to help prevent injury. NAs should also check the skin for any problems such as whiteness, redness, or warm spots, especially around bony areas, each time they reposition residents.

The following are guidelines for positioning residents in the five basic body positions:

Supine: In this position, the resident lies flat on her back. To maintain correct body position, the head and shoulders should be supported with a pillow (Fig. 10-1). Pillows, rolled towels, or washcloths can also be used to support her arms (especially a weak or immobilized arm) or hands. A pillow should be placed under the calves so the heels are elevated ("floating"). Pillows or a footboard (padded board placed against the resident's feet) can keep the feet positioned properly.

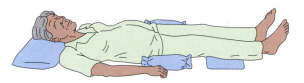

Fig. 10-1. A person in the supine position is lying flat on her back.

Lateral/side: A resident in the lateral position is lying on either side (Fig. 10-2). There are many variations of this position. Pillows can support the arm and leg on the upper side, the back, and the head. Ideally, the knee on the upper side of the body should be flexed. The leg is brought in front of the body and supported on a pillow. There should be a pillow under the bottom foot so that the toes and ankles are not touching the bed. If the top leg cannot be brought forward, it should be placed slightly behind the bottom leg, not resting directly on it. Pillows should be used between the two legs and ankles to relieve pressure and avoid skin breakdown.

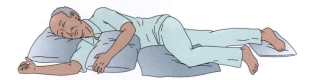

Fig. 10-2. A person in the lateral position is lying on his side.

Prone: A resident in the prone position is lying on the stomach, or front side of the body (Fig. 10-3). This is not comfortable for many people, especially elderly people. A nursing assistant should not leave a resident in the prone position for very long. In this position, the arms are either placed at the sides, raised above the head, or one is raised and one is by the side. The head is turned to one side. A small pillow may be used under the head and legs. This keeps the feet from touching the bed.

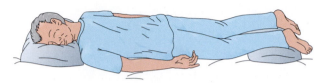

Fig. 10-3. A person lying in the prone position is lying on his stomach.

Fowler's: A resident in the Fowler's position is in a semi-sitting position (45 to 60 degrees) (Fig. 10-4). The head and shoulders are elevated. The resident's knees may be flexed and elevated using a pillow or rolled blanket as a support. The feet may be supported using a footboard or other support. The spine should be straight. In a high-Fowler's position, the upper body is sitting nearly straight up (60 to 90 degrees). In a semi-Fowler's position, the upper body is not raised as high (30 to 45 degrees).

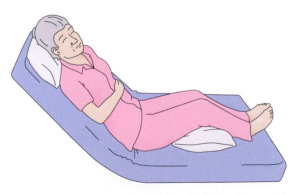

Fig. 10-4. A person in the Fowler's position is partially reclined.

Sims': The Sims' position is a left side-lying position (Fig. 10-5). The lower arm is behind the back, and the upper knee is flexed and raised toward the chest, using a pillow as support. There should be a pillow under the bottom foot so that the toes and ankle do not touch the bed.

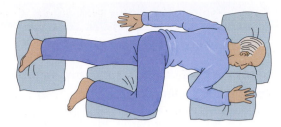

Fig. 10-5. A person in the Sims' position is lying on his left side with one leg drawn up.

Helping a resident move up in bed helps prevent skin irritation that can lead to pressure injuries. A nursing assistant should get help if she thinks it is not safe to move the resident by herself. A draw sheet, turning sheet, transfer sheet, or glide sheet should be used (Fig. 10-6). A **draw sheet** is an extra sheet placed on top of the bottom sheet when the bed is made. Draw sheets help prevent skin damage caused by shearing. **Shearing** is rubbing or friction that results from the skin moving one way and the bone underneath it remaining fixed or moving in the opposite direction. The draw sheet should lie flat under the resident's body and should not be wrinkled.

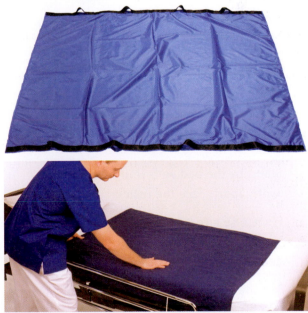

Fig. 10-6. There are different types of devices used for positioning and transferring. The top photo shows a glide sheet that is removed after use, while the bottom photo shows a draw sheet that can be left in place after the move or transfer is complete. (TOP PHOTO © MEDLINE INDUSTRIES, INC.)

Positioning, Transfers, and Ambulation

Moving a resident up in bed

Equipment: draw sheet or other device

When the resident can help you move her up in bed, take the following steps:

1. Identify yourself by name. Identify the resident by name.

2. Wash your hands.

3. Explain procedure to the resident. Speak clearly, slowly, and directly. Maintain face-to-face contact whenever possible.

4. Provide for the resident's privacy with curtain, screen, or door.

5. Adjust bed to a safe level, usually waist high. Lock bed wheels (Fig. 10-7).

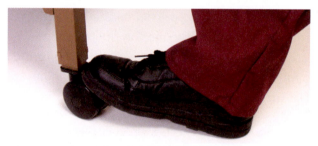

Fig. 10-7. Always lock bed wheels before positioning or transferring a resident.

6. Lower the head of the bed to make it flat. Move the pillow to the head of the bed.

7. If the bed has side rails, raise the rail on the far side of the bed.

8. Stand by the bed with your feet shoulder-width apart. Face the resident.

9. Place one arm under the resident's shoulder blades. Place the other arm under the resident's thighs. Use proper body mechanics.

10. Ask the resident to bend her knees, place her feet firmly on the mattress, and push with her feet and hands on the count of three.

11. On three, shift your body weight to help move the resident while she pushes with her feet (Fig. 10-8).

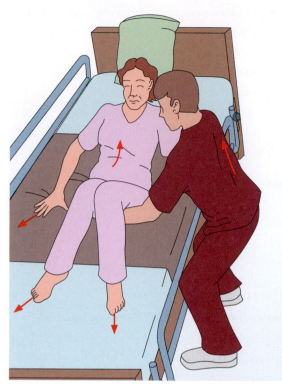

Fig. 10-8. Keep your back straight and your knees bent.

12. Make the resident comfortable. Put the pillow back under the resident's head and arrange the blankets for her.

13. Return bed to lowest position. Return side rails to ordered position. Remove privacy measures.

14. Place call light within resident's reach.

15. Wash your hands.

16. Report any changes in resident to the nurse. Document procedure using facility guidelines.

When you have help from another person, you can modify the procedure as follows:

1. Follow steps 1 through 6 above.

2. Stand on the opposite side of the bed from your helper. Each of you should be turned slightly toward the head of the bed. For each of you, the foot that is closest to the head of the bed should be pointed in that direction. Stand with your feet about shoulder-width apart. Bend your knees. Keep your back straight.

3. Roll the draw sheet up to the resident's side. Have your helper do the same on her side of the bed. Grasp the sheet with your palms up, and have your helper do the same.

4. Shift your weight to your back foot (the foot closer to the foot of the bed), and have your helper do the same (Fig. 10-9). On the count of three, you and your helper both shift your weight to the forward foot. Slide the draw sheet and resident toward the head of the bed.

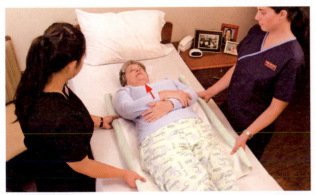

Fig. 10-9. *Both people shift their weight to their back foot and prepare to move.*

5. Make the resident comfortable. Put the pillow back under the resident's head and arrange the blankets for her. Unroll the draw sheet and leave it in place for the next repositioning (Fig. 10-10).

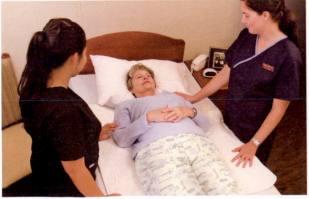

Fig. 10-10. *Unroll the draw sheet and leave it in place.*

6. Return bed to lowest position. Remove privacy measures.

7. Place call light within resident's reach.

8. Wash your hands.

9. Report any changes in resident to the nurse. Document procedure using facility guidelines.

Moving a resident to the side of the bed

Equipment: draw sheet

1. Identify yourself by name. Identify the resident by name.

2. Wash your hands.

3. Explain procedure to the resident. Speak clearly, slowly, and directly. Maintain face-to-face contact whenever possible.

4. Provide for the resident's privacy with curtain, screen, or door.

5. Adjust bed to a safe level, usually waist high. Lock bed wheels.

6. Lower the head of the bed.

7. Stand on the side of the bed to which you are moving the resident. Stand with feet shoulder-width apart, and bend your knees.

8. Gently slide your hands under the resident's head and shoulders and move them toward you (Fig. 10-11).

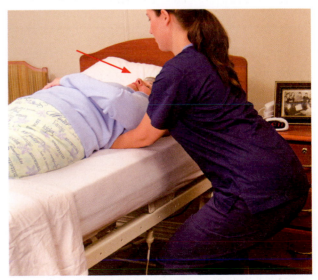

Fig. 10-11. *Gently move the resident's head and shoulders toward you.*

9. Gently slide your hands under the resident's midsection and move it toward you.

10. Gently slide your hands under the resident's hips and legs and move them toward you (Fig. 10-12).

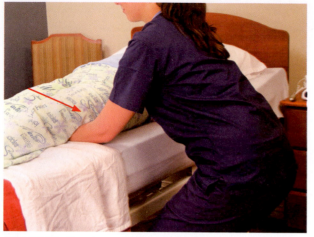

Fig. 10-12. *Gently move the resident's hips and legs toward you.*

11. Make the resident comfortable.

12. Return bed to lowest position. Remove privacy measures.

13. Place call light within resident's reach.

14. Wash your hands.

15. Report any changes in resident to the nurse. Document procedure using facility guidelines.

Residents may be turned on their sides in preparation for sitting up or to change position and to take pressure off their backs. This helps prevent skin irritation and pressure injuries.

Positioning a resident on the left side

1. Identify yourself by name. Identify the resident by name.

2. Wash your hands.

3. Explain procedure to the resident. Speak clearly, slowly, and directly. Maintain face-to-face contact whenever possible.

4. Provide for the resident's privacy with curtain, screen, or door.

5. Adjust bed to a safe level, usually waist high. Lock bed wheels.

6. Lower the head of the bed.

7. Move the resident toward the right side of the bed, using the previous procedure.

8. If the bed has side rails, raise the side rail on the left side of the bed.

9. Cross the resident's right arm over his chest. Move the left arm out of the way. Cross the right leg over the left leg.

10. Stand with feet shoulder-width apart. Bend your knees.

11. Place one hand on the resident's right shoulder. Place the other hand on the resident's right hip.

12. While supporting the body, gently roll the resident onto his left side as one unit, toward the raised side rail. (You may need to roll the resident toward you without using a raised side rail. In this scenario, you would use your body to block the resident to prevent him from rolling out of bed. Follow facility policy.)

13. Position the resident properly and comfortably. Proper positioning includes the following:

    - Head supported by a pillow (resident's face should not be obstructed by the pillow)

    - Shoulder adjusted so the resident is not lying on his arm or hand

    - Top arm supported by pillow

    - Back supported by supportive device

    - Top knee flexed

    - Supportive device between legs with top knee flexed; knee and ankle supported

• Pillow under bottom foot so that toes and ankle are not touching the bed

14. Return bed to lowest position. Return side rails to ordered position. Remove privacy measures.

15. Place call light within resident's reach.

16. Wash your hands.

17. Report any changes in resident to the nurse. Document procedure using facility guidelines.

Some residents' spinal columns must be kept in alignment. To turn these residents in bed, they have to be logrolled. **Logrolling** means moving a resident as a unit, without disturbing the alignment of the body. The head, back, and legs must be kept in a straight line. This is necessary in cases of neck or back problems, spinal cord injuries, or after back or hip surgeries. It is safer for two people to perform this procedure together. A draw sheet helps with moving.

Logrolling a resident

Equipment: draw sheet, coworker

1. Identify yourself by name. Identify the resident by name.

2. Wash your hands.

3. Explain procedure to the resident. Speak clearly, slowly, and directly. Maintain face-to-face contact whenever possible.

4. Provide for the resident's privacy with curtain, screen, or door.

5. Adjust bed to a safe level, usually waist high. Lock bed wheels.

6. Lower the head of the bed.

7. Both people stand on the same side of the bed. One person stands at the resident's head and shoulders. The other stands near the resident's midsection.

8. Place a pillow under the resident's head to support the neck during the move.

9. Place the resident's arms across his chest. Place a pillow between the knees.

10. Stand with your feet shoulder-width apart. Bend your knees.

11. Grasp the draw sheet on the far side (Fig. 10-13).

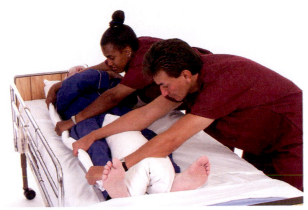

Fig. 10-13. *Both workers should grasp the draw sheet on the far side.*

12. On the count of three, gently roll the resident toward you. Turn the resident as a unit (Fig. 10-14). Use your bodies to block the resident to prevent him from rolling out of bed.

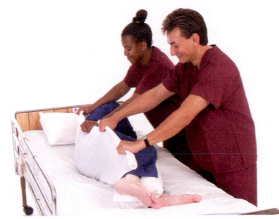

Fig. 10-14. *On the count of three, both workers should roll the resident toward them, turning the person as a unit.*

13. Make resident comfortable. Arrange pillows and covers for comfort.

14. Return bed to lowest position. Remove privacy measures.

15. Place call light within resident's reach.

16. Wash your hands.

17. Report any changes in resident to the nurse. Document procedure using facility guidelines.

Before a resident who has been lying down stands up, he should dangle. To **dangle** means to sit up on the side of the bed with the legs hanging over the side. This helps residents regain balance before standing up and allows blood pressure to stabilize. It helps prevent dizziness and lightheadedness that can cause fainting. For some residents who are unable to walk, sitting up and dangling the legs for a few minutes may be ordered in the care plan.

Assisting a resident to sit up on side of bed: dangling

1. Identify yourself by name. Identify the resident by name.

2. Wash your hands.

3. Explain procedure to the resident. Speak clearly, slowly, and directly. Maintain face-to-face contact whenever possible.

4. Provide for the resident's privacy with curtain, screen, or door.

5. Adjust bed to lowest position. Lock bed wheels.

6. Raise the head of bed to a sitting position. Fanfold (fold into pleats) the top covers to the foot of the bed. Ask the resident to turn onto his side, facing you. Assist as needed (see earlier procedure).

7. Tell the resident to reach across his chest with his top arm and place his hand on the edge of the bed near his opposite shoulder. Ask him to push down on that hand to raise his shoulders up while swinging his legs over the side of the bed (Fig. 10-15).

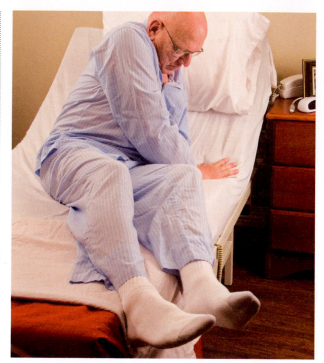

Fig. 10-15. Have the resident push himself up while swinging his legs over the side of the bed.

8. Always allow the resident to do all he can for himself. However, if the resident needs assistance, follow these steps:

a. Stand with your legs shoulder-width apart. Bend your knees. Keep your back straight.

b. Place one arm under the resident's shoulder blades. Place the other arm under the resident's thighs (Fig. 10-16).

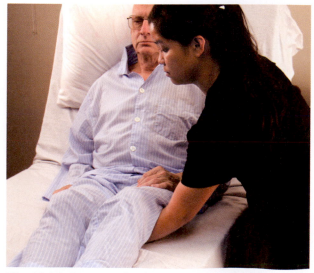

Fig. 10-16. One arm should be under the resident's shoulder blades and the other arm should be under the thighs.

c. On the count of three, slowly move the resident into a sitting position with the legs dangling over the side of the bed. The weight of the resident's legs hanging down from the bed helps the resident sit up (Fig. 10-17).

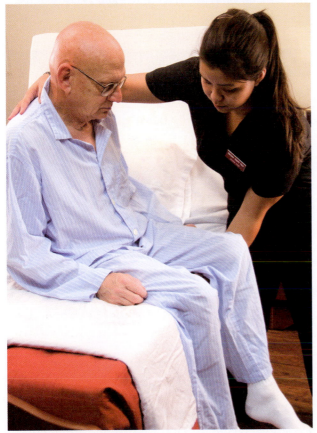

Fig. 10-17. The weight of the resident's legs hanging down from the bed helps the resident sit up.

9. Ask the resident to sit up as straight as possible and to hold onto the edge of the mattress with both hands. Help the resident to put on nonskid shoes or slippers if he is going to get out of bed.

10. Have the resident dangle as long as ordered. The care plan may direct you to allow the resident to dangle for several minutes and then assist him to lie down again, or it may direct you to allow the resident to dangle in preparation for walking or a transfer. Follow the care plan. Do not leave the resident alone. If the resident is dizzy for more than a minute, have him lie down again. Count his pulse and respiration rates and report to the nurse (you will learn how to measure vital signs in Chapter 14).

11. Remove slippers or shoes.

12. Gently assist the resident back into bed. Place one arm around the resident's shoulders and the other arm under his knees. Slowly swing the resident's legs onto the bed.

13. Make resident comfortable.

14. Leave bed in its lowest position. Remove privacy measures.

15. Place call light within resident's reach.

16. Wash your hands.

17. Report any changes in resident to the nurse. Document procedure using facility guidelines.

Residents' Rights

Positioning and Moving

When positioning and moving residents, nursing assistants should make sure residents are not unnecessarily exposed. They should be kept properly covered, dressed, or draped to protect their privacy and to promote dignity. NAs should pull the privacy curtain around the bed when moving residents in bed.

3. Describe how to safely transfer residents

Transferring a resident means that a nursing assistant is moving him from one place to another. Transfers can move residents from a bed to a chair or wheelchair, from a wheelchair to a shower or toilet, and so on.

Safety is one of the most important factors to consider during transfers. The Occupational Safety and Health Administration (OSHA, osha.gov) set specific ergonomic guidelines to help avoid injuries during transfers. **Ergonomics** is the science of designing equipment, areas, and work tasks to make them safer and to suit the worker's abilities. A person's back is more prone to injury. OSHA's ergonomic guidelines address ways to help avoid these work-related injuries. OSHA states that manual lifting and transferring of residents should be reduced and eliminated when possible. Manual lifting, transferring, and repositioning of residents may increase risk of injury.

To reduce the risk of injury, many facilities have adopted *no-lift, zero-lift,* or *lift-free* policies. These policies set strict guidelines for lifting and trans-ferring residents. Lift-free polices vary; facili-ties decide how they want to address the goal of reducing lifting and transferring of residents. Some do not allow any lifting at all and require that equipment always be used when lifting and moving residents.

The more restrictions placed on lifting, the less chance there is of injury. The amount and type of equipment available also factor into reduc-ing workplace injuries. This learning objective teaches procedures for manual lifting and trans-ferring of residents. It is important for nursing assistants to carefully follow facility policies on lifting and to use equipment properly. If NAs are unsure how to use equipment, they should ask for help and always get help when they need it.

A **transfer belt** is a safety device used to trans-fer residents who are weak, unsteady, or un-coordinated. It is called a **gait belt** when it is used to help residents walk. The belt is made of canvas or other heavy material. It has a buckle and sometimes has handles. It fits around the resident's waist, outside the clothing. It should never be placed on bare skin. It is important for the NA to check female residents to make sure their breasts are not caught under the belt.

The transfer belt is a safety device that gives the NA something firm to hold on to when assist-ing with transfers. The NA should grasp the belt securely on both sides, with hands in an upward position. Transfer belts cannot be used if a resi-dent has fragile bones, fractures, or has had cer-tain kinds of surgery recently.

Communicate!

Any time an NA helps a resident transfer, she should talk to the resident about what she would like to do. The NA can promote independence by letting the resident do what he can. The NA and resident must work together, especially during transfers.

Applying a transfer belt

Equipment: transfer belt, nonskid footwear

1. Identify yourself by name. Identify the resi-dent by name.

2. Wash your hands.

3. Explain procedure to the resident. Speak clearly, slowly, and directly. Maintain face-to-face contact whenever possible.

4. Provide for the resident's privacy with curtain, screen, or door.

5. Adjust bed to lowest position. Lock bed wheels.

6. Assist the resident to a sitting position with feet flat on the floor.

7. Put nonskid footwear on the resident and se-curely fasten.

8. Place the transfer belt over the resident's clothing and around the waist. Do not put it over bare skin.

9. Tighten the buckle until it is snug. Leave enough room to insert flat fingers/hand com-fortably under the belt.

10. Check to make sure that skin or skin folds (for example, breasts) are not caught under the belt.

11. Position the buckle slightly off-center in the front or back for comfort.

A **slide board**, or transfer board, may be used to transfer residents who are unable to bear weight on their legs. Slide boards can be used for al-most any transfer that involves moving from one sitting position to another (for example, from bed to chair) (Fig. 10-18). Slide boards should not be used against bare skin. Before beginning the transfer, the NA should make sure that the resident's fingers are not under the board.

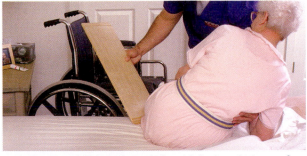

Fig. 10-18. *A slide board can help with bed-to-chair transfers.*

Guidelines: Wheelchairs

G   Learn how each wheelchair works. Residents may use manual (requiring human power to move) or electric wheelchairs. Know how to apply and release the brake and how to operate the armrests and footrests. Always lock a wheelchair before helping a resident into or out of it (Fig. 10-19). After a transfer, unlock the wheelchair.

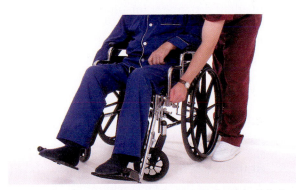

Fig. 10-19. *You must always lock the wheelchair before a resident gets into or out of it.*

G   To unfold a standard wheelchair, tilt the chair slightly to raise the wheels on the opposite side. Press down on one or both seat rails until the chair opens and the seat is flat. To fold a standard wheelchair, lift up under the center edge of the seat.

G   To remove an armrest, release the arm lock by the armrest, and lift the arm from the cen-

ter. To replace the armrest, simply reverse the procedure.

G   To move a footrest out of the way, press or pull the release lever. Swing the footrest out toward the side of the wheelchair. To remove the footrest, lift it off when it is toward the side of the wheelchair (Fig. 10-20). To replace a footrest, simply put it back in the side position, then swing it back to the front position. It should lock into place.

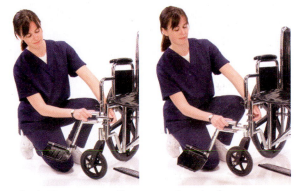

Fig. 10-20. *To remove a footrest, swing the footrest toward the side of the wheelchair and lift it off.*

G   To lift or lower a footrest, support the leg or foot. Squeeze the lever and pull up or push down.

G   To transfer to or from a wheelchair, the resident must use the side of the body that can bear weight to support and lift the side that cannot bear weight. Residents who can bear no weight with their legs may use leg braces or overhead trapezes to support themselves.

G   Before any transfer, make sure the resident is wearing nonskid footwear that is securely fastened. This promotes residents' safety and reduces the risk of falls.

G   During wheelchair transfers, make sure the resident is safe and comfortable. Ask the resident how you can help. Some may only want you to bring the chair to the bedside. Others may want you to be more involved. Always be sure the chair is as close as possible to the resident and is locked in place. Use a transfer belt if you are going to assist with the transfer. Be sure the transfer is done slowly, allowing time for the resident to rest. Upon standing, check to see if the resident is dizzy. If he is, help him sit back down. Measure vital signs as ordered and report to the nurse.

G   Check the resident's alignment in the chair once the transfer is complete. The resident's body must be in proper alignment while in a wheelchair or chair. Special cushions and pillows can be used for support. The hips should be well-positioned back in the chair. If the resident needs to be moved back in the wheelchair, lock wheelchair wheels. Stand in front of the wheelchair and ask the resident to grasp the armrests while his feet are flat on the floor. Brace one or both knees against the resident's knee(s). On the count of three, ask the resident to push with his feet into the floor and move himself toward the back of the chair. Gently assist as needed.

G   When a resident is in a wheelchair or any chair, he or she should be repositioned at least every hour. The reasons for doing this are as follows:

- It promotes comfort.
- It reduces pressure.
- It increases circulation.
- It exercises the joints.
- It promotes muscle tone.

Falls

If a resident starts to fall during a transfer or while walking, the NA should do the following:

- Widen her stance
- Bring the resident's body close to her to break the fall
- Bend her knees and support the resident as she lowers the resident to the floor
- If necessary, the NA can drop to the floor with the resident to avoid injury to herself or the resident

The NA should not try to reverse or stop a fall because she or the resident can suffer worse injuries if she tries to stop, rather than break, a fall. If a resident has fallen, the NA should call for help. She should not try to get the resident up after the fall.

Some residents have one-sided weakness due to paralysis or stroke. When transferring a resident with one-sided weakness, the NA should move the stronger side first. The weaker (also called *involved* or *affected*) side follows.

Transferring a resident from bed to wheelchair

Equipment: wheelchair, transfer belt, nonskid footwear, and robe or folded blanket

1. Identify yourself by name. Identify the resident by name.

2. Wash your hands.

3. Explain procedure to the resident. Speak clearly, slowly, and directly. Maintain face-to-face contact whenever possible.

4. Provide for the resident's privacy with curtain, screen, or door. Check the area to be certain it is uncluttered and safe.

5. Place the wheelchair at the head of the bed, facing the foot of the bed, or at the foot of the bed, facing the head of the bed. The arm of the wheelchair should be almost touching the bed. The wheelchair should be placed on the resident's stronger, or unaffected, side.

6. Remove both wheelchair footrests close to the bed.

7. Lock wheelchair wheels.

8. Raise the head of the bed. Adjust bed to lowest position. Lock bed wheels.

9. Assist the resident to sitting position with feet flat on the floor. Let resident sit for a few minutes to adjust to the change in position.

10. Put nonskid footwear on the resident and fasten securely.

11. Stand in front of the resident with your feet about shoulder-width apart. Bend your knees. Keep your back straight.

12. Place the transfer belt around the resident's waist over clothing (not on bare skin).

Tighten the buckle until it is snug. Grasp the belt securely on both sides, with hands in an upward position.

13. Provide instructions to allow the resident to help with the transfer. Instructions may include: "When you start to stand, push with your hands against the bed." "Once standing, if you're able, you can take small steps in the direction of the chair." "Once standing, reach for the chair with your stronger hand."

14. With your legs, brace (support) the resident's lower legs to prevent slipping (Fig. 10-21). This can be done by placing one or both of your knees against the resident's knees.

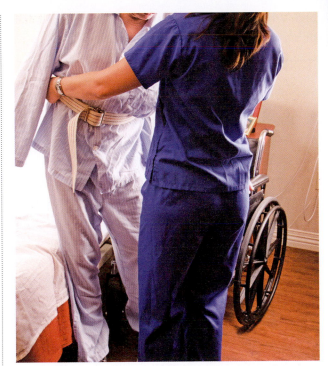

Fig. 10-22. Help the resident pivot to the front of the wheelchair. Pivoting is safer than twisting.

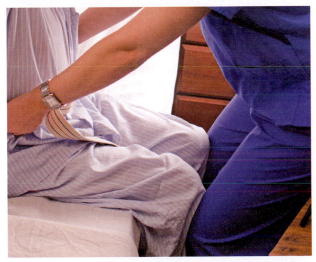

Fig. 10-21. Brace the resident's lower legs to prevent slipping by placing either one or two knees (shown) against the resident's knees.

15. Count to three to alert the resident. If possible, have the resident rock while counting to three. On three, with hands still grasping the transfer belt on both sides and moving upward, slowly help the resident to stand.

16. Tell the resident to take small steps in the direction of the wheelchair while turning his back toward the chair. If more help is needed, help the resident pivot (turn) to stand in front of the wheelchair with the back of the resident's legs against the wheelchair (Fig. 10-22). Always allow the resident to do all he can for himself.

17. Ask the resident to put his hands on the wheelchair armrests if he is able. When the chair is touching the back of the resident's legs, help him lower himself into the chair.

18. Reposition the resident so that his hips touch the back of the wheelchair seat.

19. Attach footrests and place the resident's feet on the footrests. Check that the resident is in proper alignment. Gently remove the transfer belt. Make resident comfortable. Place a robe or folded blanket over the resident's lap as appropriate.

20. Remove privacy measures.

21. Place call light within resident's reach.

22. Wash your hands.

23. Report any changes in resident to the nurse. Document procedure using facility guidelines.

When transferring back to bed from a wheelchair, the height of the bed should be equal to or slightly lower than the chair. Help the resident pivot to the

Positioning, Transfers, and Ambulation

bed. When the resident feels the bed with the back of his legs, help him sit down slowly.

Stretchers

A stretcher, also called a *gurney*, is a medical device used to move injured or ill persons from one place to another. Stretchers may be used for serious injuries and illnesses and/or when a person cannot or should not walk but needs to be transported somewhere. Stretchers transfer residents within facilities or to other facilities.

Guidelines: Safe Use of Stretchers

G Lock the stretcher's wheels before transferring a resident onto or off of a stretcher.

G Secure the resident with the safety belts while in the stretcher.

G Raise the safety rails.

G Cover the resident with a sheet. Hands, feet, fingers, etc., should remain inside the sheet during transport.

G Keep the wheels locked at all times except when moving the stretcher.

G Get help if you cannot move the stretcher alone.

G Move slowly and carefully.

G Push the stretcher from the head end.

G Go through doorways by opening the door, entering first, and pulling the stretcher through.

G Avoid hitting walls or doorways.

G Be cautious going down sloping areas.

G Stay with the resident at all times.

A draw sheet is used to transfer a resident to a stretcher. The procedure below shows how to transfer a resident to a stretcher from a bed using four staff members. At least three people are necessary to safely transfer a resident to a stretcher.

Transferring a resident from bed to stretcher

Equipment: stretcher, blanket, draw sheet

1. Identify yourself by name. Identify the resident by name.

2. Wash your hands.

3. Explain procedure to the resident. Speak clearly, slowly, and directly. Maintain face-to-face contact whenever possible.

4. Provide for the resident's privacy with curtain, screen, or door.

5. Lower the head of bed so that it is flat. Lock bed wheels.

6. Fold linens to the foot of the bed. Cover the resident with a blanket.

7. Move the resident to the side of the bed. Have your coworkers help you do this. Refer to the procedure *Moving a resident to the side of the bed* earlier in this chapter.

8. Place the stretcher solidly against the bed, and lock stretcher wheels. Bed height should be equal to or slightly above the height of the stretcher. Move the stretcher's safety belts out of the way.

9. Two workers should be on one side of the bed opposite the stretcher. Two more workers should be on the other side of the stretcher.

10. Each worker should roll up the sides of the draw sheet and prepare to move the resident (Fig. 10-23). Protect the resident's arms and legs during the transfer.

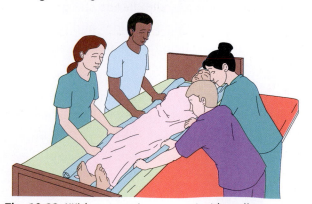

Fig. 10-23. *With two workers on each side, roll up the sides of the draw sheet and prepare to move the resident.*

11. On the count of three, the workers lift and move the resident to the stretcher. All should move at once. Make sure the resident is centered on the stretcher (Fig. 10-24).

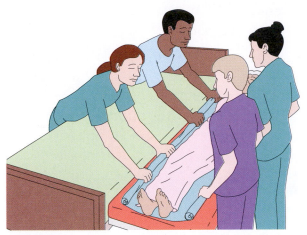

Fig. 10-24. *On the count of three, all workers should lift and move at once.*

12. Raise the head of the stretcher or place a pillow under the resident's head. Make sure the resident is still covered with the blanket.

13. Secure the safety straps across the resident. Raise side rails on the stretcher.

14. Unlock the stretcher's wheels. Move the resident to the proper place, staying with him until another staff member takes over.

15. Wash your hands.

16. Report any changes in resident to the nurse. Document procedure using facility guidelines.

To return the resident to bed, the bed height should be equal to or slightly below the stretcher.

Mechanical Lifts

Facilities often have mechanical (also called *hydraulic, power,* or *standing*) lifts available to transfer residents. This equipment helps prevent injury to residents and staff members. Nursing assistants may assist residents with many types of transfers using a mechanical or hydraulic lift. Using these lifts requires special training. Nursing assistants should not use equipment they have not been trained to use, as doing this could cause injury.

There are many different types of mechanical lifts (Fig. 10-25). Using these devices helps prevent common workplace injuries and may be mandatory at facilities that have no-lift policies. Nursing assistants should always ask for help if there is anything that they do not understand about the provided lift equipment.

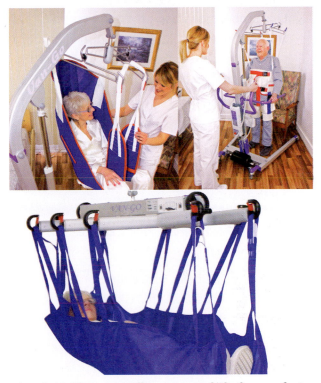

Fig. 10-25. *There are different types of lifts for transferring both completely dependent residents and residents who can bear some weight.* (PHOTOS COURTESY OF VANCARE INC., VANCARE.COM, 800-694-4525)

Guidelines: Mechanical or Hydraulic Lifts

G   Be careful when moving a resident using a mechanical lift. Have another person assist you when transferring with these lifts. It is safer for at least two people to do these types of transfers.

G   Keep the chair to which the resident is to be moved close to the bed so that the resident is only moved a short distance in the lift.

G   Check that the valves on the lift are working before using it.

G Use the correct sling for the lift that is being used. Using an incorrect sling may result in serious injury or death. If you have questions about the sling, talk to the nurse.

G Check the sling and straps for any fraying or tears. Do not use the lift if there are tears or holes.

G Open the legs of the stand to the widest position before helping the resident into the lift.

G Once the resident is in the sling and the straps are connected, pump up the lift only to the point where the resident's body clears the bed or chair.

G Electric/battery-powered lifts have emergency releases. Be aware of where the release is located and how to operate this function. Talk to the nurse if you do not know how to do this.

Transferring a resident using a mechanical lift

Equipment: wheelchair or chair, coworker, mechanical or hydraulic lift

The following is a basic procedure for transferring using a mechanical lift. Ask someone to help you before starting.

1. Identify yourself by name. Identify the resident by name.

2. Wash your hands.

3. Explain procedure to the resident. Speak clearly, slowly, and directly. Maintain face-to-face contact whenever possible.

4. Provide for the resident's privacy with curtain, screen, or door.

5. Lock bed wheels.

6. Position wheelchair next to bed. Lock brakes.

7. Help the resident turn to one side of the bed. Position the sling under the resident, with the edge next to the resident's back. Fanfold if necessary. Adjust the bottom of the sling so that it is even with the resident's knees. Help the resident roll back to the middle of the bed, and then spread out the fanfolded edge of the sling.

8. Roll the mechanical lift to bedside. Make sure the base is opened to its widest point. Push the base of the lift under the bed.

9. Position the overhead bar directly over the resident (Fig. 10-26).

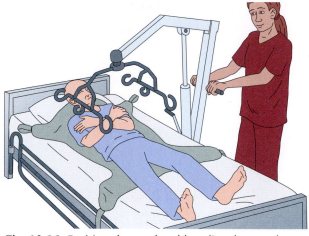

Fig. 10-26. *Position the overhead bar directly over the resident.*

10. With the resident lying on his back, attach one set of straps to each side of the sling. Attach one set of straps to the overhead bar. If available, have a coworker support the resident's head, shoulders, and knees while being lifted. The resident's arms should be folded across his chest (Fig. 10-27). If the device has S hooks, they should face away from the resident. Make sure all straps are connected properly and are smooth and straight.

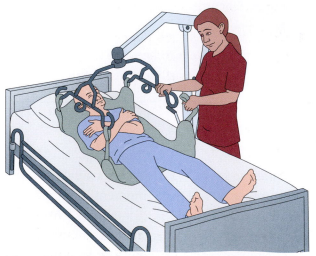

Fig. 10-27. *With the resident's arms folded across his chest, attach the straps to the sling.*

11. Following manufacturer's instructions, raise the resident two inches above the bed. Pause a moment for the resident to gain balance.

12. If available, a lifting partner can help support and guide the resident's body while you roll the lift so that the resident is positioned over the chair or wheelchair (Fig. 10-28).

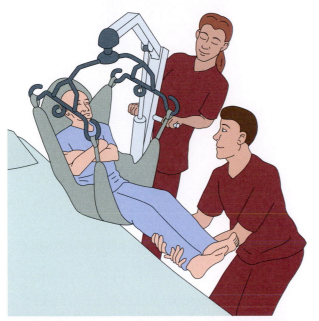

Fig. 10-28. Having another person help to support and guide the resident promotes safety during the transfer and lessens the chance of injury.

13. Slowly lower the resident into the chair or wheelchair. Push down gently on the resident's knees to help the resident into a sitting, rather than reclining, position.

14. Undo the straps from the overhead bar to the sling. Remove sling or leave in place for transfer back to bed.

15. Be sure the resident is seated comfortably and correctly in the chair or wheelchair. Remove privacy measures.

16. Place call light within resident's reach.

17. Wash your hands.

18. Report any changes in resident to the nurse. Document procedure using facility guidelines.

A stand-up, or standing, lift is used when a person can bear some weight on his legs, but has poor leg strength and/or balance (Fig. 10-25, image at top right). The resident must be able to stand and have some arm strength in order to use this lift. There are different types of stand-up lifts, including manual and battery-powered. The stand-up lift consists of both user and operator support bars (the user support bars may consist of two vertical bars or one crossbar), padded swivel swing-out seats (and/or straps, vest, or belt for some models), knee pads, a platform base with foot plate, and four small wheels with locking brakes.

If using a stand-up lift, the nursing assistant should be sure that the brakes are locked before beginning the transfer. The resident should begin in a sitting position and place his feet firmly on the foot plate of the platform, with knees pressing against the knee pads. The resident should grasp the support bar(s) and gently pull himself to a standing position, using his own strength. Then the NA can lower both sides of the padded swing-out seat into position. The NA should adjust straps, vest, or belt if these are used. The resident should slowly lower himself onto the seat while holding the support bars and pressing knees against knee pads. The NA should unlock the wheel brakes and use the operator bars to transfer the resident to the location desired and then perform these steps in reverse order to release the resident from the lift.

Toilet Transfers

The bladder empties more efficiently when a person is able to use the toilet. This is due to the person's position over the toilet. In order to use the toilet, residents must be able to bear some weight on their legs.

Nursing assistants should offer trips to the bathroom often and respond to call lights quickly. Chapter 16 has more information on bedpan and urinal use.

Transferring a resident onto and off of a toilet

Equipment: 2 pairs of gloves, toilet paper or disposable wipes, transfer belt, wheelchair

1. Identify yourself by name. Identify the resident by name.

2. Wash your hands.

3. Explain procedure to the resident. Speak clearly, slowly, and directly. Maintain face-to-face contact whenever possible. Make sure the resident is wearing nonskid shoes.

4. Provide for the resident's privacy with curtain, screen, or door.

5. Position the wheelchair at a right angle to the toilet to face the hand bar/wall rail. Place wheelchair on the resident's stronger side.

6. Remove wheelchair footrests. Lock wheels.

7. Put on gloves.

8. Apply a transfer belt around the resident's waist over clothing (not on bare skin). Grasp belt securely on both sides, with hands in an upward position.

9. Ask the resident to push against the armrests of the wheelchair and stand, reaching for and grasping the hand bar with her stronger arm. Move wheelchair out of the way (Fig. 10-29).

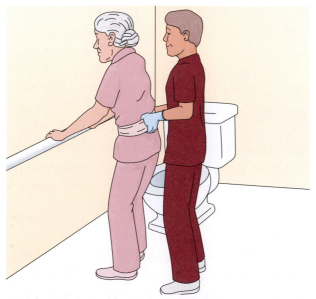

Fig. 10-29. The resident should be standing while grasping the hand bar for support.

10. Ask the resident to pivot her foot and back up so that she can feel the front of the toilet with the back of her legs (Fig. 10-30).

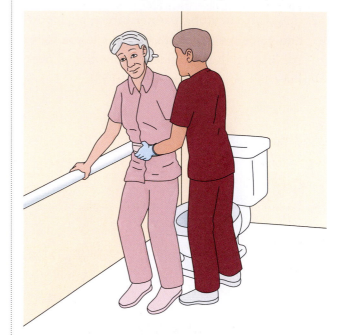

Fig. 10-30. Have the resident pivot and feel the toilet with the back of her legs. Assist as needed.

11. Help the resident to pull down pants and underwear. You may need to keep one hand on the transfer belt while helping to remove clothing.

12. Help the resident slowly sit down onto the toilet. Ask her to pull the emergency cord if she needs help. Remove and discard gloves. Wash your hands. Leave the bathroom and close the door.

13. When called, return and wash your hands. Don clean gloves. Assist with perineal care as necessary (Chapter 13). Ask the resident to stand and reach for the hand bar.

14. Use disposable wipes to clean the resident. Make sure she is clean and dry before pulling up clothing. Remove and discard gloves.

15. Help the resident to the sink to wash her hands.

16. Wash your hands.

17. Help the resident back into the wheelchair. Be sure the resident is seated comfortably

and correctly in the wheelchair. Remove transfer belt. Replace footrests.

18. Help the resident to leave the bathroom. Make sure resident is comfortable. Remove privacy measures.

19. Place call light within resident's reach.

20. Wash your hands again.

21. Report any changes in resident to the nurse. Document procedure using facility guidelines.

Vehicle Transfers

When a resident is leaving a facility, he or she may need help getting into a vehicle. The front seat is wider and is usually easier to get into.

Transferring a resident into a vehicle

Equipment: wheelchair

1. Identify yourself by name. Identify the resident by name.

2. Wash your hands.

3. Explain procedure to the resident. Speak clearly, slowly, and directly. Maintain face-to-face contact whenever possible.

4. Place wheelchair close to the vehicle at a 45-degree angle. Open the door on the resident's stronger side if possible.

5. Lock wheelchair wheels.

6. Ask the resident to push against the armrests of the wheelchair to stand, grasp the vehicle, and pivot his foot so the side of the seat touches the back of his legs.

7. The resident should then sit in the seat and lift one leg, and then the other, into the vehicle (Fig. 10-31). Assist as needed.

8. Carefully position the resident comfortably in the vehicle. Help fasten seat belt.

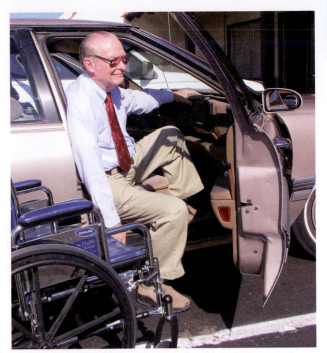

Fig. 10-31. *After the resident sits in the vehicle seat, he should put his legs in one at a time.*

9. Safely shut the door.

10. Return the wheelchair to the appropriate place for cleaning.

11. Wash your hands.

12. Document procedure using facility guidelines.

4. Discuss how to safely ambulate residents

Ambulation means walking. A resident who is **ambulatory** is one who can get out of bed and walk. Many older residents are ambulatory, but need assistance to walk safely. Several tools, including gait belts, canes, walkers, and crutches, assist with ambulation.

The nursing assistant should check the care plan before helping a resident ambulate. It is important to know the resident's abilities, limitations, and disabilities. Any time an NA helps a resident, she should communicate what she would like to do and allow the resident to do what he can.

Assisting a resident to ambulate

Equipment: gait belt, nonskid shoes for resident

1. Identify yourself by name. Identify the resident by name.

2. Wash your hands.

3. Explain procedure to resident. Speak clearly, slowly, and directly. Maintain face-to-face contact whenever possible.

4. Provide for resident's privacy with curtain, screen, or door.

5. Adjust bed to its lowest position so that the feet are flat on the floor. Lock bed wheels.

6. Before ambulating, put nonskid footwear on the resident and fasten securely.

7. Stand in front of and face the resident. Stand with your feet about shoulder-width apart. Bend your knees. Keep your back straight.

8. Place the gait belt around the resident's waist over his clothing (not on bare skin). Grasp belt securely on both sides, with hands in an upward position.

9. Always allow the resident to do whatever he is able to do for himself. If the resident is unable to stand without help, brace (support) the resident's lower extremities. This can be done by placing one of your knees against the resident's knee, or it can also be done by placing both of your knees against both of the resident's knees (Fig. 10-32). Bend your knees. Keep your back straight.

10. Hold the resident close to your center of gravity. Provide instructions to allow the resident to help with standing. Tell the resident to lean forward, push down on the bed with his hands, and stand on the count of three. When you start to count, begin to rock. On three, with hands still grasping the gait belt on both sides and moving upward, rock your weight onto your back foot and slowly help the resident to stand.

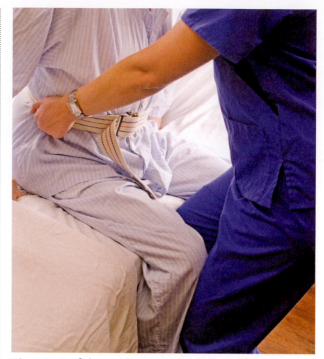

Fig. 10-32. *If the resident has a weak knee, brace it against your knee.*

11. Walk slightly behind and to one side of the resident for the full distance, while holding on to the gait belt (Fig. 10-33). If the resident has a weaker side, stand on the weaker side. Use the hand that is not holding the belt to offer support on the weak side. Ask the resident to look forward, not down at the floor, during ambulation.

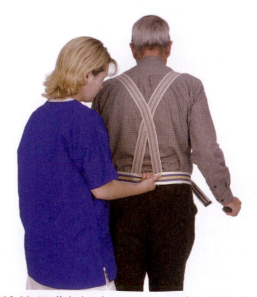

Fig. 10-33. *Walk behind and stand on the resident's weaker side, while holding onto the gait belt, when assisting with ambulation.*

12. Observe the resident's strength while you walk together. Provide a chair if the resident becomes dizzy or tired.

13. After ambulation, remove the gait belt. Help resident to the bed or chair and check that the resident is in proper alignment. Make resident comfortable.

14. Leave bed in its lowest position. Remove privacy measures.

15. Place call light within resident's reac'.

16. Wash your hands.

17. Report any changes in resident to nurse. Document procedure using facility guidelines.

When helping a resident who is visually impaired walk, the NA should let the resident walk beside and slightly behind her as he rests a hand on the NA's elbow. The NA should walk at a normal pace. She should let the resident know when they are about to turn a corner, or when a step is approaching, and whether they will be stepping up or down.

Residents who have difficulty walking may use adaptive or assistive devices, such as canes, walkers, or crutches to help themselves. Canes help with balance. Residents using canes should be able to bear weight on both legs. If one leg is weaker, the cane should be held in the hand on the stronger side.

Types of canes include the C cane, the functional grip cane, and the quad cane. The **C cane** is a straight cane with a curved handle at the top. It has a rubber-tipped bottom to prevent slipping. A C cane is used to improve balance. A **functional grip cane** is similar to the C cane, except that it has a straight grip handle rather than a curved handle. The grip handle helps improve grip control and provides a little more support than the C cane. A **quad cane**, with four rubber-tipped feet and a rectangular base, is designed to bear more weight than the other canes (Fig. 10-34).

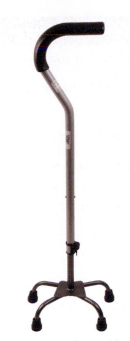

Fig. 10-34. A quad cane has four rubber-tipped feet and can bear more weight than other canes.

A **walker** is a type of walking aid used when the resident can bear some weight on both legs. The walker provides stability for residents who are unsteady or lack balance. The metal frame of the walker may have rubber-tipped feet and/or wheels (Fig. 10-35). Other types of walkers are designed with a seat in the back to allow a person to rest during ambulation (Fig. 10-36). The walker is moved first, then the weak leg, then the stronger leg.

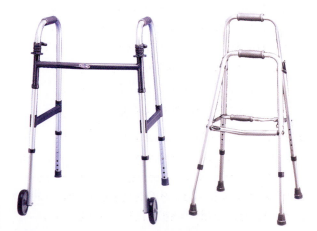

Fig. 10-35. The photo on the left shows a standard walker, and the photo on the right shows a "Hemi Walker," which is designed for people who have difficulty using an arm or a hand. (© INVACARE CORPORATION. USED WITH PERMISSION. WWW.INVACARE.COM)

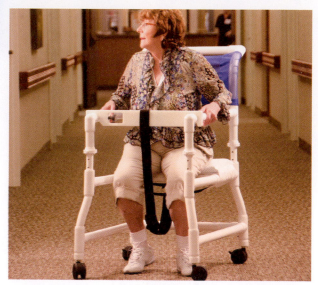

Fig. 10-36. There are different types of walkers. This type has a posterior seat to allow the person to sit and rest when necessary.

Crutches are used by residents who can bear no weight or limited weight on one leg. Crutches have rubber-tipped feet to prevent sliding. Some people use one crutch, and some use two.

Whichever device is being used, the nursing assistant's role is to ensure safety. The NA should stay near the resident, on the weaker side. The equipment must be in proper condition. It should be sturdy, and it must have rubber tips or wheels on the bottom.

Guidelines: Cane or Walker Use

G Be sure the walker or cane is in good condition. It must have rubber tips on the bottom. The tips should not be cracked. Walkers may have wheels. If so, roll the walker to make sure the wheels are moving properly.

G Be sure the resident is wearing securely fastened, nonskid shoes before ambulating.

G When using a cane, the resident should place it on his stronger side.

G When using a walker, have the resident place both hands on the walker. The walker should not be overextended; it should be placed no more than six inches in front of the resident.

G Stay near the resident on the weaker side.

G Do not hang purses or clothing on the walker.

G If the height of the cane or walker does not appear to be correct (too short, too tall, etc.), inform the nurse.

Assisting with ambulation for a resident using a cane, walker, or crutches

Equipment: gait belt, nonskid shoes for the resident, cane, walker, or crutches

1. Identify yourself by name. Identify resident by name.

2. Wash your hands.

3. Explain procedure to resident. Speak clearly, slowly, and directly. Maintain face-to-face contact whenever possible.

4. Provide for resident's privacy with curtain, screen, or door.

5. Adjust bed to lowest position so that the feet are flat on the floor. Lock bed wheels.

6. Before ambulating, put nonskid footwear on the resident and fasten securely.

7. Stand in front of and face the resident. Stand with your feet about shoulder-width apart. Bend your knees. Keep your back straight.

8. Place the gait belt around the resident's waist over clothing (not on bare skin). Grasp belt securely on both sides, with hands in an upward position.

9. If the resident is unable to stand without help, brace (support) the resident's lower extremities. This can be done by placing one of your knees against the resident's knee or by placing both of your knees against both of the resident's knees. Bend your knees. Keep your back straight. Help the resident to stand as described in the previous procedure.

10. Help as needed with ambulation.

a. **Cane**: Resident places the cane about six inches, or a comfortable distance, in front of his stronger leg. He brings his weaker leg even with the cane. He then brings his stronger leg forward slightly ahead of the cane (Fig. 10-37). Repeat.

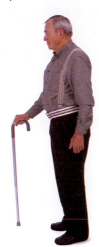

Fig. 10-37. The cane moves in front of the stronger leg first.

b. **Walker**: Resident picks up or rolls the walker and places it about six inches, or a comfortable distance, in front of him. All four feet or wheels of the walker should be on the ground before the resident steps forward to the walker. The walker should not be moved again until the resident has moved both feet forward and is steady (Fig. 10-38). The resident should never put his feet ahead of the walker.

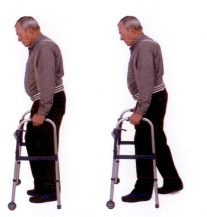

Fig. 10-38. The walker can be moved after the resident is steady and both feet are forward.

c. **Crutches**: Resident should be fitted for crutches and taught to use them correctly by a physical therapist or a nurse. The resident may use the crutches several different ways, depending on his weakness. No matter how they are used, the resident's weight should be on his hands and arms. Weight should not be on the underarm area (Fig. 10-39).

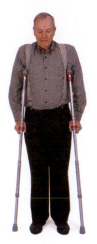

Fig. 10-39. When using crutches, weight should be on the hands and arms, not on the underarms.

11. Walk slightly behind and to one side of the resident for the full distance, while holding on to the gait belt. If the resident has a weaker side, stand on the weaker side.

12. Watch for obstacles in the resident's path. Ask the resident to look forward, not down at the floor, during ambulation.

13. Encourage the resident to rest if he is tired. When a person is tired, it increases the chance of a fall. Let the resident set the pace. Discuss how far he plans to go based on the care plan.

14. After ambulation, remove the gait belt. Help the resident to the bed or chair and check that the resident is in proper alignment. Make resident comfortable.

15. Leave bed in its lowest position. Remove privacy measures.

16. Place call light within resident's reach.

17. Wash your hands.

18. Report any changes in resident to nurse. Document procedure using facility guidelines.

Chapter Review

1. List nine guidelines for using proper body mechanics.

2. What is positioning?

3. How often should bedbound residents be repositioned?

4. In which position is a resident lying on his side?

5. In which position is a resident lying on his stomach?

6. In which position is a resident lying flat on his back?

7. In which position is a resident lying on his left side with the lower arm behind the back and the upper knee flexed and raised toward the chest?

8. In which position is a resident in a semi-sitting position (45 to 60 degrees) with the head and shoulders elevated?

9. What is a draw sheet?

10. What is shearing?

11. When is logrolling necessary?

12. How does dangling benefit a resident?

13. Describe how a transfer belt is applied.

14. Before helping a resident into or out of a wheelchair, what should a nursing assistant do?

15. If a resident has a weaker side, which side should move first in a transfer—the weaker or stronger side?

16. When may stretchers be used for residents?

17. List five guidelines for using a mechanical lift.

18. What is one benefit of using the toilet rather than a bedpan or urinal?

19. Define ambulation.

20. What is the purpose of canes?

21. How many feet does a quad cane have?

22. Which type of adaptive device for walking can be used when a resident can bear no weight on one leg—cane, walker, or crutches?

23. Which side should a nursing assistant stand near when a resident is using adaptive equipment—the weaker or stronger side?

11

Admitting, Transferring, and Discharging

1. Describe how residents may feel when entering a facility

Chapter 8 described some of the many feelings residents may be having as they make the transition into a care facility. Losses such as the loss of a familiar environment or the loss of independence can cause a person to feel scared, angry, sad, lonely, worried, helpless, or depressed. A new resident may yell at caregivers or may cry often. He may refuse to join in activities and want to be left alone. A new resident may want to talk to staff members as much as possible until he becomes more comfortable. These are just a few of the ways that new residents may show their emotions.

Moving always requires an adjustment, but as a person ages, it can be even harder (Fig. 11-1). This is especially true if illness, disability, and/or mobility problems are present. Perhaps at age 50 a new resident started living alone as his children left the house. Then he lived alone, happily, for 20 years before having a stroke. He was no longer able to live alone safely, and his children did not live nearby to help him with his daily care. Living with his children was not an option, so he had to move into a care facility. He might feel worried and scared because he has never known any other home than the one he lived in for so many years. He might feel angry or depressed about moving into a new place filled with people he does not know. When independence is restricted and health declines, people are faced with difficult decisions about care. Moving into a facility is not an easy choice to make, and it is important for staff to remember this and empathize with residents.

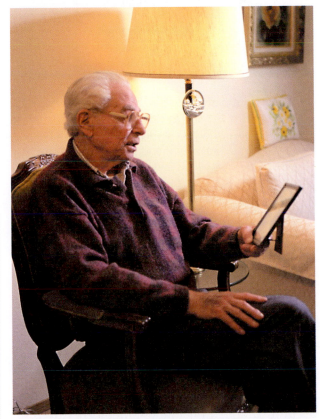

Fig. 11-1. *A new resident must leave familiar places and things. He may have just lost someone very close to him. He may be experiencing other losses as well. Nursing assistants should be supportive and welcoming.*

Nursing assistants play an important role in helping residents make a successful transition to long-term care facilities. By giving emotional support such as listening, as well as being kind, compassionate, and helpful, NAs can help residents feel better about their new homes. Guidelines for assisting new residents are found in the next learning objective.

Residents' Rights

New LGBTQ Residents

Entering a long-term care facility can be especially difficult for residents who are lesbian, gay, bisexual, transgender, or queer (LGBTQ). In addition to the challenges all residents face when giving up the independence of living in their own homes, these residents may fear that they will not be accepted by staff or other residents. They may worry that their partners will not receive the same welcome the spouse or partner of a heterosexual resident would receive.

In addition, paperwork, such as the admission form, is usually written with the assumption that a resident is heterosexual. If a resident is not legally married but has a partner of the same gender, there may be no way for him to indicate this on the form. Staff can help residents by asking questions like, "Who is important in your life?"

More and more communities are recognizing aging issues specific to LGBTQ elders. Organizations offering training to workers may exist in the community. A nursing assistant might suggest to a supervisor that staff at her facility receive such training. It is essential that NAs not judge residents. Every resident deserves professional, caring service from facility staff. The facility is the resident's home, and all staff members should make every effort to make all residents feel comfortable and welcome.

2. Explain the nursing assistant's role in the admission process

When a new resident is admitted, he is first directed to the admitting office. Paperwork is signed. The admission staff member makes copies of insurance information, Medicare cards, and other types of information. Both parties sign an agreement or contract agreeing to the services provided and the costs for them. Emergency contact information and names of doctors are obtained. The Patient Self-Determination Act (PSDA), an amendment to the Omnibus Budget Reconciliation Act (OBRA), requires staff to explain information about advance directives and

to find out if the resident has advance directives in place or wants to create them. A copy of the resident's rights is given to the new resident and his family. The rights are explained in language the resident can understand. A facility handbook of policies and procedures may be given. The procedure on how to file grievances and complaints is explained. Pictures of new residents may be taken. These photos are used to identify residents and may be posted outside of their rooms.

Admission is often the first time a nursing assistant meets a new resident. This is a time of first impressions. The NA should try to make sure the resident has a positive impression of her and her facility. Because change is difficult, staff must communicate with new residents. NAs can explain what to expect during the process and answer any questions that are within their scope of practice. If residents have questions that an NA cannot answer, she should find the nurse. It is a good idea for the NA to ask a new resident questions to find out her personal preferences and routines. NAs can also ask residents' families about personal preferences if residents are not able to respond.

Each facility will have a procedure for admitting residents to their new home. These general guidelines will help make the experience pleasant and successful:

Guidelines: Admission

G   Prepare the room before the resident arrives. This helps her to feel expected and welcome. Make sure the bed is made and the room is tidy. Restock supplies that are low. Make sure there is an admission kit available if used. Admission kits often contain personal care items, such as a bath basin, an emesis basin, a water pitcher and drinking glass, toothpaste, soap, a comb, lotion, and tissues (Fig. 11-2). Admission kits may also contain a urine specimen cup, label, and transport bag.

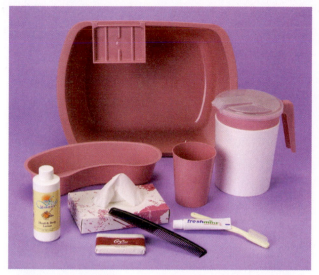

Fig. 11-2. *An admission kit is usually placed in a resident's room before he or she is admitted. It may contain personal care items that the resident will need.* (REPRINTED WITH PERMISSION OF BRIGGS CORPORATION, 800-247-2343, WWW.BRIGGSCORP.COM)

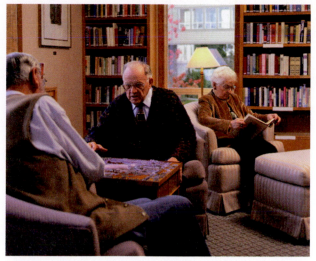

Fig. 11-3. *During the tour, be sure to introduce new residents to all other residents you see.*

G When a new resident arrives at the facility, note the time and her condition. Is she using a wheelchair, is she on a stretcher, or is she walking? Who is with her? Observe the new resident for level of consciousness and signs of confusion. She will probably be feeling anxious; look for signs of nervousness. Note any tubes she has, such as IVs or catheters.

G Introduce yourself and state your position. Smile and be friendly. Always call the person by her formal name until she tells you what she wants to be called.

G Never rush the process or the new resident. She should not feel like she is an inconvenience. Make sure that the new resident feels welcome and wanted.

G Explain day-to-day life in the facility. Offer to take the resident and her family on a tour. Show the resident the dining room, the activity room, the salon, the chapel, and any other important areas. When showing the resident where the dining room is, review the posted dining schedules. During the tour, introduce the resident to other residents and staff members you see (Fig. 11-3). Introduce the roommate if there is one.

G Handle personal items with care and respect. A resident has a legal right to have her personal items treated carefully. These are the items she has chosen to bring with her. Some items may be stored in bags marked specifically for personal belongings. Ask the new resident if she brought any valuables with her. If so, offer to have them safely stored according to your facility's policy. If she refuses, follow the procedure to write an inventory and get the necessary signatures.

G When setting up the room, place personal items where the resident wants them (Fig. 11-4).

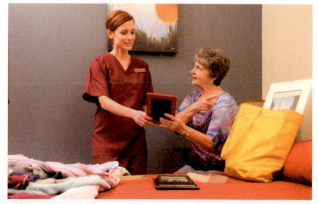

Fig. 11-4. *Handle personal items carefully, and set up the room as the resident prefers.*

G Admission is a stressful time. Observe the resident, as she could have a problem or issue that is missed during the process of transporting, paperwork, etc. It is important to observe the new resident's condition in order to recognize any changes that may take place later. Report to the nurse if you notice any of the following:

- Disconnected tubing

- Resident seems confused, combative, and/or unaware of surroundings

- Resident is having difficulty breathing or any other signs of distress

- Resident has bruises or wounds

- Resident has missed a meal during the admission process

- Resident has valuables, medications, hearing aids, eyeglasses, or dentures

G   Follow facility policy about any other required tasks during the admission process.

G   New residents may have good days followed by not-so-good days. Let residents adapt to their new home at their own pace. Everyone is different. Getting used to a new home may take weeks or months. However, do report signs of confusion or depression to the nurse.

Residents' Rights

Admission

OBRA requires that on admission, residents must be told of their legal rights. They must be provided with a written copy of these rights. This includes rights about their funds and the right to file a complaint with the state survey agency.

Admitting a resident

Equipment: may include admission paperwork (checklist and inventory form), gloves, and vital signs equipment

1. Identify yourself by name. Identify the resident by name.

2. Wash your hands.

3. Explain procedure to resident. Speak clearly, slowly, and directly. Maintain face-to-face contact whenever possible.

4. Provide for the resident's privacy with curtain, screen, or door (Fig. 11-5). If the family is present, ask them to step outside until the admission process is over. Show them where they can wait, and let them know approximately how long the process will take.

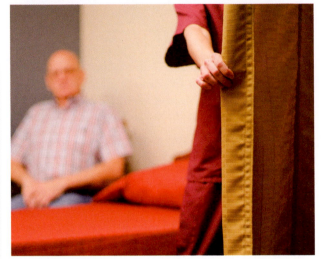

Fig. 11-5. All residents have a legal right to privacy, and providing privacy is part of doing your job professionally. Your professional, respectful behavior can help put a new resident at ease.

5. If part of facility policy, do these things:

- Measure the resident's height and weight (see procedures that follow).

- Measure the resident's baseline vital signs (see Chapter 14). **Baseline** signs are initial values that can then be compared to future measurements.

- Obtain a urine specimen if required (see Chapter 16).

- Complete the paperwork. Take an inventory of all the personal items.

- Help the resident put personal items away. Label personal items according to facility policy.

- Provide fresh water (Fig. 11-6).

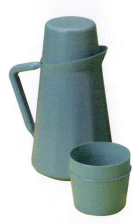

Fig. 11-6. Providing fresh water is something you should do every time you leave a resident's room, unless he is on a fluid restriction. Doing this helps prevent dehydration. Make sure the pitcher and glass are light enough for the resident to lift. Provide ice if requested. (REPRINTED WITH PERMISSION OF BRIGGS CORPORATION, 800-247-2343, WWW.BRIGGSCORP.COM)

6. Show the resident the room and bathroom. Explain how to work the bed controls and the call light. Show the resident the telephone, lights, and television controls.

7. Introduce the resident to his roommate if there is one. Introduce other residents and staff.

8. Make sure resident is comfortable. Remove privacy measures. Bring the family back inside if they were outside.

9. Place call light within resident's reach.

10. Wash your hands.

11. Document procedure using facility guidelines.

A resident's weight and height will be checked at admission. Nursing assistants also measure weight and height as part of regular care. Height is checked less often than weight. Weight changes can be signs of illness, so NAs must report any weight loss or gain, no matter how small. Weight will be measured using pounds or kilograms. A pound is a unit of weight equal to 16 ounces. A kilogram is a unit of mass equal to 1000 grams; one kilogram equals 2.2 pounds.

Measuring and recording weight of an ambulatory resident

Equipment: standing/upright scale, pen and paper

1. Identify yourself by name. Identify the resident by name.

2. Wash your hands.

3. Explain procedure to the resident. Speak clearly, slowly, and directly. Maintain face-to-face contact whenever possible.

4. Provide for resident's privacy with curtain, screen, or door.

5. Make sure the resident is wearing nonskid shoes that are securely fastened before walking to the scale.

6. Start with the scale balanced at zero before weighing the resident.

7. Help the resident to step onto the center of the scale. Be sure she is not holding, touching, or leaning against anything. This interferes with weight measurement. Do not force someone to let go. If you are unable to obtain a weight, notify the nurse.

8. Determine the resident's weight. Balance the scale by making the balance bar level. Move the small and large weight indicators until the bar balances. Read the two numbers shown (on the small and large weight indicators) when the bar is balanced. Add these two numbers together. This is the resident's weight (Fig. 11-7).

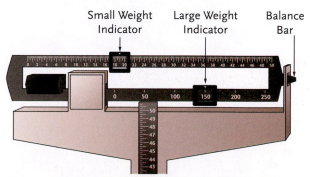
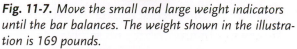

Fig. 11-7. Move the small and large weight indicators until the bar balances. The weight shown in the illustration is 169 pounds.

9. Help the resident to safely step off the scale before recording weight.

10. Wash your hands.

11. Record the resident's weight.

12. Remove privacy measures.

13. Place call light within resident's reach.

14. Report any changes in the resident's weight (when weighing resident after admission) to the nurse.

When residents are not able to get out of wheelchairs easily, they are weighed using a wheelchair scale. With this scale, wheelchairs are rolled directly onto the scale (Fig. 11-8). On some wheelchair scales, the nursing assistant will need to subtract the weight of the wheelchair from a resident's weight. If the wheelchair's weight is not listed on the chair, the NA should weigh the empty wheelchair first. The footrests should be attached if they will be attached when the resident is in the chair. Then the NA should subtract the wheelchair's weight from the total.

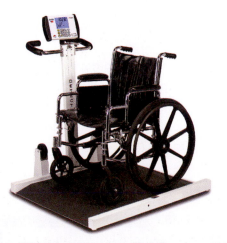

Fig. 11-8. *Wheelchairs can be rolled directly onto wheelchair scales to determine weight.* (PHOTO COURTESY OF DETECTO, WWW.DETECTO.COM, 800-641-2008)

When residents are not able to get out of bed, they are weighed on special bed scales (Fig. 11-9). Before using a bed scale, the NA should know how to use it properly and safely.

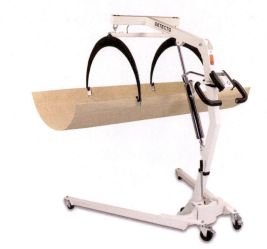

Fig. 11-9. *A type of bed scale.* (PHOTO COURTESY OF DETECTO, WWW.DETECTO.COM, 800-641-2008)

For measuring height, the rod measures in inches and fractions of inches. The nursing assistant should record the total number of inches. If inches need to be converted into feet, there are 12 inches in one foot.

Measuring and recording height of an ambulatory resident

For residents who can get out of bed, you will measure height using a standing scale.

Equipment: standing scale, pen and paper

1. Identify yourself by name. Identify the resident by name.

2. Wash your hands.

3. Explain procedure to the resident. Speak clearly, slowly, and directly. Maintain face-to-face contact whenever possible.

4. Provide for resident's privacy with curtain, screen, or door.

5. Make sure the resident is wearing nonskid shoes that are securely fastened before walking to scale.

6. Help the resident to step onto the scale, facing away from the scale.

7. Ask the resident to stand straight if possible. Help as needed.

8. Pull up the measuring rod from the back of the scale and gently lower the rod until it rests flat on the resident's head (Fig. 11-10).

9. Determine the resident's height.

10. Help the resident to safely step off the scale before recording height. Make sure that the measuring rod does not hit the resident in the head while helping the resident off the scale.

11. Wash your hands.

12. Record the resident's height.

13. Remove privacy measures.

14. Place call light within resident's reach.

15. Document procedure using facility guidelines.

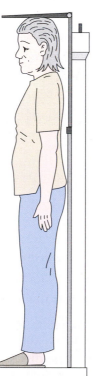

Fig. 11-10. *To determine height on a standing scale, gently lower the measuring rod until it rests flat on the resident's head.*

Some residents will be unable to get out of bed. Height can be measured by using a tape measure and making two pencil marks on the sheet

that is underneath the resident. The NA makes a mark at the top of the resident's head and one at his feet and measures the distance between the marks (Figs. 11-11 and 11-12). The height of a resident who is bedridden can also be measured using other methods. Nursing assistants should follow the procedures used at their facilities.

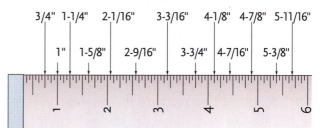

Fig. 11-11. *Height can be measured in bed using a tape measure.*

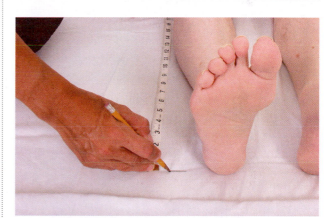

Fig. 11-12. *One way that height of a resident who is bedridden can be measured is by making marks on the sheet at the resident's head and heel. Then the distance between the marks is measured.*

3. Explain the nursing assistant's role during an in-house transfer of a resident

Residents may be transferred to a different area of the facility. In cases of acute illness, they may be transferred to a hospital. Change is difficult, and this is especially true when a person has an illness or her condition gets worse. Staff should make the transfer as smooth as possible for the resident. A resident should be informed of the transfer as soon as possible so that she can begin to adjust to the idea. The nurse will inform the resident about the transfer, and should explain how, where, when, and why the transfer will occur. Any questions the resident has should be answered.

Nursing assistants help residents pack their personal items before transferring. Because residents often worry about losing their belongings, NAs can involve them in the packing process. For example, the NA can let the resident see the empty closet, drawers, etc.

The resident may be transferred in a bed, stretcher, or wheelchair. To aid with planning, the NA should find out how the resident will be transferred beforehand. After the resident is in her new room or area, the NA should introduce her to all staff members she sees. The goal is to make the resident feel welcome, settled, and comfortable.

Transferring a resident

Equipment: may include a wheelchair, cart for belongings, the medical record, all of the resident's personal care items and packed personal items

1. Identify yourself by name. Identify the resident by name.

2. Wash your hands.

3. Explain procedure to the resident. Speak clearly, slowly, and directly. Maintain face-to-face contact whenever possible.

4. Collect the items to be moved onto the cart. Take them to the new location. If the resident is going into the hospital, they may be placed in temporary storage.

5. Help the resident into the wheelchair (or stretcher if one is used). Take him or her to the proper area.

6. Introduce new residents and staff.

7. Help the resident to put personal items away.

8. Make sure that the resident is comfortable.

9. Place call light within resident's reach.

10. Wash your hands.

11. Report any changes in resident to the nurse.

12. Document procedure using facility guidelines.

When residents are being transferred out of the facility, nursing assistants should make sure residents' clothing is clean and appropriate for the weather. In addition, NAs should observe and report the following to the nurse:

- How the resident left the facility

- Who was with the resident

- Whether the resident left by stretcher or wheelchair

- If the resident understood where she was going

- The belongings the resident took with her

- The resident's vital signs before the transfer

If the resident will be returning soon, the nursing assistant should change the bed linens, tidy the room, and restock supplies.

4. Explain the nursing assistant's role in the discharge of a resident

To discharge a resident from a facility, a doctor must give the discharge order. The nurse then completes instructions for the resident to follow after discharge. The nurse will review these instructions and important information with the resident and her family and friends. Some of the following areas may be discussed:

- Future doctor or physical, speech, and occupational therapy appointments

- Home care, skilled nursing care

- Medications

- Ambulation instructions

- Medical equipment needed

- Medical transportation

- Any restrictions on activities

- Special exercises to keep the resident functioning at the highest level (Fig. 11-13)

- Special nutrition or dietary requirements

- Community resources

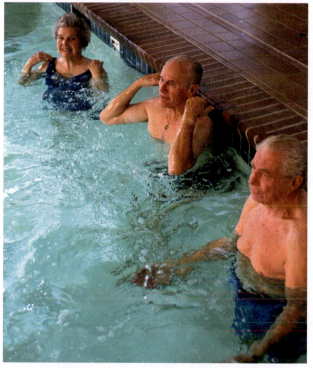

Fig. 11-13. *When a resident is discharged, she may receive instructions to exercise.*

Nursing assistants help by collecting the resident's belongings and personal care items and packing them carefully. The NA should know what the resident's condition is at the time of discharge and find out if the resident will be using a wheelchair or stretcher.

The day of discharge is often a happy day for residents who are going home. However, some residents may experience uncertainty or fear about leaving the facility. They may be concerned that their health will suffer. Nursing assistants can help by being positive and reassuring. They can remind residents that their doctors believe they are ready to leave. However, if a resident has specific questions about care, the NA should inform the nurse.

Residents' Rights

Transfers or Discharges

OBRA requires that residents have the right to receive advance notice before being transferred or discharged from a facility. The written notice must contain the specifics of where and why they are being transferred or discharged, and it must be in language residents can understand. The staff must provide adequate preparation for the transfer or discharge.

Discharging a resident

Equipment: may include a wheelchair, cart for belongings, discharge paperwork, including the inventory list from admission, the resident's care items, vital signs equipment

1. Identify yourself by name. Identify the resident by name.

2. Wash your hands.

3. Explain procedure to the resident. Speak clearly, slowly, and directly. Maintain face-to-face contact whenever possible.

4. Provide for resident's privacy with curtain, screen, or door.

5. Measure the resident's vital signs.

6. Compare the inventory checklist to the items there. If all items are there, ask the resident to sign.

7. Put the personal items to be taken onto the cart and take them to pickup area.

8. Help the resident dress and then into the wheelchair or onto the stretcher if used.

9. Help the resident to say his goodbyes to the staff and residents.

10. Take resident to the pick-up area. Help him into the vehicle. You are responsible for the resident until he is safely in the car and the door is closed.

11. Wash your hands.

12. Document procedure using facility guidelines. Include the following:

- The vital signs at discharge
- Time of discharge
- Method of transport
- Who was with the resident
- What items the resident took with him (inventory checklist)

5. Describe the nursing assistant's role in physical exams

Some residents need a physical exam when arriving at a facility to help determine their needs and to provide important information for the care plan. Others need a physical exam periodically after they have been at the facility for a while. Doctors or nurses will perform the exam. Nursing assistants may help by bringing the resident to the proper area, gathering equipment, and providing emotional support.

Exams can make people fearful or anxious. They may fear what the examiner will do or what he or she will find. Exams can cause discomfort and embarrassment. Nursing assistants can provide support during this process by being comforting and by listening and answering questions within their scope of practice.

Nursing assistants are often responsible for gathering equipment for the nurse or doctor. Examples of equipment that may be needed include the following:

- Sphygmomanometer (for blood pressure)
- Stethoscope
- Alcohol wipes
- Flashlight
- Thermometer
- Tongue depressor
- Eye chart for vision screening
- Tuning fork (tests hearing with vibrations)
- Reflex hammer (taps body parts to test reflexes) (Fig. 11-14)
- Otoscope (lighted instrument that examines the outer ear and eardrum)
- Ophthalmoscope (lighted instrument that examines the eye)
- Specimen containers
- Lubricant
- Hemoccult card (tests for blood in stool)
- Vaginal speculum for females (opens the vagina so that it and the cervix can be examined)
- Gloves
- Drape

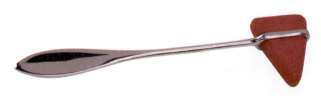

Fig. 11-14. *A reflex hammer is used to test reflexes.*
(REPRINTED WITH PERMISSION OF BRIGGS CORPORATION, 800-247-2343, WWW.BRIGGSCORP.COM)

Nursing assistants may need to place residents in the correct position and drape them for the exam. Drapes cover the parts of the body that are not being examined. Some exam positions are embarrassing and uncomfortable. The nursing assistant can help by explaining why the position is needed and how long the resident can expect to stay in the position. In addition to draping the resident, the NA should close the door to the room and/or pull the privacy curtain to protect the resident's privacy. The NA should explain to the resident that he or she will not be exposed more than necessary during the exam. Common positions used during exams include the following:

The **dorsal recumbent** position is used to examine the breasts, chest, abdomen, and perineal area. A resident in the dorsal recumbent position is flat on her back with her knees flexed and feet flat on the bed. The drape is put over the resident, covering her body. Her head remains uncovered (Fig. 11-15).

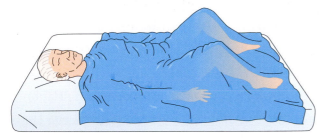

Fig. 11-15. The dorsal recumbent position.

The **lithotomy** position is used to examine the vagina. The resident lies on her back, and her hips are brought to the edge of the exam table. Her legs are flexed, and her feet are in padded stirrups. The drape is put over the resident, covering her body. Her head remains uncovered. The drape is also brought down to cover the perineal area and tops of the thighs (Fig. 11-16).

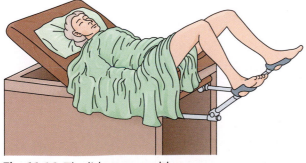

Fig. 11-16. The lithotomy position.

The **knee-chest** position may be used to examine the rectum or the vagina. A resident in the knee-chest position is lying on her abdomen. The knees are pulled toward the abdomen, and

the legs are separated. The arms are pulled up and flexed. The head is turned to one side. In the knee-chest position, the resident will be wearing a gown and possibly socks. The drape should be applied in a diamond shape to cover the back, buttocks, and thighs (Fig. 11-17).

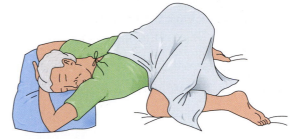

Fig. 11-17. The knee-chest position.

Guidelines: Physical Exams

G   Wash your hands before and after the exam.

G   Ask the resident to urinate before the exam. Collect any urine needed for a specimen at this time.

G   Provide privacy throughout the exam. Use drapes and privacy screens. Expose only the body part being examined.

G   Listen to and reassure the resident throughout the exam.

G   Follow the directions of the examiner.

G   Help the resident into the proper positions as needed.

G   Protect the resident from falling.

G   Provide enough light for the examiner.

G   Put instruments in the proper place for the examiner. Hand instruments to the examiner as needed.

G   Take and label specimens as needed.

G   Follow Standard Precautions.

G   For vision screenings, you may be asked to check that needed equipment is in place. Follow directions. Assist the screener to set up any equipment, such as the eye chart. If you transport residents to the site for screening, make sure to take their current eyeglasses or contact lenses with them. The screener will instruct you where to seat the residents or to have them stand. Operate the light switch as instructed. Make sure that the residents have their eyeglasses and other belongings when returning to their rooms.

G After the exam, the NA's responsibilities include the following:

- Help the resident clean up and get dressed. Help the resident safely back to his or her room.

- Dispose of any trash and disposable equipment in the exam area.

- Bring all reusable equipment to the appropriate cleaning room. Clean and store reusable equipment according to facility policy.

- Label and bring any specimens to the lab.

Residents' Rights

Exams

Residents have the right to know why exams are being done and who is doing them. Residents have the right to choose examiners and to have family members present during the exam.

Chapter Review

1. What is one way that nursing assistants help residents make a successful transition to long-term care facilities?

2. List eight guidelines for nursing assistants to follow to help residents during the admission process.

3. Why is it important for nursing assistants to report any weight loss or gain that a resident has, no matter how small?

4. How many inches are in a foot?

5. What is one nursing assistant responsibility when assisting a resident with an in-house transfer?

6. List eight types of information that the nurse may cover with the resident and her family and friends during the discharge process.

7. What are two ways that nursing assistants can provide emotional support to residents who are having physical exams?

8. In which position is a resident lying on her abdomen with her knees pulled toward the abdomen, with her arms pulled up and flexed, and her head turned to one side?

9. Which position involves placing the woman's feet in padded stirrups and is generally used to examine the vagina?

10. In which position is a resident lying flat on her back with her knees flexed and feet flat on the bed?

12

The Resident's Unit

1. Explain why a comfortable environment is important for the resident's well-being

Illness and disability cause great stress. It helps residents feel better physically and psychologically if their environments are clean and comfortable. A comfortable and clean environment aids in relaxation and helps to reduce stress. A soothing environment may also help relieve pain and promote healing. Many things affect residents' comfort within their rooms. The more nursing assistants try to improve residents' environments, the more positive impact it may have on residents' health and well-being.

Many things can affect comfort level, such as noise, odors, temperature, lighting, diet, medications, illness, fear, and anxiety. Nursing assistants can use the following guidelines to avoid problems and promote comfort:

Guidelines: Promoting Comfort

G   Common noises in facilities can upset and/ or irritate residents. Help keep the noise level low by doing the following:

- Do not bang equipment or meal trays.

- Keep your voice low.

- Promptly answer ringing telephones and call lights.

- Close doors when residents ask you to.

- Turn off televisions when they are not in use.

G   Odors may be caused by urine, feces, vomit, certain diseases, and wound drainage. Body and breath odors may be offensive, too. Help control odors by doing the following:

- Promptly clean up after episodes of incontinence.

- Change incontinence briefs as soon as they are soiled, and dispose of them properly.

- Empty and clean bedpans, urinals, commodes, and emesis basins promptly.

- Change soiled bed linens and clothing as soon as possible.

- Give regular oral care and personal care to help avoid body and breath odors.

G   Temperature can affect comfort. OBRA requires that long-term care facilities have comfortable and safe environments by maintaining a temperature range of 71–81°F. As people age and lose protective fatty tissue, they may feel cold often. Illness can also cause a person to feel cold. Help residents stay comfortable by doing the following:

- Layer clothing and bed covers for warmth.

- Keep residents away from drafty areas, such as near doors and windows.

- Offer blankets to residents in wheelchairs.

- Keep residents covered while giving personal care.

- If residents control the heat and air conditioning in their rooms, do not change the temperature for your comfort.

G Adequate lighting is important to promote safety and prevent falls. It also helps make a room pleasant. Residents may prefer darker rooms when they are ill, have a headache, or are sleeping. Keep lighting controls within the resident's reach.

G Foods ordered in special diets for residents may cause them discomfort. Heavy meals can also cause discomfort. Report resident complaints about food to the nurse. Chapter 15 contains information about nutrition and special diets.

G Foods and drinks that contain caffeine can prevent sleep or interfere with sleeping well. Caffeine may need to be decreased to promote better rest (Fig. 12-1).

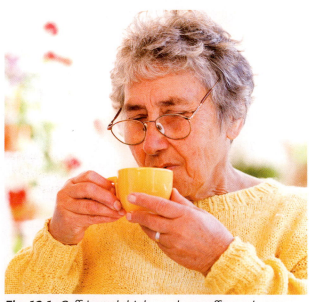

Fig. 12-1. Caffeinated drinks, such as coffee and some teas, can prevent sleep and cause fatigue and irritability.

G If residents seem sad, anxious, or fearful, help them by talking with them and listening to their concerns. Provide emotional support. If you think residents require more assistance than you can give, discuss this with the nurse.

2. Describe a standard resident unit

A resident's unit is the room or area where the resident lives. It contains the resident's furniture and personal possessions. The unit is the resident's home and must be treated with respect. Nursing assistants should always knock and wait to receive permission before entering. However, this may not always be possible. Certain residents, such as those who are confused or who have problems speaking, may not be able to give this permission.

Residents' units must be kept neat and clean. After providing care for a resident, the nursing assistant will clean the area and put equipment away. Providing a clean, safe, and orderly environment is an essential part of the NA's job.

Standard equipment that is generally found in each resident's unit includes the following:

Bed: Electric beds, also called hospital beds, are adjustable and can be raised and lowered (Fig. 12-2). Electric beds are operated by controls that hang on or near the side of the bed (Fig. 12-3). Buttons are used to raise and lower the head of the bed, the foot of the bed, sections of the bed, and the bed height. Most electric beds have a way to insert a crank so that they can be adjusted if there is a power failure. Manual beds have cranks to adjust height. The left crank usually raises and lowers the head of the bed. The right crank raises and lowers the foot of the bed. If the bed has a center crank, it will adjust the bed height. Normally beds are kept in their lowest horizontal position. Lowering the bed provides for residents' safety and helps reduce the risk of falls. Cranks should be placed back under the bed after a manual bed has been moved to reduce the risk of injury.

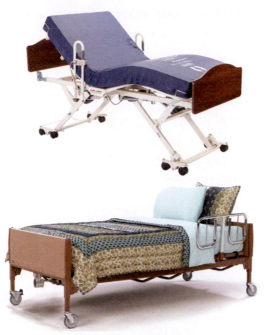

Fig. 12-2. *The top photo shows a general type of electric bed, while a bariatric bed is shown in the bottom photo. A bariatric bed can be used for people who are overweight or obese.* (© INVACARE CORPORATION. USED WITH PERMISSION. WWW.INVACARE.COM)

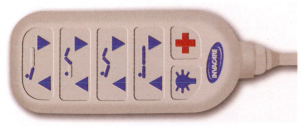

Fig. 12-3. *Controls for an electric bed may look like this.* (© INVACARE CORPORATION. USED WITH PERMISSION. WWW.INVACARE.COM)

Bedside stand: Small items are usually stored in bedside stands. The water pitcher and cup are often placed on top of the bedside stand. A telephone, radio, and other items, such as photos, may also be placed there (Fig. 12-4).

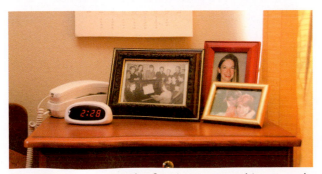

Fig. 12-4. *Bedside stands often have personal items, such as photos, as well as things like telephones and remote controls placed on top of them.*

These items may be stored inside the bedside stand:

- Wash basin
- Emesis basin (Fig. 12-5)
- Soap dish and soap
- Bath blanket
- Toilet paper
- Personal hygiene items

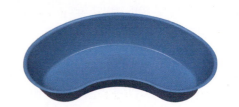

Fig. 12-5. *An emesis basin is a kidney-shaped basin often used when giving mouth care.* (REPRINTED WITH PERMISSION OF BRIGGS CORPORATION, 800-247-2343, WWW.BRIGGSCORP.COM)

Overbed table: The overbed table may be used for meals or personal care. It is considered a clean area and must be kept clean and free of clutter (Fig. 12-6). Bedpans, urinals, soiled linen, and other contaminated items should not be placed on overbed tables.

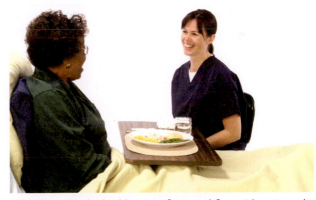

Fig. 12-6. *Overbed tables are often used for residents' meals; they must be kept clean. Nursing assistants should never place bedpans, urinals, or soiled linens on overbed tables.*

Call light: The intercom system is the most common call system used. When the resident presses the button, a light will be seen and/or a bell will be heard at the nurses' station. The call light allows the resident to communicate with staff whenever necessary. It is important for nursing assistants to always place the call light within the resident's reach and to answer all call lights immediately.

Privacy curtain: All residents in a facility have a legal right to personal privacy. This means that they must always be protected from public view when receiving care. Each bed usually has a privacy curtain that extends all the way around the bed (Fig. 12-7). Curtains keep others from seeing a resident undressed or while having care procedures done. To protect each resident's privacy, nursing assistants must keep this curtain closed when giving care. Although curtains and screens block vision, they do not block sound. NAs should keep their voices low and not discuss a resident's care near others. Closing the door when possible provides more complete privacy.

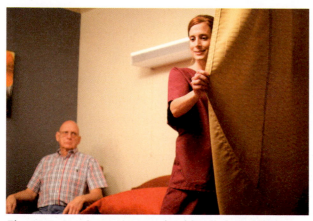

Fig. 12-7. Nursing assistants should pull the privacy curtain around the bed before giving care.

Bed Positions

Nursing assistants may be asked to position electric beds in specific positions. To position the bed in the Fowler's position, the head of the bed should be raised 45 to 60 degrees. To position the bed in the semi-Fowler's position, the head of the bed should be raised 30 to 45 degrees.

3. Discuss how to care for and clean unit equipment

There are many types of equipment in a care facility, and nursing assistants must know how to use and care for all equipment properly. This helps prevent infection and injury. If a nursing assistant does not know how to use a particular piece of equipment, she should ask for assis-

tance. An NA should not try to use equipment that she does not know how to use.

Equipment that is discarded after one use is called disposable, or single-use, equipment. Disposable razors and nitrile gloves are examples of this type of equipment. Disposable equipment is used to prevent the spread of microorganisms. Nursing assistants should discard disposable equipment in the proper containers.

Some equipment, such as bedpans, urinals, and basins, needs to be cleaned after each use. When handling this equipment, nursing assistants must wear gloves so that they do not come into contact with infectious wastes. NAs may need to clean and disinfect this equipment themselves or place it in the proper area for cleaning.

Guidelines: Resident's Unit

G   Keep residents' units neat and clean. Clean the overbed table after use. Place the table within the resident's reach before leaving.

G   Keep the call light within the resident's reach. Check to see that it is within reach before you leave the room.

G   Keep equipment clean and in good condition. If any equipment appears broken or damaged, report it to the nurse and/or file the proper paperwork to get it repaired. Do not use broken or damaged equipment.

G   Remove meal trays right after meals. Check to make sure that there are no crumbs in the bed. Straighten bed linens as needed. Change linens if they become wet, soiled, or wrinkled.

G   Restock supplies. Make sure the resident has fresh drinking water and a clean cup within reach and is able to lift the pitcher and the cup. Make sure that tissues, paper towels, toilet paper, soap, and other supplies that are used daily are stocked before you leave.

G   If trash needs to be emptied or the bathroom needs to be cleaned, notify the housekeeping department. Trash should be emptied at least daily. Remove the trash when you leave the room if housekeeping staff is not available.

G   Report signs of insects or pests immediately.

G   Do not move a resident's belongings or discard any personal items. Respect the resident's things. Ask residents where they want items stored. Offer to help residents arrange their space in a way that is pleasing to them.

G   Clean equipment and return it to proper storage. Tidy the area. Providing a clean, safe, and orderly environment is part of your job.

4. Explain the importance of sleep and factors affecting sleep

Sleep is a natural period of rest for the mind and body. As a person sleeps, the mind and body's energy is restored. During sleep, vital functions are performed. These include repairing and renewing cells, processing information, and organizing memory. Sleep is essential to a person's health and well-being.

The circadian rhythm is an important factor in determining sleep patterns of humans. The **circadian rhythm** is the 24-hour day-night cycle. It also affects body temperature and hormone production, among other things.

When a person is sleep-deprived or suffers from **insomnia** (inability to fall asleep or remain asleep) or other sleep disorders, problems result. These include decreased mental function, reduced reaction time, and irritability. Sleep deprivation also decreases immune system function.

The elderly may take longer to go to sleep and can have more irregular sleep patterns. Some take short naps during the day. Many elderly persons, especially those who are living away from home, have sleep problems. Many factors can affect sleep, such as fear, stress, noise, diet, medications, and illness. Sharing a room with another person can also disturb sleep.

Observing and Reporting: Sleep Issues

When a resident complains that he or she is not sleeping well, observe and report the following:

O/R   Sleeping too much during the day

O/R   Eating or drinking items that contain too much caffeine late in the day

O/R   Wearing nightclothes during the day

O/R   Eating heavy meals late at night

O/R   Refusing to take medication ordered for sleep

O/R   Taking new medications

O/R   Having the TV, radio, computer, phone, or light on late at night

O/R   Experiencing pain

5. Describe bedmaking guidelines and perform proper bedmaking

When residents spend much or all of their time in bed, careful bedmaking is essential to their comfort, cleanliness, and health (Fig. 12-8). Linens should always be changed after personal care procedures such as bed baths, or any time bedding or sheets are damp, soiled, or in need of straightening. Bed linens should be changed often for these reasons:

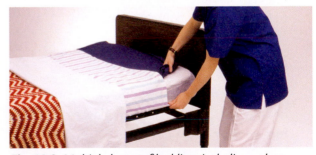

Fig. 12-8. Multiple layers of bedding, including a draw sheet, are used for residents who spend a lot of time in bed.

• Sheets that are damp, wrinkled, or bunched up under a resident are uncomfortable. They may prevent the resident from sleeping well.

• Microorganisms thrive in moist, warm places. Bedding that is damp or unclean encourages infection and disease.

- Residents who spend long hours in bed are at risk for pressure injuries. Sheets that do not lie flat under the resident's body increase the risk of pressure injuries because they cut off circulation.

Guidelines: Bedmaking

G Keep linen wrinkle-free and tidy. Change linen whenever it is wet, damp, wrinkled, or dirty.

G Wash your hands before handling clean linen (Fig. 12-9).

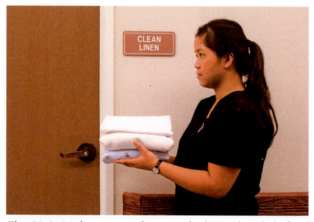

Fig. 12-9. Make sure you have washed your hands before gathering clean linen.

G Place clean linen on a clean surface within reach, such as a bedside stand, overbed table, or chair. Do not place clean linen on the floor or on a contaminated area.

G Don (put on) gloves before removing bed linen from the bed.

G Look for personal items, such as dentures, hearing aids, jewelry, and eyeglasses, before removing linen.

G When removing linen, fold or roll linen so that the dirtiest area is inside. Rolling puts the dirtiest surface of the linen inward. This lessens contamination.

G Do not shake linen or clothes. It may spread airborne contaminants.

G Bag soiled linen at the point of origin. Do not take it to other residents' rooms.

G Sort soiled linen away from resident care areas.

G Place wet linen in leakproof bags.

G Wear gloves when handling soiled linen. Hold soiled linen away from your body and place it in the proper container or area immediately. If dirty linen touches your uniform, your uniform becomes contaminated.

G Disposable pads are used for residents who are incontinent. Change disposable pads whenever they become soiled or wet, and discard them in the proper container. Put a clean pad on the bed when you change linen (Fig. 12-10).

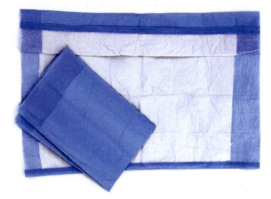

Fig. 12-10. Disposable absorbent pads help protect sheets from sweat, urine, feces, and other fluids.

If a resident cannot get out of bed, a nursing assistant must change the linens with the resident in bed. An **occupied bed** is a bed made while the resident is still in the bed. When making the bed, the NA should use a wide stance and bend her knees to avoid injury. Bending from the waist should also be avoided, especially when tucking sheets or blankets under the mattress. The height of the bed should be raised to make it easier and safer.

Making an occupied bed

Equipment: clean linen—mattress pad, fitted or flat bottom sheet, disposable absorbent pad (if needed), cotton draw sheet, flat top sheet, blanket(s), bedspread (if used), bath blanket, pillowcase(s), gloves

1. Identify yourself by name. Identify the resident by name.

2. Wash your hands.

3. Explain procedure to the resident. Speak clearly, slowly, and directly. Maintain face-to-face contact whenever possible.

4. Provide for resident's privacy with curtain, screen, or door.

5. Place clean linen on clean surface within reach (e.g., bedside stand, overbed table, or chair).

6. Adjust bed to a safe working level, usually waist high. Lower the head of the bed. Lock bed wheels.

7. Put on gloves.

8. Loosen top linen from the end of the bed on the working side.

9. Unfold the bath blanket over the top sheet to cover the resident, and remove the top sheet. Keep the resident covered at all times with the bath blanket.

10. You will make the bed one side at a time. Go to the far side of the bed. Raise the side rail (if the bed has them). This protects the resident from falling out of the bed. Help the resident to turn onto her side, toward you and the raised side rail (see Chapter 10). Then go to the other side of the bed.

11. Loosen the bottom soiled linen, mattress pad, and absorbent pad, if present, on the working side.

12. Roll the bottom soiled linen toward the resident, soiled side inside. Tuck it snugly against the resident's back.

13. Place the mattress pad (if used) on the bed, attaching elastic at corners on working side.

14. Place the clean bottom linen or fitted bottom sheet, finishing with bottom sheet free of wrinkles. If a flat sheet is used, leave enough overlap on each end to tuck under the mat-

tress. If the sheet is only long enough to tuck in at one end, tuck it in securely at the top of the bed. Make hospital, or mitered, corners to keep the bottom sheet wrinkle-free (Fig. 12-11). If a fitted sheet is used, tightly pull the two fitted corners on the working side.

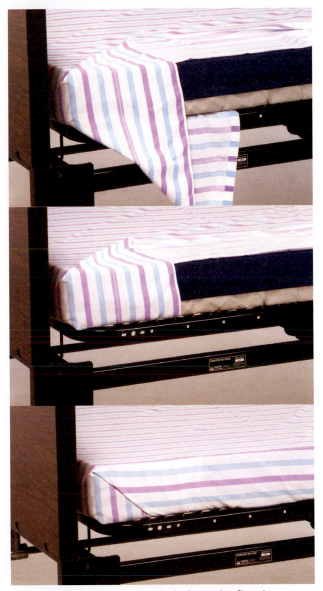

Fig. 12-11. Hospital corners help keep the flat sheet smooth under the resident. They help prevent a resident's feet from being restricted by or tangled in linen when getting in and out of bed.

15. Smooth the bottom sheet out toward the resident. Be sure there are no wrinkles in the mattress pad. Roll the extra material toward the resident. Tuck it under the resident's body (Fig. 12-12).

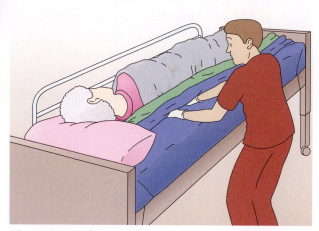

Fig. 12-12. *Tuck extra material under the resident's body.*

16. If using a disposable absorbent pad, unfold it and center it on the bed. Tuck the side near you under the mattress. Smooth it out toward the resident. Tuck as you did with the sheet.

17. If using a draw sheet, place it on the bed. Tuck in on your side, smooth it out, and tuck as you did with the other bedding.

18. Raise side rail on the working side. Help the resident roll or turn onto the clean bottom sheet, toward you. Explain that she will be moving over a pile of linen. Protect the resident from any soiled matter on the old linens.

19. Go to the other side of the bed and lower that side rail. Loosen the soiled linen. Check for any personal items. Roll the linen from head to foot of the bed. Avoid contact with your skin or clothes. Place it in a hamper or bag. Never put it on the floor or furniture. Do not shake it. Soiled bed linens are full of microorganisms that should not be spread to other parts of the room.

20. Pull the clean linen through as quickly as possible. Start with the mattress pad and wrap it around corners. Pull and tuck in the clean bottom linen, just like you did on the other side. Pull and tuck in the disposable absorbent pad and draw sheet if used. Make hospital corners with bottom sheet. Finish with the bottom sheet free of wrinkles.

21. Ask the resident to turn onto her back. Help as needed. Keep the resident covered and comfortable, with a pillow under her head. Raise the side rail nearest you.

22. Unfold the top sheet. Place it over the resident and center it. Ask the resident to hold the top sheet. Slip the bath blanket from underneath (Fig. 12-13). Put it in the hamper or bag.

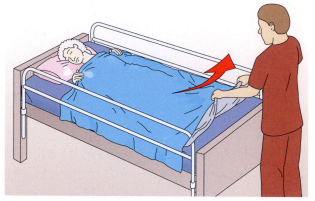

Fig. 12-13. *With the resident holding on to the top sheet, pull the bath blanket out.*

23. Place a blanket over the top sheet, matching the top edges. Place the bedspread over the blanket (if used), matching the top edges. Tuck the bottom edges of the top sheet, blanket, and bedspread under the foot of the bed. Make hospital corners on each side. Loosen the top linens over the resident's feet. This prevents pressure on the feet. At the top of the bed, fold the top sheet over the blanket about six inches.

24. Remove the pillow. Do not hold it near your face. Remove the soiled pillowcase by turning it inside out. Place it in the hamper or bag.

25. Remove and discard gloves. Wash your hands.

26. With one hand, grasp the clean pillowcase at the closed end. Turn it inside out over your arm. Next, using the same hand that has the pillowcase over it, grasp the center of the end of the pillow. Pull the pillowcase over it with your free hand (Fig. 12-14). Do the same for any other pillows. Place them under the resident's head with the open end away from door.

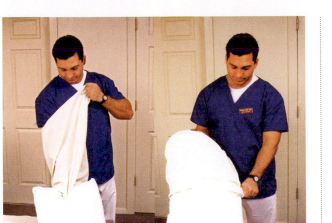

Fig. 12-14. After the pillowcase is turned inside out over your arm, grasp one end of the pillow. Pull the pillowcase over the pillow.

27. Make resident comfortable.

28. Return bed to lowest position. Leave side rails in the ordered position. Remove privacy measures.

29. Place call light within resident's reach.

30. Take laundry bag or hamper to proper area.

31. Wash your hands.

32. Report any changes in resident to the nurse.

33. Document procedure using facility guidelines.

Mattresses can be heavy. It is easier to make an empty bed than one with a resident in it. An **unoccupied bed** is a bed made while no resident is in the bed. If the resident can be moved, the NA's job will be easier.

Making an unoccupied bed

Equipment: clean linen—mattress pad, fitted or flat bottom sheet, disposable absorbent pad (if needed), cotton draw sheet, flat top sheet, blanket(s), bedspread (if used), bath blanket, pillowcase(s), gloves

1. Wash your hands.

2. Place clean linen on clean surface within reach (e.g., bedside stand, overbed table, or chair).

3. Adjust bed to a safe working level, usually waist high. Put bed in flattest position. Lock bed wheels.

4. Put on gloves.

5. Loosen soiled linen. Roll soiled linen (soiled side inside) from head to foot of bed. Avoid contact with your skin or clothes. Place it in a hamper or bag. Remove pillows and pillowcases, and place pillowcases in the hamper. Do not put linen on the floor or furniture.

6. Remove and discard gloves. Wash your hands.

7. Remake the bed. Place the mattress pad (if used) on the bed, attaching elastic at corners on working side. Place a clean bottom sheet or fitted bottom sheet, finishing with the bottom sheet free of wrinkles. If a flat sheet is used, leave enough overlap on each end to tuck under the mattress. If the sheet is only long enough to tuck in at one end, tuck it in securely at the top of the bed. Make hospital corners to keep the bottom sheet wrinkle-free. If a fitted sheet is used, tightly fit corners over all four corners of the bed.

8. Put on a disposable absorbent pad and then draw sheet if used. Place them in the center of the bed on the bottom sheet. Smooth and tightly tuck the bottom sheet and draw sheet together under the sides of the bed.

9. Place the top sheet over the bed and center it. Place the blanket over the bed and center it. Place the bedspread (if used) over the bed and center it. Tuck the bottom edges of the top sheet, blanket, and bedspread under the foot of the bed, making hospital corners on each side.

10. Fold down the top sheet over the blanket about six inches. Fold both the top sheet and blanket down so resident can easily get into bed. If the resident will not be returning to bed immediately, leave bedding up.

11. Put on clean pillowcases (as described in previous procedure). Replace pillows.

12. Return bed to lowest position.

13. Take laundry bag or hamper to proper area.

14. Wash your hands.

15. Document procedure using facility guidelines.

A **closed bed** is a bed completely made with the bedspread and blankets in place. It is made for residents who will be out of bed most of the day. It is also made when a resident is discharged. A closed bed is converted to an **open bed** by folding the linen down to the foot of the bed. An open bed is a bed that is ready to receive a resident who has been out of bed all day or who is being admitted to the facility.

A **surgical bed** is made to accept residents who are returning to bed on stretchers, or gurneys. These residents may be coming from a hospital or returning from a test or procedure. A surgical bed is opened to receive residents by loosening the linens on one side and folding them to the other side. This leaves one side open. Chapter 10 contains information about transferring residents into bed from a stretcher.

Making a surgical bed

Equipment: clean linen, gloves

1. Wash your hands.

2. Place clean linen on clean surface within reach (e.g., bedside stand, overbed table, or chair).

3. Adjust bed to a safe working level, usually waist high. Lock bed wheels.

4. Put on gloves.

5. Remove all soiled linen, rolling it (soiled side inside) from head to foot of bed. Avoid contact with your skin or clothes. Place it in a hamper or bag.

6. Remove and discard gloves. Wash your hands.

7. Make an unoccupied, closed bed. See procedure: *Making an unoccupied bed.*

8. Loosen linens on the side of the bed that is away from the door (where the stretcher will be).

9. Fanfold linens lengthwise to the side away from the door (Fig. 12-15). Fanfolded means folded several times into pleats.

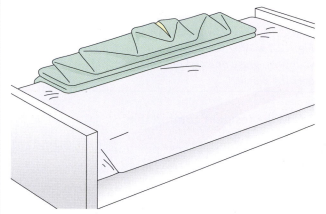

Fig. 12-15. *Fanfold the linen so that it is in pleated layers and position linen opposite the stretcher side of the bed.*

10. Put on clean pillowcases. Replace pillows.

11. Leave bed in its locked position with both side rails down.

12. Make sure the pathway to the bed is clear.

13. Take the laundry bag or hamper to proper area.

14. Wash your hands.

15. Document procedure using facility guidelines.

Chapter Review

1. What are three ways that nursing assistants can keep the noise level low in facilities?

2. What are three ways that nursing assistants can help control odors in facilities?

3. What temperature range for long-term care facilities is required by OBRA?

4. Why are beds usually kept in their lowest positions?

5. What is the overbed table used for? Can bedpans and soiled linen be placed on an overbed table?

6. Where should call lights always be placed?

7. How do privacy curtains help protect residents' privacy?

8. What is disposable equipment? Why is it used?

9. List two functions that sleep performs for the body.

10. What problems can result from a lack of sleep?

11. When should bed linens be changed?

12. List three reasons why it is important to change bed linens frequently.

13. Which way should pillows face while under residents' heads?

13

Personal Care Skills

1. Explain personal care of residents

Personal care is different from other tasks that nursing assistants may perform for residents, such as measuring vital signs or tidying a unit. The term *personal* refers to tasks that are concerned with the person's body, appearance, and hygiene, and suggests privacy may be important. **Hygiene** is the term used to describe practices that keep bodies clean and healthy. Bathing and brushing teeth are two examples. **Grooming** refers to practices like caring for fingernails and hair, shaving, and applying makeup. Hygiene and grooming activities, as well as dressing, eating, transferring, and eliminating, are called **activities of daily living (ADLs)**.

Some people who are recovering from an illness or an accident may not have the energy to care for themselves. They may also need help with personal care due to any of the following:

- A person has a long-term, chronic condition
- A person is frail because of advanced age
- A person is permanently disabled
- A person is dying

These residents may need assistance with their personal care, or they may need nursing assistants to provide it for them entirely. NAs may provide or help with any or all of this personal care: bathing, **perineal care** (care of the genital and anal area), elimination, mouth care, shampooing and combing the hair, nail care, shaving,

dressing, eating, walking, and transferring. NAs will assist residents with these tasks every day. These activities are often referred to as *a.m. care* or *p.m. care*, which refers to the time of day that they are done.

Assisting with a.m. care includes the following:

- Offering a bedpan or urinal or helping the resident to the bathroom
- Helping the resident wash face and hands
- Assisting with hair care, dressing, and shaving
- Assisting with mouth care before or after breakfast

Assisting with p.m. care includes the following:

- Offering a bedpan or urinal or helping the resident to the bathroom
- Helping the resident wash face and hands
- Giving a snack
- Assisting with mouth care
- Assisting with changing into nightclothes
- Giving a back rub

Some residents may never be able to care for themselves, while other residents will regain strength and be able to perform their own personal care. An important part of a nursing assistant's job is to help residents be as independent as possible. This means showing residents with disabilities how to care for themselves and encouraging other residents to perform self-care as soon as they are able. Promoting independence is an important part of care.

All people have routines for personal care and activities of daily living. They also have preferences for how they are done. These routines remain important even when people are elderly, sick, or disabled. NAs should be aware of residents' individual preferences concerning their personal care. Residents may prefer certain soaps or skin care products. They may choose to bathe in the morning or at night. It is important for NAs to ask residents about their routines and preferences, which is part of providing person-centered care.

Many people have been doing personal care tasks for themselves their entire lives. They may feel uncomfortable about having anyone, especially a person they do not know well, assist them with these tasks. Some residents may not like to be touched by someone else. It may be stressful for some people to have help with personal care, and NAs should be sensitive to these issues.

Before beginning any task, the NA should explain to the resident exactly what she will be doing. Explaining care to a resident is not only his legal right, but it may also help lessen anxiety. The NA should ask if he would like to use the bathroom or bedpan first. She should also provide privacy and let the resident make as many decisions as possible about when, where, and how a procedure will be done (Fig. 13-1). This encourages independence. In order to promote respect, dignity, and privacy, nursing assistants must do the following:

- Encourage residents to do as much as they are able to do and be patient.

- Knock and wait for permission to enter the resident's room if the resident is able to give permission.

- Not interrupt residents while they are in the bathroom.

- Leave the room when residents receive or make phone calls.

- Respect residents' private time and personal things.

- Not interrupt residents while they are dressing.

- Keep residents covered whenever possible when helping with dressing.

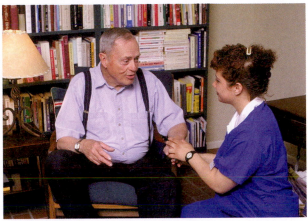

Fig. 13-1. Nursing assistants should let residents make as many decisions as possible about personal care.

Personal care provides an opportunity for the NA to observe a resident's skin, mental state, mobility, flexibility, comfort level, and ability to perform activities of daily living. While assisting with personal care, the NA should look for any problems or changes that have occurred. Communication is especially important during personal care. Some residents will talk about symptoms they are experiencing during personal care. They may say that they have been itching or that their skin feels dry. They may complain of numbness and tingling in a certain part of the body. The NA should keep a small notepad in a pocket to note exactly how the resident describes these symptoms. These comments should be reported to the nurse and documented immediately after the procedure.

During personal care, the NA can also observe the resident's mental and emotional state. Is the resident depressed or confused? Can the resident concentrate on the activity or hold a conversation? Is the resident short of breath? Does the resident tremble or shake? The focus should be on changes from the resident's normal state. Is there a change in behavior, level of activity, skin color, movement, or anything else? NAs are in the best position to observe, report, and document any small change in residents. No matter what care task is assigned, performing it is only half the job.

During the procedure, if the resident appears tired, the NA should stop and take a short break. The resident should never be rushed. After care, the NA should always ask if the resident would like anything else. She should leave the resident's area clean and tidy and make sure that the call light is within reach. Before leaving, the NA must check to see that the room has proper lighting and is a comfortable temperature. There should not be any electrical cords or other objects in the walkways. The bed should be left in its lowest position unless the care plan indicates otherwise.

Observing and Reporting: Personal Care

- o/R Skin color, temperature, redness (more information is listed in next Learning Objective)
- o/R Mobility
- o/R Flexibility
- o/R Comfort level, or pain or discomfort
- o/R Strength and the ability to perform ADLs
- o/R Mental and emotional state
- o/R Resident's complaints

2. Identify guidelines for providing skin care and preventing pressure injuries

Immobility reduces the amount of blood that circulates to the skin. Residents who have restricted mobility are at an increased risk of skin deterioration at pressure points. **Pressure points** are areas of the body that bear much of the body weight.

Pressure points are mainly located at bony prominences. **Bony prominences** are areas of the body where the bone lies close to the skin. The skin here is at a much higher risk for skin breakdown. These areas include elbows, shoulder blades, the sacrum (tailbone), hips and knees (inner and outer parts), ankles, heels, toes, and the back of the head. Other areas at risk for breakdown are the ears, the area under the breasts or scrotum, the area between the folds of the buttocks or abdomen, and the skin between the legs (Fig. 13-2).

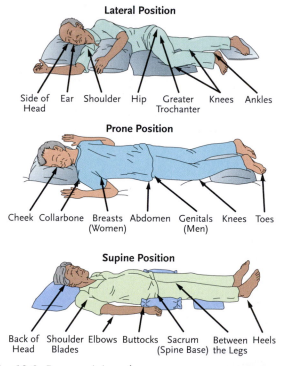

Fig. 13-2. Pressure injury danger zones.

Pressure on these areas reduces circulation, decreasing the amount of oxygen the cells receive. Warmth and moisture also contribute to skin breakdown. Once the surface of the skin has broken down and is weakened, injuries can occur and may become infected, causing damage to the underlying tissue. When infection occurs, the healing process slows down. The injuries or wounds that result from skin deterioration and shearing are called **pressure injuries**. Shearing is rubbing or friction resulting from the skin moving one way and the bone underneath it remaining fixed or moving in the opposite direction.

Pressure Injuries

Pressure injuries are also called *pressure ulcers, pressure sores, decubitus ulcers,* or *bed sores.* In 2016, the National Pressure Ulcer Advisory Panel (NPUAP, npuap.org) replaced the term *pressure ulcer* with *pressure injury.* The reason for this change in terminology is that the new term more accurately describes pressure injuries to both intact and non-intact skin. Definitions of the stages of pressure injuries were also updated. NPUAP is an independent, nonprofit organization whose board of directors is made up of a variety of healthcare experts. NPUAP is committed to preventing and managing pressure injuries through education, advocacy, and research.

If caught early, a break or tear in the skin can heal fairly quickly without other complications. However, if not caught early, a pressure injury can get bigger, deeper, and infected. Pressure injuries are painful and are difficult to heal. They can lead to life-threatening infections. Prevention is very important and is the key to skin health. Stages of pressure injuries are (Fig. 13-3):

- **Stage 1**: Skin is intact, but it may look red, and the redness is not relieved after removing pressure. Darker skin may not look red, but may appear to be a different color than the surrounding area. The area may be swollen, painful, firm, soft, and warmer or cooler when compared to the area around it.

- **Stage 2**: There is partial-thickness skin loss involving the outer and/or inner layers of skin. The injury is pink or red and moist, and may also look like a blister.

- **Stage 3**: There is full-thickness skin loss in which fat is visible in the ulcer. Slough and/or eschar may be present. *Slough* is yellow, tan, gray, green, or brown tissue that is usually moist. *Eschar* is dead tissue that is hard or soft in texture and black, brown, or tan, and may be similar to a scab. The damage may extend down to, but not through, the tissue that covers muscle.

- **Stage 4**: There is full-thickness skin loss extending through all layers of the skin, tissue, muscle, bone, and other structures, such as tendons. The ulcer will look like a deep crater and slough and/or eschar may be visible.

- **Unstageable Pressure Injury**: There is full-thickness skin and tissue loss but the extent of the damage cannot be determined because it is covered with slough or eschar. Once the slough and/or eschar is removed, the injury can then be staged (either Stage 3 or Stage 4).

- **Deep Tissue Pressure Injury**: The skin area is intact or non-intact and is deep red, purple, or maroon. The wound may appear as a blood-filled blister. The area may be painful and may be warmer or cooler than the surrounding tissue. Discoloration may be different in darker skin.

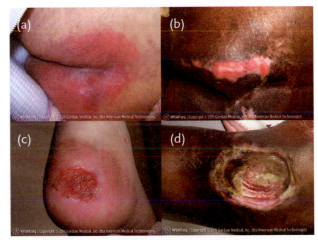

Fig. 13-3. Pressure injury stages as described by the National Pressure Ulcer Advisory Panel (NPUAP). (a) Stage 1 photo of a pressure injury on the buttocks. (b) Stage 2 photo of a pressure injury on the buttocks. (c) Stage 3 photo of a pressure injury on the heel. (d) Stage 4 photo of a pressure injury on the foot. (PHOTOS COPYRIGHT © NATIONAL PRESSURE ULCER ADVISORY PANEL, NPUAP.ORG, USED WITH PERMISSION.)

Observing and Reporting: Resident's Skin

Report any of these to the nurse:

- O/R Pale, white, reddened, gray, or purple skin
- O/R Blisters, bruises, or wounds on the skin
- O/R Differences in temperature of the skin when compared to the area around it
- O/R Complaints of tingling, warmth, or burning of the skin

O/R Dry, cracked, or flaking skin

O/R Itching or scratching

O/R Rash or any skin discoloration

O/R Swelling

O/R Fluid or blood draining from the skin

O/R Broken skin anywhere on the body, including between the toes or around the toenails

O/R Changes in existing injury, including size, depth, drainage, color, or odor

Breaks in the skin can cause serious, even life-threatening, complications. It is much better to prevent skin problems and keep the skin healthy than it is to treat skin problems.

Guidelines: Basic Skin Care

G Report any changes you observe in a resident's skin.

G Provide regular, daily care for skin to keep it clean and dry. Check the skin daily, even when complete baths are not given or taken every day.

G Reposition immobile residents often (at least every two hours).

G Give frequent, thorough skin care as often as needed for residents who are incontinent. Change clothing and linens often as well. Check on residents at least every two hours.

G Do not scratch or irritate the skin in any way. Keep rough, scratchy fabrics away from the resident's skin. Report to the nurse if a resident wears shoes that cause blisters or sores.

G Massage the skin often. Use light, circular strokes to increase circulation. Use little or no pressure on bony areas. Do not massage a white, red, or purple area or put any pressure on it. Massage the healthy skin and tissue around the area.

G Elderly residents may have very fragile, thin skin. This makes the skin more susceptible to injury. Be gentle during transfers. Avoid pulling or tearing fragile skin.

G Residents who are overweight may have poor circulation and extra folds of skin. The skin under the folds may be difficult to clean and to keep dry. Pay careful attention to these areas and give regular skin care. Report signs of skin irritation.

G Encourage residents to eat well-balanced meals. Proper nutrition is important for keeping skin healthy. Nutrition affects the color and texture of the skin. Very thin residents may be malnourished, which puts them at risk for skin injuries and poor wound healing. Be gentle when moving and positioning them. Chapter 15 contains more information about nutrition.

G Keep plastic or rubber materials from coming into contact with the resident's skin. These materials prevent air from circulating, which causes the skin to sweat.

G The care plan may include instructions on giving special skin care for dry, closed wounds or other conditions. The skin may have to be washed with a special soap or a brush may have to be used on the skin. Follow the care plan and nurse's instructions.

For residents who are immobile or who cannot change positions easily:

G Keep the bottom sheet tight and free from wrinkles. Keep the bed free from crumbs. Keep clothing or gowns free of wrinkles, too.

G Do not pull the resident across sheets during transfers or repositioning. This causes shearing, which can lead to skin breakdown.

G Place an absorbent bed pad under the back and buttocks to absorb moisture or perspiration that may build up. This also protects the skin from irritating bed linens. Absorbent pads are also available for wheelchairs.

G Relieve pressure under bony prominences. Use pillows and other positioning devices to keep elbows and heels from resting on the surface of the bed (Fig. 13-4).

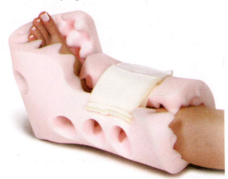

Fig. 13-4. *This foam boot suspends the heel to help reduce pressure.* (© MEDLINE INDUSTRIES, INC.)

G A bed or chair can be made softer with flotation cushions or special foam overlays.

G Use a bed cradle to keep top sheets from rubbing the resident's skin.

G Residents seated in chairs or wheelchairs need to be repositioned often, too. Reposition residents every 15 minutes if they are in a wheelchair or chair and cannot change positions easily.

Applying Nonprescription Ointments, Lotions, or Powders

Nursing assistants may need to apply ointments, lotions, or powders to a resident's skin (Fig. 13-5). However, not all nursing assistants are allowed to do this, so they should make sure they understand the rules in their facility. If instructed to apply an ointment, lotion, or powder by the nurse, the NA should follow these rules and ask questions if anything is unclear:

- Read the directions.
- Know exactly where it is to be applied.
- Know if it should be rubbed in or left on the top of the skin.
- Wash her hands before and after application.
- Wear gloves.
- Avoid getting any on clothing, as it may stain.

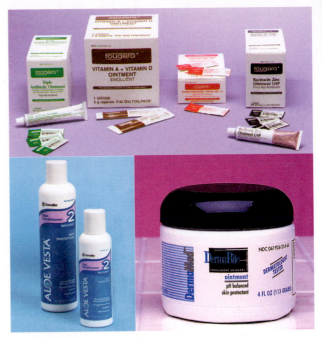

Fig. 13-5. *There are many types of ointments, creams, and lotions that are used to treat, soften, and protect the skin.* (REPRINTED WITH PERMISSION OF BRIGGS CORPORATION, 800-247-2343, WWW.BRIGGSCORP.COM)

Many positioning devices are available to help make residents safer and more comfortable.

Guidelines: Positioning Devices

G Backrests provide support and comfort for the back. They can be regular pillows or special wedge-shaped foam pillows.

G Bed cradles or foot cradles are used to keep the bed covers from resting on residents' legs and feet (Fig. 13-6). Sometimes even light pressure of a sheet draped over the toes can eventually lead to pressure injuries.

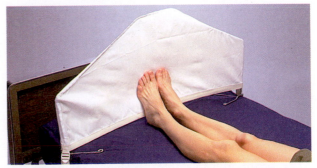

Fig. 13-6. *Bed cradles help prevent bed covers from resting on the legs and feet.* (REPRINTED WITH PERMISSION OF BRIGGS CORPORATION, 800-247-2343, WWW.BRIGGSCORP.COM)

G   A draw sheet may be placed under a resident who is unable to assist with turning, lifting, or moving up in bed. Draw sheets help prevent skin damage that can be caused by shearing. A regular bed sheet folded in half can be used as a draw sheet.

G   Footboards are padded boards placed against the resident's feet to keep them properly aligned. They help prevent foot drop. **Foot drop** is a weakness of muscles in the feet and ankles that causes difficulty with the ability to flex the ankles and walk normally. Foot splints may also be used to help prevent foot drop. Footboards are also used to keep bed covers off the feet. Rolled blankets or pillows can also be used as footboards.

G   Handrolls are cloth-covered or rubber items that keep the hand and/or fingers in a normal, natural position (Fig. 13-7). A rolled washcloth, gauze bandage, or a rubber ball placed inside the palm may be used to keep the hand in a natural position. Handrolls can help prevent finger, hand, or wrist contractures.

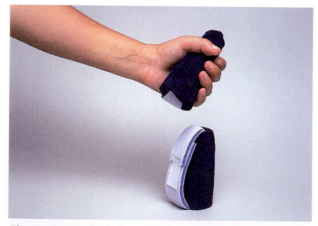

Fig. 13-7. *Handrolls keep the fingers and hand in a natural position, helping to prevent contractures.* (REPRINTED WITH PERMISSION OF BRIGGS CORPORATION, 800-247-2343, WWW.BRIGGSCORP.COM)

G   An **orthotic device**, or **orthosis**, is a device that helps support and align a limb and improve its functioning (Fig. 13-8). It may be prescribed by a doctor to keep a resident's joints in the correct position. Orthoses also help prevent or correct deformities. Splints are a type of orthotic device. Splints and the skin area around them should be cleaned at least once daily and as needed.

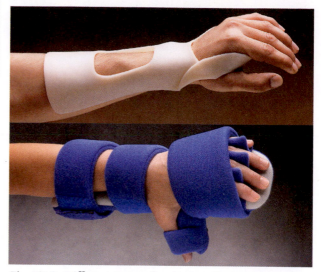

Fig. 13-8. *Different types of orthotic splints.* (PHOTO COURTESY OF NORTH COAST MEDICAL, INC., WWW.NCMEDICAL.COM, 800-821-9319)

G   Trochanter rolls are rolled towels or blankets used to keep a resident's hips and legs from turning outward (Fig. 13-9).

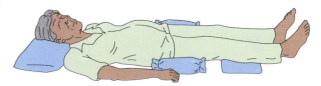

Fig. 13-9. *Trochanter rolls help keep the hips in their proper position.*

G   Abduction pillows/wedges/splints/pads (hip wedges) keep hips in proper position after hip surgery.

3. Explain guidelines for assisting with bathing

Bathing promotes health and well-being. It removes perspiration, dirt, oil, and dead skin cells that collect on the skin. It helps to prevent skin irritation and body odor. Bathing can also be relaxing. The bed bath is an excellent time for moving arms and legs and increasing circulation. Bathing gives nursing assistants an opportunity to observe residents' skin carefully.

Residents may be given a complete bath in bed, or they may take a shower or have a tub bath. They may have a **partial bath**, which is a bath given on days when a complete bed bath, tub bath, or shower is not done. It includes washing the face, hands, **axillae** (underarms), and perineum. The **perineum** is the genital and anal area.

Most people have specific preferences for bathing. Some like to take long, hot baths, while others prefer a quick shower. Usually they have been bathing the same way most of their lives. Doctors must consider a number of factors before honoring residents' personal preferences regarding bathing. These factors include the resident's capabilities and his or her safety, as well as the safety of the caregiver. The doctor, along with the resident, will decide which type of bath is appropriate.

A doctor may order a special bath using an additive. An **additive** is a substance added to another substance that changes its effect. Examples of some common bath additives and their purpose include the following:

- Bran helps to relieve itching.

- Oatmeal baths are used for inflamed skin. Oatmeal helps to relieve itching and irritation and is soothing.

- Sodium bicarbonate (baking soda) is used to treat psoriasis (non-contagious skin disorder that causes red, scaly patches on the skin) and helps relieve itching.

- Epsom salt baths or soaks reduce pain and swelling and relax muscles.

- Pine products help refresh, calm, and cool.

- Tar coal baths are used to treat eczema and other skin conditions.

- Sulfur baths may be used for skin rashes and eczema, and to help relieve inflammation related to arthritis.

Guidelines: Bathing

G The face, hands, underarms, and perineum should be washed every day. A complete bath or shower can be taken every other day or less often.

G Older skin produces less perspiration and oil. Elderly people with dry and fragile skin should bathe only once or twice a week. This prevents further dryness. Be gentle with the skin when bathing residents.

G Use only products approved by the facility and that the resident prefers.

G Before bathing a resident, make sure the room is warm enough.

G Be familiar with available safety and assistive devices.

G Gather supplies before giving a bath so that the resident is not left alone.

G Before bathing, make sure the water temperature is safe and comfortable. Test the water temperature with a thermometer or against the inside of your wrist to make sure it is not too hot. Then have the resident test the water temperature. The resident is best able to choose a comfortable water temperature.

G Wear gloves while bathing a resident and change your gloves before performing perineal care.

G Make sure all soap is removed from the skin before completing the bath.

G Keep a record of the bathing schedule for each resident. Follow the care plan.

Giving a complete bed bath

Equipment: bath blanket, bath basin, soap, bath thermometer (if available), 2–4 washcloths, 2–4 bath towels, clean gown or clothes, 2 pairs of gloves, orangewood stick, lotion, deodorant, brush or comb

When bathing, move the resident's body gently and naturally. Avoid force and overextension of limbs and joints.

1. Identify yourself by name. Identify the resident by name.

2. Wash your hands.

3. Explain procedure to the resident. Speak clearly, slowly, and directly. Maintain face-to-face contact whenever possible.

4. Provide for the resident's privacy with curtain, screen, or door. Be sure the room is a comfortable temperature and there are no drafts.

5. Adjust bed to a safe level, usually waist high. Lock bed wheels.

6. Place a bath blanket or towel over the resident (Fig. 13-10). Ask him to hold on to it as you remove or fold back the top bedding to the foot of the bed. Remove top clothing, while keeping resident covered with the bath blanket (or top sheet). Place top clothing in the proper container.

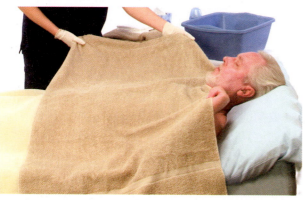

Fig. 13-10. *Cover the resident with a bath blanket before removing top bedding.*

7. Fill the basin with warm water. Test water temperature with a bath thermometer or against the inside of your wrist. Water temperature should be no higher than 105°F. Have the resident check the water temperature to see if it is comfortable. Adjust if necessary. The water will cool quickly. During the bath, change the water when it becomes too cool, soapy, or dirty.

8. Put on gloves.

9. Ask the resident to participate in washing. Help him do this whenever needed.

10. Uncover only one part of the body at a time. Place a towel under the part being washed.

11. Wash, rinse, and dry one part of the body at a time. Start at the head, work down, and complete the front first. Fold the washcloth over your hand like a mitt and hold it in place with the thumb (Fig. 13-11). When washing, use a clean area of the washcloth for each stroke.

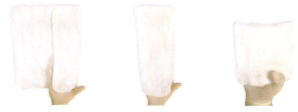

Fig. 13-11. *Make a mitt with the washcloth.*

Eyes, Face, Ears, and Neck: Wash face with wet washcloth (no soap). Begin with the eye farther away from you. Wash inner area to outer area (Fig. 13-12). Use a different area of the washcloth for each stroke. Wash the face from the middle outward using firm but gentle strokes. Wash the ears and behind the ears. Wash the neck. Rinse and pat dry.

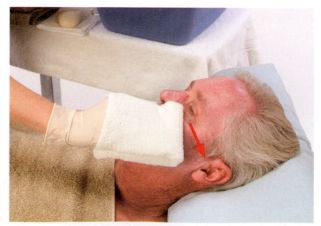

Fig. 13-12. *Wash the eye from the inner to outer area, using a different area of the washcloth for each stroke.*

Arms and Axillae: Remove one arm from under the towel. With a soapy washcloth, wash the upper arm and the underarm. Use long strokes from the shoulder down to the wrist (Fig. 13-13). Rinse and pat dry. Repeat for the other arm.

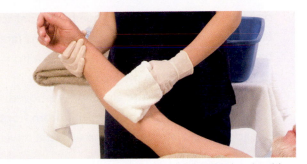

Fig. 13-13. *Support the wrist while washing the shoulder, arm, underarm, and elbow.*

Hands: Wash one hand in a basin. Clean under the nails with an orangewood stick. Rinse and pat dry. Make sure to dry between the fingers. Give nail care (see procedure later in this chapter). Repeat for the other hand. Put lotion on the resident's elbows and hands.

Chest: Place the towel again across the resident's chest. Pull the blanket down to the waist. Lift the towel only enough to wash the chest, rinse it, and pat dry. For a female resident, wash, rinse, and dry breasts and under breasts. Check the skin in this area for signs of irritation.

Abdomen: Keep the towel across chest. Fold the blanket down so that it still covers the pubic area. Wash the abdomen, rinse, and pat dry. If the resident has an ostomy, or opening in the abdomen for getting rid of body wastes, give skin care around the opening (Chapter 17 contains information about ostomies). Cover with the towel. Pull the bath blanket up to the resident's chin. Remove the towel.

Legs and Feet: Expose one leg and place a towel under it. Wash the thigh. Use long, downward strokes when washing. Rinse and pat dry. Do the same from the knee to the ankle (Fig. 13-14).

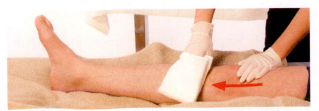

Fig. 13-14. *Use long, downward strokes when washing the legs.*

Place another towel under the foot. Move the basin to the towel. Place the foot into the basin. Wash the foot and between the toes (Fig. 13-15). Rinse the foot and pat dry, making sure the area between the toes is dry. Give nail care (see procedure later in this chapter) if it has been assigned. Never clip a resident's toenails. Apply lotion to the foot if ordered, especially at the heels. Do not apply lotion between the toes. Remove excess lotion (if any) with a towel. Repeat the steps for the other leg and foot.

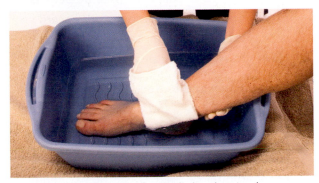

Fig. 13-15. *Washing the feet includes cleaning between the toes.*

Back: Help the resident move to the center of the bed. If the bed has rails, raise the rail on the far side for safety. Ask the resident to turn onto his side, toward the raised side rail. Return to the working side of the bed. The resident's back should be facing you. Fold the blanket away from the back. Place a towel lengthwise next to the back. Wash the neck and back with long, downward strokes (Fig. 13-16). Rinse and pat dry. Apply lotion if ordered.

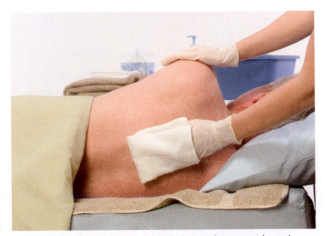

Fig. 13-16. *Wash the back with long, downward strokes.*

12. Place the towel under the buttocks and upper thighs. Help the resident turn onto his back. If the resident is able to wash his perineal area, place a basin of clean, warm water, a washcloth, and towel within reach. Hand items to the resident as needed. If the resident wants you to leave the room, remove and discard gloves. Wash your hands. Leave supplies and the call light within reach. If the resident has a urinary catheter in place, remind him not to pull it.

13. If the resident is unable to provide perineal care, you will do so. Remove and discard your gloves. Wash your hands and put on clean gloves. Provide privacy at all times.

14. **Perineal area and buttocks**: Change the bath water. Wash, rinse, and dry perineal area, working from front to back (clean to dirty).

    For a female resident: Using water and a small amount of soap, wash the perineum from front to back, using single strokes (Fig. 13-17). Use a clean area of the washcloth or a clean washcloth for each stroke.

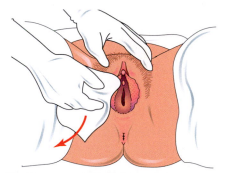

Fig. 13-17. Always work from front to back when performing perineal care. This helps prevent infection.

Working from front to back, wipe one side of the labia majora, the outside folds of perineal skin that protect the urinary meatus and the vaginal opening. Then wipe the other side, using a clean part of the washcloth. With your thumb and forefinger, gently separate the labia majora. Wipe from front to back on one side with a clean washcloth, using a single stroke. Using a clean area of the washcloth, wipe from front to back on the other side. Using another

clean area of the washcloth, wipe from front to back down the center. Clean the perineum (area between the vagina and anus) last with a front to back motion. Rinse the area thoroughly in the same way. Make sure all soap is removed. Dry the entire perineal area, moving from front to back, using a blotting motion with the towel.

Ask resident to turn on her side. Wash, rinse, and dry buttocks and anal area. Clean the anal area without contaminating the perineal area.

For a male resident: If the resident is uncircumcised, pull back the foreskin first. Gently push the skin toward the base of penis. Hold the penis by the shaft. Wash in a circular motion from the tip down to the base. Use a clean area of washcloth or clean washcloth for each stroke (Fig. 13-18).

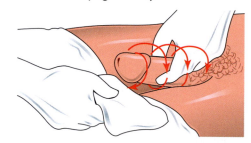

Fig. 13-18. Wash the penis in a circular motion from the tip down to the base.

Thoroughly rinse the penis and pat dry. If the resident is uncircumcised, gently return the foreskin to normal position. Then wash the scrotum and groin. The **groin** is the area from the pubis (area around the penis and scrotum) to the upper thighs. Rinse thoroughly and pat dry. Ask the resident to turn on his side. Using a clean washcloth, wash, rinse, and dry buttocks and anal area. Clean the anal area without contaminating the perineal area.

15. Cover the resident with the bath blanket.

16. Empty, rinse, and dry bath basin. Place basin in designated dirty supply area or return to storage, depending on facility policy.

17. Place soiled clothing and linens in proper containers.

18. Remove and discard gloves.

19. Wash your hands.

20. Provide the resident with deodorant. Place a towel over the pillow and brush or comb the resident's hair (see procedure later in this chapter). Help the resident put on clean clothing and get into a comfortable position with proper body alignment.

21. Return bed to lowest position. Remove privacy measures.

22. Place call light within resident's reach.

23. Wash your hands.

24. Report any changes in resident to the nurse.

25. Document procedure using facility guidelines.

Back rubs help relax tired muscles, relieve pain, and increase circulation. Back rubs are often given after baths. After giving a back rub, the nursing assistant should note any changes in a resident's skin.

Giving a back rub

Equipment: cotton blanket or towel, lotion

1. Identify yourself by name. Identify the resident by name.

2. Wash your hands.

3. Explain procedure to the resident. Speak clearly, slowly, and directly. Maintain face-to-face contact whenever possible.

4. Provide for resident's privacy with curtain, screen, or door.

5. Adjust bed to a safe working level, usually waist high. Lower the head of the bed. Lock bed wheels.

6. Position the resident so he is lying on his side (lateral position) or his stomach (prone position). Many elderly people find that lying on their stomach is uncomfortable. If so, have the resident lie on his side. Cover the resident with a cotton blanket, then fold back the bed covers. Expose the resident's back to the top of the buttocks. Back rubs can also be given with the resident sitting up.

7. Warm lotion by putting bottle in warm water for five minutes. Run your hands under warm water to warm them. Pour lotion on your hands and rub them together to spread it. Always put the lotion on your hands first, rather than directly on the resident's skin. Warn the resident that the lotion may still feel cool.

8. Place your hands on each side of the upper part of the buttocks. Use the full palm of your hand. Make long, smooth upward strokes with both hands. Move along each side of the spine, up to the shoulders (Figs. 13-19 and 13-20). Circle your hands outward. Then move back along outer edges of the back. At the buttocks, make another circle. Move your hands back up to the shoulders. Without taking your hands off the resident's skin, repeat this motion for three to five minutes.

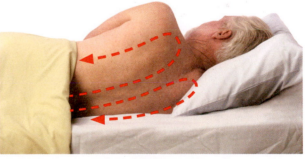

Fig. 13-19. *Move along each side of the spine, up to the shoulders.*

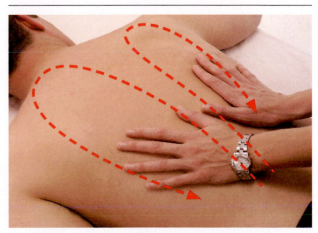

Fig. 13-20. *Long, upward strokes help release muscle tension.*

9. Knead with the first two fingers and thumb of each hand. Place them at the base of the spine. Move upward together along each side of the spine. Apply gentle downward pressure with fingers and thumbs. Follow the same direction as with the long smooth strokes, circling at shoulders and buttocks.

10. Gently massage bony areas (spine, shoulder blades, hip bones) with circular motions of your fingertips, using little or no pressure. Gentle massage stimulates circulation and helps prevent skin damage. However, do not massage a white, red, or purple area or put any pressure on it. The discoloration indicates that the skin is already irritated and fragile. Include this information in your report to the nurse.

11. Let the resident know when you are almost through. Finish with some long smooth strokes, like the ones you used at the beginning of the massage.

12. Dry the back if extra lotion remains on it.

13. Remove the blanket and towel.

14. Help the resident get dressed. Help the resident into a comfortable position.

15. Store supplies. Place soiled clothing and linens in proper containers.

16. Return bed to lowest position. Remove privacy measures.

17. Place call light within resident's reach.

18. Wash your hands.

19. Report any changes in resident to the nurse.

20. Document procedure using facility guidelines.

Hair care is an important part of cleanliness. Shampooing the hair removes dirt, bacteria, oils, and other materials from the hair. Residents who can get out of bed may have their hair shampooed in the sink, tub, or shower. For residents who cannot get out of bed, special troughs exist for shampooing hair in bed (Fig. 13-21). Troughs fit under the resident's head and neck and have a spout or hose that drains the water into a basin at the side of the bed. There are also special types of shampoos that do not require the use of water (Fig. 13-22). Nursing assistants should follow the care plan regarding the type of shampoo to use.

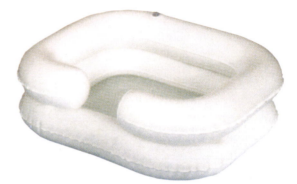

Fig. 13-21. *An inflatable bed shampoo trough can be used to shampoo hair while the person is in bed.* (REPRINTED WITH PERMISSION OF BRIGGS CORPORATION, 800-247-2343, WWW.BRIGGSCORP.COM)

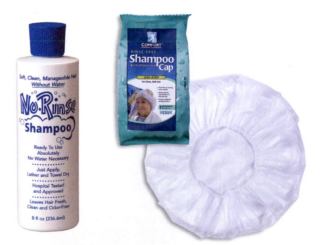

Fig. 13-22. *The left photo shows one type of shampoo that does not require water. The right photo shows a rinse-free shampoo cap that does not require the use of running water.* (LEFT PHOTO REPRINTED WITH PERMISSION OF BRIGGS CORPORATION, 800-247-2343, WWW.BRIGGSCORP.COM AND RIGHT PHOTO REPRINTED WITH PERMISSION OF SAGE PRODUCTS LLC, 800-323-2220, WWW.SAGEPRODUCTS.COM)

Shampooing hair

Equipment: shampoo, hair conditioner (if requested), 2 bath towels, washcloth, bath thermometer, pitcher or handheld shower or sink attachment, waterproof pad (for washing hair in bed), bath blanket (for washing hair in bed), trough and catch basin (for washing hair in bed), chair (for washing hair in sink), protective plastic sheet or drape (for washing hair in sink), comb and brush, hair dryer

1. Identify yourself by name. Identify the resident by name.

2. Wash your hands.

3. Explain procedure to the resident. Speak clearly, slowly, and directly. Maintain face-to-face contact whenever possible.

4. Provide for the resident's privacy with curtain, screen, or door. Be sure the room is a comfortable temperature and there are no drafts.

5. Test water temperature with bath thermometer or against the inside of your wrist. Water temperature should be no higher than 105°F. Have resident check water temperature. Adjust if necessary.

6. Position the resident and wet the resident's hair.

a. *For washing hair in the sink*, seat the resident in a chair covered with a protective plastic drape or sheet. Use a pillow under the plastic to support the head and neck. Have the resident lean her head back toward the sink. Give the resident a folded washcloth to hold over her forehead or eyes. Wet hair using a plastic cup or a handheld sink attachment (Fig. 13-23).

b. *For washing hair in bed*, arrange the supplies within reach on a nearby table. Remove all pillows, and place the resident in a flat position. Adjust bed to a safe level, usually waist high. Lock bed wheels. Place a waterproof pad beneath the resident's head and shoulders. Cover the resident with the blanket, and fold back the top sheet and regular blankets. Place the trough under the resident's head and connect the trough to the catch basin. Place one towel across the resident's shoulders. Protect the resident's eyes with a dry wash-

cloth. Using the pitcher or attachment, pour enough water on the resident's hair to make it thoroughly wet.

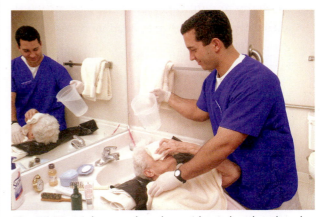

Fig. 13-23. *Make sure that the resident's head and neck are supported and her eyes are covered when washing hair in the sink.*

7. Apply a small amount of shampoo to your hands and rub them together. Using both hands, massage the shampoo to a lather in the resident's hair. With your fingertips (not fingernails), massage the scalp in a circular motion, from front to back (Fig. 13-24). Do not scratch the scalp.

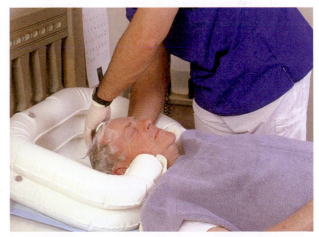

Fig. 13-24. *Use your fingertips, not your fingernails, to work shampoo into a lather. Be gentle so that you do not scratch the scalp.*

8. Rinse the hair in the same way you wet it. Rinse until water runs clear. Repeat the shampoo, rinse again, and use conditioner if the resident wants it. Be sure to rinse the hair thoroughly to prevent the scalp from getting dry and itchy.

9. Wrap the resident's hair in a clean towel. If shampooing at the sink, return the resident to an upright position. If shampooing in bed, remove the trough. Using the washcloth or towel, wipe water from the face, head, and neck.

10. Remove the hair towel and gently rub the scalp and hair with the towel. Comb or brush hair (see procedure later in the chapter).

11. Dry hair with a hair dryer on the low setting. Style hair as the resident prefers.

12. Make resident comfortable.

13. Return bed to lowest position. Remove privacy measures.

14. Place call light within resident's reach.

15. Empty, rinse, and wipe bath basin/pitcher. Take to proper area.

16. Clean the comb or brush. Return hair dryer and comb or brush to proper storage.

17. Place soiled linen in proper container.

18. Wash your hands.

19. Report any changes in resident to nurse.

20. Document procedure using facility guidelines.

Many people prefer showers or tub baths to bed baths (Fig. 13-25). It is important for a nursing assistant to check with the nurse first to make sure a shower or tub bath is allowed.

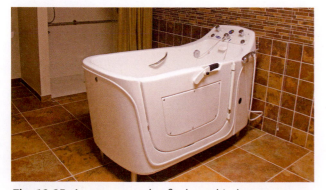

Fig. 13-25. *A common style of tub used in long-term care facilities.*

Guidelines: Safety for Showers and Tub Baths

G Clean tub or shower before and after use.

G Make sure the floor is dry.

G Be familiar with available safety and assistive devices. Check that handrails, grab bars, and lifts are in working order.

G Have the resident use safety bars to get into or out of the tub or shower.

G Place all needed items within reach.

G Do not leave the resident alone.

G Do not use bath oils, lotions, or powders in showers or tubs. They make surfaces slippery and dangerous.

G Test water temperature with a bath thermometer or against the inside of your wrist before the resident gets into the tub or shower. Water temperature should be no higher than 105°F. Make sure temperature is comfortable for the resident.

Residents' Rights

Privacy When Bathing

Privacy is very important when residents are having a shower or tub bath. Just as with a bed bath, keep residents covered when possible. Make sure their bodies are not unnecessarily exposed.

Some residents will have whirlpool baths. In a whirlpool bath, the water moves around the tub. The water movement helps clean, stimulates circulation, and promotes wound healing. To take a whirlpool bath, a resident is first covered, placed in a chairlift, and lowered into the whirlpool. The resident may feel faint or dizzy after the bath. The nursing assistant should remain with the resident while he or she is bathing.

Giving a shower or tub bath

Equipment: bath blanket, soap, shampoo, bath thermometer, 2–4 washcloths, 2–4 bath towels, clean clothes, nonskid footwear, 2 pairs of gloves, lotion, deodorant, hair dryer

1. Wash your hands.

2. Place equipment in the shower or tub room. Put on gloves. Clean the shower or tub area and shower chair. Place a bucket under shower chair (in case the resident has a bowel movement). Turn on the heat lamp to warm the room, if available.

3. Remove and discard gloves. Wash your hands.

4. Go to the resident's room. Identify yourself by name. Identify the resident by name.

5. Wash your hands.

6. Explain procedure to the resident. Speak clearly, slowly, and directly. Maintain face-to-face contact whenever possible.

7. Provide for resident's privacy with curtain, screen, or door.

8. Help the resident to put on nonskid footwear. Transport resident to shower or tub room.

9. Wash your hands. Put on clean gloves.

10. Help the resident remove clothing and shoes.

For a shower:

11. If using a shower chair, place it close to the resident and lock its wheels (Fig. 13-26). Safely transfer the resident into shower chair.

12. Turn on water. Test water temperature with the thermometer or against the inside of your wrist. Water temperature should be no higher than 105°F. Have resident check water temperature. Adjust if necessary. Check temperature throughout the shower.

13. Unlock the shower chair and move it into the shower stall. Lock the wheels.

14. Stay with the resident during the procedure.

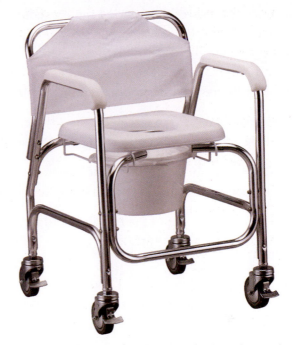

*Fig. 13-26. A **shower chair** is a sturdy chair designed to be placed in a bathtub or shower. It is water- and slip-resistant. The chair or bench enables a person who is unable to get into a tub or is too weak to stand in a shower to bathe in the tub or shower, rather than in bed. A shower chair must be locked before transferring a resident into it.* (PHOTO COURTESY OF NOVA MEDICAL PRODUCTS, WWW.NOVAMEDICALPRODUCTS.COM)

15. Let the resident wash as much as possible. Help to wash his or her face.

16. Help the resident shampoo and rinse hair.

17. Using soap, help to wash and rinse the entire body. Move from head to toe (clean to dirty).

18. Turn off water. Unlock shower chair wheels. Roll the resident out of the shower.

For a tub bath:

11. Residents may need help to get into the bath, depending on their level of mobility. Safely transfer the resident onto chair or tub lift, or help the resident into the bath.

12. Fill the tub halfway with warm water. Test water temperature with thermometer or against the inside of your wrist. Water temperature should be no higher than 105°F. Have resident check water temperature. Adjust if necessary.

13. Stay with the resident during the procedure.

14. Let the resident wash as much as possible. Help to wash his or her face.

15. Help the resident shampoo and rinse hair.

16. Using soap, help to wash and rinse the entire body. Move from head to toe (clean to dirty).

17. Drain the tub. Cover the resident with the bath blanket while the tub drains.

18. Help resident out of the tub and onto a chair.

Remaining steps for either procedure:

19. Give the resident towel(s) and help to pat dry. Pat dry under the breasts, between skin folds, in the perineal area, and between toes.

20. Apply lotion and deodorant as needed.

21. Place soiled clothing and linens in proper containers.

22. Remove and discard gloves.

23. Wash your hands.

24. Help the resident dress and comb hair before leaving shower or tub room. Put on nonskid footwear. Return resident to room.

25. Make sure resident is comfortable.

26. Place call light within resident's reach.

27. Report any changes in resident to nurse.

28. Document procedure using facility guidelines.

After a resident showers or bathes, the nursing assistant may need to return to the shower room and clean the shower, shower chair, chair lift, or the tub. She should follow facility policy.

4. Explain guidelines for assisting with grooming

Grooming affects the way people feel about themselves and how they appear to others. A well-groomed person is more likely to feel better physically and emotionally (Fig. 13-27). When helping with grooming, nursing assistants should always let residents do all they can for themselves. Residents should make as many choices as possible. Some residents may be embarrassed, depressed, or anxious because they need help with grooming tasks that they have performed for themselves all their lives. Nursing assistants should be sensitive to this. Being professional and respectful helps residents maintain self-respect and promotes person-centered care.

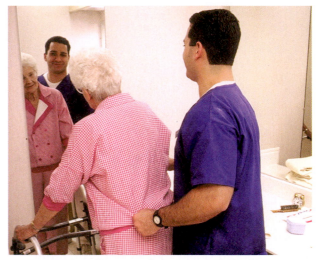

Fig. 13-27. *A well-groomed appearance helps a person feel good about herself.*

Fingernail Care

Fingernails can harbor bacteria. It is important to keep hands and nails clean to help prevent infection. Nail care should be given when nails are dirty or have jagged edges and whenever it has been assigned. Some facility's policies do not allow nursing assistants to cut a resident's fingernails or toenails. For some residents, poor circulation can lead to infection if skin is accidentally cut while caring for nails. For a resident who has compromised circulation due to a disease such as diabetes, an infection can lead to a severe wound or even amputation. Chapter 18 contains more information on diabetes. If directed to provide nail care, the NA should know exactly what care to provide. In addition, the same nail equipment should not be used on more than one resident.

Providing fingernail care

Equipment: orangewood stick, emery board, basin, soap, washcloth, 2 towels, bath thermometer, lotion, gloves

1. Identify yourself by name. Identify the resident by name.

2. Wash your hands.

3. Explain procedure to the resident. Speak clearly, slowly, and directly. Maintain face-to-face contact whenever possible.

4. Provide for resident's privacy with curtain, screen, or door.

5. If resident is in bed, adjust bed to a safe level, usually waist high. Lock bed wheels.

6. Fill the basin halfway with warm water. Test water temperature with the bath thermometer or against the inside of your wrist to ensure it is safe. Water temperature should be no higher than 105°F. Have resident check the water temperature. Adjust if necessary. Place basin at a comfortable level for the resident.

7. Put on gloves.

8. Soak the resident's hands and nails in the basin of water. Soak all 10 fingertips for at least five minutes.

9. Remove hands from water. Wash hands with a soapy washcloth. Rinse. Pat hands dry with a towel, including between the fingers. Remove the hand basin.

10. Place the resident's hands on the towel. Gently clean under each fingernail with the orangewood stick (Fig. 13-28).

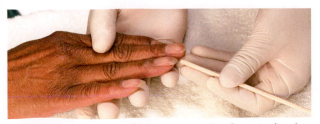

Fig. 13-28. *Be gentle when removing dirt from under the nails with an orangewood stick.*

11. Wipe the orangewood stick on the towel after cleaning under each nail. Wash the hands again. Dry them thoroughly, especially between the fingers.

12. Shape fingernails with an emery board or nail file, moving in one direction only (not back and forth). File in a curve. Finish with nails smooth and free of rough edges.

13. Apply lotion from fingertips to wrists.

14. Empty, rinse, and dry basin. Place basin in designated dirty supply area or return to storage, depending on facility policy.

15. Place soiled clothing and linens in proper containers.

16. Remove and discard gloves. Wash your hands.

17. Make resident comfortable.

18. Return bed to lowest position. Remove privacy measures.

19. Place call light within resident's reach.

20. Wash your hands.

21. Report any changes in resident to the nurse.

22. Document procedure using facility guidelines.

Foot Care

Careful foot care is extremely important; it should be a part of daily care of residents. For residents with diabetes, which causes poor circulation, a small sore on the foot can grow into a much larger wound that may take months to heal, or may not heal at all. It can result in amputation. Long, thickened toenails contribute to pressure injuries and problems with balance, which contribute to falls. Falls can lead to hospitalization and further complications.

As mentioned earlier, a nursing assistant should not trim a resident's toenails unless allowed and directed to do so. Often a podiatrist (a doctor who specializes in care of the feet, ankles, and related structures of the legs) is the person who cares for a resident's toenails. When NAs provide foot care, they should observe the feet for any of the following:

Observing and Reporting: Foot Care

Report any of these to the nurse:

O/R Dry, flaking skin

O/R Non-intact or broken skin

O/R Discoloration of the feet, such as reddened, gray, white, or black areas

O/R Blisters

O/R Bruises

O/R Blood or drainage

O/R Long, ragged toenails

O/R Ingrown toenails

O/R Swelling

O/R Soft, fragile, or reddened heels

O/R Differences in temperature of the feet

Providing foot care

Equipment: basin, bath mat, 2 towels, washcloth, soap, lotion, bath thermometer, clean socks, gloves

1. Identify yourself by name. Identify the resident by name.

2. Wash your hands.

3. Explain procedure to the resident. Speak clearly, slowly, and directly. Maintain face-to-face contact whenever possible.

4. Provide for resident's privacy with curtain, screen, or door.

5. If resident is in bed, adjust bed to a safe level, usually waist high. Lock bed wheels.

6. Fill the basin halfway with warm water. Test water temperature with thermometer or against the inside of your wrist to ensure it is

safe. Water temperature should be no higher than 105°F. Have resident check water temperature. Adjust if necessary.

7. Place the basin on a bath mat or towel on the floor (if the resident is in a chair) or on a towel at the foot of the bed (if the resident is in bed). Make sure the basin is in a comfortable position for the resident. Support the foot and ankle throughout the procedure.

8. Put on gloves.

9. Remove the resident's socks. Completely submerge the resident's feet in the water. Soak the feet for 10 to 20 minutes. Add warm water to the basin as necessary.

10. Put soap on a wet washcloth. Remove one foot from the water. Wash the entire foot, including between the toes and around the nail beds (Fig. 13-29).

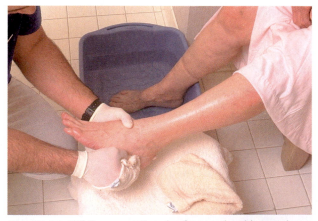

Fig. 13-29. *While supporting the foot and ankle, wash the entire foot with a soapy washcloth.*

11. Rinse the entire foot, including between the toes.

12. Using the towel, pat the entire foot dry, especially between the toes.

13. Repeat steps 10 through 12 for the other foot.

14. Put lotion in one hand and warm lotion by rubbing hands together. Massage lotion into entire foot (top and bottom), except between the toes. Remove excess, if any, with a towel.

15. Help the resident put on clean socks.

16. Empty, rinse, and dry basin. Place basin in designated dirty supply area or return to storage, depending on facility policy.

17. Place soiled clothing and linens in proper containers.

18. Remove and discard gloves. Wash your hands.

19. Make resident comfortable.

20. Return bed to lowest position. Remove privacy measures.

21. Place call light within resident's reach.

22. Wash your hands.

23. Report any changes in resident to the nurse.

24. Document procedure using facility guidelines.

Shaving

The NA should make sure the resident wants her to shave him or help him shave before beginning. Personal preferences for shaving must be respected. NAs must wear gloves when shaving residents due to the risk of being exposed to blood. This is part of following Standard Precautions; it helps prevent infection.

If a resident has a beard or mustache, it will need daily care. Washing and combing a beard or mustache every day is usually enough. The NA can ask the resident how he would like it done. She should not trim or shave a beard or mustache without a resident's permission.

There are different types of razors. NAs should check with the nurse to know which type of razor the resident uses:

- A **safety razor** has a sharp blade, which comes with a special safety casing to help prevent cuts. This type of razor requires shaving cream or soap.

- A **disposable razor** requires shaving cream or soap. The NA should not attempt to recap a disposable razor. It should be discarded in a biohazard container for sharps after use.

- An **electric razor** is the safest and easiest type of razor to use. It does not require soap or shaving cream. Some residents who take blood thinners may be told to use an electric razor to avoid nicks and cuts. An electric razor should not be used near water or any water source or when oxygen is in use.

Shaving a resident

Equipment: razor, basin filled halfway with warm water (if using a safety or disposable razor), shaving cream or soap (if using a safety or disposable razor), 2 towels, washcloth, mirror, aftershave lotion, gloves

1. Identify yourself by name. Identify the resident by name.

2. Wash your hands.

3. Explain procedure to the resident. Speak clearly, slowly, and directly. Maintain face-to-face contact whenever possible.

4. Provide for resident's privacy with curtain, screen, or door.

5. If resident is in bed, adjust bed to safe level, usually waist high. Lock bed wheels.

6. Raise the head of the bed so that the resident is sitting up. Place a towel across the resident's chest, under his chin.

7. Put on gloves.

Shaving using a safety or disposable razor:

8. If using a safety or disposable razor, use a blade that is sharp. A dull blade can irritate the skin. Soften the beard with a warm, wet washcloth on the face for a few minutes before shaving. Lather the face with shaving cream or soap and warm water. Warm water and lather make shaving more comfortable.

9. Hold skin taut. Shave in the direction of hair growth. Shave beard in short, downward, and even strokes on the face and upward strokes

on the neck (Fig. 13-30). Rinse the blade often in the basin to keep it clean and wet.

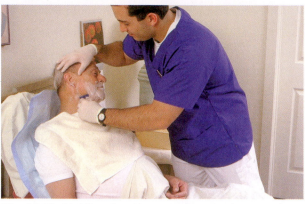

Fig. 13-30. Holding the skin taut, shave in downward strokes on the face and upward strokes on the neck.

10. When you have finished, wash and rinse the resident's face with a warm, wet washcloth. If he is able, let him use the washcloth himself. Use the towel to dry the resident's face. Offer a mirror to the resident.

Shaving using an electric razor:

8. Use a small brush to clean the razor. Do not use an electric razor near any water source or when oxygen is in use. Electricity near water may cause electrocution. Electricity near oxygen may cause an explosion.

9. Turn on the razor and hold skin taut. Shave with smooth, even movements (Fig. 13-31). If using a foil shaver, shave the beard with a back and forth motion in the direction of beard growth. If using a three-head shaver, shave the beard in circular motion. Shave the chin and under the chin.

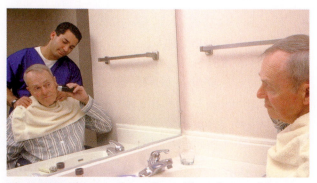

Fig. 13-31. Shave, or have the resident shave, with smooth, even movements.

10. When you have finished, offer a mirror to the resident.

Final steps:

11. If the resident wants aftershave lotion, moisten your palms with the lotion and pat it onto the resident's face.

12. Remove the towel. Place the towel and washcloth in proper container.

13. Clean the equipment and store it. Follow facility policy for a safety razor. For a disposable razor, dispose of it in a biohazard container for sharps. For an electric razor, clean head of razor. Remove whiskers, recap shaving head, and return razor to case.

14. Remove and discard gloves. Wash your hands.

15. Make resident comfortable.

16. Return bed to lowest position. Remove privacy measures.

17. Place call light within resident's reach.

18. Wash your hands.

19. Report any changes in resident to the nurse.

20. Document procedure using facility guidelines.

Hair Care

Nursing assistants help keep residents' hair clean and styled. Hair ornaments should be used only as requested, and residents' hair should never be combed or brushed into childish styles. Because hair thins as people age, pieces of hair can be accidentally pulled out of the head while combing or brushing it. Nursing assistants must handle residents' hair very gently.

Pediculosis is the medical term for an infestation of lice. Lice are tiny parasites that bite into the skin and suck blood to live and grow. Three types of lice are head lice, body lice, and crab or pubic lice.

Head lice are usually found on the scalp. Lice are usually difficult to see. Symptoms include itching, bite marks on the scalp, skin sores, and matted, bad-smelling hair and scalp. Lice eggs may be visible on the hair, behind the ears, and on the neck. They are small and round and may be brown or white. Lice droppings look like a fine black powder. They may be seen on sheets or pillows.

If an NA notices any of these symptoms, she should report to the nurse immediately. Lice can spread very quickly. Special creams, shampoos, lotions, sprays, or special combs may be used to treat lice. People who have lice can spread it to others. To help prevent the spread of lice, a resident's combs, brushes, clothes, wigs, and hats should not be shared with anyone else.

Dandruff is an excessive shedding of dead skin cells from the scalp. It is a result of the normal growing process of the skin cells of the scalp. The most common symptom is the flaking of small, round, white patches from the head. Itching can also occur. Dandruff is a natural process. It cannot be stopped; it can only be controlled. Residents who have dandruff may use a special medicated shampoo to help control it.

Combing or brushing hair

Equipment: comb, brush, towel, mirror, hair care items requested by resident

Use hair care products that the resident prefers for his or her type of hair.

1. Identify yourself by name. Identify the resident by name.

2. Wash your hands.

3. Explain procedure to the resident. Speak clearly, slowly, and directly. Maintain face-to-face contact whenever possible.

4. Provide for resident's privacy with curtain, screen, or door.

5. If the resident is in bed, adjust bed to a safe level, usually waist high. Raise the head of the bed so that the resident is sitting up. Lock bed wheels. If resident is ambulatory, provide a chair.

6. Place a towel under the resident's head or around the shoulders.

7. Remove any hair pins, hair ties, or clips.

8. If the hair is tangled, work on the tangles first. Remove tangles by dividing hair into small sections. Hold the lock of hair just above the tangle so you do not pull at the scalp. Gently comb or brush through the tangle. If the resident agrees, use a small amount of detangler or leave-in conditioner.

9. After tangles are removed, brush two-inch sections of hair at a time (Fig. 13-32).

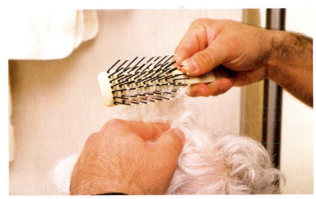

Fig. 13-32. *Gently brush hair after tangles are removed.*

10. Neatly style hair as the resident prefers (Fig. 13-33). Each resident may prefer different styles and hair products. Avoid childish hairstyles. Offer the mirror to the resident.

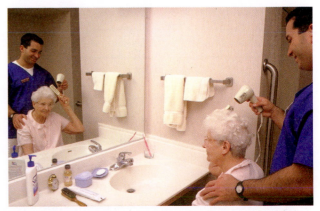

Fig. 13-33. *Assist the resident in styling her hair as she prefers.*

11. Return supplies to proper storage. Clean hair from comb or brush. Clean comb or brush.

12. Dispose of soiled linen in the proper container.

13. Make resident comfortable.

14. Return bed to lowest position. Remove privacy measures.

15. Place call light within resident's reach.

16. Wash your hands.

17. Report any changes in resident to nurse.

18. Document procedure using facility guidelines.

5. List guidelines for assisting with dressing

Dressing and undressing residents is an important part of daily care. When helping with dressing, the NA should know what limitations the resident has. Residents may have one side of the body that is weaker than the other side due to stroke or injury. This side is called the weaker, **affected**, or **involved side**. The NA should not refer to the weaker side as the "bad side" or talk about the "bad" leg or arm. When dressing residents, the NA should begin with the weaker side of the body to reduce the risk of injury. The weaker arm is placed through a sleeve first (Fig. 13-34). When a leg is weak, it is easier if the resident sits down to pull the pants over both legs.

Guidelines: Dressing and Undressing

G   As with all care, ask about and follow the resident's preferences. This is part of promoting person-centered care. Performing resident-directed care is the resident's legal right and your responsibility.

G   Let the resident choose clothing for the day. However, check to see if it is clean, appropriate for the weather, and in good condition.

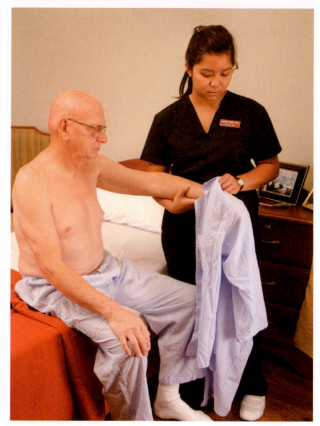

Fig. 13-34. *When dressing, the NA should start with the affected (weaker) side first.*

G   Encourage the resident to dress in regular clothes rather than nightclothes. Wearing regular daytime clothing encourages more activity and out-of-bed time. Clothing with elastic waistbands and clothing that is a larger size than normal are easier to put on. Be sure the elastic waistband of underpants, slip, stockings, tights, pants, or skirt fits comfortably at the waist.

G   The resident should do as much to dress or undress himself as possible. It may take longer, but it helps him maintain independence and regain self-care skills. Ask where your help is needed.

G   Provide privacy. If the resident has just had a bath, cover him with the bath blanket. Put on undergarments first. Never expose more than what is needed.

G   When putting on socks or stockings, roll or fold them down. They can then be slipped over the toes and foot, then unrolled up into place. Make sure the toes, heels, and seams of socks or stockings are in the right place.

G   For a female resident, make sure bra cups fit over the breasts. A front-fastening bra is easier for residents to work by themselves. A bra that fastens in the back can be put around the waist and fastened first. After fastening, rotate the bra around and move it up, putting arms through the straps last. This can be done in reverse for undressing.

G   For residents who have weakness or paralysis on one side, place the weaker arm or leg through the garment first, then the strong arm or leg. When undressing, do the opposite—start with the stronger, or unaffected, side.

G   Several types of adaptive or assistive devices for dressing are available to help residents maintain independence in dressing themselves (Fig. 13-35). An occupational therapist may teach residents to perform activities of daily living (ADLs) using adaptive equipment.

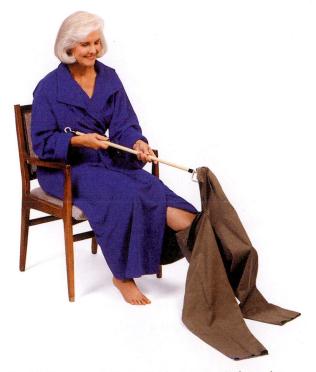

Fig. 13-35. *Special dressing aids promote independence by helping residents dress themselves.* (PHOTO COURTESY OF NORTH COAST MEDICAL, INC., WWW.NCMEDICAL.COM, 800-821-9319)

Dressing a resident

Equipment: bath blanket, clean clothes of resident's choice, nonskid footwear, gloves

When putting on all items, move the resident's body gently and naturally. Avoid force and over-extension of limbs and joints.

1. Identify yourself by name. Identify the resident by name.

2. Wash your hands.

3. Explain procedure to the resident. Speak clearly, slowly, and directly. Maintain face-to-face contact whenever possible.

4. Provide for resident's privacy with curtain, screen, or door.

5. Adjust bed to a safe level, usually waist high. Lock bed wheels.

6. Raise the head of the bed so that the resident is sitting up.

7. Ask the resident what she would like to wear. Dress her in the outfit she chooses.

8. Put on gloves if the resident has non-intact (broken) skin.

9. Place a bath blanket over the resident. Ask her to hold onto it as you remove or fold back the top bedding to the foot of the bed. Remove the gown or top clothing, while keeping the resident covered with the bath blanket. Take clothes off the stronger, or unaffected, side first when undressing. Then remove from the weaker side. Place top clothing in the proper container. Move the bath blanket down to cover the lower body.

10. If the resident wears a bra, put the strap over the weaker hand first, then the stronger hand. Move the straps up the arms and place on the shoulders. Make sure the breasts are inside the cups of the bra, then fasten the bra.

11. Help the resident put on the top. If the top goes over the head, slide the top over the

head first. Then place the weaker/affected arm through the sleeve before placing the garment on the stronger/unaffected arm. Help the resident lean forward and smooth the top down. If the top fastens in the front, slide your hand through one sleeve and grasp the resident's hand on the weaker side, pulling it through. Help the resident lean forward and arrange the top across the back. Pull the second sleeve on the stronger side as you did with the first one. Fasten the top.

12. Remove the bath blanket and place in the proper container. Help the resident put on skirt or pants. Put the weaker/affected leg through the skirt or pants first. Then place the stronger/unaffected leg through the skirt or pants. Have the resident raise her buttocks or turn the resident from side to side to pull the pants over the buttocks up to the waist. Fasten the pants or skirt if needed and make sure the clothing is comfortable.

13. Roll one sock over the weaker foot, making sure the heel of the sock is over the heel of the foot. Make sure there are no twists or wrinkles in the sock after it is on. Repeat for the other foot.

14. Starting with the weaker foot, slip on nonskid footwear, using an assistive device if needed. Fasten one shoe securely and then put on the other shoe.

15. Finish with the resident dressed appropriately. Make sure clothing is right-side-out and zippers and buttons are fastened.

16. Make resident comfortable.

17. Return bed to lowest position. Remove privacy measures.

18. Place call light within resident's reach.

19. Wash your hands.

20. Report any changes in resident to the nurse.

21. Document procedure using facility guidelines.

6. Identify guidelines for proper oral care

Oral care, or care of the mouth, teeth, and gums, is performed at least twice each day to clean the mouth. Oral care should be done after breakfast and after the last meal or snack of the day. It may also be done before a resident eats. Oral care includes brushing the teeth, tongue, and gums; flossing teeth with dental floss; caring for lips; and caring for dentures (Fig. 13-36). **Dental floss** is a special kind of string used to clean between teeth. When giving oral care, nursing assistants must wear gloves and follow Standard Precautions.

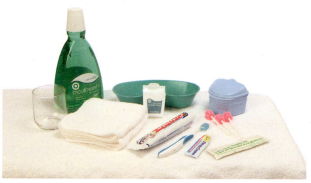

Fig. 13-36. Some supplies needed for oral care.

Proper, regular oral care can help prevent disease and bad breath (**halitosis**). Regular oral care also promotes a healthy appetite. Cleaning the mouth removes particles and leftover food, which makes eating more pleasant. Residents who are unconscious, are on oxygen, or have tubes in their noses or mouths need frequent oral care. Also, if they are not taking any fluids by mouth or are taking medications that dry their mouths, they will need oral care more often. When an NA performs oral care, he should observe the resident's mouth carefully.

Observing and Reporting: Oral Care

Report any of these to the nurse:

O/R Irritation

O/R Raised areas

O/R Coated or swollen tongue

O/R Ulcers, such as canker sores or small, painful, white sores

O/R Flaky, white spots

O/R Dry, cracked, bleeding, or chapped lips

O/R Loose, chipped, broken, or decayed teeth

O/R Swollen, irritated, bleeding, or whitish gums

O/R Breath that smells bad or fruity

O/R Resident reports of mouth pain

Providing oral care

Equipment: toothbrush, toothpaste, emesis basin, clothing protector or towel, glass of water, lip moisturizer, gloves

1. Identify yourself by name. Identify the resident by name.

2. Wash your hands.

3. Explain procedure to the resident. Speak clearly, slowly, and directly. Maintain face-to-face contact whenever possible.

4. Provide for resident's privacy with curtain, screen, or door.

5. If the resident is in bed, adjust bed to a safe level, usually waist high. Raise the head of the bed to have the resident in an upright sitting position. Lock bed wheels.

6. Put on gloves.

7. Place a clothing protector or towel across the resident's chest.

8. Wet toothbrush and put on a small amount of toothpaste.

9. Clean entire mouth, including the tongue and all surfaces of teeth and the gumline, using gentle strokes. First brush inner, outer, and chewing surfaces of the upper teeth, then do the same with the lower teeth. Use short strokes. Brush back and forth. Brush the tongue.

10. Give the resident the glass of water to rinse the mouth. Place the emesis basin under the

resident's chin, with the inward curve under the chin. Have resident spit water into emesis basin (Fig. 13-37). Wipe resident's mouth and remove the towel. Apply lip moisturizer.

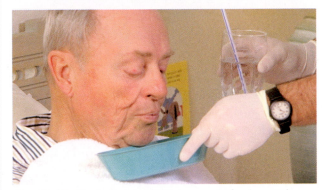

Fig. 13-37. *Rinsing and spitting removes food particles and toothpaste.*

11. Rinse the toothbrush and place in proper container. Empty, rinse, and dry basin. Place basin in designated dirty supply area or return to storage, depending on facility policy.

12. Place soiled clothing and linens in proper containers.

13. Remove and discard gloves. Wash your hands.

14. Make resident comfortable.

15. Return bed to lowest position. Remove privacy measures.

16. Place call light within resident's reach.

17. Wash your hands.

18. Report any problems with teeth, mouth, tongue, and lips to the nurse. This includes odor, cracking, sores, bleeding, and any discoloration.

19. Document procedure using facility guidelines.

Oral care does not just involve taking care of the teeth. Residents who do not have teeth will need oral care performed, too. **Edentulous** means having no teeth. For residents who have no teeth, NAs will clean the mouth, tongue, and gums using mouthwash or other solution on sponge swabs.

Even though a person who is unconscious cannot eat, breathing through the mouth causes saliva to dry in the mouth. Oral care needs to be performed more frequently to keep the mouth clean and moist. For a resident who is unconscious, the NA must use as little liquid as possible when giving mouth care. Because the person's swallowing reflex is weak, he is at risk for aspiration. **Aspiration** is the inhalation of food, fluid, or foreign material into the lungs. Aspiration can cause pneumonia or death. Turning an unconscious resident on his side before giving oral care can also help prevent aspiration. Only swabs soaked in tiny amounts of fluid should be used to clean the mouth.

Providing oral care for the unconscious resident

Equipment: sponge swabs, tongue depressor, towel, emesis basin, gloves, glass of water, lip moisturizer, cleaning solution (check the care plan)

1. Identify yourself by name. Identify the resident by name. Even residents who are unconscious may be able to hear you. Always speak to them as you would to any resident.

2. Wash your hands.

3. Explain procedure to the resident. Speak clearly, slowly, and directly. Maintain face-to-face contact whenever possible.

4. Provide for resident's privacy with curtain, screen, or door.

5. Adjust bed to a safe level, usually waist high. Lock bed wheels.

6. Put on gloves.

7. Turn the resident onto his side or turn his head to the side. Place a towel under his cheek and chin. Place an emesis basin next to the cheek and chin so that excess fluid flows into the basin.

8. Hold the mouth open with the tongue depressor.

9. Dip the sponge swab in the cleaning solution. Squeeze excess solution to prevent aspiration. Wipe the teeth, gums, tongue, and inside surfaces of mouth. Remove debris with the swab. Change the swab often. Repeat this until the mouth is clean.

10. Rinse with a clean swab dipped in water. Squeeze swab first to remove excess water.

11. Remove the towel and basin. Pat lips or face dry if needed. Apply lip moisturizer.

12. Empty, rinse, and dry basin. Place basin in designated dirty supply area or return to storage, depending on facility policy.

13. Place soiled linens in the proper container.

14. Remove and discard gloves. Wash your hands.

15. Return bed to lowest position. Remove privacy measures.

16. Place call light within resident's reach.

17. Wash your hands.

18. Report any problems with teeth, mouth, tongue, and lips to nurse. This includes odor, cracking, sores, bleeding, and any discoloration.

19. Document procedure using facility guidelines.

Flossing the teeth removes plaque and tartar buildup around the gumline and between the teeth. Teeth may be flossed immediately after or before they are brushed, as the resident prefers. Nursing assistants should follow the care plan's instructions regarding flossing.

Flossing teeth

Equipment: dental floss, glass of water, emesis basin, towel, gloves

1. Identify yourself by name. Identify the resident by name.

2. Wash your hands.

3. Explain procedure to the resident. Speak clearly, slowly, and directly. Maintain face-to-face contact whenever possible.

4. Provide for resident's privacy with curtain, screen, or door.

5. If the resident is in bed, adjust bed to a safe level, usually waist high. Raise the head of the bed to have the resident in an upright sitting position. Lock bed wheels.

6. Put on gloves.

7. Wrap the ends of the floss securely around each index finger (Fig. 13-38).

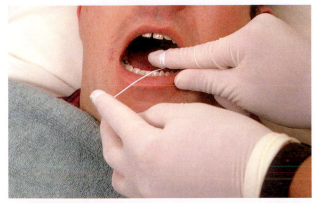

Fig. 13-38. Before beginning, wrap floss securely around each index finger.

8. Starting with the back teeth, place the floss between the teeth. Move it down the surface of the tooth using a gentle sawing motion (Fig. 13-39).

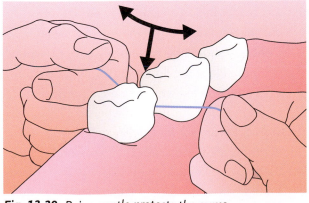

Fig. 13-39. Being gentle protects the gums.

Continue to the gumline. At the gumline, curve the floss. Slip it gently into the space

between the gum and tooth, then go back up, scraping that side of the tooth (Fig. 13-40). Repeat this on the side of the other tooth.

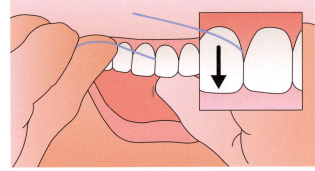

Fig. 13-40. Floss in the space between the gum and tooth. This removes food and helps prevent tooth decay.

9. After every two teeth, unwind the floss from your fingers. Move it so you are using a clean area. Floss all teeth.

10. Occasionally offer water so that the resident can rinse debris from the mouth into the emesis basin.

11. Offer the resident a face towel when done flossing all teeth.

12. Discard the floss. Discard the water and rinse and dry the basin. Place basin in designated dirty supply area or return to storage, depending on facility policy.

13. Place soiled linens in the proper container.

14. Remove and discard gloves. Wash your hands.

15. Make resident comfortable.

16. Return bed to lowest position. Remove privacy measures.

17. Place call light within resident's reach.

18. Wash your hands.

19. Report any problems with the teeth, mouth, tongue, and lips to the nurse. This includes odor, cracking, sores, bleeding, and any discoloration.

20. Document procedure using facility guidelines.

7. Define *dentures* and explain how to care for dentures

Dentures are artificial teeth. They are expensive, so they must be handled carefully to avoid breaking or chipping them. If a resident's dentures break, he or she cannot eat. The NA should notify the nurse if a resident's dentures do not fit properly, are chipped, or are missing.

The nursing assistant must wear gloves when handling and cleaning dentures. Dentures and denture brushes should not be placed on contaminated surfaces. Once dentures are cleaned, they should either be returned to the resident or stored in denture solution or in clean, moderate/cool water (not hot water) so that they do not dry out and warp. Dentures may crack if left uncovered. Dentures should be stored in a denture cup labeled with the resident's name and room number when not being worn.

Each person has his own preference about when and how denture care should be done. The NA should ask the resident how she can assist with denture care.

Residents' Rights

Denture Care

Each person has her own preference about when and how denture care should be done. To promote person-centered care, the NA should ask the resident how she can assist with denture care. In addition, promoting privacy is important. The NA should pull the privacy curtain and close the door before beginning. Many people who have dentures do not want to be seen without their teeth in place. After the teeth are removed, they should be cleaned and returned immediately.

Cleaning and storing dentures

Equipment: denture brush or toothbrush, denture cleanser or tablet, labeled denture cup, 2 towels, gloves

1. Wash your hands.

2. Put on gloves.

3. Line the sink or a basin with one or two towels and partially fill the sink with water. The towel and water will prevent the dentures from breaking if they slip from your hands and fall into the sink.

4. Rinse the dentures in clean, moderate/cool running water before brushing them. Do not use hot water, or dentures may warp.

5. Apply toothpaste or cleanser to the denture brush or toothbrush.

6. Brush dentures on all surfaces (Fig. 13-41). These include the inner, outer, and chewing surfaces of the dentures, as well as the groove that will touch gum surfaces.

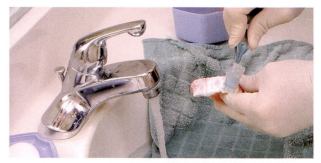

Fig. 13-41. *Brush dentures on all surfaces to properly clean them.*

7. Rinse all surfaces of dentures under clean, moderate/cool running water. Do not use hot water.

8. Rinse the denture cup before placing clean dentures in the cup.

9. Place dentures in a clean, labeled denture cup with solution or moderate/cool water. Dentures should be completely covered with solution. Place the lid on the cup. Make sure the cup is labeled with resident's name and room number. Put the cup where it is normally stored. Some residents will want to wear their dentures all of the time. They will only remove them for cleaning. If the resident wants to continue wearing dentures, return them to him or her. Do not place them in the denture cup.

10. Rinse the denture brush or toothbrush and place it in the proper container. Clean, dry,

and return the equipment to proper storage. Drain the sink. Place soiled linens in the proper container.

11. Remove and discard gloves. Wash your hands.

12. Document procedure using facility guidelines. Report any changes in appearance of dentures to the nurse.

Removing and Reinserting Dentures

If a resident cannot remove her dentures, the NA must do it if trained and allowed to do so. The resident should be sitting upright before beginning. The NA should first don gloves. The lower denture should be removed first. The lower denture is easier to remove because it floats on the gumline of the lower jaw. The NA should grasp the lower denture with a gauze square (for a good grip) and remove it. She should place it in a denture cup filled with solution or moderate/cool temperature water.

The upper denture is sealed by suction. The NA should firmly grasp the upper denture with a gauze square and give a slight downward pull to break the suction. She should turn it at an angle to take it out of the mouth.

When inserting dentures, the NA should ask the resident to sit upright, then she should don gloves. If needed, she should apply denture cream or adhesive to the dentures. When the resident's mouth is open, the upper denture should be placed into the mouth by turning it at an angle. The NA should straighten it and press it onto the upper gumline firmly and evenly (Fig. 13-42). She should insert the lower denture onto the gumline of the lower jaw and press firmly.

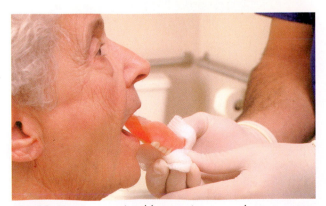

Fig. 13-42. *The NA should press the upper denture onto the upper gumline firmly and evenly.*

Chapter Review

1. List four examples of activities of daily living.

2. Give four examples of how to promote dignity while giving personal care.

3. What are five observations that a nursing assistant can make about a resident during personal care?

4. Why is preventing pressure injuries extremely important?

5. At a minimum, how often should residents be repositioned?

6. List four examples of positioning devices and explain how they can help.

7. Why is it unnecessary for many elderly people to have a complete bath every day?

8. Why should residents, as well as NAs, test the water temperature before bathing?

9. Why should the nursing assistant wipe from front to back when giving perineal care?

10. List two benefits of back rubs.

11. Why should bath oils, lotions, or powders not be used in showers or tubs?

12. Explain why NAs must be careful while giving nail care to residents who have diabetes.

13. Why should an NA wear gloves while shaving residents?

14. If a resident has an affected side due to a stroke, how should the NA refer to that side?

15. When dressing a resident with a weaker side, which arm is usually placed through the sleeve first—the weaker or stronger arm?

16. How can NAs help prevent aspiration during oral care of residents who are unconscious?

17. Why should hot water not be used on dentures?

14
Basic Nursing Skills

1. Explain the importance of monitoring vital signs

Nursing assistants monitor, document, and report residents' **vital signs**. Vital signs are important. They show how well the vital organs of the body, such as the heart and lungs, are working. They consist of the following:

• Measuring the body temperature

• Counting the pulse rate

• Counting the rate of respirations

• Measuring the blood pressure

• Observing and reporting the level of pain

Watching for changes in vital signs is very important. Changes can indicate that a resident's condition is worsening. Nursing assistants do not make diagnoses based on vital signs, but they do record accurate measurements and report changes and observations to the nurse. An NA should always notify the nurse if

• The resident has a fever (temperature is above average for the resident or outside the normal range)

• The resident has a respiratory or pulse rate that is too rapid or too slow

• The resident's blood pressure changes

• The resident's pain is worse or is not relieved by pain management

Ranges for Adult Vital Signs

Temp. Site	Fahrenheit	Celsius
Mouth (oral)	97.6°–99.6°	36.5°–37.5°
Rectum (rectal)	98.6°–100.6°	37.0°–38.1°
Armpit (axilla)	96.6°–98.6°	36.0°–37.0°
Ear (tympanic)	96.6°–99.7°	35.8°–37.6°
Temporal Artery (forehead)	97.2°–100.1°	36.2°–37.8°

Normal Pulse Rate: 60–100 beats per minute
Normal Respiratory Rate: 12–20 respirations per minute

Blood Pressure

Normal	Systolic–less than 120 Diastolic–less than 80
Low	Less than 90/60
Prehypertensive	Systolic 120–139 Diastolic 80–89
High	140/90 or above

Residents' Rights

Vital Signs

Nursing assistants should protect residents' privacy while checking vital signs by not exposing them. If blood pressure needs to be measured or clothing moved out of the way, the NA should pull the privacy curtain around the bed and close the door. Care team members should not discuss residents' vital signs measurements when near other people. The NA should report the information to the nurse.

2. List guidelines for measuring body temperature

Body temperature is normally very close to 98.6°F (Fahrenheit) or 37°C (Celsius). Body temperature reflects a balance between the heat created by the body and the heat lost to the environment. Many factors affect body temperature: age, illness, stress, environment, exercise, and the circadian rhythm can all cause changes in body temperature. The circadian rhythm is the 24-hour day-night cycle. Average temperature readings change throughout the day. People tend to have lower temperatures in the morning. Increases in body temperature may indicate an infection or disease.

There are different sites for measuring the body's temperature: the mouth (oral), the rectum (rectal), the armpit (axilla), the ear (tympanic), and the temporal artery (the artery just under the skin of the forehead). The different sites require different thermometers. There are several types of thermometers, including the following:

- Digital
- Electronic
- Disposable
- Tympanic
- Temporal artery
- Mercury-free

A digital thermometer can be used to measure an oral, rectal, or axillary temperature (Figure 14-1). This thermometer displays the results digitally and registers the temperature quickly, usually within two to 60 seconds. The thermometer will beep or flash when the temperature has registered. A digital thermometer is battery-operated and requires battery replacement periodically. This thermometer may require a disposable plastic sheath to cover the probe to help prevent infection.

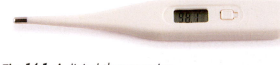

Fig. 14-1. *A digital thermometer.*

An electronic thermometer can be used to measure an oral, rectal, or axillary temperature. This thermometer registers the results digitally in two to 60 seconds. The thermometer flashes or makes a sound when the temperature is displayed. An electronic thermometer is battery-operated and is stored in a wall unit for recharging when it is not in use (Fig. 14-2). A probe cover is applied before use.

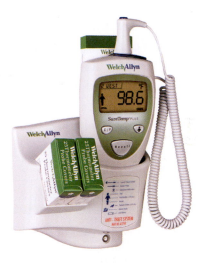

Fig. 14-2. *An electronic thermometer.* (PHOTO COURTESY OF WELCH ALLYN, WWW.WELCHALLYN.COM, 800-535-6663)

A disposable thermometer can be used to measure an oral or axillary temperature. This thermometer registers the temperature in about 60 seconds. Usually a colored dot shows the temperature (Fig. 14-3). A disposable thermometer is often individually wrapped. It is only used once and is then discarded in the proper container. Disposable, or single-use, equipment helps prevent infection.

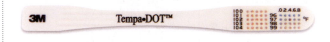

Fig. 14-3. *A disposable thermometer.*

The tympanic thermometer is used to measure the temperature reading in the ear (Fig. 14-4). This thermometer registers the temperature in seconds. However, this thermometer may require more practice to be able to use it accurately.

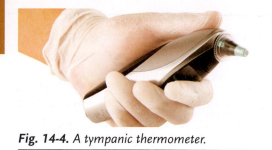

Fig. 14-4. *A tympanic thermometer.*

A temporal artery thermometer determines the temperature reading by measuring the heat from the skin over the temporal artery, the artery under the skin of the forehead. This is done by a gentle stroke or scan across the forehead, and the reading is registered in about three seconds (Fig. 14-5). A temporal artery thermometer is noninvasive, which means that it does not need to be inserted into the body.

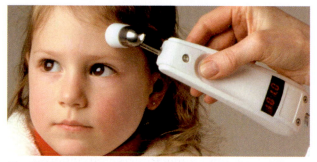

Fig. 14-5. *A temporal artery thermometer.* (PHOTO COURTESY OF EXERGEN CORPORATION, 800-422-3006, WWW.EXERGEN.COM)

A mercury-free thermometer can be used to measure an oral, rectal, or axillary temperature. Thermometers are usually color-coded. Oral thermometers are usually green or blue. Rectal thermometers are usually red (Fig. 14-6).

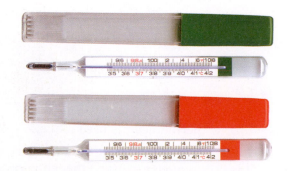

Fig. 14-6. *A mercury-free oral thermometer and a mercury-free rectal thermometer. Oral thermometers are usually green or blue; rectal thermometers are usually red.* (PHOTOS COURTESY OF RG MEDICAL DIAGNOSTICS OF WIXOM, MI, RGMD.COM)

Numbers on the thermometer allow the temperature to be read after it registers. Most thermometers show the temperature in degrees Fahrenheit (F). Each long line represents one degree and each short line represents two-tenths of a degree. Some thermometers show the temperature in degrees Celsius (C), with the long lines representing one degree and the short lines representing one-tenth of a degree. Small arrows or highlighted numbers show the normal temperature: 98.6°F and 37°C (Fig. 14-7).

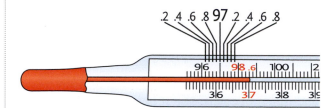

Fig. 14-7. *This shows a normal temperature reading: 98.6°F and 37°C.*

There is a range of normal temperatures. Some people's temperatures normally run low. Others in good health will run slightly higher temperatures. Normal temperature readings also vary by the method used to take the temperature. A rectal temperature is considered to be the most accurate. However, measuring a rectal temperature on an uncooperative person, such as a resident with dementia, can be dangerous. An axillary temperature is considered the least accurate.

A nursing assistant should not measure an oral temperature on a person who:

- Is unconscious

- Has recently had facial or oral surgery

- Is younger than 5 years old

- Is confused or disoriented

- Is heavily sedated

- Is likely to have a seizure

- Is coughing

- Is using oxygen

- Has facial paralysis

- Has a nasogastric tube (a feeding tube that is inserted through the nose and goes into the stomach)

- Has sores, redness, swelling, or pain in the mouth

- Has an injury to the face or neck

Measuring and recording an oral temperature

Equipment: clean mercury-free, digital, or electronic thermometer, gloves, disposable sheath/cover for thermometer, tissues, pen and paper

Do not take an oral temperature if the resident has smoked, eaten food or drunk fluids, chewed gum, or exercised in the last 10–20 minutes.

1. Identify yourself by name. Identify the resident by name.

2. Wash your hands.

3. Explain procedure to the resident. Speak clearly, slowly, and directly. Maintain face-to-face contact whenever possible.

4. Provide for resident's privacy with curtain, screen, or door.

5. Put on gloves.

6. **Digital thermometer**: Put on the disposable sheath. Turn on the thermometer and wait until *ready* sign appears.

   Electronic thermometer: Remove the probe from the base unit. Put on probe cover.

   Mercury-free thermometer: Hold the thermometer by the stem. Before inserting it in the resident's mouth, shake the thermometer down to below the lowest number (at least below 96°F or 35°C). To shake the thermometer down, hold it at the end opposite the bulb with the thumb and two fingers. With a snapping motion of the wrist, shake the thermometer (Fig. 14-8). Stand away from furniture and walls while doing so.

7. **Digital thermometer**: Insert the end of digital thermometer into the resident's mouth, under the tongue and to one side.

Electronic thermometer: Insert the end of the electronic thermometer into the resident's mouth, under the tongue and to one side.

Mercury-free thermometer: Put on disposable sheath if available. Insert the bulb end of the thermometer into the resident's mouth, under the tongue and to one side.

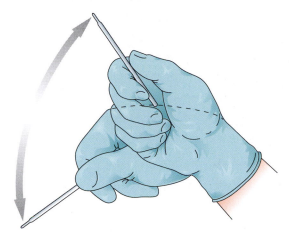

Fig. 14-8. Shake the thermometer down to below the lowest number before inserting in a resident's mouth.

8. **For all thermometers:** Tell the resident to hold the thermometer in her mouth with her lips closed (Fig. 14-9). Assist as necessary. The resident should breathe through her nose. Ask the resident not to bite down or talk.

   Digital thermometer: Leave in place until the thermometer blinks or beeps.

   Electronic thermometer: Leave in place until you hear a tone or see a flashing or steady light.

   Mercury-free thermometer: Leave the thermometer in place for at least three minutes.

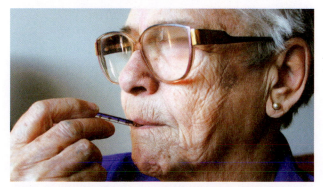

Fig. 14-9. While the thermometer is in the resident's mouth, she should keep her lips closed.

9. **Digital thermometer**: Remove the thermometer. Read the temperature on the display screen. Remember the temperature reading.

   Electronic thermometer: Read the temperature on the display screen. Remember the temperature reading. Remove the probe.

   Mercury-free thermometer: Remove the thermometer. Wipe with a tissue from the stem to bulb or remove the sheath. Discard the tissue or sheath. Hold the thermometer at eye level. Rotate until the line appears, rolling the thermometer between your thumb and forefinger. Read the temperature. Remember the temperature reading.

10. **Digital thermometer**: Using a tissue, remove and discard the sheath. Replace the thermometer in the case.

    Electronic thermometer: Press the eject button to discard the cover. Return the probe to the holder.

    Mercury-free thermometer: Clean thermometer according to facility guidelines. Rinse with clean water and dry. Return it to case.

11. Remove and discard gloves.

12. Wash your hands.

13. Immediately record the temperature, date, time, and method used (oral).

14. Place call light within resident's reach.

15. Report any changes in resident to the nurse.

Rectal temperatures can be necessary for residents who are unconscious, residents with poorly fitting dentures or missing teeth, and anyone having trouble breathing through the nose. Rectal thermometers should be lubricated and inserted one-half to one inch for adults. The nursing assistant must always explain what she will do before starting this procedure. The NA needs the resident's cooperation to take a rectal temperature. She should ask the resident to hold still and reassure him that the procedure will only take a few minutes. It is important to hold on to the thermometer at all times while the thermometer is in the rectum.

Measuring and recording a rectal temperature

Equipment: clean rectal mercury-free, digital, or electronic thermometer, lubricant, gloves, tissues, disposable sheath/cover, pen and paper

1. Identify yourself by name. Identify the resident by name.

2. Wash your hands.

3. Explain procedure to the resident. Speak clearly, slowly, and directly. Maintain face-to-face contact whenever possible.

4. Provide for resident's privacy with curtain, screen, or door.

5. Adjust bed to a safe level, usually waist high. Lock bed wheels.

6. Help the resident to the left-lying (Sims') position (Fig. 14-10).

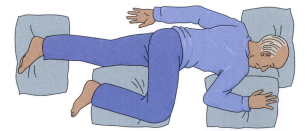

Fig. 14-10. *The resident must be in the left-lying (Sims') position.*

7. Fold back the linens to expose only the rectal area.

8. Put on gloves.

9. **Digital thermometer**: Put on the disposable sheath. Turn on the thermometer and wait until *ready* sign appears.

   Electronic thermometer: Remove the probe from the base unit. Put on the probe cover.

   Mercury-free thermometer: Hold the thermometer by the stem. Shake the thermometer down to below the lowest number.

10. Apply a small amount of lubricant to the tip of the bulb or probe cover (or apply pre-lubricated cover).

11. Separate the buttocks. Gently insert the thermometer into the rectum 1/2 to 1 inch. Stop if you meet resistance. Do not force the thermometer into the rectum (Fig. 14-11).

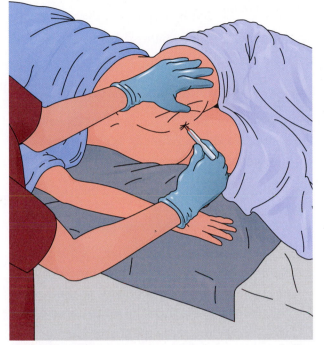

Fig. 14-11. Gently insert a rectal thermometer one-half to one inch into the rectum.

12. Replace the sheet over the buttocks while holding on to the thermometer at all times.

13. **Digital thermometer**: Leave in place until the thermometer blinks or beeps.

    Electronic thermometer: Leave in place until you hear a tone or see a flashing or steady light.

    Mercury-free thermometer: Leave the thermometer in place for at least three minutes.

14. Gently remove the thermometer. Wipe with tissue from stem to bulb or remove sheath. Discard the tissue or sheath.

15. Read the thermometer at eye level as you would for an oral temperature. Remember the temperature reading.

16. **Digital thermometer**: Clean the thermometer according to facility guidelines. Replace the thermometer in the case.

    Electronic thermometer: Press the eject button to discard the cover. Return the probe to the holder.

    Mercury-free thermometer: Clean thermometer according to facility guidelines. Rinse with clean water and dry. Return it to case.

17. Remove and discard gloves.

18. Assist the resident to a position of safety and comfort. Return bed to lowest position.

19. Wash your hands.

20. Immediately record the temperature, date, time, and method used (rectal).

21. Place call light within resident's reach.

22. Report any changes in resident to the nurse.

Tympanic thermometers can be used to take a fast temperature reading. The nursing assistant should explain to the resident that she will be placing a thermometer in the ear canal. She should reassure the resident that the procedure is painless. The short tip of the thermometer will only go into the ear one-quarter to one-half inch, following the manufacturer's instructions.

Measuring and recording a tympanic temperature

Equipment: tympanic thermometer, gloves, disposable probe sheath/cover, pen and paper

1. Identify yourself by name. Identify the resident by name.

2. Wash your hands.

3. Explain procedure to the resident. Speak clearly, slowly, and directly. Maintain face-to-face contact whenever possible.

4. Provide for resident's privacy with curtain, screen, or door.

5. Put on gloves.

6. Put a disposable sheath over the earpiece of the thermometer.

7. Position the resident's head so that the ear is in front of you. Straighten the ear canal by gently pulling up and back on the outside edge of the ear (Fig. 14-12). Insert the covered probe into the ear canal and press the button.

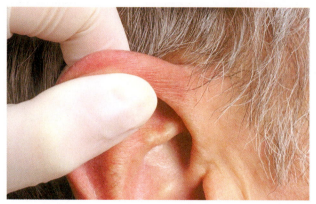

Fig. 14-12. *Straighten the ear canal by gently pulling up and back on the outside edge of the ear.*

8. Hold the thermometer in place until it blinks or beeps.

9. Read the temperature. Remember the temperature reading.

10. Dispose of the sheath. Return the thermometer to storage or to the battery charger if the thermometer is rechargeable.

11. Remove and discard gloves.

12. Wash your hands.

13. Immediately record the temperature, date, time, and method used (tympanic).

14. Place call light within resident's reach.

15. Report any changes in resident to the nurse.

Axillary temperatures are not as accurate as temperatures measured at other sites. However, they can be safer if a resident is confused, dis-

oriented, uncooperative, or has dementia. The axillary area must be clean and dry before measuring the temperature.

Measuring and recording an axillary temperature

Equipment: clean mercury-free, digital, or electronic thermometer, gloves, tissues, disposable sheath/ cover, pen and paper

1. Identify yourself by name. Identify the resident by name.

2. Wash your hands.

3. Explain procedure to the resident. Speak clearly, slowly, and directly. Maintain face-to-face contact whenever possible.

4. Provide for resident's privacy with curtain, screen, or door.

5. Put on gloves.

6. Remove the resident's arm from the sleeve of gown to allow skin contact with the end of the thermometer. Wipe the axillary area with tissues before placing the thermometer.

7. **Digital thermometer**: Put on the disposable sheath. Turn on the thermometer and wait until *ready* sign appears.

   Electronic thermometer: Remove the probe from the base unit. Put on the probe cover.

   Mercury-free thermometer: Hold the thermometer by the stem. Shake the thermometer down to below the lowest number.

8. Position the thermometer (bulb end for mercury-free) in the center of the armpit. Fold the resident's arm over his chest.

9. **Digital thermometer**: Leave in place until the thermometer blinks or beeps.

   Electronic thermometer: Leave in place until you hear a tone or see a flashing or steady light.

Mercury-free thermometer: Leave the thermometer in place, with the arm close against the side, for eight to 10 minutes (Fig. 14-13).

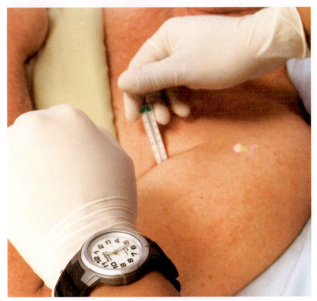

Fig. 14-13. *After inserting the thermometer, fold the resident's arm over his chest and hold it in place for eight to 10 minutes.*

10. **Digital thermometer**: Remove the thermometer. Read the temperature on the display screen. Remember the temperature reading.

    Electronic thermometer: Read the temperature on the display screen. Remember the temperature reading. Remove the probe.

    Mercury-free thermometer: Remove the thermometer. Wipe with a tissue from the stem to bulb or remove the sheath. Discard the tissue or sheath. Read the thermometer at eye level as you would for an oral temperature. Remember the temperature reading.

11. **Digital thermometer**: Using a tissue, remove and discard the sheath. Replace the thermometer in the case.

    Electronic thermometer: Press the eject button to discard the cover. Return the probe to the holder.

    Mercury-free thermometer: Clean thermometer according to facility guidelines. Rinse with clean water and dry. Return it to case.

12. Remove and discard gloves.

13. Wash your hands.

14. Put resident's arm back into sleeve of gown.

15. Immediately record the temperature, date, time, and method used (axillary).

16. Place call light within resident's reach.

17. Report any changes in resident to the nurse.

3. List guidelines for measuring pulse and respirations

The pulse is the number of heartbeats per minute. The beat that is felt at certain pulse points in the body represents the wave of blood moving as a result of the heart pumping. The most common site for monitoring the pulse is on the inside of the wrist, where the radial artery runs just beneath the skin. This is called the **radial pulse**. The procedure for counting this pulse is located later in this chapter. The **brachial pulse** is the pulse inside the elbow, about one to one-and-a-half inches above the elbow. The radial and brachial pulses are involved in measuring blood pressure, which is explained later in this chapter. Common pulse sites are shown below.

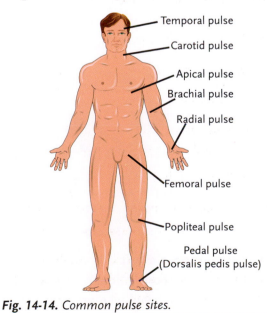

Fig. 14-14. *Common pulse sites.*

For adults, the normal pulse rate is 60 to 100 beats per minute. Small children have more rapid pulses, in the range of 100 to 120 beats per minute. A newborn baby's pulse rate may be as high as 120 to 180 beats per minute. Many things can affect pulse rate, including exercise, fear, anger, anxiety, heat, infection, illness, medications, and pain. A high or low rate does not necessarily indicate disease. However, sometimes the pulse rate can signal that illness exists. For example, a rapid pulse may result from fever, dehydration, or heart failure. A slow or weak pulse may indicate infection.

The **apical pulse** is heard by listening directly over the heart with a stethoscope. A **stethoscope** is an instrument designed to listen to sounds within the body, such as the heart beating or air moving through the lungs (Fig. 14-15). This is often the easiest method for measuring the pulse in infants and small children because their pulse points are harder to find.

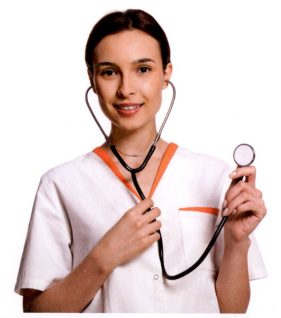

Fig. 14-15. *The diaphragm (the larger side) of the stethoscope is used to hear a pulse and to measure blood pressure.*

The apical pulse is on the left side of the chest, just below the nipple. For adult residents, the apical pulse may be checked when the person has heart disease or takes medication that affects the heart. It may also be checked if residents have a weak radial pulse or an irregular pulse.

Counting and recording apical pulse

Equipment: stethoscope, watch with second hand, alcohol wipes, pen and paper

1. Identify yourself by name. Identify the resident by name.

2. Wash your hands.

3. Explain procedure to the resident. Speak clearly, slowly, and directly. Maintain face-to-face contact whenever possible.

4. Provide for resident's privacy with curtain, screen, or door.

5. Before using the stethoscope, wipe the diaphragm and earpieces with alcohol wipes.

6. Fit the earpieces of the stethoscope snugly into your ears. Place the flat metal diaphragm on the left side of the chest, just below the nipple. Listen for the heartbeat.

7. Use the second hand of your watch. Count the heartbeats for one minute (Fig. 14-16). Each *lubdub* that you hear is counted as one beat. A normal heartbeat is rhythmical. Leave the stethoscope in place to count respirations (see procedure later in this chapter).

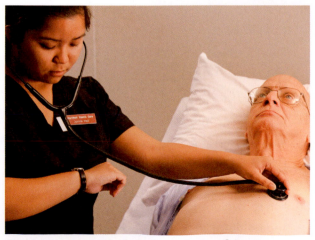

Fig. 14-16. *Count the heartbeats for one full minute to measure the apical pulse.*

8. Wash your hands.

9. Immediately record the pulse rate, date, time, and method used (apical). Note any irregularities in the rhythm.

10. Clean earpieces and diaphragm of stethoscope with alcohol wipes. Store stethoscope.

11. Wash your hands.

12. Place call light within resident's reach.

13. Report any changes in resident to the nurse.

Respiration is the process of inhaling air into the lungs, or **inspiration**, and exhaling air out of the lungs, or **expiration**. Each respiration consists of an inspiration and an expiration. The chest rises during inspiration and falls during expiration.

The normal respiration rate for adults ranges from 12 to 20 breaths per minute. Infants and children have a faster respiratory rate. Infants normally breathe at a rate of 30 to 40 respirations per minute. Different types of respirations include the following:

- **Apnea**: the absence of breathing

- **Dyspnea**: difficulty breathing

- **Eupnea**: normal breathing

- **Orthopnea**: shortness of breath when lying down that is relieved by sitting up

- **Tachypnea**: rapid breathing

- **Bradypnea**: slow breathing

- **Cheyne-Stokes**: alternating periods of slow, irregular breathing and rapid, shallow breathing, along with short periods of apnea

The respiratory rate is usually counted directly after counting the pulse rate because people tend to breathe more quickly if they know they are being observed. The nursing assistant should keep his fingers on the resident's wrist or on the stethoscope over the heart. He should not make it obvious that he is observing the resident's breathing and should not mention he is counting respirations.

Counting and recording radial pulse and counting and recording respirations

Equipment: watch with a second hand, pen and paper

1. Identify yourself by name. Identify the resident by name.

2. Wash your hands.

3. Explain procedure to the resident. Speak clearly, slowly, and directly. Maintain face-to-face contact whenever possible.

4. Provide for resident's privacy with curtain, screen, or door.

5. Place the fingertips of your index finger and middle finger on the thumb side of the resident's wrist to locate the radial pulse (Fig. 14-17).

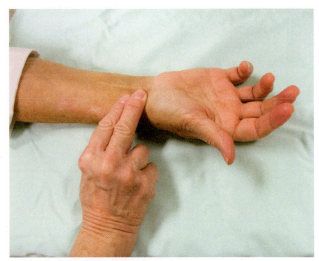

Fig. 14-17. *Measure the radial pulse by placing the fingertips of your index finger and middle finger on the thumb side of the resident's wrist.*

6. Using your watch, count the beats for one full minute.

7. Keeping your fingertips on the resident's wrist, count respirations for one full minute (Fig. 14-18). Observe the pattern and character of the resident's breathing. Normal breathing is smooth and quiet. If you see signs of difficult, shallow, or noisy breathing, such as wheezing, report it to the nurse.

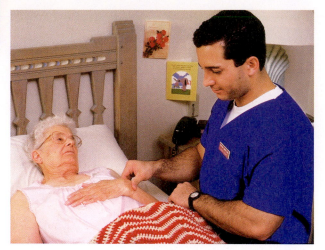

Fig. 14-18. Count the respiratory rate directly after counting the radial pulse rate. Do not make it obvious that you are watching the resident's breathing.

8. Wash your hands.

9. Immediately record the pulse rate, date, time, and method used (radial). Record the respiratory rate and the pattern or character of breathing.

10. Place call light within resident's reach.

11. Report to the nurse if the pulse is less than 60 beats per minute, over 100 beats per minute, if the rhythm is irregular, or if breathing is irregular.

4. Explain guidelines for measuring blood pressure

Blood pressure is an important indicator of a person's health. The measurement shows how well the heart is working. Blood pressure is measured in millimeters of mercury (mm Hg) and is recorded as a fraction—for example, 120/80. There are two parts of blood pressure: the systolic measurement and the diastolic measurement.

In the **systolic** phase, which is the top number of the blood pressure reading, the heart is at work, contracting and pushing the blood from the left ventricle of the heart. The reading shows the pressure on the walls of the arteries as blood is pumped through the body. The normal range for systolic blood pressure is less than 120 mm Hg.

The second measurement reflects the **diastolic** phase, which is the bottom number of the reading. This phase is when the heart relaxes. The diastolic measurement is always lower than the systolic measurement. It shows the pressure in the arteries when the heart is at rest. The normal range for adults is less than 80 mm Hg.

People with consistently high blood pressure, or **hypertension**, have elevated systolic and/or diastolic blood pressures. A blood pressure level of 140/90 mmHg or above is considered high and should be reported to the nurse.

Blood pressure that is too low (less than 90/60) is called **hypotension**. A loss of blood or slowed blood flow can cause hypotension, which can be life-threatening if not corrected.

If blood pressure is between 120/80 mm Hg and 139/89 mm Hg, it is called **prehypertension**. This means that the person does not have high blood pressure now but is likely to develop it in the future.

Blood pressure is affected by many factors. These include aging, exercise, stress, pain, medications, illness, obesity, alcohol intake, tobacco products, and the volume of blood in circulation.

Blood pressure is measured with either a manual or digital **sphygmomanometer**. An aneroid sphygmomanometer is a type of manual sphygmomanometer (Fig. 14-19). This sphygmomanometer consists of a cuff, a bulb, and a pressure gauge. Inside the cuff is an inflatable balloon that expands when air is pumped into the cuff. Two pieces of tubing are connected to the cuff. One leads to a rubber bulb that pumps air into the cuff. A pressure control button allows the release of air from the cuff after it is inflated. The other piece of tubing is connected to a pressure gauge with numbers that shows the blood pressure. Manual sphygmomanometers require the use of a stethoscope to determine the blood pressure reading.

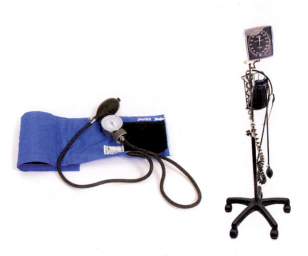

Fig. 14-19. *Two types of aneroid sphygmomanometers.*

With a digital sphygmomanometer, the systolic and diastolic pressure readings are displayed digitally. In addition to blood pressure, a digital sphygmomanometer may also measure other vital signs, such as pulse rate, respiratory rate, and temperature (Fig. 14-20). Some units have automatic inflation and deflation. The use of a stethoscope is not required with digital sphygmomanometers.

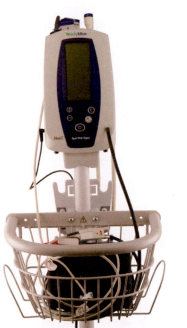

Fig. 14-20. *This type of digital sphygmomanometer measures blood pressure, as well as other vital signs.*

When measuring blood pressure, the first sound heard is the systolic pressure (top number). When the sound changes to a soft muffled

thump or disappears, this is the diastolic pressure (bottom number).

Blood pressure should not be measured on an arm that has an IV, a dialysis shunt, or any medical equipment. A side that has a cast, recent trauma, paralysis, burns, or has had breast surgery (mastectomy) should be avoided.

It is important to use a cuff that is the correct size when measuring blood pressure. Available sizes for adults include small adult, adult, large adult, and thigh. There are also sizes available for infants and children.

Measuring and recording blood pressure (one-step method)

Equipment: sphygmomanometer, stethoscope, alcohol wipes, pen and paper

1. Identify yourself by name. Identify the resident by name.

2. Wash your hands.

3. Explain procedure to the resident. Speak clearly, slowly, and directly. Maintain face-to-face contact whenever possible.

4. Provide for resident's privacy with curtain, screen, or door.

5. Before using the stethoscope, wipe the diaphragm and earpieces with alcohol wipes.

6. Ask the resident to roll up his sleeve so that his upper arm is exposed. Do not measure blood pressure over clothing.

7. Position the resident's arm with the palm up. The arm should be level with the heart.

8. With the valve open, squeeze the cuff to make sure it is completely deflated.

9. Place the blood pressure cuff snugly on the resident's upper arm. The center of the cuff with sensor/arrow is placed over the brachial artery (1 to 1½ inches above the elbow, toward the inside of the elbow) (Fig. 14-21).

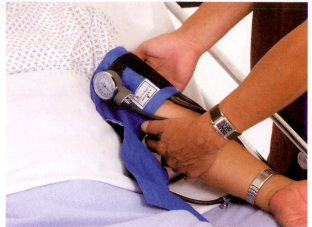

Fig. 14-21. Place the center of the cuff over the brachial artery.

10. Locate the brachial pulse with your fingertips.

11. Place the earpieces of the stethoscope in your ears.

12. Place the diaphragm of the stethoscope over the brachial artery.

13. Close the valve (clockwise) until it stops. Do not overtighten it (Fig. 14-22).

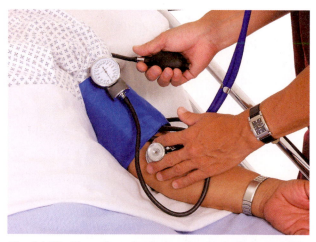

Fig. 14-22. Close the valve by turning it clockwise until it stops. Do not overtighten it.

14. Inflate the cuff to between 160 mm Hg to 180 mm Hg. If a beat is heard immediately upon cuff deflation, completely deflate the cuff. Reinflate the cuff to no more than 200 mm Hg.

15. Open the valve slightly with the thumb and index finger. Deflate the cuff slowly. Releas-

ing the valve slowly allows you to hear beats accurately.

16. Watch the gauge and listen for the sound of the pulse.

17. Remember the reading at which the first pulse sound is heard. This is the systolic pressure.

18. Continue listening for a change or muffling of pulse sound. The point of change or the point at which the sound disappears is the diastolic pressure. Remember this reading.

19. Open the valve to deflate the cuff completely. Remove the cuff.

20. Wash your hands.

21. Immediately record both the systolic and diastolic pressures. Record the numbers like a fraction, with the systolic reading on top and the diastolic reading on the bottom (for example: 120/80). Note which arm was used. Write *RA* for right arm and *LA* for left arm.

22. Clean earpieces and diaphragm of stethoscope with alcohol wipes. Store equipment.

23. Place call light within resident's reach.

24. Wash your hands.

25. Report any changes in resident to the nurse.

Orthostatic Blood Pressures

Nursing assistants may be asked by the nurse to take an orthostatic blood pressure measurement. To do this, the resident must first lie down, and the nursing assistant should record the systolic and diastolic pressures. Next, the resident should sit up. The NA should wait two minutes and measure blood pressure again, recording the systolic and diastolic pressures. Finally, the resident should stand up. The NA should wait two minutes and measure blood pressure again, recording both pressures. Orthostatic blood pressures must be checked in this order: lying down, sitting, and standing up. All three blood pressure measurements should be reported to the nurse.

5. Describe guidelines for pain management

Pain is sometimes referred to as the fifth vital sign because it is as important to monitor as the other vital signs. However, pain is different in that it is a subjective experience (something reported by the person). The other vital signs are objective measurements (information collected by using the senses). Pain is also a personal experience, which means it is different for each person.

Pain is uncomfortable. It can greatly affect a resident's quality of life and the ability to perform self care. It can drain energy and hope. Because nursing assistants spend the most time with residents, they play an important role in pain monitoring, management, and prevention. Care plans are made and adjusted based on NAs' reports.

Pain is not a normal part of aging. Sustained pain may lead to withdrawal, depression, and isolation. Nursing assistants must treat residents' complaints of pain seriously (Fig. 14-23). They should listen to what residents are saying about the way they feel. They should take action to help them by reporting to the nurse immediately. The following are questions that nurses may ask residents to assess their pain. Depending on facility policy, a nurse may ask an NA to ask these questions and then immediately report the information to the nurse:

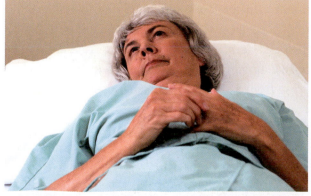

Fig. 14-23. Nursing assistants should believe residents when they say they are in pain and take quick action to help them. Being in pain is unpleasant. NAs should be empathetic.

- Where is the pain?

- When did the pain start?

- How long does the pain last, and how often does it occur?

- How severe is the pain? To help assess this, the resident may be asked to rate the pain on a scale of 0 to 10, with 0 being no pain and 10 being the worst pain the resident can imagine.

- Can you describe the pain? For example, is it a dull, aching, sharp, piercing, or stabbing pain? The NA should use the resident's words when reporting to the nurse.

- What makes the pain better? What makes the pain worse?

- Do you remember what were you doing when the pain started?

Residents may have concerns about their pain. These concerns may make them hesitant to report their pain. Barriers to managing pain include the following:

- Fear of addiction to pain medication

- Feeling that pain is a normal part of aging

- Worrying about constipation and fatigue from pain medication

- Feeling that caregivers are too busy to deal with their pain

- Feeling that too much pain medication will cause death

NAs should be patient and caring when helping residents who are in pain. If residents are worried about the effects of pain medication or if they have questions about it, the NA should report to the nurse. Some people do not feel comfortable saying that they are in pain. A person's culture affects how he or she responds to pain. In some cultures, there is a belief that it is best not to react to pain. In other cultures, people are encouraged to express pain freely. Body language or other messages that a resident may be in pain are important for the NA to observe.

Observing and Reporting: Pain

Report any of these to the nurse:

O/R Increased pulse, respirations, blood pressure

O/R Sweating

O/R Nausea

O/R Vomiting

O/R Tightening the jaw

O/R Squeezing eyes shut

O/R Holding or guarding a body part

O/R Frowning

O/R Grinding teeth

O/R Increased restlessness

O/R Agitation or tension

O/R Change in behavior

O/R Crying

O/R Sighing

O/R Groaning

O/R Breathing heavily

O/R Rocking

O/R Pacing

O/R Repetitive movements

O/R Difficulty moving or walking

Guidelines: Measures to Reduce Pain

G Report complaints of pain or unrelieved pain immediately.

G Gently position the body in proper alignment. Use pillows for support. Assist in frequent changes of position if the resident desires it.

G Give back rubs.

G Ask if the resident would like to take a warm bath or shower.

G Assist the resident to the bathroom or commode or offer the bedpan or urinal.

G Encourage slow, deep breathing.

G Provide a calm and quiet environment. Use soft music to distract the resident.

G Be patient, caring, gentle, empathetic, and responsive to residents who are in pain.

6. Explain the benefits of warm and cold applications

Applying heat or cold to injured areas can have several positive effects. Heat relieves pain and muscular tension. It reduces swelling, elevates the temperature in the tissues, and increases blood flow. Increased blood flow brings more oxygen and nutrients to the tissues for healing.

Cold applications can help stop bleeding. They help prevent swelling, reduce pain, and bring down high fevers. Applying ice bags or cold compresses immediately after an injury can stop bleeding and prevent swelling.

Nursing assistants must be very careful when using these applications. They should know how long the application should be performed and should use the correct temperature as given in the care plan. Using warm and cold applications for too long can cause the opposite effect of what is intended.

Residents receiving warm or cold applications should be checked often, especially those who have conditions that may make them unaware of possible injury. Paralysis, numbness, disorientation, confusion, dementia, and other conditions may make a person unable to feel, notice, or understand damage that is occurring from a warm or cold application. For example, a resident recovering from a stroke who has paralysis on one side may not be able to feel if a warm pack is burning his skin. A resident with Alzheimer's disease may not understand that he is being burned and/or be able to communicate pain clearly.

Warm and cold applications may be dry or moist. Moist applications include the following:

• Compresses (warm or cold)

- Soaks (warm or cold)

- Tub baths (warm)

- Sponge baths (warm or cold)

- Sitz baths (warm)

- Ice packs (cold)

Dry applications include the following:

- Aquamatic K-pad (warm or cold)

- Electric heating pads (warm)

- Disposable warm packs (warm)

- Ice bags (cold)

- Disposable cold packs (cold)

Nursing assistants may be allowed to prepare and apply warm and cold applications. NAs should only perform procedures that are assigned to them and that they are trained to do.

Observing and Reporting: Warm and Cold Applications

These signs indicate that the application may be causing tissue damage and should be reported:

O/R Excessive redness

O/R Pain

O/R Blisters

O/R Numbness

Residents' Rights

Warm and Cold Applications

When applying warm or cold applications, the NA should keep the resident's body covered and only expose the area that needs treatment. Doing this promotes dignity and honors a resident's legal right to privacy.

Warm Applications

A washcloth or a commercial warm compress may be used as a warm compress. There are different types of commercial compresses available (Fig. 14-24). If these are provided, the NA should follow the package directions and the nurse's instructions.

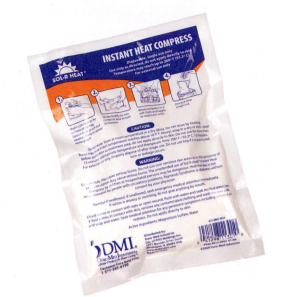

Fig. 14-24. *Disposable heat compresses are used only once and then discarded. The compress shown here must be squeezed and shaken to activate and then applied. It maintains heat for a certain amount of time, usually up to 20 minutes.* (REPRINTED WITH PERMISSION OF BRIGGS CORPORATION, 800-247-2343, WWW.BRIGGSCORP.COM)

Applying warm compresses

Equipment: washcloth or compress, plastic wrap, towel, basin, bath thermometer

1. Identify yourself by name. Identify the resident by name.

2. Wash your hands.

3. Explain procedure to the resident. Speak clearly, slowly, and directly. Maintain face-to-face contact whenever possible.

4. Provide for the resident's privacy with curtain, screen, or door.

5. Fill the basin one-half to two-thirds full with warm water. Test water temperature with thermometer or against the inside of your wrist to ensure it is safe. Water temperature should be no higher than 105°F. Have resident check water temperature. Adjust if necessary.

6. Soak the washcloth in the water and wring it out. Immediately apply it to the area. Note the time. Quickly cover the washcloth with

Basic Nursing Skills

plastic wrap and the towel to keep it warm (Fig. 14-25).

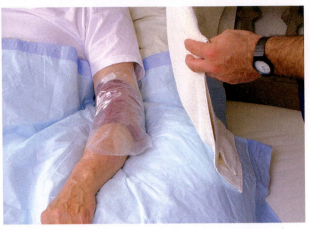

Fig. 14-25. *Cover compresses to keep them warm.*

7. Check the area every five minutes. Remove the compress if the area is red or numb or if the resident complains of pain or discomfort. Change the compress if cooling occurs. Remove the compress after 20 minutes.

8. Make resident comfortable. Remove privacy measures.

9. Discard the plastic wrap. Empty, rinse, and dry bath basin. Place the basin in designated dirty supply area or return to storage, depending on facility policy.

10. Place soiled towels in the proper container.

11. Place call light within resident's reach.

12. Wash your hands.

13. Report any changes in resident to the nurse.

14. Document procedure using facility guidelines.

Administering warm soaks

Equipment: towel, basin, bath thermometer, bath blanket, disposable absorbent pad

1. Identify yourself by name. Identify the resident by name.

2. Wash your hands.

3. Explain procedure to the resident. Speak clearly, slowly, and directly. Maintain face-to-face contact whenever possible.

4. Provide for the resident's privacy with curtain, screen, or door.

5. Fill the basin half full of warm water. Test water temperature with thermometer or against the inside of your wrist to ensure it is safe. Water temperature should be no higher than 105°F. Have resident check water temperature. Adjust if necessary.

6. Place the basin on a disposable absorbent pad (protective barrier) in a comfortable position for the resident.

7. Immerse the body part in the basin. Pad the edge of the basin with a towel (Fig. 14-26). Use a bath blanket to cover the rest of the resident, if needed, for extra warmth.

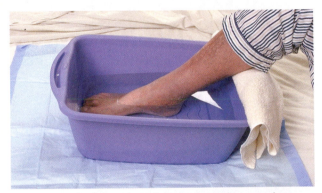

Fig. 14-26. *Pad the edge of the basin with a towel to make the resident more comfortable.*

8. Check the water temperature every five minutes. Add hot water as needed to maintain the temperature. Never add water hotter than 105°F to avoid burns. To prevent burns, ask the resident not to add hot water. Observe the area for redness. Discontinue the soak if the resident has pain or discomfort.

9. Soak for 15 to 20 minutes or as ordered.

10. Remove the basin. Use the towel to dry the resident.

11. Make resident comfortable. Remove privacy measures.

12. Discard the disposable pad. Empty, rinse, and dry bath basin. Place the basin in designated dirty supply area or return to storage, depending on facility policy.

13. Place the soiled towel in proper container.

14. Place call light within resident's reach.

15. Wash your hands.

16. Report any changes in resident to the nurse.

17. Document procedure using facility guidelines.

Applying an Aquamatic K-Pad

Equipment: K-Pad and control unit (Fig. 14-27), covering for pad, distilled water

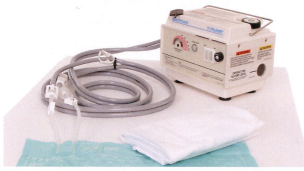

Fig. 14-27. An Aquamatic K-Pad and control unit.

---

1. Identify yourself by name. Identify the resident by name.

2. Wash your hands.

3. Explain procedure to the resident. Speak clearly, slowly, and directly. Maintain face-to-face contact whenever possible.

4. Provide for the resident's privacy during procedure with curtain, screen, or door.

5. Place the control unit on the bedside table. Make sure the cords are not frayed or damaged. Check that the tubing between the pad and unit is intact.

6. Remove the cover of the control unit to check the water level. If it is low, fill it with distilled water to the fill line.

7. Put the control unit cover back in place.

8. Plug the unit in and turn the pad on. Temperature should have been pre-set. If it was not, check with the nurse for proper temperature.

9. Place the pad in the cover. Do not pin the pad to the cover.

10. Uncover the area to be treated. Place the covered pad on the area. Note the time. Make sure the tubing is not hanging below the bed. It should be coiled on the bed. Make sure the tubing has no kinks.

11. Return and check the area every five minutes. Remove the pad if the area is red or numb or if the resident reports pain or discomfort.

12. Check the water level and refill with distilled water to the fill line when necessary.

13. Turn off the unit and remove the pad after 20 minutes.

14. Make resident comfortable.

15. Clean and store supplies.

16. Place call light within resident's reach.

17. Wash your hands.

18. Report any changes in resident to the nurse.

19. Document procedure using facility guidelines.

Another type of heat application is a **sitz bath**, or a warm soak of the perineal area. Sitz baths clean perineal wounds and reduce inflammation and pain. Sitz baths cause circulation to be increased to the perineal area. Voiding may be stimulated by a sitz bath. Residents with perineal swelling (such as hemorrhoids) or perineal wounds (such as those that occur during childbirth) may be ordered to take sitz baths. Because the sitz bath causes increased blood flow to the pelvic area, blood flow to other parts of the body is decreased. Residents may feel weak, faint, or dizzy after a sitz bath. Nursing assistants must always wear gloves when helping with a sitz bath.

A disposable sitz bath fits on the toilet seat and is attached to a rubber bag containing warm water (Fig. 14-28).

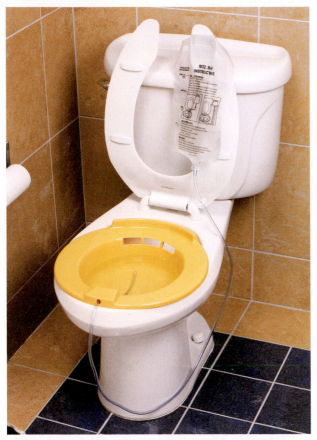

Fig. 14-28. *A disposable sitz bath.* (REPRINTED WITH PERMISSION OF BRIGGS CORPORATION, 800-247-2343, WWW.BRIGGSCORP.COM)

Assisting with a sitz bath

Equipment: disposable sitz bath, bath thermometer, towels, gloves

1. Identify yourself by name. Identify the resident by name.

2. Wash your hands.

3. Explain procedure to the resident. Speak clearly, slowly, and directly. Maintain face-to-face contact whenever possible.

4. Provide for the resident's privacy with curtain, screen, or door.

5. Put on gloves.

6. Fill the sitz bath two-thirds full with warm water. Place the sitz bath on the toilet seat. Check the water temperature using the bath thermometer. Water temperature should be no higher than 105°F. If the sitz bath is being used to help relieve pain and to stimulate circulation, the water temperature may need to be higher. Follow instructions in the care plan.

7. Help the resident undress and sit on the sitz bath. A valve on the tubing connected to the bag allows the resident or you to refill the sitz bath with warm water.

8. You may be required to stay with the resident for safety reasons. If you leave the room, check on the resident every five minutes to make sure she is not dizzy or weak. Stay with a resident who seems unsteady.

9. Help the resident off of the sitz bath after 20 minutes. Provide towels and help with dressing if needed.

10. Make sure resident is comfortable.

11. Clean and store supplies. Place soiled towels in proper container.

12. Remove and discard gloves.

13. Wash your hands.

14. Place call light within resident's reach.

15. Report any changes in resident to the nurse.

16. Document procedure using facility guidelines.

Cold Applications

There are different types of commercial packs available, which may be used instead of traditional ice packs. If these are provided, nursing assistants should follow the package directions and the nurse's instructions. Some cold packs are disposable, while others are cleaned and reused.

Applying ice packs

Equipment: cold pack or sealable plastic bag and crushed ice, towel to cover pack or bag

1. Identify yourself by name. Identify the resident by name.

2. Wash your hands.

3. Explain procedure to the resident. Speak clearly, slowly, and directly. Maintain face-to-face contact whenever possible.

4. Provide for the resident's privacy with curtain, screen, or door.

5. Fill plastic bag one-half to two-thirds full with crushed ice. Seal bag. Remove excess air. Cover bag or ice pack with towel (Fig. 14-29).

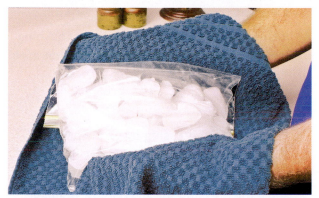

Fig. 14-29. *Seal the bag filled with ice and cover it with a towel.*

6. Apply the bag or pack to the area as ordered. Note the time. Use another towel to cover the bag if it is too cold.

7. Check the area after five minutes for blisters or pale, white, or gray skin. Stop treatment if the resident reports numbness or pain.

8. Remove bag or pack after 20 minutes or as ordered in the care plan.

9. Make resident comfortable.

10. Discard supplies or store in freezer. Place soiled towel in the proper container.

11. Place call light within resident's reach.

12. Wash your hands.

13. Report any changes in resident to the nurse.

14. Document procedure using facility guidelines.

A washcloth dipped in cold water may be used as a cold compress; disposable or reusable compresses are also available (Fig. 14-30). Nursing assistants should follow instructions on the package.

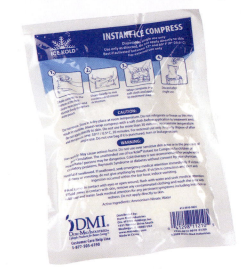

Fig. 14-30. *Disposable cold compresses are used only once and then discarded. The compress here must be squeezed to activate before being applied.* (REPRINTED WITH PERMISSION OF BRIGGS CORPORATION, 800-247-2343, WWW.BRIGGSCORP.COM)

Applying cold compresses

Equipment: basin filled with water and ice, two washcloths, disposable absorbent pad, towels

1. Identify yourself by name. Identify the resident by name.

2. Wash your hands.

3. Explain procedure to the resident. Speak clearly, slowly, and directly. Maintain face-to-face contact whenever possible.

4. Provide for the resident's privacy with curtain, screen, or door.

5. Place the absorbent pad under the area to be treated. Rinse washcloth in basin and wring it out (Fig. 14-31). Cover the area to be treated

with a towel. Apply the cold washcloth to the area as directed. Change washcloths often to keep area cold.

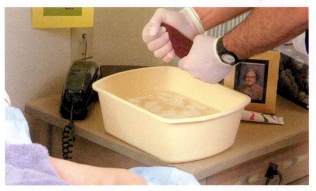

Fig. 14-31. *Wring out the washcloth before applying it to the area to be treated.*

6. Check the area after five minutes for blisters or pale, white, or gray skin. Stop treatment if resident complains of numbness or pain.

7. Remove compresses after 20 minutes or as ordered in the care plan. Give the resident towels as needed to dry the area.

8. Make resident comfortable.

9. Discard the disposable pad. Empty, rinse, and dry bath basin. Place the basin in designated dirty supply area or return to storage, depending on facility policy.

10. Place soiled towels in the proper container.

11. Place call light within resident's reach.

12. Wash your hands.

13. Report any changes in resident to the nurse.

14. Document procedure using facility guidelines.

7. Discuss non-sterile and sterile dressings

Sterile dressings cover new, open, or draining wounds. A nurse changes these dressings. Non-sterile dressings are applied to dry, closed wounds that have less chance of infection. Nursing assistants may change non-sterile dressings.

Equipment: package of square gauze dressings, adhesive tape, scissors, 2 pairs of gloves, plastic bag

1. Identify yourself by name. Identify the resident by name.

2. Wash your hands.

3. Explain procedure to the resident. Speak clearly, slowly, and directly. Maintain face-to-face contact whenever possible.

4. Provide for resident's privacy with curtain, screen, or door.

5. With scissors, cut pieces of tape long enough to secure the dressing. Hang the tape on the edge of a table within reach. Open the four-inch gauze square package without touching the gauze. Place the opened package on a flat surface.

6. Put on gloves.

7. Remove soiled dressing by gently peeling tape toward the wound. Lift dressing off the wound. Do not drag it over the wound. Observe the dressing for any odor or drainage. Notice the color and size of the wound. Discard used dressing in plastic bag.

8. Remove gloves and discard them in plastic bag. Wash your hands.

9. Put on clean gloves. Touching only the outer edges of new four-inch gauze, remove it from the package. Apply it to the wound. Tape gauze in place. Secure it firmly (Fig. 14-32).

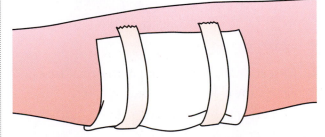

Fig. 14-32. *Tape gauze in place to secure the dressing. Do not completely cover all areas of the dressing with tape.*

10. Discard supplies.

11. Remove and discard gloves.

12. Wash your hands.

13. Make resident comfortable.

14. Place call light within resident's reach.

15. Report any changes in resident to the nurse.

16. Document procedure using facility guidelines.

Even though nursing assistants do not change sterile dressings, they can gather and store equipment and supplies and observe and report about the dressing site. They may also be allowed to clean the equipment. Duties may also include properly positioning the resident, cutting the tape, and disposing of the soiled dressing. Supplies that may be needed for changing a sterile dressing include the following:

- Special gauze has one side with a shiny, non-stick surface, which will not stick to wounds when removed.

- Abdominal pads (ABDs) are large, heavy gauze dressings that cover smaller gauze dressings and help keep them in place and provide absorbency.

- Cotton bandages (sometimes called *Kerlix* or *Kling* bandages) can stretch and mold to a body part and help hold it in place; these are often used on bony areas, such as the knees and elbows.

- Binders are stretchable pieces of fabric that can be fastened. They hold dressings in place and give support to surgical wounds. Binders can also reduce swelling and ease discomfort.

- Medical-grade adhesive tape panels (sometimes called *Montgomery Straps*) help keep frequently changed dressings in place. The adhesive is not removed with each dressing change so that the skin is less likely to become irritated.

Guidelines: Sterile Dressings

G   If the wrapper on the supply is torn, it is no longer considered sterile and cannot be used.

G   The wrapper on the supply cannot be opened and closed again. Once a wrapper is opened, the supplies inside are no longer sterile.

G   If a wrapper is wet or has wrinkles or marks that indicate it was once wet, it is no longer considered sterile.

G   If the date on the supply shows it has expired, it is no longer considered sterile. All commercially prepared supplies are dated. A sterile supply that has expired should not be used.

G   If you are unsure whether a wrapper is sterile or not, do not use it.

G   Because of the way the wound and the skin around it may look, the resident may feel embarrassed about having others see the area. Promote the resident's comfort and dignity when assisting the nurse with a sterile dressing change by being professional. Do not show discomfort, even if you are bothered by the appearance of the resident's wound or skin.

G   Observing and documenting your observations are very important parts of your job. While you are assisting with changing a sterile dressing, observe for any changes in the wound, especially the following:

- Skin that has changed color
- Scabs that have come off
- Bleeding
- Swelling
- Odor
- Drainage

8. Discuss guidelines for elastic bandages

Elastic bandages, also called *non-sterile bandages, ACE bandages,* or *ACE wraps,* are stretchy bandages that are used to hold dressings in place, secure splints, and support and protect body parts (Fig. 14-33). In addition, these bandages may decrease swelling that occurs from an injury.

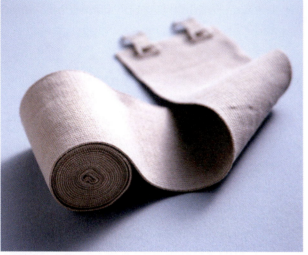

Fig. 14-33. *This is one type of elastic bandage.*

Nursing assistants may be required to assist with the use of an elastic bandage. Duties may include bringing the bandage to the resident, positioning the resident to apply the bandage, washing and storing the bandage, and documenting observations. Some states allow NAs to apply and remove elastic bandages. If allowed to assist with these bandages, the NA should follow these guidelines:

Guidelines: Elastic Bandages

G Keep the area to be wrapped clean and dry.

G Apply elastic bandages snugly enough to control bleeding and prevent movement of dressings. However, make sure that the body part is not wrapped too tightly, which can decrease circulation.

G Wrap the bandage evenly, in a figure-eight pattern, so that no part of the wrapped area is pinched.

G Do not tie the bandage because this cuts off circulation to the body part; the end is held in place with special clips, tape, or velcro.

G Remove the bandage as often as indicated in the care plan.

G Check the bandage often because it can become wrinkled or loose, which causes it to lose effectiveness, or it can become bunched up, which causes pressure and possible discomfort.

G Check the resident 10 to 15 minutes after the bandage is first applied to see if there are any signs of poor circulation. Signs and symptoms of poor circulation include the following:

* Swelling

* Pale, gray, cyanotic (bluish), or white skin

* Shiny, tight skin

* Skin that is cold to the touch

* Sores

* Numbness

* Tingling

* Pain or discomfort

Loosen the bandage if you note any signs of poor circulation, and notify the nurse immediately.

9. List care guidelines for intravenous (IV) therapy

Intravenous therapy, often called IV therapy, is the delivery of medication, nutrition, or fluids through a vein. When a doctor prescribes IV therapy, a nurse inserts a needle or tube into a vein. This allows direct access to the bloodstream. Medication, nutrition, or fluids either drip from a bag suspended on a pole or are pumped by a portable pump through a tube and into the vein (Fig. 14-34). Some residents with chronic conditions may have a permanent opening for IVs, called a *port*. This opening has been surgically created to allow easy access for IV fluids.

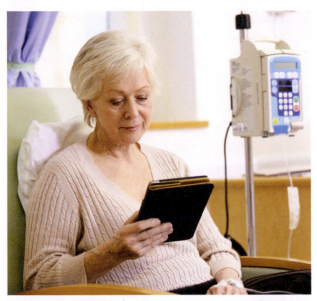

Fig. 14-34. A resident receiving intravenous medication.

Nursing assistants never insert or remove IV lines. They are not responsible for care of the IV site. Their only responsibility for IV care is to report and document any observations of changes or problems with the IV line.

Observing and Reporting: IVs

Report any of the following to the nurse:

O/R The tube/needle falls out or is removed

O/R The tubing disconnects

O/R The dressing around the IV site is loose or not intact

O/R Blood in the tubing or around the IV site

O/R The site is swollen or discolored

O/R The bag is broken, or the level of fluid does not seem to decrease

O/R The IV fluid is not dripping or is leaking

O/R The IV fluid is nearly gone

O/R The pump beeps, indicating a problem

O/R The pump is dropped

O/R The resident complains of pain or has difficulty breathing

The nursing assistant should document her observations and the care she provided. The NA should not do any of the following when caring for a resident who has an IV line:

- Measure blood pressure on an arm with an IV line

- Get the IV site wet

- Pull or catch the tubing on anything, such as clothing (special gowns with sleeves that snap and unsnap are available to lessen the risk of pulling out IV lines)

- Leave the tubing kinked

- Lower the IV bag below the IV site

- Touch the clamp

- Disconnect the IV from the pump or turn off the alarm

Assisting in changing clothes for a resident who has an IV

Equipment: clean clothes

1. Identify yourself by name. Identify the resident by name.

2. Wash your hands.

3. Explain procedure to the resident. Speak clearly, slowly, and directly. Maintain face-to-face contact whenever possible.

4. Provide for resident's privacy with curtain, screen, or door.

5. Adjust bed to lowest position. Lock bed wheels.

6. Assist the resident to sitting position with feet flat on the floor.

7. Ask the resident to remove the arm without the IV from clothing. Assist as necessary.

8. Help the resident gather the clothing on the arm with the IV. Carefully lift the clothing over the IV site and move it up the tubing toward the IV bag (Fig. 14-35).

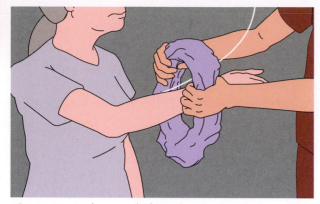

Fig. 14-35. *Make sure clothing does not catch on tubing.*

9. Lift the IV bag off of its pole, keeping it higher than the IV site. Carefully slide clothing over the bag. Place bag back on the pole.

10. Set the used clothing aside to be placed with the soiled laundry.

11. Gather the sleeve of the clean clothing.

12. Lift the IV bag off its pole and, keeping it higher than the IV site, carefully slide the clothing over the bag (Fig. 14-36). Place the IV bag back on the pole.

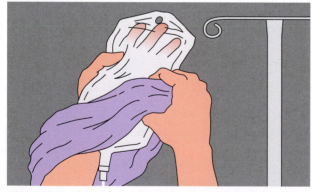

Fig. 14-36. *Always keep the IV bag higher than the IV site.*

13. Carefully move the clean clothing down the IV tubing, over the IV site, and onto the resident's arm.

14. Have the resident put her other arm in the clothing. Assist as necessary.

15. Observe the IV line for one minute to make sure it is dripping properly. If it is not dripping at all or if the drops are coming too

slowly or too rapidly, notify the nurse. Make sure none of the tubing is dislodged and that the IV site dressing is in place. Make sure the tubing is not kinked.

16. Assist the resident with changing the rest of her clothing as necessary.

17. Place soiled clothes in proper container.

18. Make resident comfortable.

19. Place call light within resident's reach.

20. Wash your hands.

21. Report any changes in resident to the nurse.

22. Document procedure using facility guidelines.

Residents' Rights

IVs

A nursing assistant can protect the rights of a resident with an IV line by helping her be as independent as possible. The NA should set up the area so the resident may still feed herself, help with bathing and hair care if able, etc. The NA can ask the nurse how to transport the resident to the activities she wants to attend.

10. Discuss oxygen therapy and explain related care guidelines

Oxygen therapy is the administration of oxygen to increase the supply of oxygen to the lungs. This increases the availability of oxygen to the body tissues. Oxygen therapy is used to treat breathing difficulties and is prescribed by a doctor. Nursing assistants should never stop, adjust, or administer oxygen for a resident.

Oxygen may be piped into a resident's room through a central system. It may be in tanks or produced by an oxygen concentrator. Compressed oxygen and liquid oxygen are stored in tanks of varying sizes (Fig. 14-37). An oxygen concentrator produces and distributes oxygen, but it does not store oxygen.

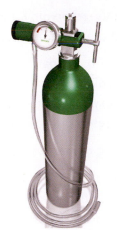

Fig. 14-37. *This is one type of oxygen tank.*

Some residents receive oxygen through a nasal cannula. A **nasal cannula** is a piece of plastic tubing that fits around the face and is secured by a strap that goes over the ears and around the back of the head. The face piece has two short prongs made of tubing. These prongs fit inside the nose, and oxygen is delivered through them. The length of the prongs (usually no more than half an inch) is adjusted for the resident's comfort. The resident can talk and eat while wearing the cannula (Fig. 14-38).

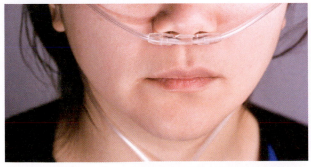

Fig. 14-38. *A nasal cannula.*

An **oxygen concentrator** is a box-like device that changes air in the room into air with more oxygen. Oxygen concentrators are quiet machines. They can be larger units or portable ones that can move or travel with the resident (Fig. 14-39). They have at least one filter that typically needs to be cleaned once per week. Oxygen concentrators run on electricity. They are plugged into wall outlets and are turned on and off by a switch. It may take a few minutes for the oxygen concentrator to reach full power after it is turned on.

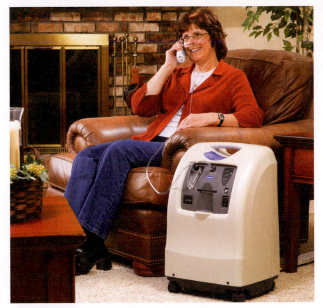

Fig. 14-39. *One type of oxygen concentrator.* (© INVACARE CORPORATION. USED WITH PERMISSION. WWW.INVACARE.COM)

Residents who do not need concentrated oxygen all the time may use a face mask when they need oxygen (Fig. 14-40). The face mask fits over the nose and mouth. It is secured by a strap that goes over the ears and around the back of the head. Plastic tubing connects the mask to the oxygen source. The mask should be checked to see that it fits snugly on the resident's face, but it should not pinch the face. It is difficult for a resident to talk when wearing an oxygen face mask. The mask must be removed for the resident to eat or drink anything.

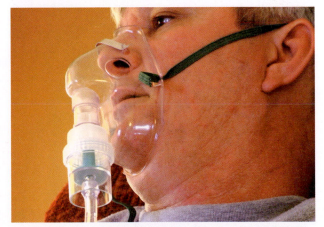

Fig. 14-40. *Residents who need oxygen only occasionally may use a face mask.*

Oxygen can be irritating to the nose and mouth. The strap of a nasal cannula or face mask can also cause irritation around the ears. NAs should wash and dry skin carefully and provide frequent mouth care. They should offer the resident plenty of fluids and report any irritation observed.

Oxygen is a very dangerous fire hazard because it makes other things burn (supports combustion). Safety guidelines for oxygen use are located in Chapter 6.

Guidelines: Oxygen Delivery Devices

For residents using oxygen tanks:

G Count and record pulse and respirations before and after the resident uses the oxygen tank to see if there are any changes.

G The flow meter shows how much oxygen is flowing out to the resident at any time. It should be set at the amount stated in the care plan. If it is not, report this to the nurse. Do not adjust the oxygen level.

G Make sure the humidifying bottle has distilled water in it and is attached correctly. Wash the humidifying bottle according to the care plan or equipment supplier's instructions.

G Change the nasal cannula when ordered. It will need to be changed when it is hard or cracked, at least once every two weeks. It should also be changed after the resident has had a cold or the flu.

G Make sure the oxygen tank is secured and will not tip over.

For residents using liquid oxygen:

G Turn off supply valves when the reservoir is not in use.

G Do not tip the reservoir on its side.

G Make sure the reservoir is not in a closet, cupboard, or other closed-in space.

G Do not cover the reservoir with bed linens or clothing.

G When lifting the reservoir, lift with two hands. Do not roll it or walk it on its edge.

G Do not touch frosted parts of the equipment, because the cold can cause frostbite. Do not touch liquid oxygen; it can cause frostbite. Report if the reservoir is leaking.

For residents using oxygen concentrators:

G Count and record pulse and respirations before and after the resident uses the oxygen concentrator to see if there are any changes.

G The oxygen concentrator dial must be set at the same rate as indicated in the care plan. If it is not, report this to the nurse. Do not adjust the oxygen level.

G Check the humidifying bottle each time the device is used to see that it has distilled water in it and that it is screwed on tightly. Distilled water, not tap water, must be used because minerals in tap water may clog the tubing.

G Make sure the concentrator is in a well-ventilated area, at least six inches from a wall.

G Because the air filter cleans the air going into the machine, brush it off daily to remove dust.

Humidifiers

A humidifier is a device that puts moisture into the air. Residents who use oxygen equipment or who have breathing problems may use humidifiers. Making the air moist or humid can make residents more comfortable.

There are different types of humidifiers; some humidifiers put warm moisture into the air and some put cool moisture into the air.

For cleaning and care of a humidifier, the NA should follow the care plan's instructions. Because pathogens grow in moist areas, the water tank of the humidifier should be washed often. Other NA responsibilities may include adding water to the humidifier when needed and possibly adding special tablets to prevent mineral buildup.

Chapter Review

1. List five vital signs that must be monitored.

2. What are the sites for measuring the body's temperature?

3. Which temperature site is considered to be the most accurate?

4. What is the most common site for monitoring the pulse? Where is it located?

5. Why should respirations be counted immediately after measuring the pulse rate?

6. List and define the two phases measured in a blood pressure reading.

7. How are blood pressure numbers written and recorded?

8. List seven ways to reduce pain.

9. What are the benefits of warm applications? What are the benefits of cold applications?

10. When are non-sterile dressings usually used?

11. List six signs of poor circulation that an NA should observe for when an elastic bandage is applied.

12. What is a nursing assistant's only responsibility as far as IV therapy is concerned?

13. What is a nasal cannula?

14. What is an oxygen concentrator?

15. Why is oxygen a dangerous fire hazard?

15
Nutrition and Hydration

1. Describe the importance of proper nutrition and list the six basic nutrients

Proper nutrition is very important. **Nutrition** is how the body uses food to maintain health. Bodies need a well-balanced diet containing essential nutrients and plenty of fluids. This helps the body grow new cells, maintain normal body function, and have energy for activities.

Proper nutrition in childhood and early adulthood helps ensure health later in life. For the ill or elderly, a well-balanced diet helps maintain muscle and skin tissues and prevent pressure injuries. A healthy diet promotes the healing of wounds. It also helps a person cope with physical and emotional stress.

A **nutrient** is a necessary substance that provides energy, promotes growth and health, and helps regulate metabolism. Metabolism is the process by which nutrients are broken down and transformed to be used by the body for energy, growth, and maintenance. The body needs the following six nutrients for healthy growth and development:

1. **Water**: Water is the most essential nutrient for life; it is needed by every cell in the body. Without water, a person can only live for a few days. Water assists in the digestion and absorption of food. It helps with the elimination of waste. Through perspiration, water also helps maintain normal body temperature. Maintaining enough fluid in the body is necessary for health.

The fluids a person drinks—water, juice, soda, coffee, tea, and milk—provide most of the water the body uses. Some foods are also sources of water, including soup, celery, lettuce, apples, and peaches.

2. **Carbohydrates**: Carbohydrates supply the body with energy and extra protein and help the body use fat efficiently. Carbohydrates also provide fiber, which is necessary for bowel elimination. Carbohydrates can be divided into two basic types: complex and simple. **Complex carbohydrates** are found in bread, cereal, potatoes, rice, pasta, vegetables, and fruits (Fig. 15-1). **Simple carbohydrates** are found in foods such as sugars, sweets, syrups, and jellies. Simple carbohydrates do not have the same nutritional value that complex carbohydrates have.

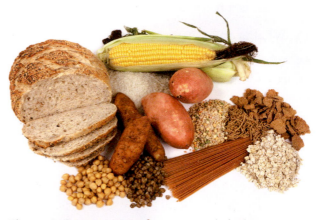

Fig. 15-1. *Some sources of complex carbohydrates.*

3. **Protein**: Proteins are part of every body cell. They are essential for tissue growth and repair. Proteins also supply energy for the body. Excess

proteins are excreted by the kidneys or stored as body fat. Sources of protein include seafood, poultry, meat, eggs, milk, cheese, nuts, nut butters, peas, dried beans or legumes, and vegetarian meat substitutes from a variety of food sources (Fig. 15-2). Whole-grain cereals, pastas, rice, and breads contain some proteins, too.

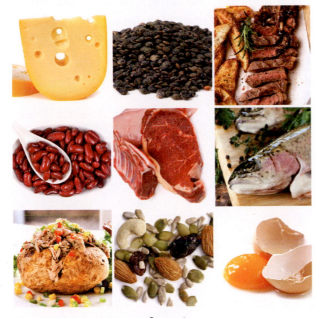

Fig. 15-2. *Some sources of protein.*

4. **Fats:** Fat helps the body store energy. Fats also add flavor to food and are important for the absorption of certain vitamins. Excess fat in the diet is stored as fat in the body.

Fat falls into four categories: saturated, trans, monounsaturated, and polyunsaturated. Saturated and trans fats can increase cholesterol levels and the risk of some diseases, such as cardiovascular disease. Monounsaturated and polyunsaturated fats can be helpful in the diet, and can decrease the risk of cardiovascular disease and type 2 diabetes.

Some fats come from animal fats, such as butter, beef, pork, fowl, fish, and dairy products. Some fats come from plant sources, such as olives, nuts, and seeds (Fig. 15-3).

5. **Vitamins:** Vitamins are substances that are needed by the body to function. The body can-

not make most vitamins; they can only be obtained by eating certain foods. Some vitamins are fat-soluble, which means they are carried and stored in body fat. Vitamins A, D, E, and K are examples. Other vitamins are water-soluble, meaning they are broken down by water in the body and cannot be stored. Vitamins B and C are examples of water-soluble vitamins.

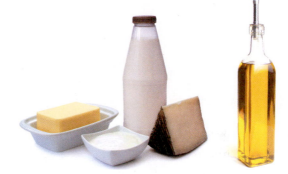

Fig. 15-3. *Some sources of fat.*

6. **Minerals:** Minerals maintain body functions. Minerals help build bones, make hormones, and help in blood formation. They provide energy and control body processes. Zinc, iron, calcium, and magnesium are examples of minerals. Minerals are found in many foods.

2. Describe the USDA's MyPlate

Most foods contain several nutrients, but no one food contains all the nutrients needed for a healthy body. That is why it is important to eat a daily diet that is well-balanced. There is not one single dietary plan that is right for everyone. People have different nutritional needs depending upon their age, gender, and activity level.

In 2011, in response to increasing rates of obesity, the United States Department of Agriculture (USDA, usda.gov) developed MyPlate to help people build a healthy plate at meal times (Fig. 15-4). The MyPlate icon emphasizes vegetables, fruits, grains, protein, and low-fat dairy products.

The goal of MyPlate is to guide people in making healthy food choices. The icon is based on scientific information about nutrition and health. It shows the amounts of each food group that should be on a person's plate.

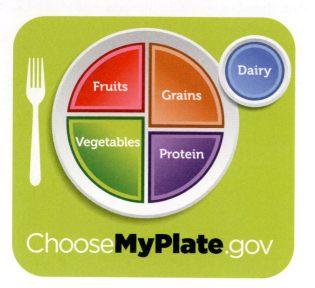

Fig. 15-4. *The U.S. Department of Agriculture developed the MyPlate icon and website (ChooseMyPlate.gov) to help promote healthy eating practices.*

MyPlate gives suggestions and tools for making healthy choices; however, it does not provide specific messages about what a person should eat. The MyPlate icon includes the following food groups:

Vegetables and fruits: Vegetables and fruits should make up half of a person's plate. Vegetables include all fresh, frozen, canned, and dried vegetables, and vegetable juices. There are five subgroups within the vegetable group, organized by their nutritional content. These are dark green vegetables, red and orange vegetables, dry beans and peas, starchy vegetables, and other vegetables. A variety of vegetables from these subgroups should be eaten every day. Dark green, red, and orange vegetables have the best nutritional content (Fig. 15-5).

Vegetables are low in fat and calories and have no cholesterol (although sauces and seasonings may add fat, calories, and cholesterol). They are good sources of dietary fiber, potassium, vitamin A, vitamin E, and vitamin C.

Fruits include all fresh, frozen, canned, and dried fruits, and 100% fruit juices. Most choices should be whole, cut-up, or pureed fruit, rather than juice, for the additional dietary fiber provided. Fruit can be added as a main dish, side dish, or dessert.

Fruits, like vegetables, are naturally low in fat, sodium, and calories and have no cholesterol. They are important sources of dietary fiber and many nutrients, including folic acid, potassium, and vitamin C. Foods containing dietary fiber help provide a feeling of fullness with fewer calories. Folic acid helps the body form red blood cells. Vitamin C is important for growth and repair of body tissues.

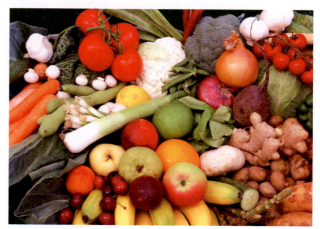

Fig. 15-5. *Eating a variety of vegetables every day, especially dark green, red, and orange vegetables, helps promote good health.*

Grains: A person should make half his grain intake whole grains. There are many different grains. Some common ones are wheat, rice, oats, cornmeal, and barley. Foods made from grains include bread, pasta, oatmeal, breakfast cereals, tortillas, and grits. Grains can be divided into two groups: whole grains and refined grains. Whole grains contain bran and germ, as well as the endosperm. Refined grains retain only the endosperm. The endosperm is the tissue within flowering plants. It surrounds and nourishes the plant embryo. Examples of whole grains include brown rice, wild rice, bulgur, oatmeal, whole-grain corn, whole oats, whole wheat, and whole rye. Consuming foods rich in fiber reduces the risk of heart disease and other diseases and may reduce constipation.

Protein: MyPlate guidelines emphasize the importance of eating a variety of protein foods every week. Meat, poultry, seafood, and eggs are animal sources of proteins. Beans, peas, soy products, vegetarian meat substitutes, nuts, and seeds are plant sources of proteins.

Seafood should be eaten twice a week in place of meat or poultry. Seafood that is higher in oils and low in mercury, such as salmon or trout, is a better choice (Fig. 15-6). Lean meats and poultry, as well as eggs and egg whites, can be eaten on a regular basis. A person should eat plant-based protein foods more often. Beans and peas, soy products (tofu, tempeh, many vegetarian products), vegetarian meat substitutes, nuts, and seeds are low in saturated fat and high in fiber. Some nuts and seeds (flax, walnuts) are excellent sources of essential fatty acids. These fatty acids may reduce the risk of cardiovascular disease. Sunflower seeds and almonds are good sources of vitamin E.

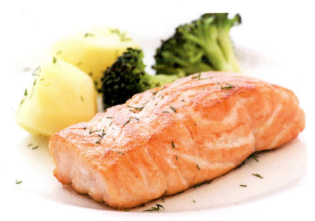

Fig. 15-6. Fish, like this salmon, contains healthy oils and is a good source of protein.

Dairy: All milk products and foods made from milk that retain their calcium content, such as yogurt and cheese, are part of the dairy category. Most dairy group choices should be fat-free (0%) or low-fat (1%). Fat-free or low-fat milk or yogurt should be chosen more often than cheese. Milk and yogurt contain less sodium than most cheeses.

Milk provides nutrients that are vital for the health and maintenance of the body. These nutrients include calcium, potassium, vitamin D, and protein. Fat-free or low-fat milk provides these nutrients without the extra calories and saturated fat (Fig. 15-7). Soy products enriched with calcium are an alternative to dairy foods.

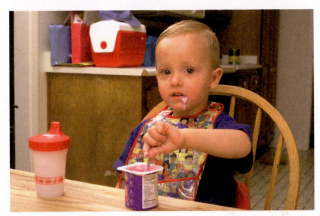

Fig. 15-7. Low-fat milk or yogurt is a good source of calcium without the added saturated fat.

The following guidelines provide additional tips for making healthy food choices:

Guidelines: Healthy Food Choices

G **Balance calories**. Calorie balance is the relationship between the calories obtained from food and fluids consumed and the calories used during normal body functions and physical activity. Proper calorie intake varies from person to person. To find the proper calorie intake, the USDA suggests visiting ChooseMyPlate.gov.

G **Enjoy your food, but eat less**. Eating too fast or eating without paying attention to your food can lead to overeating. Recognize when you feel hungry and when you are full. Notice what you are eating. Stop eating when you feel satisfied.

G **Avoid oversized portions**. Choose smaller-sized portions when eating. Portion out food before you eat it, and use smaller bowls and plates for meals. When eating out, split food with others or take part of your meal home.

G **Eat these foods more often**: vegetables, fruits, whole grains, and fat-free or 1% milk and low-fat dairy products. These foods have better nutrients for health.

G **Eat these foods less often:** foods high in solid fats, added sugars, and salt. These foods include fatty meats, like bacon and hot dogs, cheese, fried foods, ice cream, and cookies.

G **Check sodium content in foods.** Read product labels to determine if they contain salt or sodium. Foods high in sodium include the following:

- Cured meats, including ham, bacon, lunch meat, sausage, salt pork, and hot dogs

- Salty or smoked fish, including herring, salted cod, sardines, anchovies, caviar, smoked salmon, and lox

- Processed cheese and some other cheeses

- Salted foods, including nuts, pretzels, potato chips, dips, and spreads, such as salted butter and margarine

- Vegetables preserved in brine, such as pickles, sauerkraut, pickled vegetables, olives, and relishes

- Sauces with high concentrations of salt, including Worcestershire, chili, steak, and soy sauces; ketchup, mustard, and mayonnaise

- Commercially prepared foods such as breads, canned soups and vegetables, and certain breakfast cereals

Select canned foods that are labeled *sodium-free, very low-sodium, low-sodium,* or *reduced sodium.*

G Drink water instead of sugary drinks. Drinking water or unsweetened beverages reduces sugar and calorie intake. Sweetened beverages, such as soda, fruit punch, and sports drinks, are a major source of sugar and calories in diets.

3. Identify nutritional problems of the elderly or ill

Aging and illness can lead to emotional and physical problems that affect the intake of food. For example, people who are lonely or who suffer from illnesses that affect their ability to chew and swallow may have little interest in food. Weaker hands and arms due to paralysis and tremors make it hard to eat. People with illnesses that affect their ability to chew and swallow may not want to eat. In addition, people who are ill are often fatigued, nauseated, or in pain, which contributes to poor fluid and food intake. Other problems that affect nutritional intake include the following:

- Metabolism slows. Muscles weaken and lose tone, and body movement slows. Reduced activity or exercise affects appetite.

- A loss of vision may affect the way food looks, which can decrease appetite.

- Weakened senses of smell and taste affect appetite. Medication may impair these senses (Fig. 15-8).

- Less saliva production affects chewing and swallowing.

- Dentures, tooth loss, and poor dental health can make chewing difficult.

- Digestion takes longer and is less efficient.

- Certain medication, such as pain medication, and limited activity cause constipation. Constipation often interferes with appetite. Fiber, fluids, and exercise can improve this common problem.

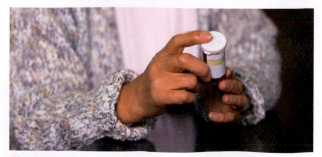

Fig. 15-8. *Many elderly people take a variety of medications, which can affect the way food smells and tastes.*

Unintended weight loss is a serious problem for the elderly. Weight loss can mean that the resident has a serious medical condition. It can lead to skin breakdown, which leads to pressure injuries. It is very important for nursing assistants to report any weight loss, no matter how small. If a resident has diabetes, chronic obstructive pulmonary disease, cancer, HIV, or other diseases, he is at a greater risk for malnutrition. (Chapter 18 contains more information on these diseases.)

Guidelines: Preventing Unintended Weight Loss

G Report observations and warning signs to the nurse.

G Food should look, taste, and smell good, particularly since the resident may have a poor sense of taste and smell.

G Encourage residents to eat. Talk about the food that is being served in a positive tone of voice, using positive words (Fig. 15-9).

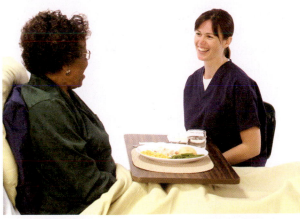

Fig. 15-9. Being friendly and positive while helping residents with eating helps promote appetite and may prevent weight loss.

G Honor residents' food likes and dislikes.

G Offer different kinds of foods and beverages.

G Help residents who have trouble feeding themselves.

G Season foods to residents' preferences.

G Allow enough time for residents to finish eating.

G Tell the nurse if residents have trouble using utensils.

G Record the meal/snack intake.

G Provide oral care before and after meals.

G Position residents sitting upright for eating.

G If a resident has had a loss of appetite and/or seems sad, ask about it.

Observing and Reporting: Unintended Weight Loss

Report any of these to the nurse:

O/R Resident needs help eating or drinking

O/R Resident eats less than 75% of meals served

O/R Resident has mouth pain

O/R Resident has dentures that do not fit properly

O/R Resident has difficulty chewing or swallowing

O/R Resident coughs or chokes while eating

O/R Resident is sad, has crying spells, or withdraws from others

O/R Resident is confused, wanders, or paces

Care must be taken in meal planning to ensure nutrition for the elderly and ill. Many illnesses require the restriction of fluids, proteins, certain minerals, or calories. Conditions that make eating or swallowing difficult include the following:

- Stroke, or CVA, which can cause facial weakness and paralysis

- Nerve and muscle damage from head and neck cancer

- Multiple sclerosis

- Parkinson's disease

- Alzheimer's disease

If a resident has trouble swallowing, soft foods and liquids that have been thickened may be easier to swallow. Thickening improves the ability to control fluid in the mouth and throat. Thickened liquids include milkshakes, sherbet, gelatin, thin hot cereal, cream soups, and fruit juices that have been frozen to a slushy consistency. There is more information about swallowing problems and thickened liquids later in the chapter.

When the digestive system does not function properly, **parenteral nutrition (PN)**, (sometimes referred to as *total parenteral nutrition* [*TPN*]) may be necessary. With parenteral nutrition, a solution of nutrients is administered directly into the bloodstream. It bypasses the digestive system. The nutrients are in their most basic forms of carbohydrates, proteins, and fats and are absorbed directly by the cells.

Nursing assistants are not responsible for parenteral nutrition. They may be assigned to measure the resident's temperature or assemble supplies. In addition, duties include observing, reporting, and documenting any changes in the resident or problems with the feeding.

When a person is unable to swallow, he or she may be fed through a tube. A **nasogastric tube** is inserted into the nose and goes to the stomach. A tube can also be placed into the stomach through the abdominal wall. This is called a **percutaneous endoscopic gastrostomy (PEG) tube**. The surgically-created opening into the stomach that allows the insertion of a tube is called a **gastrostomy** (Fig. 15-10). Tube feedings are used when residents cannot swallow but can digest food. Conditions that may prevent residents from swallowing include coma, cancer, stroke, refusal to eat, or extreme weakness. It is important to remember that residents have the legal right to refuse treatment, which includes the insertion of tubes.

Nursing assistants never insert or remove tubes, do the feeding, or irrigate (clean) the tubes. They may assemble equipment and supplies and hand them to the nurse. NAs may position residents in a sitting position for feeding. They may also discard or clean used equipment and supplies. In addition, NAs may observe, report, and document any changes in the resident or problems with the feeding.

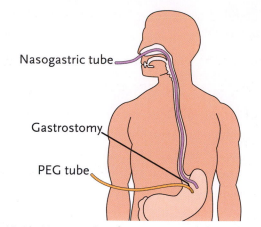

Fig. 15-10. *Nasogastric tubes are inserted through the nose, and PEG tubes are inserted through the abdominal wall into the stomach.*

Guidelines: Tube Feedings

G   Wash your hands carefully before assisting with any aspect of tube feedings.

G   Make sure the tubing is not coiled or kinked or resting underneath the resident.

G   Be aware if the resident has an order for *nothing by mouth* or *NPO*.

G   The tube is only inserted and removed by a doctor or nurse. If it comes out, report it immediately.

G   A doctor will prescribe the type and amount of feeding. The feedings should be at room temperature and in liquid form.

G   A resident with a feeding tube should always have the head of the bed elevated 30 degrees. However, during a feeding, the resident should remain in a sitting position with the head of the bed elevated at least 45 degrees. This helps prevent serious problems, such as aspiration. The elderly can develop pneumonia or even die from improper positioning during tube feedings. After the feeding, keep the resident upright for as long as ordered, at least 30 minutes.

G   If the resident must remain in bed for long periods during feedings, give careful skin care. This helps to prevent pressure injuries on the hips and sacral area.

Observing and Reporting: Tube Feedings

Report any of these to the nurse immediately:

- O/R Redness or drainage around the opening
- O/R Skin sores or bruises
- O/R Cyanotic skin
- O/R Resident complaints of pain or nausea
- O/R Choking or coughing
- O/R Vomiting
- O/R Diarrhea
- O/R Swollen abdomen
- O/R Fever
- O/R Tube falling out
- O/R Problems with equipment
- O/R Sound of feeding pump alarm
- O/R Change of resident's inclined position

4. Describe factors that influence food preferences

Culture, ethnicity, income, education, religion, and geography all affect ideas about nutrition. Food preferences may be formed by what a person ate as a child, by what tastes good, or by personal beliefs about what should be eaten (Fig. 15-11). For instance, some people choose not to eat any animals or animal products, such as steak, chicken, butter, or eggs. These people are called *vegetarians* or *vegans*, depending on what they eat.

The region or culture in which a person grows up often influences his food preference. For example, people from the southwestern United States may like spicy foods. Southern cooking may include fried foods, such as fried chicken or fried okra. Ethnic groups often share common foods. These may be eaten at certain times of the year or all the time. Religious beliefs affect diet, too. For example, some Muslims and Jewish people do not eat any pork. Mormons may not drink alcohol, tea, or coffee.

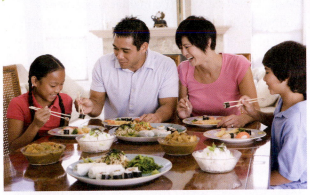

Fig. 15-11. *Food likes and dislikes are influenced by what a person ate as a child.*

Food preferences may change while a resident is living at a facility. Just as anyone may decide that he likes some foods for a time and then changes his mind, so may residents. Providing person-centered care means respecting each resident's preferences. It is never appropriate to make fun of personal preferences. If an NA notices that a certain food is not being eaten—no matter how small the amount—she should report it to the nurse.

Residents' Rights

Food Choices

Residents have the legal right to make choices about their food. They can choose what kind of food they want to eat, and they can refuse the food and drink being offered. Nursing assistants must honor a resident's personal beliefs and preferences about selecting and avoiding specific foods. Although residents have the right to refuse, it is best to ask questions when they do. Communication is the key to understanding why a resident refuses something. For example, if a resident refuses his dinner, the NA can ask if there is something wrong with the food. The resident may say he is Jewish and cannot eat a pork chop because it is not kosher. NAs should respond to requests for different food in a pleasant way. The NA can explain that she will report to the nurse and will get him another meal as quickly as possible. She should remove the tray and take it to the dietitian or dietary department so that an alternative may be offered.

5. Explain the role of the dietary department

The dietary department staff are responsible for planning meals for all residents. Residents have different nutritional needs. When planning meals, the dietary staff consider these needs, along with individual likes and dislikes. Meals must be balanced to provide proper nutrition.

In addition to planning meals, the dietary staff must prepare food in such a way that each resident can manage it. The food must also look appealing. Staff also create **diet cards** (Fig. 15-12). Diet cards list the resident's name and information about special diets, allergies, likes and dislikes, and other dietary instructions. A diet card is often included with each meal that is served to residents who do not eat in the dining room. Nursing assistants are responsible for checking that the diet card matches the correct resident.

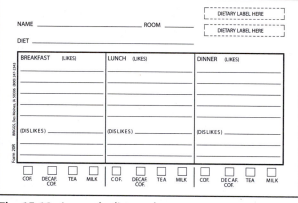

Fig. 15-12. *A sample diet card.* (REPRINTED WITH PERMISSION OF BRIGGS CORPORATION, 800-247-2343, WWW.BRIGGSCORP.COM)

The dietary department staff must follow strict procedures when preparing food in order to prevent the spread of infection. Regular surveys are performed to check for cleanliness and to ensure that staff are following proper guidelines.

6. Explain special diets

Residents who do not have any health problems that require a change in diet often eat a *regular* diet. However, residents who have certain illnesses may be placed on **therapeutic**, **modified**, or **special diets**. With special diets, certain nutrients or fluids may be restricted or eliminated. Some medications may also interact with certain foods, which then must be restricted. Residents who do not eat enough may be placed on special supplementary diets. Diets are also prescribed for weight control and food allergies.

Several types of diets are available for different illnesses. Some residents may be on a combination of restricted diets. The care plan should specify any special diets that are prescribed for a resident. It should also explain any eating problems that a resident may have and how the resident's eating habits can be improved (Fig. 15-13). Nursing assistants must never modify a resident's diet. Special diets can only be prescribed by doctors and planned by dietitians, along with residents. NAs should follow each resident's diet plan without making judgments. Observations should be reported to the nurse.

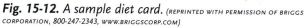

Fig. 15-13. *The care plan specifies the special diet ordered, as well as any additional dietary restrictions.*

Low-Sodium Diet: People are most familiar with sodium as one of the two components of salt. Salt is restricted first in a low-sodium diet because it is high in sodium. Excess sodium causes the body to retain more water in tissues and in the circulatory system than is necessary. This causes the heart to pump harder. This is harmful for residents who have high blood pressure, coronary artery disease, or kidney disease. A modified fluid intake may also be required for people with these conditions, because too much fluid can lead to congestive heart failure. For residents on a low-sodium diet, salt will not be used. Salt shakers or packets will not be on the diet tray. Common abbreviations for this diet are *Low Na*, which means low sodium, or *NAS*, which stands for *No Added Salt*.

Fluid-Restricted Diet: The amount of fluid consumed through food and fluids must equal the amount of fluid that leaves the body through perspiration, stool, urine, and respiration. This is fluid balance. When fluid intake is greater than fluid output, body tissues become swollen with excess fluid. In addition, people with severe heart disease and kidney disease may have trouble processing fluid. To prevent further damage, doctors may restrict a resident's fluid intake. For residents on fluid restriction, the NA will need to measure and document exact amounts of fluid intake and report excesses to the nurse. Additional fluids or foods that count as fluids, such as ice cream, puddings, gelatin, etc., should not be offered. If the resident complains of thirst or requests fluids, the NA should tell the nurse. A common abbreviation for this diet is *RF*, which stands for *Restrict Fluids*.

High-Potassium Diet: Some residents take certain blood pressure medications or **diuretics**, which are medications that reduce fluid volume. These residents may be excreting so much fluid that their bodies could be depleted of potassium. Other residents may be placed on a high-potassium diet for different reasons.

Foods high in potassium include bananas, grapefruit, oranges, orange juice, prune juice, prunes, dried apricots, figs, raisins, dates, cantaloupes, tomatoes, potatoes with skins, sweet potatoes and yams, winter squash, legumes, avocados, and unsalted nuts. *K+* is the common abbreviation for this diet.

Low-Protein Diet: People who have kidney disease may also be on low-protein diets. Protein is restricted because it breaks down into compounds that may lead to further kidney damage. The extent of the restrictions depends on the stage of the disease and whether the resident is on dialysis. Vegetables and starches, such as breads and pasta, are encouraged.

Low-Fat/Low-Cholesterol Diet: People who have high levels of cholesterol in their blood are at risk for heart attacks and heart disease. People with gallbladder disease, diseases that interfere with fat digestion, and liver disease are also placed on low-fat/low-cholesterol diets.

Low-fat/low-cholesterol diets permit skim milk, low-fat cottage cheese, fish, white meat of turkey and chicken, and vegetable fats (especially monounsaturated fats such as olive and canola oils).

Residents on this diet may need to follow these guidelines:

* Eat lean cuts of meat, including lamb, beef, and pork, and eat these only three times a week.
* Limit egg yolks to three per week (including eggs used in baking).
* Avoid organ meats, shellfish, fatty meats, processed meats such as sausage and hot dogs, cream, butter, lard, meat drippings, coconut and palm oils, and desserts and soups made with whole milk.
* Avoid fried foods and sweets.

People who have gallbladder disease or other digestive problems may be placed on a diet that restricts all fats. A common abbreviation for this diet is *Low-Fat/Low-Chol*.

Modified Calorie Diet: Some residents may need to reduce calories to lose weight or prevent additional weight gain. Other residents may need to gain weight and increase calories because of malnutrition, surgery, illness, or fever. Common abbreviations for this diet are *Low-Cal* or *High-Cal*.

Nutritional Supplements

Illness and injury may call for nutritional supplements to be added into the resident's diet. Certain medications also change the need for nutrients. For example, some medication prescribed for high blood pressure increases the need for potassium.

Nutritional supplements may come in a powdered form or liquid form. Some supplements may be pre-mixed and ready to consume. Powdered supplements need to be mixed with a liquid before being taken; the care plan will include instructions for how much liquid to add. When preparing supplements, the supplement must be mixed thoroughly.

The NA may need to make sure the resident takes the supplement at the ordered time. Residents who are ill, tired, or in pain may not have much of an appetite. It may take a long time for them to drink a large glass of a thick liquid. The NA should be patient and encouraging. If a resident does not want to drink the supplement, the NA should not insist that he do so, but should report this to the nurse.

Bland Diet: Gastric and duodenal ulcers can be irritated by foods that produce or increase levels of acid in the stomach, so these foods are eliminated. The bland diet is also used for people who have intestinal disorders, such as Crohn's disease or irritable bowel syndrome (IBS). The following foods and drinks should be avoided: alcohol; beverages containing caffeine, such as coffee, tea, and soft drinks; citrus juices; spicy foods; and spicy seasonings such as black pepper, cayenne, and chili pepper. Three meals or more per day are usually advised. If alcohol is allowed, it should be drunk with meals.

Diabetic Diet: People with diabetes must be very careful about what they eat (Fig. 15-14). Calories and carbohydrates are carefully controlled, and protein and fats are also regulated. The types and amounts of foods are determined by nutritional and energy needs. A dietitian and the resident will make up a meal plan, taking into account the person's health status, activity levels, and lifestyle. The meal plan will include all the right types and amounts of food for each day.

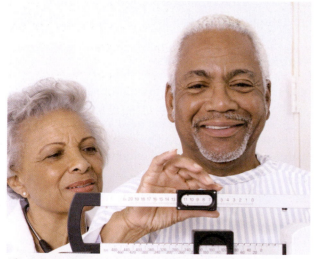

Fig. 15-14. *People who have diabetes must be very careful about what they eat and must keep their weight in a healthy range.*

The meal plan may use a counting carbohydrates approach (often called *carb counting*). After the proper amount of carbohydrates is determined by the dietitian, they need to be counted in each meal or snack. Nutrition labels need to be read, paying attention to serving size and carbohydrate content. Food portions may need to be measured.

To keep their blood glucose levels near normal, residents who have diabetes must eat the right amount of the right type of food at the right time. They must eat all that is served. Nursing assistants should encourage them to eat all of their meals and snacks. NAs should not offer other foods without the nurse's approval. Any variation in eating patterns and routine must be reported to the nurse. If a resident will not eat what is directed, does not finish meals or snacks, or is not following the diet, the NA should tell the nurse.

People who have diabetes should avoid foods that are high in sugar because sugary foods can cause problems with insulin balance. Foods and drinks high in sugar include candy, ice cream, cakes, cookies, jellies, jams, fruits canned in heavy syrup, soft drinks, sports drinks, and alcoholic beverages. Many foods are higher in sugar than they appear, such as canned vegetables, many breakfast cereals, and ketchup.

A meal tray for a resident with diabetes may have artificial sweetener, low-calorie jelly, and/or low-calorie maple syrup. Residents with diabetes should use artificial sweetener, rather than sugar, in their coffee or tea. Common abbreviations for this diet are *NCS*, which stands for *No Concentrated Sweets*, or *LCS*, which stands for *Low Concentrated Sweets*. The American Diabetic Association's (ADA) website, diabetes.org, has more information on diabetic diets.

Low-Residue (Low-Fiber) Diet: This diet decreases the amount of fiber, whole grains, raw fruits and vegetables, seeds, and other foods, such as dairy and coffee, in a person's diet. The low-residue diet is used for people with bowel disturbances.

High-Residue (High-Fiber) Diet: High-residue diets increase the intake of fiber and whole grains, such as whole-grain cereals, bread, and raw fruits and vegetables. This diet helps with problems such as constipation and bowel disorders.

Gluten-Free Diet: This diet is free of gluten, which is a protein found in wheat, rye, and barley. It is used for people with celiac disease, which is a disorder that can damage the intestines if gluten is consumed. Foods containing wheat flour, such as tortillas, crackers, breads, cakes, pastas, and cereals, are eliminated from the diet. Some sauces and dressings also have wheat in them. Other items that may contain gluten include beer, hot dogs, candy, broths, and medications.

Unlike celiac disease, gluten intolerance is a condition that does not cause damage to the intestines. It does, however, cause unpleasant symptoms such as abdominal pain, gas, and diarrhea when products containing gluten are consumed. If a person has a gluten intolerance, eliminating gluten from the diet is usually enough to manage symptoms.

Vegetarian Diet: Health problems, such as diabetes or obesity, may cause a person to require a vegetarian diet. A person may also choose to eat a vegetarian diet for religious reasons or due to a dislike of meat, a compassion for animals, a belief in nonviolence, or financial issues. There are different types of vegetarian diets, including the following:

- A lacto-ovo vegetarian diet excludes all meats, fish, and poultry, but allows eggs and dairy products.

- A lacto-vegetarian diet eliminates poultry, meats, fish, and eggs, but allows dairy products.

- An ovo-vegetarian diet omits all meats, fish, poultry, and dairy products, but allows eggs.

- A vegan diet eliminates poultry, meats, fish, eggs, and dairy products, along with all foods that are derived from animals.

A person might choose to limit his intake of animal-based foods by being a pescatarian (also spelled pescetarian). A pescatarian diet eliminates all meats and poultry, but allows fish and other seafood. Eggs and dairy products may be consumed.

Liquid Diet: A liquid diet is usually ordered for a short time due to a medical condition or before or after a test or surgery. It is ordered when a resident needs to keep the intestinal tract free of food. A liquid diet consists of foods that are in a liquid state at body temperature. Liquid diets are usually ordered as *clear* or *full*. A clear liquid diet includes clear juices, broth, gelatin, and popsicles. A full liquid diet includes all the liquids served on a clear liquid diet, with the addition of cream soups, milk, and ice cream.

Soft Diet and Mechanical Soft Diet: The soft diet is soft in texture and consists of soft or chopped foods that are easier to chew and swallow. Foods that are hard to chew and swallow, such as raw fruits and vegetables and some meats, will be restricted. High-fiber foods, fried foods, and spicy foods may also be limited to help with digestion. Doctors order this diet for residents who have trouble chewing and swallowing due to dental problems or other medical conditions. It is also ordered for people who are making the transition from a liquid diet to a regular diet.

The mechanical soft diet consists of chopped or blended foods that are easier to chew and swallow. Foods are prepared with blenders, food processors, or cutting utensils. Unlike the soft diet, the mechanical soft diet does not limit spices, fat, and fiber. Only the texture of foods is changed. For example, meats and poultry can be ground and moistened with sauces or water to ease swallowing. This diet is used for people recovering from surgery or who have difficulty chewing and swallowing.

Pureed Diet: To **puree** a food means to blend or grind it into a thick paste of baby food consistency. The food should be thick enough to hold its form in the mouth. This diet does not require a person to chew his food. A pureed diet is often used for people who have trouble chewing and/or swallowing more textured foods.

Menus

Residents may receive daily menus for their meals, and nursing assistants may need to help residents complete them. If asked to help a resident with a menu, the NA should make sure the menu offered matches the resident. When reading the menu to the resident, the NA should make the food choices sound appetizing. He should mark the selection that the resident wants if the resident is unable to do this. After completing each category on the menu, he should submit the menu to the dietary department.

7. Explain thickened liquids and identify three basic thickened consistencies

Residents with swallowing problems may be restricted to consuming only thickened liquids. Thickened liquids have a thickening powder or agent added to them, which improves the ability to control fluid in the mouth and throat. A doctor orders the necessary thickness after the resident has been evaluated by a speech-language pathologist.

Some beverages arrive already thickened and ready to consume. Other beverages must have the thickening agent added before serving. If thickening is ordered, it must be used with all liquids. This means that regular liquids, such as water or other beverages, should not be offered to residents who require thickened liquids. There are three basic thickened consistencies:

1. **Nectar Thick**: This consistency is thicker than water. It is the thickness of a thick juice, such as pear nectar or tomato juice. A resident can drink this from a cup.

2. **Honey Thick**: This consistency has the thickness of honey. It will pour very slowly. A resident will usually use a spoon to consume it.

3. **Pudding Thick**: With this consistency, the liquids have become semi-solid, much like pudding. A spoon should stand up straight in the glass when put into the middle of the drink. A resident must consume these liquids with a spoon.

8. Describe how to make dining enjoyable for residents

Mealtime is often one of the most anticipated times of a resident's day. Not only is mealtime the time for getting proper nourishment, but it is also a time for socializing. Socializing has a positive effect on eating. It can help prevent weight loss, dehydration, and malnutrition. It can also prevent loneliness and boredom. Promoting healthy eating is an important part of a nursing assistant's job. Mealtime should be pleasant and enjoyable.

Guidelines: Promoting Appetites

G   Assist residents with grooming and hygiene tasks before dining as needed.

G   Give oral care before eating if requested.

G   Offer a trip to the bathroom or help with elimination before eating.

G   Help residents wash their hands before eating.

G   Encourage the use of dentures, eyeglasses, and hearing aids. If these are damaged, notify the nurse.

G   Check the environment. The temperature should be comfortable. Address any odors. Keep noise level low. Televisions should be off. Do not shout or raise your voice. Do not bang plates or cups.

G   Seat residents next to their friends or people with like interests. Encourage conversation.

G   Properly position residents for eating. Usually the proper position is upright, at a 90-degree angle. This helps prevent swallowing problems. If residents use a wheelchair, make sure they are sitting at a table that is the right height. Most facilities have adjustable tables for wheelchairs. Residents who use *geri-chairs*—reclining chairs on wheels—should be upright, not reclined, while eating.

G   Serve food promptly to maintain the correct temperature. Keep food covered until ready to serve.

G   Plates and trays should look appetizing. If they do not, inform your supervisor.

G   Give the resident the proper eating tools. Use assistive or adaptive utensils if needed (Fig. 15-15).

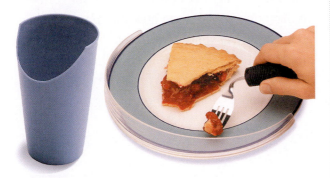

Fig. 15-15. *Special cups, plates with guards on them, and utensils with thick handles that are easier to hold are examples of adaptive devices that can help with eating.* (PHOTOS COURTESY OF NORTH COAST MEDICAL, INC., 800-821-9319, WWW.NCMEDICAL.COM)

G   Be cheerful, positive, and helpful. Make conversation if the resident wishes to talk.

G   Honor requests regarding food. Residents have the legal right to ask for and receive different food. They can also ask for additional food.

9. Explain how to serve meal trays and assist with eating

Food may be served on trays or carried to residents from the kitchen. Nursing assistants must work quickly to make sure that food is served at the proper temperature and that residents do not have to wait too long for their food.

Guidelines: Serving Meal Trays

G   Before you begin serving or helping residents, wash your hands.

G   As you learned earlier in this textbook, it is very important to identify residents before serving a meal tray. Feeding a resident the wrong food can cause serious problems, even death. Identify each resident before placing food in front of him or her.

G   Before you deliver trays or plates, check them closely. Make sure that you have the correct resident and the correct food and beverages for that person. Trays and plates should also be closely checked for added sugar and salt packets (Fig. 15-16). Be aware of residents who eat special diets. Watch for foods in residents' rooms or in the dining room that are not permitted by their doctors. Report any problems to the nurse.

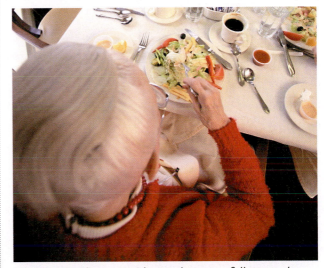

Fig. 15-16. *Observe residents' plates carefully to make sure they are receiving the correct food.*

G   Serve all residents who are sitting together at one table before serving another table. Residents will then be able to eat together and not have to watch others eat.

G   Prepare the food by following these steps, only doing what the resident cannot do for himself:

•   Remove the food and drink if it is on a tray and set it out on the table.

•   Cut food into small, bite-sized portions. Only cut meat and vegetables when necessary. If you know residents need their food cut up, cut it before bringing it to the table. This promotes dignity.

- Open milk or juice cartons. Open and insert a straw if the resident uses one. Place straws in the containers using the paper wrappers; do not touch them directly with your fingers. Some residents may not be able to use straws due to swallowing problems. This should be noted on their diet cards, and no straws should be on the tray. Residents may want you to pour the beverage into a cup. Do so if the resident wishes.

- Butter roll, bread, and vegetables as the resident prefers.

- Open any condiment packets. Offer to season food as resident prefers, including pureed food.

Residents will need different levels of assistance with eating. Some residents will not need any help. Other residents will only need help setting up; they may only need help opening cartons and cutting and seasoning their food. Once that is done, they can feed themselves. If this is the case, the NA should check in with these residents from time to time to see if they need anything else.

Other residents will be completely unable to feed themselves, and it will be the NA's job to feed them. Residents who must be fed are often embarrassed and depressed about their dependence on another person. Nursing assistants should be sensitive to this and give privacy while residents are eating. Residents should not be rushed through their meals.

NAs should only give assistance as specified, when necessary, or when residents request it. They should encourage residents to do whatever they can for themselves. For example, if a resident can hold and use a napkin, she should. If she can hold and eat finger foods, the NA should offer them. There are devices that help residents eat more independently (Fig. 15-15 on previous page). More adaptive devices are shown in Chapter 21.

Mealtime involves more than eating. It is a chance for social interaction. Residents look forward to their interactions with nursing assistants and with others. It may be the highlight of their day. To avoid weight loss and dehydration, NAs must do all that they can to increase food and drink intake. Cheerful company and conversation can greatly increase how much a resident eats and drinks. Fewer digestive problems may occur. Positive interactions also have a helpful effect on residents' attitudes. The reverse is also true. Negative attitudes and poor communication can decrease how much a resident consumes. NAs should avoid making negative comments, such as "I don't know how you can eat this" or "This looks awful." They should not judge residents' food preferences.

Guidelines: Assisting a Resident with Eating

G   Verify that you have the right resident by checking the diet card against the name listed outside the door (if available). Ask the resident to state his name. Check that the diet on the tray is correct and matches the diet card.

G   Sit at the resident's eye level. The resident should be sitting upright, at a 90-degree angle. Make eye contact with the resident.

G   If the resident wishes, allow time for prayer.

G   Never treat the resident like a child. This is embarrassing and disrespectful. It is hard for many people to accept help with feeding. Be supportive and encouraging.

G   Test the temperature of the food by putting your hand over the dish to sense the heat. Do not touch food to test its temperature. If you think the food is too hot, do not blow on it to cool it. Offer other food to give it time to cool.

G   Cut foods and pour liquids as needed. Season foods to the resident's preference.

G   Identify the foods and fluids that are in front of the resident. Call pureed foods by the correct name. For example, ask "Would you like green beans?" rather than referring to it as "some green stuff."

G   Ask the resident which food he prefers to eat first. Allow him to make the choice, even if he wants to eat dessert first.

G   Do not mix foods unless the resident requests it.

G   Do not rush the meal. Allow time for the resident to chew and swallow each bite. Be relaxed.

G   Be social and friendly. Make simple conversation if the resident wishes to do so (Fig. 15-17). Try not to ask questions that require long answers. Use appropriate topics, such as the news, weather, the resident's life, things the resident enjoys, and food preferences. Say positive things about the food being served, such as "This smells really good," and "This looks really fresh."

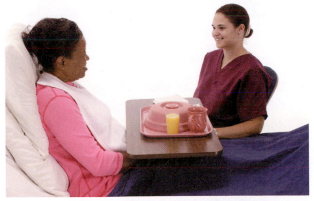

Fig. 15-17. Being friendly and social while helping residents with eating is important. Encourage residents to do whatever they can for themselves.

G   Give the resident your full attention while he or she is eating. Do not talk to other staff members while helping a resident eat.

G   Alternate offering food and drink. Alternating cold and hot foods or bland foods and sweets can help increase appetite.

G   If the resident wants a different food from what is being served, inform the dietitian so that an alternative may be offered.

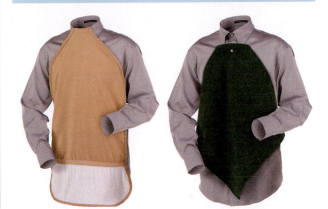

Fig. 15-18. Residents have the right to choose whether or not to use a clothing protector. Each resident's decision should be respected. (PHOTOS COURTESY OF STANDARD TEXTILE, STANDARDTEXTILE.COM, 800-999-0400)

Feeding a resident

Equipment: meal, eating utensils, clothing protector, washcloths or wipes

1.   Identify yourself by name. Identify the resident by name.

2.   Wash your hands.

3.   Explain procedure to the resident. Speak clearly, slowly, and directly. Maintain face-to-face contact whenever possible.

4.   Provide for resident's privacy with curtain, screen, or door.

5.   Look at diet card or menu, and ask the resident to state her name. If the resident is unable to state her name, check identification another way, such as looking at a photo ID or an armband. Verify that the resident has the right tray.

6.   Raise the head of the bed. Make sure the resident is in an upright sitting position (at a 90-degree angle).

7. Adjust bed height to where you will be to able to sit at the resident's eye level. Lock bed wheels.

8. Place meal tray where it can be easily seen by the resident, such as on the overbed table.

9. Help the resident clean her hands with hand wipes if resident cannot do it herself.

10. Help the resident put on clothing protector if desired.

11. Sit facing the resident at the resident's eye level (Fig. 15-19). Sit on the stronger side if the resident has one-sided weakness.

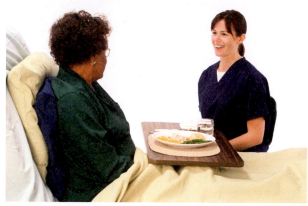

Fig. 15-19. The resident should be sitting upright, and the nursing assistant should be sitting at her eye level.

12. Tell the resident what foods are on the plate. Offer a drink of beverage and ask what the resident would like to eat first.

13. Check the temperature of the food. Using utensils, offer the food in bite-sized pieces. Tell the resident the content of each bite of food offered (Fig. 15-20). Alternate types of food offered, allowing for resident's preferences. Do not feed all of one type before offering another type. Make sure the resident's mouth is empty before next bite or sip is offered. Report any swallowing problems to the nurse immediately.

14. Offer sips of beverage throughout the meal. If you are holding the cup, touch it to the resident's lips before you tip it. Give small, frequent sips.

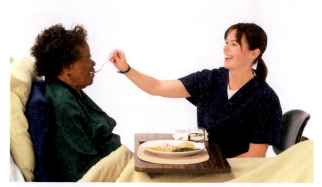

Fig. 15-20. Offer the food in bite-sized pieces. Tell the resident the content of each bite of food.

15. Talk with the resident during the meal. It makes mealtime more enjoyable (Fig. 15-21). Do not rush the resident.

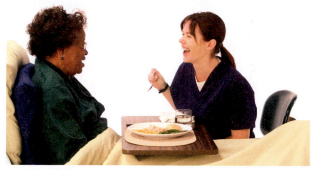

Fig. 15-21. Socializing during mealtime makes eating more enjoyable and may promote a healthy appetite.

16. Use washcloths or wipes to wipe food from the resident's mouth and hands as needed during the meal. Wipe again at the end of the meal (Fig. 15-22).

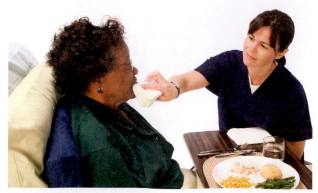

Fig. 15-22. Wiping food from the mouth during the meal helps to maintain the resident's dignity.

17. When the resident is finished eating, remove the clothing protector if used. Place the protector in the proper container.

18. Remove the food tray. Check for eyeglasses, dentures, or any personal items before removing the tray. Place tray in the proper area.

19. Make resident comfortable. Keep the resident in the upright position for at least 30 minutes if ordered in the care plan. Make sure the bed is free from crumbs.

20. Return bed to lowest position. Remove privacy measures.

21. Place call light within resident's reach.

22. Wash your hands.

23. Report any changes in resident to the nurse.

24. Document procedure using facility guidelines.

Food trays and plates should also be observed after the meal. This helps to identify residents with poor appetites. It may also signal illness, a problem, such as dentures that do not fit properly, or a change in food preferences.

10. Describe how to assist residents with special needs

Residents with specific diseases or conditions, such as Parkinson's disease, Alzheimer's disease or other dementias, head trauma, blindness, confusion, or those recovering from a stroke, may need special assistance when eating.

Guidelines: Dining Techniques

G   Use assistive devices such as utensils with built-up handle grips and plate guards. Assistive devices for eating are designed to help people feed themselves. These devices should be included on the meal tray.

G   Residents may benefit from physical and verbal cues, which promote independence. A cue is something that signals that a person should do something. The hand-over-hand

approach is an example of a physical cue. The resident lifts a utensil if he is able, and you put your hand over his to help with eating (Fig. 15-23). With your hand placed over the resident's hand, help him get food on the utensil. Steer the utensil from the plate to the mouth and back. Repeat this until the resident is finished with his meal.

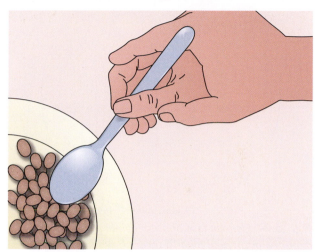

Fig. 15-23. The hand-over-hand approach is used when a resident can help by lifting utensils. It helps promote independence.

G   Verbal cues must be short and clear so that they are easily understood, and they should prompt the resident to do something. Give verbal cues one at a time. Wait until one task is finished before asking the resident to do another. Repeat the cues until the resident is done eating. Examples of cues include:

• "Pick up your spoon."

• "Put some carrots on your spoon."

• "Raise the spoon to your lips."

• "Open your mouth."

• "Place the spoon in your mouth."

• "Close your mouth."

• "Take the spoon out of your mouth."

• "Chew."

• "Swallow."

• "Drink some water."

G For residents who are visually impaired, read menus to them if needed. When helping with eating, place the plate or tray directly in front of residents. Use the face of an imaginary clock to explain the position of what is in front of them (Fig. 15-24).

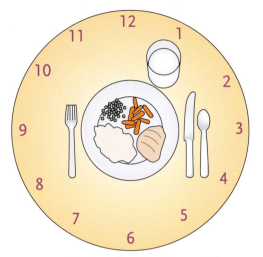

Fig. 15-24. Use the face of an imaginary clock to explain the position of food to residents who are visually impaired.

G For residents who have had a stroke and have a paralyzed or weaker side, place food in the stronger side of the mouth. Make sure food is swallowed before offering another bite.

G Place food in the resident's field of vision. The nurse will determine a resident's field of vision.

G For residents who have Parkinson's disease, tremors or shaking can make it very difficult to eat. Help by using physical cues. Place food and drinks close so that the resident can easily reach them. Use assistive devices as needed.

G If a resident has poor sitting balance, seat him in a regular dining room chair with armrests, rather than in a wheelchair. Proper position in the chair means hips are at a 90-degree angle, knees are flexed, and feet and arms are fully supported. Push the chair under the table. Place forearms on the table. If a resident tends to lean to one side, ask him to keep his elbows on the table.

G If a resident has poor neck control, a neck brace may be used to stabilize the head. Use assistive devices as needed. If the resident is in a geri-chair, a wedge cushion behind the head and shoulders may be used.

G If the resident bites down on utensils, ask him to open his mouth. Do not pull the utensil out of his mouth. Wait until his jaw relaxes.

G If the resident pockets food in his cheeks, ask him to chew and swallow the food. Touch the side of his cheek. Ask him to use his tongue to get the food. Using your fingers on the cheek (near the lower jaw), gently push the food toward his teeth.

G If the resident holds food in his mouth, ask him to chew and swallow the food. You may need to trigger swallowing. To do this, gently press down on the tongue when taking the spoon out of the mouth. You can also try to gently press down on the top of his head with your hand. Make sure the resident has swallowed the food before offering more.

11. Define *dysphagia* and identify signs and symptoms of swallowing problems

Residents may have conditions that make eating or swallowing difficult. **Dysphagia** means difficulty in swallowing. A stroke, or CVA, can cause weakness and paralysis on one side of the body. Nerve and muscle damage from head and neck cancer, multiple sclerosis, Parkinson's disease, or Alzheimer's disease can contribute to dysphagia. If a resident has trouble swallowing, soft foods and thickened liquids will probably be served. A special cup will help make swallowing easier.

Nursing assistants need to be able to recognize and report signs that a resident has a swallowing problem. Signs and symptoms of swallowing problems include the following:

- Coughing during or after meals

- Choking during meals

- Dribbling saliva, food, or fluid from the mouth

- Having food residue inside the mouth or cheeks during and after meals

- Gurgling during or after meals or losing voice

- Eating slowly

- Avoiding eating

- Spitting out pieces of food

- Swallowing several times per mouthful

- Clearing the throat frequently during and after meals

- Watering of the eyes when eating or drinking

- Food or fluid coming up into the nose

- Making a visible effort to swallow

- Breathing rapidly or with shorter breaths while eating or drinking

- Difficulty chewing food

- Difficulty swallowing medications

Swallowing problems put residents at high risk for choking on food or drink. Inhaling food, fluid, or foreign material into the lungs is called **aspiration**. Aspiration can cause pneumonia or death. An NA should alert the nurse immediately if he notices any signs of swallowing problems.

Guidelines: Preventing Aspiration

G   Position residents properly for eating and drinking. They must sit upright at a 90-degree angle. Do not feed residents in a reclining position.

G   Offer small pieces of food or small spoonfuls of pureed food.

G   Feed residents slowly; do not rush them.

G   Place food in the unaffected, or stronger, side of the mouth.

G   Make sure the mouth is empty before offering another bite of food or sip of drink.

G   If possible, keep residents in the upright position for about 30 minutes after eating and drinking.

12. Explain intake and output (I&O)

To maintain health, the body must take in a certain amount of fluid each day. Fluid comes in the form of liquids that a person drinks and is also found in semi-liquid foods like gelatin, soup, ice cream, pudding, and yogurt. Generally, a healthy person needs about 64 ounces (oz) of fluid each day. The fluid a person consumes is called **intake**, or **input**. If a person's intake is not in a healthy range, he can become dehydrated. Dehydration is a serious medical condition that requires immediate attention. More information on dehydration is in the next learning objective.

All fluid taken in each day cannot remain in the body. It must be eliminated as **output**. Output includes urine, feces (including diarrhea), and vomitus, as well as perspiration, moisture in the air that a person exhales, and wound drainage. If a person's intake exceeds his output, fluid builds up in body tissues. This fluid retention can cause medical problems and discomfort.

Fluid balance is maintaining equal input and output, or taking in and eliminating equal amounts of fluid. Most people do this naturally. But some residents must have their intake and output, or I&O, monitored and documented due to illness or special diets. To monitor this, the nursing assistant will need to measure and document all food and fluids that the resident takes in by mouth, as well as all urine and vomitus produced. This information is recorded on an Intake and Output (I&O) sheet (Fig. 15-25).

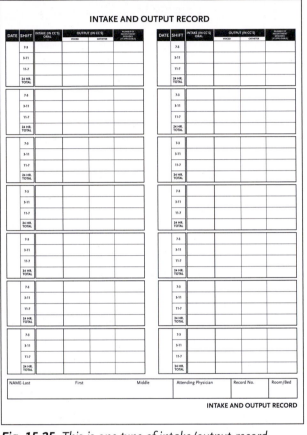

INTAKE AND OUTPUT RECORD

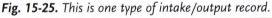

Fig. 15-25. *This is one type of intake/output record.*

Fluids are usually measured in milliliters (mL). Milliliters are units of measurement in the metric system. One milliliter is 1/1000 of a liter. Ounces (oz) are converted to milliliters. One ounce equals 30 milliliters, so to convert ounces to milliliters, the number of ounces must be multiplied by 30.

For example, an NA serves a resident an eight-ounce carton of milk. The resident finishes about half of the milk, and the NA estimates the resident drank four ounces of milk. To convert ounces to milliliters, the number of ounces must be multiplied by 30. Four ounces multiplied by 30 equals 120 milliliters (mL). The NA would document 120 mL milk on her input sheet.

Graduates are containers that measure fluid in milliliters and may also measure in ounces (Fig. 15-26). Some common conversions are listed in the orange box.

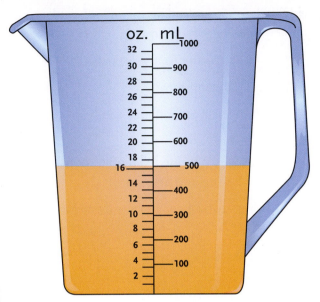

Fig. 15-26. *A graduate is a measuring container for measuring fluid volume.*

Conversions

One ounce equals 30 milliliters. To convert ounces to milliliters, the number of ounces must be multiplied by 30.

1 oz = 30 mL

2 oz = 60 mL

3 oz = 90 mL

4 oz = 120 mL

5 oz = 150 mL

6 oz = 180 mL

7 oz = 210 mL

8 oz = 240 mL

¼ cup = 2 oz = 60 mL

½ cup = 4 oz = 120 mL

1 cup = 8 oz = 240 mL

Before beginning, the NA should explain to the resident that she needs to keep track of his intake. The resident should be asked to let the NA know when he drinks something (if it is not something she served to him) and how much it was.

Measuring and recording intake and output

Equipment: I&O sheet, graduate, pen and paper

Measure intake first.

1. Identify yourself by name. Identify the resident by name.

2. Wash your hands.

3. Explain procedure to the resident. Speak clearly, slowly, and directly. Maintain face-to-face contact whenever possible.

4. Provide for resident's privacy with curtain, screen, or door.

5. Note the amount of fluid a resident is served on paper. The amount of fluid is often marked on the container that is served.

6. When the resident has finished a meal or snack, measure any leftover fluids with the graduate. Note this amount on paper.

7. Subtract the leftover amount from the amount served. If you have measured in ounces, convert to milliliters (mL) by multiplying by 30.

8. Document the amount of fluid consumed (in mL) in the input column on I&O sheet, as well as the time and the type of fluid consumed. Report anything unusual, such as the resident refusing to drink, drinking very little, or feeling nauseated.

9. Wash your hands.

Measuring output is the other half of monitoring fluid balance.

Equipment: I&O sheet, graduate, gloves, pen and paper

1. Wash your hands.

2. Put on gloves before handling the bedpan or urinal.

3. Pour the contents of the bedpan or urinal into the graduate. Do not spill or splash any of the urine.

4. Place the graduate on flat surface. Measure the amount of urine at eye level. Keep the container level (Fig. 15-27). Note the amount on paper, converting to mL if necessary.

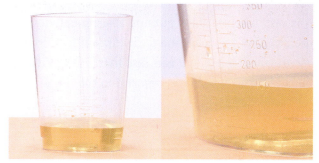

Fig. 15-27. Keep the container on a flat surface while measuring output.

5. After measuring urine, empty the graduate into the toilet without splashing.

6. Turn on the faucet, using a paper towel. Rinse the graduate with cold water and pour rinse water into the toilet.

7. Rinse the bedpan/urinal with cold water and pour rinse water into toilet. Flush the toilet.

8. Place graduate and bedpan in area for cleaning or clean and store according to policy.

9. Remove and discard gloves.

10. Wash hands before recording output.

11. Document the time and amount of urine in output column on sheet. For example: 1545 hours, 200 mL urine. To measure vomitus, pour from basin into measuring container, then discard in the toilet. If resident vomits on the bed or floor, estimate the amount. Document emesis and amount on the I&O sheet.

12. Report any changes in resident to the nurse.

All facilities keep track of how much food and fluid a resident consumes. Percentages are often used to document food intake, but the method can vary (Fig. 15-28). The dietician calculates the percentages for meals. The NA may be asked to document how much of the entire meal a resident ate. For example, if the resident ate the entire meal served, the NA would document that 100% was eaten. If the resident ate about half of the meal, the NA would document 50% eaten, and so on.

It is very important for nursing assistants to follow their facility's policies and to document food intake accurately. If a resident eats less than 75% of his or her meal, the NA should report it to the nurse.

13. Identify ways to assist residents in maintaining fluid balance

Water is an essential nutrient for life. Proper fluid intake is important. Drinking at least 64 ounces of water or other fluids per day can help prevent constipation and urinary incontinence.

Without enough fluid, urine becomes concentrated. More concentrated urine creates a higher risk for infection. Proper fluid intake also helps to dilute wastes and flush out the urinary system. It may even help prevent confusion.

The sense of thirst can lessen as people age. Infection, fever, diarrhea, and some medications will also increase the need for fluid intake. Nursing assistants should remind residents to drink fluids often (Fig. 15-29). Some residents will drink more fluids if they are offered them in smaller amounts, rather than in one large glassful.

Some residents may have an order to encourage or restrict fluids because of medical conditions. When a resident has an order to restrict fluids, she must limit the daily amount of fluid intake to a level set by the doctor. The NA should not give the resident any extra fluids or a water pitcher unless the nurse approves it.

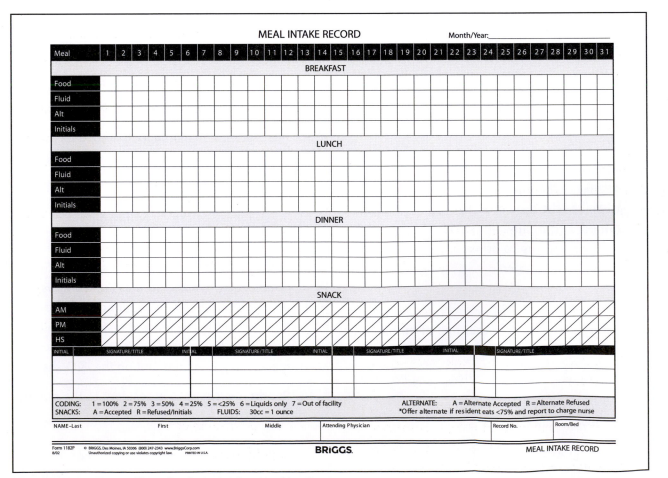

Fig. 15-28. *One type of form for documenting meal intake.* (REPRINTED WITH PERMISSION OF BRIGGS CORPORATION, 800-247-2343, WWW.BRIGGSCORP.COM)

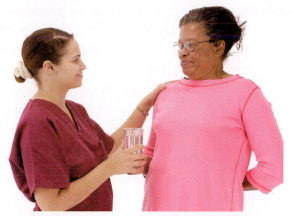

Fig. 15-29. Drinking enough water and other fluids promotes good health. NAs should encourage residents to drink fluids often.

The abbreviation **NPO** stands for *nothing by mouth*. This means that a resident is not allowed to have anything to eat or drink. Some residents have such a severe problem with swallowing that it is unsafe to give them anything by mouth. These residents will receive nutrition through a feeding tube or intravenously. Some residents may not be able to eat or drink for a short time before a medical test or surgery. Nursing assistants need to know this abbreviation and should never offer any food or drink, even water, to a resident with this order.

Dehydration occurs when a person does not have enough fluid in the body. Dehydration is a serious condition and is a major problem among the elderly. People can become dehydrated if they do not drink enough or if they have diarrhea or are vomiting. Preventing dehydration is very important.

Guidelines: Preventing Dehydration

G Report observations and warning signs to the nurse immediately.

G Encourage residents to drink every time you see them.

G Offer fresh water or other fluids often. Offer drinks that the resident enjoys. Some residents may prefer water or sparkling water (seltzer water). Some residents may not like water and prefer other types of beverages, such as juice, soda, tea, or milk. Some residents do not want ice in their drinks. As always, it is important to provide person-centered care and to honor personal preferences. Report to the nurse if the resident tells you he does not like the fluids being served.

G Ice chips, frozen flavored ice sticks, and gelatin are also forms of liquids. Offer them often. Do not offer ice chips or sticks if a resident has a swallowing problem.

G If appropriate, offer sips of liquid between bites of food during meals and snacks.

G Make sure pitcher and cup are nearby and are light enough for the resident to lift.

G Offer assistance if resident cannot drink without help. Use adaptive cups as needed.

G Record fluid intake and output.

Observing and Reporting: Dehydration

Report any of the following immediately:

O/R Resident drinks less than six eight-ounce glasses of liquid per day

O/R Resident drinks little or no fluids at meals

O/R Resident needs help drinking from a cup or glass

O/R Resident has trouble swallowing liquids

O/R Resident has frequent vomiting, diarrhea, or fever

O/R Resident is easily confused or tired

Report if the resident has any of the following:

O/R Dry mouth

O/R Cracked lips

O/R Sunken eyes

O/R Dark urine

O/R Strong-smelling urine

O/R Weight loss

O/R Complaints of abdominal pain

Serving fresh water

Equipment: water pitcher, ice scoop, cup, straw, gloves

1. Identify yourself by name. Identify the resident by name.

2. Wash your hands.

3. Put on gloves.

4. Scoop ice into the water pitcher without touching the ice scoop to the pitcher. Add fresh water. Do not touch the pitcher to the spout or faucet.

5. Use and store the ice scoop properly. Do not allow the ice to touch your gloved hand and fall back into the container. Place the scoop in the proper receptacle after each use.

6. Take the pitcher to the resident.

7. Pour water into the resident's cup. Offer the resident a drink of water. Leave the pitcher and cup at the bedside.

8. Make sure that the pitcher and cup are light enough for the resident to lift. Leave a straw if the resident desires and is allowed to use one (if he does not have swallowing problems).

9. Place call light within resident's reach.

10. Remove and discard gloves.

11. Wash your hands.

Residents' Rights

Fluid Intake

Offering fresh fluids often helps prevent dehydration and promotes health. Nursing assistants should encourage, but not force, fluids. NAs can ask residents which beverages they prefer and arrange for those to be available. They should respond to drink requests promptly unless there is a doctor's order restricting fluid intake. If this is the case, the NA should inform the resident about the order, and report the request to the nurse. If fluid intake is increased, additional trips to the bathroom should be offered. It is important for the NA to give plenty of privacy. If urine is being measured, it should be done with the door closed.

Fluid overload occurs when the body cannot handle the amount of fluid consumed. This condition often affects people with heart or kidney disease.

Observing and Reporting: Fluid Overload

Report any of the following to the nurse:

O/R Swelling/edema of extremities (ankles, feet, fingers, hands); **edema** is swelling caused by excess fluid in body tissues

O/R Weight gain (daily weight gain of one to two pounds)

O/R Decreased urine output

O/R Shortness of breath

O/R Increased heart rate

O/R Anxiety

O/R Skin that appears tight, smooth, and shiny

Chapter Review

1. List the six basic nutrients and identify which nutrient is the most essential for life.

2. According to MyPlate's suggestions, what should make up half of a person's plate?

3. List some examples of plant-based proteins.

4. According to MyPlate, what should most dairy group choices be?

5. List four problems that may affect an elderly person's nutritional intake.

6. Why is it important for an NA to report any weight loss, no matter how small?

7. What are two ways a resident may be fed if he has a digestive system that does not function properly or he cannot swallow?

8. List two factors that influence food preferences.

9. What information do diet cards contain?

10. What is the first item to be restricted in a low-sodium diet?

11. Why might a resident be placed on a low-fat/low-cholesterol diet?

12. What is the difference between a clear liquid diet and a full liquid diet?

13. How is the mechanical soft diet different from the soft diet?

14. List five reasons that a person may choose to be a vegetarian.

15. How can thickened liquids help a person with swallowing problems?

16. What is the proper position to place a resident in for eating?

17. How might being cheerful and positive during mealtimes affect the amount of food a resident consumes?

18. How can a nursing assistant verify that she has the correct resident for the meal tray that she is serving?

19. How should a nursing assistant test the temperature of food?

20. What should the nursing assistant do if a resident wants a different food than what is being served?

21. When feeding a resident, how should the bed height be adjusted?

22. How do verbal cues assist a resident with eating?

23. When assisting a resident who is visually impaired, how should the nursing assistant explain the position of food and objects to the resident?

24. To which side of the mouth should food be directed if a resident has a weaker side—the weaker (affected) or stronger (unaffected) side?

25. What is the medical term for difficulty swallowing?

26. Describe five guidelines to help prevent aspiration.

27. How many ounces of fluid does a healthy person need each day?

28. What is fluid balance?

29. How many milliliters (mL) equal one ounce (oz)?

30. What counts as output?

31. What does the abbreviation *NPO* stand for?

32. Describe six ways that a nursing assistant can help prevent dehydration.

33. List four signs of fluid overload that a nursing assistant should report.

16

Urinary Elimination

1. List qualities of urine and identify signs and symptoms about urine to report

Urination, also known as *micturition* or *voiding*, is the act of passing urine from the bladder through the urethra to the outside of the body. Urine is made up of water and waste products filtered from the blood by the kidneys. Normal urine output varies with age and the amount and type of liquids consumed. Adults usually produce about 1200 to 1500 milliliters (mL) of urine per day, although elderly adults may produce less.

Urine is normally light, pale yellow, or amber in color (Fig. 16-1). However, there are many factors that can cause urine to change color, such as medications, certain foods or food dyes, and vitamins and supplements. For example, beets can make urine appear pink or red, and B vitamins can make urine very bright yellow. Unusual urine color can also be a sign of illness.

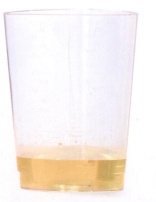

Fig. 16-1. *Urine is normally light or pale yellow in color. It should be clear, not cloudy.*

Normal urine should be clear or transparent when freshly voided and should have a faint smell. Urine that is cloudy or murky or that smells bad or fruity can be a sign of infection or illness.

Observing and Reporting: Urine

Report any of the following to the nurse:

- **O/R** Cloudy urine
- **O/R** Dark or rust-colored urine
- **O/R** Strong-, offensive-, or fruity-smelling urine
- **O/R** Resident complaints of pain, burning, or pressure when urinating
- **O/R** Blood, pus, mucus, or discharge in urine
- **O/R** Protein or glucose in urine (there is more information about this later in the chapter)
- **O/R** Urinary incontinence (the inability to control the bladder, which leads to an involuntary loss of urine)

2. List factors affecting urination and demonstrate how to assist with elimination

There are many factors that can affect normal urination, including the following:

Normal changes of aging: As a person ages, the ability of the kidneys to filter blood decreases.

The bladder muscle tone weakens. The bladder is not able to hold the same amount of urine as it once did, which can cause elderly people to urinate more frequently. Many awaken several times during the night to urinate. The bladder may not empty completely, causing susceptibility to infection.

To promote normal urination, the nursing assistant should offer frequent trips to the bathroom or bedpans and urinals. The NA should respond to call lights immediately. Toileting schedules should be followed. The best position for women to have normal urination is sitting. For men, it is standing. The supine (lying on the back) position should be avoided because it does not put pressure on the bladder and works against gravity.

When helping with perineal care, the NA should wipe from front to back to prevent infection. The NA should assist the resident with handwashing after urination as needed.

Psychological factors: A lack of privacy, new environments, stress, anxiety, and depression can all affect urination. To promote normal urination, it is very important for the NA to provide plenty of privacy for elimination. She should close the bathroom door if a resident is in the bathroom. If the resident needs to use a bedpan or urinal, the NA should pull the privacy curtain and close the door. Residents should not be rushed or interrupted when they are in the bathroom. It is important for an NA to report signs of depression and anxiety (Chapter 20), as well as any changes in output.

Fluid intake: The sense of thirst lessens as a person ages. When a person drinks fewer fluids, urinary output decreases, and dehydration may result. Some beverages, such as those containing alcohol and caffeine, increase urine output.

To promote normal urination, NAs should encourage residents to drink fluids often. Because a healthy person needs to take in at least 64 ounces of fluid each day, the NA should provide fresh water and juices often (Fig. 16-2). The pitcher and cup should be left close to the resident and they should be light enough for the resident to lift. Beverages that are high in vitamin C are especially good for preventing urinary tract infections. The NA must follow any fluid restrictions that a resident has.

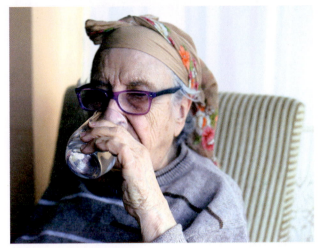

Fig. 16-2. *Drinking plenty of fluids is important to promoting a healthy urinary system.*

Medications: Medications can affect urinary output. For example, a resident who is taking diuretics (medications that reduce fluid in the body) will need to urinate frequently. To promote normal urination, the NA should regularly offer a trip to the bathroom or offer a bedpan or urinal. Fluid intake should be encouraged and the NA should report any changes in output or discoloration of urine.

Disorders: Many disorders and illnesses, such as bladder disease, infections, arthritis, congestive heart disease, neurological diseases, and diabetes, affect urination. Chapter 18 contains more information about these diseases.

Assisting with Elimination

Residents who are unable to get out of bed to use the toilet may be given a standard bedpan, a fracture pan, or a urinal. A **fracture pan** is a bedpan that is flatter than a regular bedpan. It is used for residents who cannot assist with raising their hips onto a regular bedpan (Fig. 16-3). Women will generally use a bedpan for urination and bowel movements. Men will generally use a bedpan for bowel movements and a urinal for urination (Fig. 16-4).

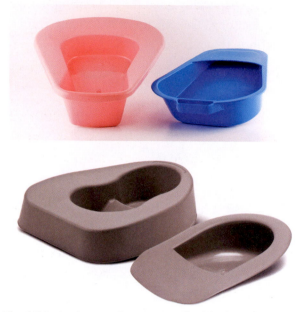

Fig. 16-3. *In the top photo, a standard bedpan is on the left side, and a fracture pan is on the right. In the bottom photo, a bariatric standard bedpan is in back, and a bariatric fracture pan is in front. Bariatric bedpans can be used for people who are overweight or obese.* (BOTTOM PHOTO © MEDLINE INDUSTRIES, INC.)

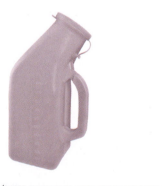

Fig. 16-4. *A urinal.* (PHOTO COURTESY OF NOVA MEDICAL PRODUCTS, WWW.NOVAMEDICALPRODUCTS.COM)

Elimination equipment is usually kept in the bathroom between uses. Residents who share bathrooms may need to have urinals and bedpans labeled. Nursing assistants should never place this equipment on overbed tables or on top of side tables.

Urine and feces are considered infectious wastes. Nursing assistants must always wear gloves when handling bedpans, urinals, or basins that contain wastes, including dirty bath

water. NAs should be careful not to spill or splash wastes, and wastes should be discarded in the toilet. Immediately after use, containers used for elimination should be placed in the proper area for cleaning, or they should be cleaned and stored according to facility policy.

Residents' Rights

Rights with Elimination

Residents may be embarrassed about needing help with elimination. Nursing assistants should be professional when giving assistance and provide as much privacy as possible. To help promote dignity, NAs should treat residents as adults. When assisting with elimination needs, proper terms for bodily functions should be used; childish words should be avoided.

Assisting a resident with the use of a bedpan

Equipment: bedpan, bedpan cover, disposable bed protector, bath blanket, toilet paper, disposable wipes, 2 towels, supplies for perineal care, 2 pairs of gloves

1. Identify yourself by name. Identify the resident by name.

2. Wash your hands.

3. Explain procedure to the resident. Speak clearly, slowly, and directly. Maintain face-to-face contact whenever possible.

4. Provide for resident's privacy with curtain, screen, or door.

5. Adjust bed to a safe working level, usually waist high. Before placing bedpan, lower the head of the bed. Lock bed wheels.

6. Put on gloves.

7. Cover the resident with the bath blanket and ask him to hold it while you pull down the covers underneath. Do not expose more of the resident than you need to. Keeping him covered, ask the resident to remove his undergarments, or help him do so.

8. Ask the resident to raise his hips by pushing with his feet and hands at the count of three. If he needs help, place your arm under the small of his back and tell him to push with his heels

and hands on your signal as you raise his hips. Place the bed protector under the resident's buttocks and hips. Slide the bedpan in the correct position under his hips (Fig. 16-5). A **standard bedpan** should be positioned with the wider end aligned with the resident's buttocks. A **fracture pan** should be positioned with the handle toward the foot of bed.

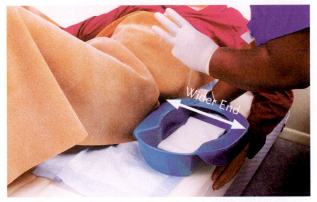

Fig. 16-5. On the count of three, slide the bedpan under the buttocks after placing the bed protector. The wider end of the bedpan should be aligned with the buttocks.

If the resident cannot assist in getting on the bedpan, raise the side rail on the working side. Ask the resident to turn toward you or turn him toward you (see Chapter 10). Move to the empty side of the bed and place the protective pad on the area where the resident will lie on his back. Place the bedpan firmly against the resident's buttocks (Fig. 16-6). Holding the bedpan securely, gently roll the resident back onto the bedpan. Keep the bedpan centered underneath.

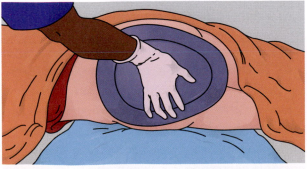

Fig. 16-6. Placing the bedpan firmly against the resident's buttocks, gently roll him back onto the bedpan.

9. Remove and discard gloves. Wash your hands.

10. Raise the head of the bed. Prop the resident into a semi-sitting position using pillows. Leave the side rails up if used.

11. Make sure the bath blanket is still covering the resident. Place toilet paper and disposable wipes within the resident's reach. Ask the resident to clean his hands with a wipe when finished if he is able.

12. Place the call light within the resident's reach. Wash your hands. Ask the resident to signal when done. Leave the room and close the door.

13. When called by the resident, return and wash your hands. Put on clean gloves.

14. Lower the head of the bed. Make sure the resident is still covered. Do not overexpose the resident.

15. Remove the bedpan carefully and cover the bedpan with a bedpan cover or towel.

16. Give perineal care if help is needed. Wipe from front to back. Dry perineal area with a towel. Help resident put on undergarment. Cover the resident and remove bath blanket.

17. Remove and discard the bed protector. Discard disposable supplies. Place the towel and bath blanket in a hamper or bag.

18. Take the bedpan to the bathroom. Note color, odor, and consistency of contents. Empty contents into the toilet unless a specimen is needed or urine is being measured for intake/output monitoring. If you notice anything unusual about the stool or urine (for example, the presence of blood), do not discard it. You will need to inform the nurse.

19. Turn the faucet on with a paper towel. Rinse the bedpan with cold water and empty it into the toilet. Flush the toilet. Place the bedpan in the proper area for cleaning or clean and disinfect it according to facility policy.

20. Remove and discard gloves.

21. Wash your hands.

22. Make resident comfortable.

23. Return bed to lowest position. Remove privacy measures.

24. Place call light within resident's reach.

25. Report any changes in resident to the nurse.

26. Document procedure using facility guidelines.

Assisting a male resident with a urinal

Equipment: urinal, disposable bed protector, disposable wipes, 2 pairs of gloves

1. Identify yourself by name. Identify the resident by name.

2. Wash your hands.

3. Explain procedure to the resident. Speak clearly, slowly, and directly. Maintain face-to-face contact whenever possible.

4. Provide for resident's privacy with curtain, screen, or door.

5. Adjust bed to a safe working level, usually waist high. Lock bed wheels.

6. Put on gloves.

7. Place the bed protector under the resident's buttocks and hips, as in earlier procedure.

8. Hand the urinal to the resident. If the resident is not able to help himself, place urinal between his legs and position the penis inside the urinal (Fig. 16-7). Replace covers.

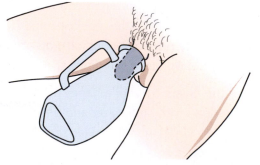

Fig. 16-7. *Position the penis inside the urinal if the resident cannot do it himself.*

9. Remove and discard gloves. Wash your hands.

10. Raise the head of the bed. Place disposable wipes within the resident's reach. Ask the resident to clean his hands with a hand wipe when finished if he is able.

11. Place the call light within reach while resident is using urinal. Ask resident to signal when done. Leave the room and close the door.

12. When called by the resident, return and put on clean gloves.

13. Discard disposable wipes.

14. Remove urinal or have resident hand it to you. Empty contents into toilet unless specimen is needed or the urine is being measured for intake/output monitoring. Note color, odor, and qualities (for example, cloudiness) of contents.

15. Turn the faucet on with a paper towel. Rinse the urinal with cold water and empty it into the toilet. Flush the toilet. Place the urinal in the proper area for cleaning or clean and disinfect it according to facility policy.

16. Remove and discard gloves.

17. Wash your hands.

18. Make resident comfortable.

19. Return bed to lowest position. Remove privacy measures.

20. Place call light within resident's reach.

21. Report any changes in resident to the nurse.

22. Document procedure using facility guidelines.

Some residents are able to get out of bed, but may still need help walking to the bathroom and using the toilet. Others who are able to get out of bed but cannot walk to the bathroom may use a portable commode (also called a *bedside commode* [*BSC*]). A **portable commode** is a chair with a toilet seat and a removable container underneath (Fig. 16-8). The removable container must be cleaned after each use. Toilets can be fitted with raised seats to make it easier for residents to get up and down. Hand rails can also be installed next to the toilet (Fig. 16-9). If these assistive devices are needed but are not present, nursing assistants should report this to the nurse. The NA should offer to help residents get to the bathroom or commode often. This can avoid accidents and embarrassment.

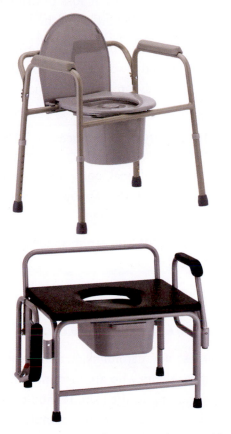

Fig. 16-8. *The top photo shows a regular portable commode and the bottom photo shows a bariatric portable commode, which can be used for people who are overweight or obese.* (PHOTO COURTESY OF NOVA MEDICAL PRODUCTS, WWW.NOVAMEDICALPRODUCTS.COM)

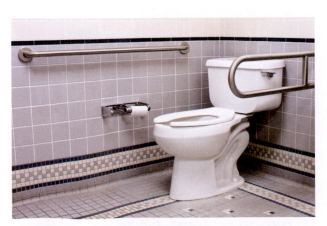

Fig. 16-9. *Hand rails can be installed next to toilets to promote safety.*

Assisting a resident to use a portable commode or toilet

Equipment: portable commode with basin, toilet paper, disposable wipes, towel, supplies for perineal care, 3 pairs of gloves

1. Identify yourself by name. Identify the resident by name.

2. Wash your hands.

3. Explain procedure to the resident. Speak clearly, slowly, and directly. Maintain face-to-face contact whenever possible.

4. Provide for resident's privacy with curtain, screen, or door.

5. Lock commode wheels. Adjust bed to lowest position. Lock bed wheels. Make sure resident is wearing nonskid shoes and that the laces are tied. Help resident out of bed and to the portable commode or bathroom.

6. Put on gloves.

7. If needed, help the resident remove clothing and sit comfortably on toilet seat. Put toilet paper and disposable wipes within reach. Ask resident to clean his hands with a wipe when finished if he is able.

8. Remove and discard your gloves. Wash your hands.

9. Provide privacy. Place call light within reach while resident is using commode. Ask resident to signal when done. Leave the room and close the door.

10. When called by the resident, return and wash your hands. Put on clean gloves. Provide perineal care if help is needed. Remember to wipe from front to back. Dry the perineal area with a towel. Help the resident put on clothing.

11. Place the towel in a hamper or bag, and discard disposable supplies.

12. Remove and discard gloves. Wash your hands.

13. Help resident back to bed. Make resident comfortable.

14. Put on clean gloves.

15. When using a portable commode, remove the waste container. Note color, odor, and consistency of contents. Empty it into the toilet unless a specimen is needed or the urine is being measured for intake/output monitoring.

16. Turn the faucet on with a paper towel. Rinse the container with cold water and empty it into the toilet. Flush the toilet. Place the container in proper area for cleaning or clean and disinfect it according to facility policy.

17. Remove and discard gloves.

18. Wash your hands.

19. Make sure bed is in lowest position. Remove privacy measures.

20. Place call light within resident's reach.

21. Report any changes in resident to the nurse.

22. Document procedure using facility guidelines.

3. Describe common diseases and disorders of the urinary system

Urinary Incontinence

Urinary incontinence is the inability to control the bladder, which leads to an involuntary loss of urine. Incontinence can occur in residents who are confined to bed, ill, elderly, paralyzed, or who have circulatory or nervous system diseases or injuries. There are different types of incontinence:

- Stress incontinence is the loss of urine due to an increase in intra-abdominal pressure, for example, when sneezing or coughing.

- Urge incontinence is involuntary voiding from a sudden urge to void.

- Mixed incontinence is a combination of both urge incontinence and stress incontinence.

- Functional incontinence is urine loss caused by environmental, cognitive, or physical reasons.

- Overflow incontinence is loss of urine due to overflow or over-distention of the bladder.

Incontinence is *not* a normal part of aging. Nursing assistants should always report incontinence. It may be a sign or symptom of an illness.

Guidelines: Urinary Incontinence

G Offer a bedpan, urinal, commode, or trip to the bathroom often. Follow the toileting schedules in the care plan.

G Answer call lights and requests for help immediately.

G Urinary incontinence is a major risk factor for pressure injuries. Document all episodes of incontinence carefully and accurately.

G Cleanliness and careful skin care are important for residents who are incontinent. Urine is very irritating to the skin. It should be washed off immediately and completely. Keep residents clean, dry, and free from odor. Observe the skin carefully when bathing and giving perineal care.

G Change wet or soiled clothing immediately. Change bed linen any time it is wet or soiled. Use absorbent pads under bed linen for residents who are incontinent.

G Some residents will wear disposable incontinence pads or briefs for adults. They keep body wastes away from the skin (Fig. 16-10). Assist residents as needed with changing wet briefs immediately. Do not refer to an incontinence brief as a diaper. Residents are not children, and using that term is disrespectful.

G Encourage residents to drink plenty of fluids.

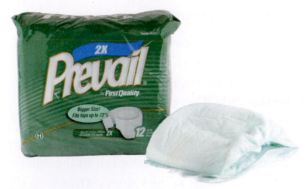

Fig. 16-10. *A type of incontinence brief.*

G Residents who are incontinent need reassurance and understanding. Be professional and kind when dealing with incontinence. Doing so may help put residents at ease.

Changing Incontinence Briefs

When changing an incontinence brief, the NA should make sure to assemble all needed items beforehand, including a protective pad, perineal care supplies, disposable wipes, gloves, and a clean brief. She should put on gloves before handling the brief. When removing the soiled brief, the NA should roll it inward, soiled side inside, without spilling its contents. Working from front to back, she should carefully remove all urine and/or feces from the skin. After cleaning the area thoroughly, she should blot it dry, and apply the clean brief.

Urinary Tract Infection (UTI)

A **urinary tract infection (UTI)** is a bacterial infection of the urethra, bladder, ureter, or kidney. This results in painful burning during urination and the frequent feeling of needing to urinate. The infection is commonly caused by *Escherichia coli* (*E. coli*), which is a type of bacteria usually found in the gastrointestinal tract.

Urinary tract infections are more common in women. This is due, in part, to the female urethra being shorter (three to four inches) than the male urethra (seven to eight inches). In addition, because the female urethra is located directly in front of the vagina and anus, it is closer to potential sources of bacteria. Bacteria can reach a woman's bladder more easily.

Guidelines: Preventing UTIs

G Encourage residents to wipe from front to back after elimination (Fig. 16-11). When you give perineal care, make sure you do this too.

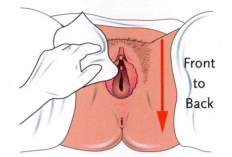

Fig. 16-11. *After elimination, wipe from front to back to prevent infection.*

G Give careful perineal care when changing incontinence briefs.

G Encourage plenty of fluids. Drinking water and other fluids helps prevent UTIs. Cranberry, orange, and blueberry juices, which are rich in vitamin C, help to acidify urine, which can prevent infection.

G Offer a bedpan or a trip to the toilet at least every two hours. Answer call lights promptly.

G Taking showers, rather than baths, helps prevent urinary tract infections.

G Report cloudy, dark, or foul-smelling urine, or if a resident urinates often and in small amounts.

Kidney Stones

Kidney stones, also called *renal calculi*, form when urine crystallizes in the kidneys. The stones can block the kidneys and ureters, causing severe pain. Kidney stones often have no single cause, but may be the result of lack of fluid intake, diet, infection, disorders, or certain genetic factors.

Signs and symptoms of kidney stones may not be noticeable until they begin to move down the

ureter, causing pain. Signs and symptoms include the following:

- Abdominal pain
- Flank or back pain
- Groin pain
- Burning during urination, painful urination
- Frequent urination
- Blood in the urine
- Nausea, vomiting
- Chills, fever

Urine straining is the process of pouring all urine through a fine filter to catch any particles. This is done to detect the presence of kidney stones that can develop in the urinary tract. The stones can be as small as grains of sand or as large as golf balls. If any stones are found, they are saved and then sent to a laboratory for examination.

If straining urine is listed on an assignment sheet, the nursing assistant will first need to collect a routine urine specimen. Then he will go into the bathroom and pour the specimen through a strainer or a 4x4-inch piece of gauze into a specimen container. Any stones that are found are wrapped in the filter and are placed in the specimen container to go to the lab.

Kidney stones are treated with increased water intake, as well as pain relievers and other medications. Larger stones may need to be treated with surgery or a procedure that uses sound waves to break up the stones.

Renovascular Hypertension

Renovascular hypertension is a condition in which a blockage of arteries in the kidneys causes high blood pressure. Treatment of this condition includes medications to help control blood pressure, as well as sometimes surgery. More information about hypertension and its symptoms, treatment, and related care is in Chapter 18.

Chronic Renal Failure

Chronic renal failure (CRF), also called *chronic kidney failure,* occurs because the kidneys become unable to eliminate certain waste products from the body. This disease can develop as the result of chronic urinary tract infections, high blood pressure, inflammation of the kidneys (nephritis), or diabetes. Excessive salt in the diet can also cause damage to the kidneys. Over time, the disease becomes worse. Signs and symptoms include the following:

- High blood pressure
- Decreased urine output or no urine output
- Dark urine
- Anemia
- Nausea, vomiting
- Loss of appetite
- Weight changes
- Fatigue and weakness
- Headaches
- Difficulty sleeping
- Back pain
- Edema
- Stool that is bloody or black

Kidney **dialysis**, an artificial means of removing the body's waste products, can improve and extend life for several years. Residents will be on fluid restrictions of different degrees. Chronic renal failure can progress to end-stage renal disease, which is fatal without kidney dialysis or a kidney transplant.

4. Describe guidelines for urinary catheter care

Some residents may have a urinary catheter. A **catheter** is a thin tube inserted into the body that is used to drain fluids or inject fluids. A **urinary catheter** is used to drain urine from the bladder. A **straight catheter** is a type of

catheter that is inserted to drain urine from the bladder. It is removed immediately after urine is drained. It does not remain inside the person. An **indwelling catheter** (also called a *Foley catheter*) remains inside the bladder for a period of time (Fig. 16-12). The urine drains into a bag.

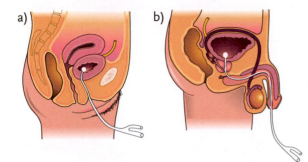

Fig. 16-12. An illustration of a) an indwelling catheter (female) and b) an indwelling catheter (male).

Another type of catheter that is used for males is an external, or **condom catheter** (also called a *Texas catheter*). It has an attachment on the end that fits onto the penis and is fastened with special tape. Urine drains through the catheter into the tubing, then into the drainage bag. A smaller bag, called a *leg bag*, attaches to the leg and collects the urine (Fig. 16-13). The condom catheter is changed daily or as needed.

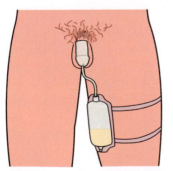

Fig. 16-13. An illustration of a condom catheter with a leg bag.

Nurses or doctors insert urinary catheters. Nursing assistants do not insert, irrigate, or remove catheters. NAs may be asked to give daily catheter care, clean the area around the urethral opening, and empty the drainage bag. The bag is emptied into a measuring container (a graduate).

Guidelines: Catheters

G Thoroughly wash your hands before giving catheter care.

G Keep the genital area clean to prevent infection. Because the catheter goes all the way into the bladder, bacteria can enter the bladder more easily. Daily care of the genital area is especially important.

G Make sure that the drainage bag always hangs lower than the hips or bladder. Urine must never flow from the bag or tubing back into the bladder. This can cause infection.

G Keep the drainage bag off the floor. Make sure the catheter tubing does not touch the floor.

G To help keep the urine draining properly, keep the tubing as straight as possible. Make sure there are no kinks in the tubing and that the resident is not sitting or lying on the tubing.

Observing and Reporting: Catheters

Report any of the following to the nurse:

O/R Blood in the urine or urine that looks unusual in any way

O/R Catheter bag does not fill after several hours

O/R Catheter bag fills suddenly

O/R Catheter is not in place

O/R Urine leaks from the catheter

O/R Resident reports pain or pressure

O/R Odor is present

Providing catheter care

Equipment: bath blanket, disposable bed protector, bath basin with warm water, soap, bath thermometer, 2–4 washcloths or disposable wipes, towel, gloves

1. Identify yourself by name. Identify the resident by name.

2. Wash your hands.

3. Explain procedure to the resident. Speak clearly, slowly, and directly. Maintain face-to-face contact whenever possible.

4. Provide for resident's privacy with curtain, screen, or door.

5. Adjust bed to a safe working level, usually waist high. Lock bed wheels.

6. Lower the head of the bed. Position the resident lying flat on her back.

7. Remove or fold back top bedding, keeping the resident covered with the bath blanket.

8. Test water temperature with bath thermometer or against the inside of your wrist. Water temperature should be no higher than 105°F. Have the resident check the water temperature to see if it is comfortable. Adjust if necessary.

9. Put on gloves.

10. Ask the resident to flex her knees and raise her buttocks off the bed by pushing against the mattress with her feet. If she needs help, place your arm under the small of her back and tell her to push with her heels and hands on your signal as you raise her hips. Place a clean bed protector under her buttocks.

11. Expose only the area necessary to clean the catheter. Avoid overexposing the resident.

12. Place towel under catheter tubing before washing.

13. Wet washcloth in basin and apply soap to a washcloth. Clean the area around the meatus. Use a clean area of the washcloth for each stroke.

14. Hold the catheter near the meatus. Avoid tugging the catheter throughout the procedure.

15. Clean at least four inches of catheter nearest the meatus. Move in only one direction, away

from the meatus (Fig. 16-14). Use a clean area of the cloth for each stroke.

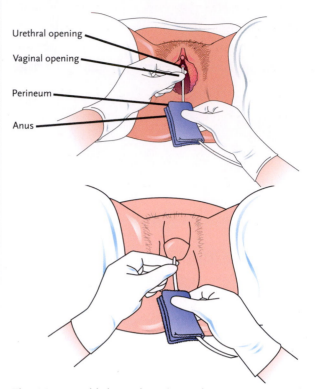

Urethral opening
Vaginal opening
Perineum
Anus

Fig. 16-14. *Hold the catheter near the meatus to avoid tugging the catheter. Moving in only one direction, away from the meatus, helps prevent infection. Use a clean area of the washcloth for each stroke.*

16. Dip a clean washcloth in the water. Rinse the area around the meatus, using a clean area of the washcloth for each stroke. With a towel, dry the area around the meatus.

17. Dip a clean washcloth in the water. Rinse at least four inches of catheter nearest the meatus. Move in only one direction, away from the meatus. Use a clean area of the washcloth for each stroke.

18. With a towel, dry at least four inches of the catheter nearest the meatus. Move in only one direction, away from the meatus.

19. Remove and discard bed protector. Remove towel from under catheter tubing and place in proper container.

20. Place linen and used washcloths in proper containers.

21. Empty the basin into the toilet and flush toilet. Place basin in proper area for cleaning or clean and store it according to facility policy.

22. Remove and discard gloves.

23. Wash your hands.

24. Remove bath blanket and replace top covers. Make resident comfortable. Check that the catheter tubing is free from kinks and twists and that it is securely fastened to the leg.

25. Return bed to lowest position. Remove privacy measures.

26. Place call light within resident's reach.

27. Report any changes in resident to the nurse.

28. Document procedure using facility guidelines.

Emptying the catheter drainage bag

Equipment: graduate (measuring container), alcohol wipes, paper towels, gloves

1. Identify yourself by name. Identify the resident by name.

2. Wash your hands.

3. Explain procedure to the resident. Speak clearly, slowly, and directly. Maintain face-to-face contact whenever possible.

4. Provide for resident's privacy with curtain, screen, or door.

5. Put on gloves.

6. Place paper towel on the floor under the drainage bag. Place the graduate on the paper towel.

7. Open the clamp on the drainage bag so that the urine flows out of the bag and into the graduate (Fig. 16-15). Do not let the spout or clamp touch the graduate.

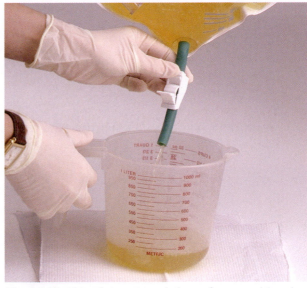

Fig. 16-15. Keep the spout and clamp from touching the graduate while draining urine.

8. When the urine has drained out of the bag, close the clamp. Using alcohol wipes, clean the drain spout. Replace the drain spout in its holder on the bag.

9. Go into the bathroom. Place the graduate on a flat surface and measure at eye level. Note amount and characteristics of urine. Empty into the toilet and flush toilet.

10. Clean and store graduate. Discard paper towels.

11. Remove and discard gloves.

12. Wash your hands.

13. Document procedure and amount of urine.

Changing a condom catheter

Equipment: condom catheter and collection bag, catheter tape, plastic bag, bath blanket, disposable bed protector, supplies for perineal care, gloves

1. Identify yourself by name. Identify the resident by name.

2. Wash your hands.

3. Explain procedure to the resident. Speak clearly, slowly, and directly. Maintain face-to-face contact whenever possible.

4. Provide for resident's privacy with curtain, screen, or door.

5. Adjust bed to a safe level, usually waist high. Lock bed wheels.

6. Lower the head of the bed. Position the resident lying flat on his back.

7. Remove or fold back top bedding, keeping the resident covered with the bath blanket.

8. Put on gloves.

9. Place a clean bed protector under the resident's buttocks.

10. Adjust bath blanket to only expose the genital area.

11. Gently remove the condom catheter. Place condom and tape in the plastic bag.

12. Assist as necessary with perineal care.

13. Move pubic hair away from the penis so it does not get rolled into the condom.

14. Hold the penis firmly. Place the condom at tip of penis and roll toward base of penis. Leave space (at least one inch) between the drainage tip and glans of penis to prevent irritation. If the resident is not circumcised, be sure that the foreskin is in normal position.

15. Gently secure the condom to penis with special tape provided (Fig. 16-16). Apply tape in a spiral manner. Never wrap tape all the way around the penis because it can impair circulation.

16. Connect the catheter tip to drainage tubing. Do not touch the tip to any object but the drainage tubing. Make sure tubing is not twisted or kinked.

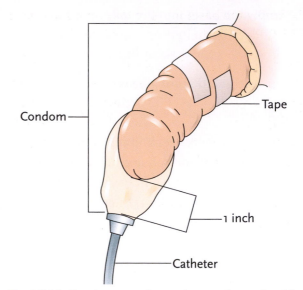

Fig. 16-16. *Gently secure the condom to the penis with provided tape, applying it in a spiral.*

17. Check to see if collection bag is secured to leg. Make sure drain is closed.

18. Remove and discard bed protector. Discard used supplies in plastic bag. Place soiled clothing and linens in proper containers. Clean and store supplies.

19. Remove and discard gloves.

20. Wash your hands.

21. Remove bath blanket and replace top covers. Make resident comfortable.

22. Return bed to lowest position. Remove privacy measures.

23. Place call light within resident's reach.

24. Report any changes in resident to the nurse.

25. Document procedure using facility guidelines.

5. Identify types of urine specimens that are collected

Nursing assistants may need to collect a specimen from a resident. A **specimen** is a sample that is used for analysis in order to try to make a diagnosis. Different types of specimens are used for different tests.

There are several factors to consider when collecting specimens. Body wastes and elimination needs are very private matters for most people. Having another person handle their body wastes may make residents embarrassed and uncomfortable. Nursing assistants should be sensitive to this, and should empathize with residents. When collecting specimens, the NA should behave professionally. If she feels that this is an unpleasant task, she should not make it known to the resident. She should not make faces, frown, or use words that let the resident know she feels uncomfortable. Remaining professional when collecting specimens can help put residents at ease.

Urine specimens may be categorized as routine, clean-catch (mid-stream), or 24-hour. A **routine urine specimen** is collected any time the resident voids, or urinates. The resident will void into a bedpan, urinal, commode, or hat. A **hat** is a plastic collection container sometimes put into a toilet bowl to collect and measure urine or stool (Fig. 16-17). Some residents will be able to collect their own urine specimens. Others will need help. The NA should be sure to explain exactly how the specimen must be collected (Fig. 16-18).

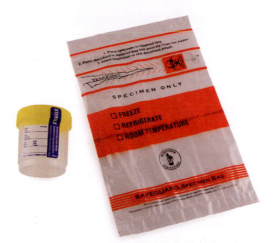

Fig. 16-18. *Specimens must always be labeled with the resident's name, date of birth, room number, and the date and time before being taken to the lab. A specimen may need to be placed in a clean specimen bag before transporting it.*

Collecting a routine urine specimen

Equipment: urine specimen container and lid, completed label (labeled with resident's name, date of birth, room number, date, and time), specimen bag, 2 pairs of gloves, bedpan or urinal (if resident cannot use a portable commode or toilet), hat for toilet (if resident uses portable commode or toilet), plastic bag, toilet paper, disposable wipes, paper towels, supplies for perineal care, laboratory slip

1. Identify yourself by name. Identify the resident by name.

2. Wash your hands.

3. Explain procedure to the resident. Speak clearly, slowly, and directly. Maintain face-to-face contact whenever possible.

4. Provide for resident's privacy with curtain, screen, or door.

5. Put on gloves.

6. Fit hat to toilet or commode, or provide resident with bedpan or urinal.

7. Ask resident to void into hat, urinal, or bedpan. Ask resident not to put toilet paper in with the sample. Provide a plastic bag to discard toilet paper separately.

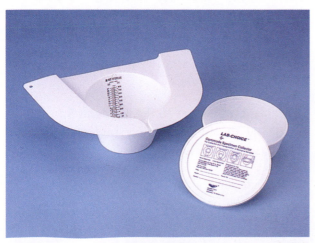

Fig. 16-17. *A hat is a container that is sometimes placed under the toilet seat to collect a specimen. Hats should be labeled and must be cleaned after each use.*

8. Place toilet paper and disposable wipes within resident's reach. Ask resident to clean his hands with a wipe when finished if he is able.

9. Remove and discard gloves. Wash your hands.

10. Place the call light within resident's reach. Ask resident to signal when done. Leave the room and close the door.

11. When called by the resident, return and wash your hands. Put on clean gloves. Provide perineal care if help is needed.

12. Take bedpan, urinal, or hat to the bathroom.

13. Pour urine into the specimen container. Specimen container should be at least half full.

14. Cover the urine container with its lid. Do not touch the inside of the container. Wipe off the outside with a paper towel and discard the paper towel.

15. Apply label, place the container in a clean specimen bag, and seal the bag.

16. Discard extra urine in the toilet. Turn the faucet on with a paper towel. Rinse the bedpan, urinal, or hat with cold water and empty it into the toilet. Flush the toilet. Place equipment in the proper area for cleaning or clean it according to facility policy.

17. Remove and discard gloves.

18. Wash your hands.

19. Make resident comfortable.

20. Return bed to lowest position if adjusted. Remove privacy measures.

21. Place call light within resident's reach.

22. Report any changes in resident to the nurse.

23. Take specimen and lab slip to proper area. Document procedure using facility guidelines. Note amount and characteristics of urine.

Residents' Rights

Specimens

When collecting specimens, the nursing assistant should first explain how she will collect the specimen. The NA should do this in private, keeping her voice low. She should also close the door to the bathroom or bedroom and pull the privacy curtain. In addition, the NA should be discreet when removing the specimen from the room.

The **clean-catch specimen**, or mid-stream specimen (CCMS), does not include the first and last urine voided in the sample. First the perineal area is cleaned and then the resident urinates a small amount into the toilet to clear the urethra. Then the resident begins urinating again into a clean or sterile container, stopping before urination is complete. The container is removed, and the resident finishes urinating into the toilet. This specimen is collected to detect bacteria in the urine.

Collecting a clean-catch (mid-stream) urine specimen

Equipment: specimen kit with container and lid, completed label (labeled with resident's name, date of birth, room number, date, and time), specimen bag, cleansing wipes, gloves, bedpan or urinal (if resident cannot use a portable commode or toilet), plastic bag, toilet paper, disposable wipes, paper towels, supplies for perineal care, laboratory slip

1. Identify yourself by name. Identify the resident by name.

2. Wash your hands.

3. Explain procedure to the resident. Speak clearly, slowly, and directly. Maintain face-to-face contact whenever possible.

4. Provide for resident's privacy with curtain, screen, or door.

5. Put on gloves.

6. Open the specimen kit. Do not touch the inside of the container or the inside of the lid.

7. If the resident cannot clean his or her perineal area, you will need to do it. Use the cleansing wipes to do this. Be sure to use a clean area of the wipe or a clean wipe for each stroke. See bed bath procedure in Chapter 13 for a reminder on how to give perineal care.

8. Ask the resident to urinate a small amount into the bedpan, urinal, or toilet, and to stop before urination is complete.

9. Place the container under the urine stream and have the resident start urinating again. Fill the container at least half full. Ask the resident to stop urinating and remove the container. Have the resident finish urinating in the bedpan, urinal, or toilet.

10. After urination, provide a plastic bag so the resident can discard toilet paper. Give perineal care if help is needed. Ask resident to clean his hands with a wipe if he is able.

11. Cover the urine container with its lid. Do not touch the inside of the container. Wipe off the outside with a paper towel and discard paper towel.

12. Apply label, place the container in a clean specimen bag, and seal the bag.

13. Discard extra urine in the toilet. Turn the faucet on with a paper towel. Rinse the bedpan or urinal with cold water and empty it into the toilet. Flush the toilet. Place equipment in the proper area for cleaning or clean it according to facility policy.

14. Remove and discard gloves.

15. Wash your hands.

16. Make resident comfortable.

17. Return bed to lowest position if adjusted. Remove privacy measures.

18. Place call light within resident's reach.

19. Report any changes in resident to the nurse.

20. Take specimen and lab slip to proper area. Document procedure using facility guidelines. Note amount and characteristics of urine.

A **24-hour urine specimen** collects all the urine voided by a resident in a 24-hour period. It is used to test for certain chemicals and hormones. Usually the collection begins at 7 a.m. and continues until 7 a.m. the next day. When beginning a 24-hour urine specimen collection, the resident must void and discard the first urine so that the collection begins with an empty bladder. All urine must be collected and stored properly. If any is accidentally thrown away or improperly stored, the collection will have to be started over.

Collecting a 24-hour urine specimen

Equipment: 24-hour specimen container with lid, completed label (labeled with resident's name, date of birth, room number, date, and time), bedpan or urinal (for residents confined to bed), hat for toilet (if resident can use portable commode or toilet), gloves, toilet paper, disposable wipes, supplies for perineal care, sign to alert other team members that a 24-hour urine specimen is being collected, form for recording output, laboratory slip

1. Identify yourself by name. Identify the resident by name.

2. Wash your hands.

3. Explain procedure to the resident. Speak clearly, slowly, and directly. Maintain face-to-face contact whenever possible. Emphasize that all urine must be saved.

4. Provide for resident's privacy with curtain, screen, or door.

5. Place a sign on the resident's bed to let all care team members know that a 24-hour specimen is being collected. Sign may read "Save all urine for 24-hour specimen."

6. When starting the collection, have the resident completely empty the bladder. Discard the urine. Note the exact time of this voiding. The collection will run until the same time the next day (Fig. 16-19).

INTAKE-OUTPUT RECORD

Resident/Patient Name   Room No.

	FLUID INTAKE	URINE	EMESIS or DRAINAGE
7:00 A.M. to 3:00 P.M.			
8-Hour Total			
3:00 P.M. to 11:00 P.M.			
8-Hour Total			
11:00 P.M. to 7 A.M.			
8-Hour Total			

Form 3039 © Briggs, Des Moines, IA 50306 PRINTED IN U.S.A. R404

DON'T BREAK THE LAW   Save   1-800-247-2343
MAKE THE CALL   13%   www.BriggsCorp.com
*savings on buying vs. copying

Fig. 16-19. *One type of form for recording urine output over 24 hours.* (REPRINTED WITH PERMISSION OF BRIGGS CORPORATION, 800-247-2343, WWW.BRIGGSCORP.COM)

7. Label the container with the resident's name, date of birth, room number, and dates and times the collection period began and ended.

8. Wash hands and put on gloves each time the resident voids.

9. Pour urine from bedpan, urinal, or hat into the container. The container may be stored at room temperature, in the refrigerator, or on ice. Follow the nurse's instructions.

10. After each voiding, help as necessary with perineal care. Ask the resident to clean his hands with a wipe after each voiding.

11. After each voiding, place equipment in proper area for cleaning or clean it according to facility policy.

12. Remove and discard gloves.

13. Wash your hands.

14. After the last void of the 24-hour period, re-move the sign. Take the specimen and lab slip to proper area. Document procedure using facility guidelines. Make sure to include the time of the last void before the 24-hour collection period began and the last void of the 24-hour collection period.

6. Explain types of tests performed on urine

Different types of tests can be used to detect different things in urine. Dip strips can be used to test for such things as pH level, glucose, ketones, blood, nitrite, and specific gravity. These strips, called *reagent strips*, have different sections that change color when they react with urine (Fig. 16-20).

Testing pH levels: The pH scale ranges from 0 to 14. The lower the number, the more acidic the fluid. The higher the number, the more alkaline the fluid. The normal pH range for urine is 4.6–8.0. A pH imbalance may be due to medication, food, or illness.

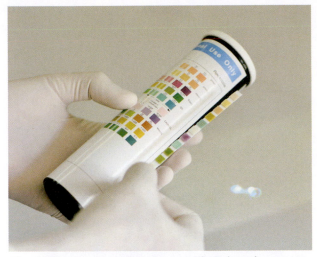

Fig. 16-20. *Reagent strips change color when they react with urine. The color is then compared to a color chart to determine levels of each chemical factor.*

Testing for glucose and ketones: In diabetes, the pancreas does not produce enough insulin or does not produce any insulin (Chapter 18). Insulin is the hormone that works to move glucose, or natural sugar, from the blood and into the cells for energy for the body. Without enough insulin to process glucose, these sugars collect in the blood. Some sugar appears in the urine.

People who have diabetes may also have ketones in the urine. Ketones are chemical substances produced when the body burns fat for energy or fuel. They are produced when there is not enough insulin to help the body use sugar for energy. Without enough insulin, glucose builds up in the blood. Since the body cannot use glucose for energy, it breaks down fat instead. When this occurs, ketones build up in the blood and spill into the urine.

In addition to strip testing, a double-voided (also called *fresh-fractional*) urine specimen may be used to test for glucose. A double-voided specimen is a urine specimen that is collected after first emptying the bladder and then waiting until another specimen can be collected. This may be ordered because testing urine that has been in the bladder for some time may not accurately reflect the amount of glucose present. With a double-voided specimen, after the person

has voided, he is encouraged to drink fluids. Then approximately 30 minutes later, a second (double-voided) specimen is collected and tested.

Testing for blood: In normal urine, blood should not be present. Illness and disease can cause blood to appear in urine. Some blood is hidden, or occult. This blood can be detected by testing the urine.

Testing for nitrite: This test may be performed to determine if the person has a urinary tract infection. Nitrite is a substance produced by many urinary tract infections.

Testing specific gravity: A specific gravity (also called *urine density*) test is performed to measure the concentration of chemical particles in the urine. The test evaluates the body's water balance and urine concentration by showing how the density of urine compares to water. Normal values range from 1.002 to 1.028. Certain disorders increase or decrease specific gravity. For example, kidney failure can decrease it. This test usually requires a clean-catch urine specimen.

Testing urine with reagent strips

Equipment: urine specimen as ordered, reagent strip, gloves, paper towel

1. Wash your hands.

2. Put on gloves.

3. Take a strip from the bottle and recap bottle. Close it tightly.

4. Dip the strip into the specimen.

5. Follow manufacturer's instructions for when to remove strip from the specimen. Remove the strip at the correct time.

6. Follow manufacturer's instructions for how long to wait after removing the strip. After the proper time has passed, compare the strip with the color chart on the bottle. Do not touch the bottle with the strip.

7. Read results.

8. Store strips. Discard used items. Discard specimen in the toilet. Flush the toilet.

9. Remove and discard gloves.

10. Wash your hands.

11. Document procedure using facility guidelines.

7. Explain guidelines for assisting with bladder retraining

Injury, illness, or inactivity may cause a loss of normal bladder function. Residents may need help in reestablishing a regular routine and normal function. Problems with elimination can be embarrassing or difficult to discuss. Nursing assistants should be sensitive to this and always remain professional when handling incontinence or working to reestablish routines. It is hard enough for residents to handle incontinence without having to worry about caregivers' reactions.

Guidelines: Bladder Retraining

G Follow Standard Precautions. Wear gloves when handling body wastes.

G Explain the bladder training schedule to the resident. Follow the schedule carefully.

G Keep a record of the resident's bladder habits. When you see a pattern of elimination, you can predict when the resident will need a bedpan or a trip to the bathroom.

G Offer a bedpan or a trip to the bathroom before beginning long procedures. (Fig. 16-21).

G Encourage the resident to drink plenty of fluids. Do this even if urinary incontinence is a problem. About 30 minutes after fluids are taken, offer a trip to the bathroom or a bedpan or urinal.

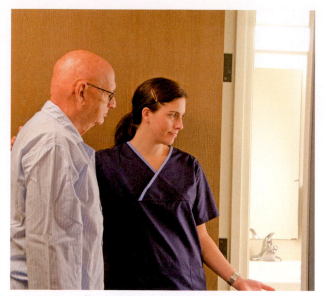

Fig. 16-21. *Offer regular trips to the bathroom.*

G Answer call lights promptly. Residents cannot wait long when the urge to go to the bathroom occurs. Leave call lights within reach.

G Provide privacy for elimination—both in the bed and in the bathroom.

G If a resident has trouble urinating, try running water in the sink. Have her lean forward slightly to put pressure on the bladder.

G Do not rush the resident during urination.

G Help residents with careful perineal care. This helps prevent skin breakdown and promotes proper hygiene. Carefully observe for skin changes.

G Discard wastes according to your facility's policies.

G Discard clothing protectors and incontinence briefs properly. Double-bag these items if ordered. This stops odors from collecting.

G Some facilities use washable bed pads or briefs. Follow Standard Precautions when rinsing before placing these items in the laundry.

G Keep an accurate record of urination. This includes any episodes of incontinence (Fig. 16-22).

BOWEL & BLADDER RETRAINING PROGRAM

DATE																					
DATE STARTED	INCONTINENT	VOIDED	BM	INCONTINENT	VOIDED	BM	INCONTINENT	VOIDED	BM	INCONTINENT	VOIDED	BM	INCONTINENT	VOIDED	BM	INCONTINENT	VOIDED	BM	INCONTINENT	VOIDED	BM
7 am																					
8 am																					
9 am																					
10 am																					
11 am																					
12 noon																					
1 pm																					
2 pm																					
3 pm																					
4 pm																					
5 pm																					
6 pm																					
7 pm																					
8 pm																					
9 pm																					
10 pm																					
11 pm																					
12 midnight																					
1 am																					
2 am																					
3 am																					
4 am																					
5 am																					
6 am																					
SIGNATURE 7-3																					
3 - 11																					
11 - 7																					

S – SUPPOSITORY INSERTED
BM – BOWEL MOVEMENT

LICENSED NURSES INSTRUCTIONS: _____

_____

_____

_____

NAME – LAST	FIRST	MIDDLE	ROOM NO.	ATTENDING PHYSICIAN	HOSP. NO.

Form 609   Briggs, Des Moines, IA 50306 (800) 247-2343
PRINTED IN U.S.A.

BOWEL & BLADDER RETRAINING PROGRAM

Fig. 16-22. *A sample bowel and bladder retraining record.* (REPRINTED WITH PERMISSION OF BRIGGS CORPORATION, 800-247-2343, WWW.BRIGGSCORP.COM)

G Offer positive words for successes or even attempts to control the bladder. However, do not talk to residents as if they were children. Keep your voice low and do not draw attention to any aspect of retraining.

G Never show frustration or anger toward residents who are incontinent. The problem is out of their control. Your negative reactions will only make things worse. Be kind, supportive, and professional.

G When the resident is incontinent or cannot urinate when asked, be positive. Never make the resident feel like a failure. Praise and encouragement are essential for a successful program. Remember that each resident has different needs and may respond to different types of encouragement. Finding out each resident's needs and preferences is part of providing person-centered care.

G Some residents will always be incontinent. Be patient. Offer these residents extra care and attention. Skin breakdown may lead to pressure injuries without proper care. Always report changes in skin.

Chapter Review

1. What is the normal color of urine?

2. List five things to observe and report to the nurse about urine.

3. What is the best position for women to be in to urinate normally? What is the best position for men?

4. When performing perineal care, in what direction should the nursing assistant wipe the resident?

5. How should a standard bedpan be positioned? How should a fracture pan be positioned?

6. Is urinary incontinence a normal part of aging?

7. Why should a nursing assistant never refer to an incontinence brief as a diaper?

8. What are four ways that nursing assistants can help prevent urinary tract infections?

9. Why should the catheter drainage bag always be kept lower than the hips or the bladder?

10. Why should catheter tubing be kept as straight as possible?

11. What is a clean-catch urine specimen?

12. How can nursing assistants help reduce discomfort and embarrassment when assisting with specimen collection?

13. List four things reagent strips can detect in urine.

14. Why do residents who are incontinent need careful skin care?

15. About how long after fluids are taken should the NA offer to take a resident to the bathroom?

16. List two guidelines for bladder retraining that help promote dignity.

17

Bowel Elimination

1. List qualities of stool and identify signs and symptoms about stool to report

Defecation, or bowel elimination, is the act of passing feces from the large intestine out of the body through the anus. Feces, also called *stool* or *bowel movements*, are semi-solid material made up of water, solid waste material, bacteria, and mucus. The number of bowel movements a person has varies with age and with the amount and type of foods consumed.

Stool is normally brown, soft, and formed in a tubular shape from its passage through the colon. However, food, medications, and supplements, as well as illness, can cause a change in the normal color of stool. For example, iron supplements can cause stool to appear black. Red food coloring, beets, and tomato juice can make stool red.

Observing and Reporting: Stool

Report any of these to the nurse:

O/R Whitish, black, red, or hard stools

O/R Liquid stools (diarrhea)

O/R Constipation (the inability to have a bowel movement or the infrequent, difficult, and often painful elimination of a hard, dry stool)

O/R Flatulence/gas

O/R Pain when having a bowel movement

O/R Blood, pus, mucus, or discharge in stool

O/R Fecal incontinence (inability to control the bowels, leading to an involuntary passage of stool)

2. List factors affecting bowel elimination

There are many factors that can affect normal bowel elimination, including the following:

Normal changes of aging: As a person ages, peristalsis slows. **Peristalsis** are involuntary contractions that move food through the gastrointestinal system. Digestion takes longer and is less efficient. Proteins, vitamins, and minerals are not absorbed as well. Decreased saliva production affects the ability to chew and swallow, as does tooth loss. Medication use and a dulled sense of taste may result in poor appetite.

To help promote normal bowel elimination, nursing assistants should encourage fluids and nutritious, appealing meals and should help make mealtimes enjoyable. Dentures should fit properly and be cleaned regularly. Oral care should be given regularly as well. Residents who have trouble chewing and swallowing are at risk for choking. NAs can assist by providing plenty of fluids with meals and cutting food into smaller pieces if ordered. NAs should follow a toileting schedule for residents if there is one.

Residents who have fecal incontinence or diarrhea must be kept clean and dry. When assisting with perineal care, NAs should wipe from front to back to prevent infection. They should help residents wash their hands after having bowel movements.

Psychological factors: Stress, anger, fear, and depression all affect gastrointestinal function. Stress, anger, and fear can increase peristalsis and elimination, while depression may decrease it. A lack of privacy can greatly affect elimination, too.

To promote normal bowel elimination, it is very important for an NA to provide plenty of privacy. She should close the bathroom door if a resident is in the bathroom. If the resident needs to use a bedpan, the NA should pull the privacy curtain and close the door. Residents should not be rushed or interrupted during elimination. It is important for an NA to report signs of depression and anxiety (Chapter 20), as well as any changes in frequency of elimination.

Food and fluids: What a person consumes greatly affects bowel elimination. Fiber intake improves bowel elimination. Foods high in fiber include fruits, whole grains, and raw vegetables (Fig. 17-1). Some high-fiber foods cause flatulence, or gas, which can aid elimination, but can also cause discomfort. Foods that may cause gas include the following:

- Beans
- Fruits (e.g., pears, apples, peaches)
- Whole grains
- Vegetables (e.g., broccoli, cabbage, onions, asparagus)
- Dairy products
- Carbonated drinks

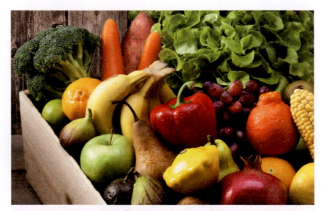

Fig. 17-1. Many raw fruits and vegetables are high in fiber, which helps with bowel elimination.

Some foods can cause constipation, such as foods high in animal fats (dairy products, meats, and eggs) or foods high in refined sugar but low in fiber. Inadequate fluid intake not only contributes to dehydration, but also can cause constipation.

To promote normal bowel elimination, residents should eat a diet that contains fiber and drink plenty of fluids to help prevent constipation. NAs should offer drinks to residents every time they see them, as long as they are not on fluid restrictions. A healthy person needs at least 64 ounces of fluid each day.

Physical activity: Regular physical activity helps bowel elimination (Fig. 17-2). It strengthens the abdominal and pelvic muscles, which helps peristalsis. Immobility and a lack of exercise weakens these muscles and may slow elimination.

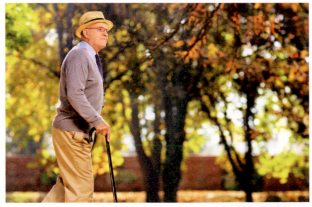

Fig. 17-2. Regular exercise and activity is important for promoting normal bowel elimination.

To promote normal bowel elimination, the NA should encourage regular activity and assist as needed. She can try to make it fun for the resident. A walk can be something that the resident enjoys and looks forward to.

Personal habits: The time of day that bowel movements occur varies from person to person. For example, one person may have a bowel movement early in the day, while another has one in the early afternoon. Another person may have a few bowel movements throughout the day. This depends on the person, his habits, and the amount and type of food and drink consumed. Elimination usually occurs after meals.

The position of the body affects elimination. A person who is supine (flat on his back) will have the most trouble with bowel elimination. It is very difficult to contract muscles in this position.

To promote normal bowel elimination, residents should be allowed to have an opportunity to have a bowel movement at the time of day that is normal for them. The best position for elimination is squatting and leaning forward. If the person cannot get out of bed, the NA can raise the head of the bed for elimination. That way the resident does not have to work against gravity.

Medications: Medications affect bowel elimination. Laxatives are used to cause bowel movements and may cause excessive elimination. Other medications, such as pain relievers, can slow elimination. Antibiotics may cause diarrhea. To promote normal bowel elimination, the NA can offer a trip to the bathroom or a bedpan often. Any changes in appearance of stool or frequency of bowel elimination should be reported.

Disorders and illnesses affect bowel elimination, and there is more information about them in the next Learning Objective.

3. Describe common diseases and disorders of the gastrointestinal system

Constipation

Constipation is the inability to eliminate stool (have a bowel movement), or the infrequent, difficult, and often painful elimination of a hard, dry stool. Constipation occurs when the feces move too slowly through the intestine. This can result from decreased fluid intake, poor diet, inactivity, medications, aging, certain diseases, or ignoring the urge to eliminate. Signs of constipation include abdominal swelling, gas, irritability, and a record of no recent bowel movement.

Treatment often includes increasing the amount of fiber eaten and fluids consumed, increasing the activity level, and possibly medication. Accurate

documentation of bowel movements is important. An enema or rectal suppository may be ordered to help with constipation. An **enema** is a specific amount of water, with or without an additive, that is introduced into the colon to stimulate the elimination of stool. A rectal suppository is a medication given rectally to cause a bowel movement.

Fecal Impaction

A **fecal impaction** is a hard stool that is stuck in the rectum and cannot be expelled. It results from unrelieved constipation. Symptoms include no stool for several days, oozing of liquid stool, cramping, abdominal swelling, and rectal pain. When an impaction occurs, a nurse or doctor will insert one or two gloved fingers into the rectum and break the mass into fragments so that it can be passed. Prevention of fecal impactions often includes the same measures as those used for preventing constipation, i.e., high-fiber diet, plenty of fluids, an increase in activity level, and possibly medication. Early assessments of constipation may also help prevent impactions.

Hemorrhoids

Hemorrhoids are enlarged veins in the rectum. They may also be visible outside the anus. Chronic constipation, obesity, pregnancy, chronic diarrhea, overuse of laxatives and enemas, and straining during bowel movements are common causes of hemorrhoids. Rectal itching, burning, pain, and bleeding during bowel elimination are signs and symptoms of hemorrhoids. Treatment includes adding more fiber into the diet and increasing fluid intake. Medications, compresses, and sitz baths are also used to treat hemorrhoids. Surgery may be necessary. When cleaning the anal area, the nursing assistant should be very careful to avoid causing pain and bleeding.

Diarrhea

Diarrhea is the frequent elimination of liquid or semi-liquid feces. Abdominal cramps, urgency, nausea, and vomiting can accompany diarrhea, depending on the cause. Bacterial and viral infections, microorganisms in food and water, irritating foods, and medications can cause diarrhea. Treatment of diarrhea usually involves medication, an increase in certain fluids, and a change of diet.

Fecal Incontinence

Fecal incontinence is the inability to control the bowels, leading to an involuntary passage of stool. Common causes are constipation, muscle and nerve damage, loss of storage capacity in the rectum, and diarrhea. Treatment includes a change in diet, medication, bowel training, or surgery.

Flatulence

Flatulence, also called *flatus* or *gas*, is air in the intestine that is passed through the rectum, which can result in cramping or abdominal pain. Flatulence may have any of the following causes:

- Swallowing air while eating

- Eating high-fiber foods

- Eating foods that a person cannot tolerate, for example, when a person who has lactose intolerance eats dairy products (**Lactose intolerance** is the inability to digest lactose, a type of sugar found in milk and other dairy products. It is caused by a deficiency of lactase enzyme.)

- Antibiotics

- Irritable bowel syndrome (IBS), which is a chronic condition of the large intestine that gets worse from stress

- **Malabsorption**, which means that the body cannot absorb or digest a particular nutrient properly; it is often accompanied by diarrhea

Excessive flatulence, depending on the cause, is often treated with change of diet, medication, and reducing the amount of air swallowed.

Gastroesophageal Reflux Disease

Gastroesophageal reflux disease, commonly referred to as **GERD**, is a chronic condition in which the liquid contents of the stomach back up into the esophagus. The liquid can inflame and damage the lining of the esophagus. It can cause bleeding or ulcers. In addition, scars from tissue damage can narrow the esophagus and make swallowing difficult.

Heartburn is the most common symptom of GERD. **Heartburn** is the result of a weakening of the sphincter muscle that joins the esophagus and the stomach. When healthy, this muscle prevents the leaking of stomach acid and other contents back into the esophagus. Stomach acid causes a burning sensation, commonly called *heartburn*, in the esophagus. If heartburn occurs frequently and remains untreated, it can cause **ulceration**.

Heartburn must be reported to the nurse. Heartburn and GERD are usually treated with medications. Serving the evening meal three to four hours before bedtime may help. The resident should not lie down until at least two to three hours after eating. Providing residents with extra pillows so the body is more upright during sleep can help. Serving the largest meal of the day at lunchtime, serving several meals of small portions throughout the day, and reducing fast foods, fatty foods, and spicy foods may also help. Stopping smoking, not drinking alcohol, and wearing loose-fitting clothing are often helpful as well.

Peptic Ulcers

Peptic ulcers are raw sores in the stomach. A dull or burning pain occurs one to three hours after eating, accompanied by belching or vomiting. Peptic ulcers can cause bleeding, and stool may appear black (tarry). Ulcers are caused by excessive acid secretion. Treatment includes antacids and other medications, as well as a change in diet. A bland diet may be ordered (Chapter 15). Residents with peptic ulcers should avoid smoking and drinking too much alcohol and caffeine, which increase the production of gastric acid.

Ulcerative Colitis

Ulcerative colitis is a chronic inflammatory disease of the large intestine. Symptoms include cramping, diarrhea, pain occurring on one side of the lower abdomen, rectal bleeding, loss of appetite, and weight loss. Ulcerative colitis is a serious illness that can cause intestinal bleeding and death if left untreated.

Medications can relieve symptoms, but they cannot cure ulcerative colitis. Surgical treatment may include a colostomy, which is the diversion of waste to an artificial opening (**stoma**) through the abdomen. Stool is diverted through the stoma instead of the anus. There is more information on colostomy care later in the chapter.

Colorectal Cancer

Colorectal cancer, also known as *colon cancer*, is cancer of the gastrointestinal tract. Signs and symptoms include changes in normal bowel patterns, cramps, abdominal pain, and rectal bleeding. Colorectal cancer must be treated with surgery. Chapter 18 contains more information on cancer.

4. Discuss how enemas are given

Putting fluid into the rectum in order to eliminate stool or feces is called an enema. Enemas may be given prior to surgery or a medical test, or when a person cannot eliminate stool on his own. Nursing assistants may be trained to give enemas, depending upon the state and facility in which they work. If NAs are allowed to give enemas, they must make sure to follow policies and procedures. Any questions an NA may have should be discussed with the nurse before giving an enema.

Doctors will write an enema order. There are four different types of enemas:

- Tap water enema (TWE): 500–1000 milliliters (mL) of water from a faucet

- Soapsuds enema (SSE): 500–1000 mL water with 5 mL of mild castile soap added

- Saline enema: 500–1000 mL water with two teaspoons of salt added

- Commercially-prepared enema (also called *commercial enema* or *pre-packaged enema*): 120 mL solution; may have oil or other additive

Tap water, soapsuds, and saline enemas are all considered cleansing enemas. They all require more fluid than commercially-prepared enemas do. Equipment used for giving cleansing enemas includes an IV pole, the enema solution, tubing, and a clamp.

Guidelines: Enemas

G Provide plenty of privacy for this procedure.

G Keep the bedpan nearby or make sure that the bathroom is vacant before assisting with an enema.

G The resident will be placed in Sims' (left side-lying) position (Fig. 17-3). If the person is positioned on the left side, the water does not have to flow against gravity.

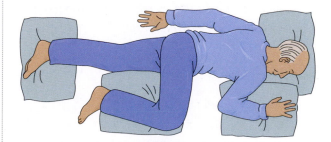

Fig. 17-3. *The Sims' position (left side-lying position) is the proper position for an enema.*

G The enema solution should be warm, not hot or cold.

G The enema bag should not be raised to more than the height listed in the care plan.

G   The tip of the tubing should be lubricated with lubricating jelly.

G   Unclamp the tube. Allow a small amount of solution to run through the tubing, then re-clamp the tube. This gets rid of the air before it is inserted (the air could cause cramping).

G   The solution should flow in slowly; the resident will be less likely to have cramps.

G   Hold the enema tubing in place while giving the enema. Stop immediately if the resident has pain or if you feel resistance. Report to the nurse if this happens.

G   The resident should take slow deep breaths when taking an enema to help hold the solution longer.

G   Report any of the following to the nurse:

   • Resident could not tolerate enema because of cramping.

   • The enema had no results.

   • The amount of stool was very small.

   • Stool was hard, streaked with red, very dark, or black.

Giving a cleansing enema

Equipment: bath blanket, IV pole, enema solution, tubing and clamp, disposable bed protector, bedpan, bedpan cover, lubricating jelly, bath thermometer, tape measure, toilet paper, disposable wipes, towel, robe, nonskid footwear, supplies for perineal care, paper towel, 2 pair of gloves

1. Identify yourself by name. Identify the resident by name.

2. Wash your hands.

3. Explain procedure to the resident. Speak clearly, slowly, and directly. Maintain face-to-face contact whenever possible.

4. Provide for resident's privacy with curtain, screen, or door.

5. Adjust bed to a safe level, usually waist high. Lock bed wheels.

6. Put on gloves.

7. Place the bed protector under the resident. Ask the resident to remove undergarments or help him do so.

8. Help the resident into a left-sided Sims' position. Place the bedpan close to resident's body. Cover with a bath blanket.

9. Place the IV pole beside the bed.

10. Clamp the enema tube. Prepare the enema solution. Fill bag with 500–1000 mL of warm water (105°F), and mix the solution. Check water temperature with bath thermometer.

11. Unclamp the tube. Let a small amount of solution run through the tubing to release the air. Re-clamp the tube.

12. Hang the bag on the IV pole. Using the tape measure, make sure the bottom of the enema bag is not more than 12 inches above the resident's anus (Fig. 17-4).

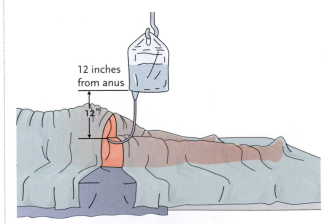

12 inches from anus

12"

Fig. 17-4. *The bottom of the bag should not be more than 12 inches above the anus.*

13. Lubricate tip of tubing with lubricating jelly.

14. Ask the resident to breathe deeply to relieve cramps during procedure.

15. Place one hand on the upper buttock. Lift to expose the anus. Ask the resident to take a deep breath and exhale (Fig. 17-5). Using the other hand, gently insert the tip of the tubing two to four inches into the rectum. Stop

immediately if you feel resistance or if the resident complains of pain. If this happens, clamp the tubing. Tell the nurse immediately.

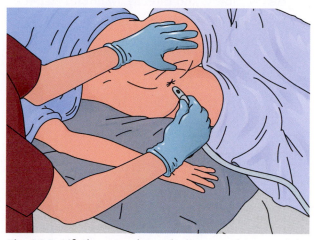

Fig. 17-5. Lift the upper buttock to expose the anus. Ask the resident to take a deep breath before inserting the tubing.

16. Unclamp the tubing. Allow the solution to flow slowly into the rectum. Ask the resident to take slow, deep breaths. If the resident complains of cramping, clamp the tubing and stop for a couple of minutes. Encourage him to take as much of the solution as possible.

17. Clamp the tubing before the bag is empty, when the solution is almost gone. Gently remove the tip from the rectum. Place the tip into the enema bag. Do not contaminate yourself, the resident, or the bed linens.

18. Ask the resident to hold the solution inside as long as possible.

19. Help the resident to use bedpan, commode, or get to the bathroom. Raise the head of the bed if the resident is using the bedpan. If the resident uses a commode or toilet, put on the robe and nonskid footwear. Lower the bed to its lowest position before the resident gets up.

20. Remove and discard gloves. Wash your hands.

21. Place toilet paper and wipes within the resident's reach. Ask the resident to clean his

hands with a hand wipe when finished if he is able. If the resident is using the toilet, ask him not to flush it when finished.

22. Place the call light within the resident's reach. Ask resident to signal when done. Leave the room and close the door.

23. When called by the resident, return and wash your hands. Put on clean gloves.

24. Lower the head of the bed if raised. Make sure the resident is still covered.

25. Remove the bedpan carefully and cover it with a bedpan cover or towel.

26. Give perineal care if help is needed. Wipe from front to back. Dry the perineal area with a towel. Help the resident put on his undergarments. Cover the resident and remove the bath blanket.

27. Remove and discard the bed protector. Place the towel and bath blanket in a hamper or bag, and discard disposable supplies.

28. Take bedpan to the bathroom. Call the nurse to observe the enema results. Empty the contents of bedpan carefully into the toilet.

29. Turn the faucet on with a paper towel. Rinse the bedpan with cold water and empty it into the toilet. Flush the toilet. Place bedpan in the proper area for cleaning or clean it according to facility policy.

30. Remove and discard gloves.

31. Wash your hands.

32. Make resident comfortable.

33. Return bed to lowest position. Remove privacy measures.

34. Place call light within resident's reach.

35. Report any changes in resident to the nurse.

36. Document procedure using facility guidelines.

Giving Enemas

Protecting a resident's rights when giving an enema includes providing plenty of privacy during this procedure. The NA should keep the resident covered with a bath blanket or sheet, only exposing the anal area. She should pull the privacy curtain around the bed and close the door. The NA should answer any questions that the resident has about the procedure. However, if any questions are not within the NA's scope of practice to answer, she should refer them to the nurse before beginning.

A commercially-prepared enema usually has 120 mL solution and may have an additive (Fig. 17-6). An oil retention enema has a type of oil in it that softens the stool to allow it to pass more easily. It is often used when a person has been constipated for a long time, resulting in a stool that is very hard, or when a person has a fecal impaction. Commercially-prepared enemas do not require an IV pole, tubing, or clamp, because they are prepackaged and pre-mixed.

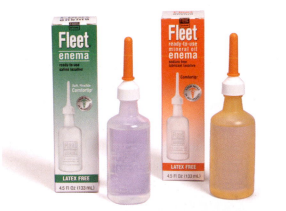

Fig. 17-6. Commercially prepared enemas may come with additives, such as saline and mineral oil. (REPRINTED WITH PERMISSION OF BRIGGS CORPORATION, 800-247-2343, WWW.BRIGGSCORP.COM)

Giving a commercial enema

Equipment: bath blanket, standard or oil retention commercial enema kit, disposable bed protector, bedpan, bedpan cover, lubricating jelly, toilet paper, disposable wipes, robe, nonskid footwear, towel, supplies for perineal care, 2 pairs of gloves

1. Identify yourself by name. Identify the resident by name.

2. Wash your hands.

3. Explain procedure to the resident. Speak clearly, slowly, and directly. Maintain face-to-face contact whenever possible.

4. Provide for resident's privacy with curtain, screen, or door.

5. Adjust bed to a safe level, usually waist high. Lock bed wheels.

6. Put on gloves.

7. Place bed protector under resident. Ask resident to remove undergarments or help him do so.

8. Help resident into a left-sided Sims' position. Place the bedpan close to resident's body. Cover with a bath blanket.

9. Uncover resident enough to expose anus only.

10. Lubricate tip of bottle with lubricating jelly.

11. Ask the resident to breathe deeply to relieve cramps during procedure.

12. Place one hand on the upper buttock. Lift to expose the anus. Ask the resident to take a deep breath and exhale. Using the other hand, gently insert the tip of the tubing about one and a half inches into the rectum. Stop if you feel resistance or if the resident complains of pain. Tell the nurse immediately.

13. Slowly squeeze and roll the enema container so that the solution runs inside the resident. Stop when the container is almost empty.

14. Gently remove the tip from the rectum, and place the bottle inside the box upside down (Fig. 17-7).

15. Ask the resident to hold the solution inside as long as possible.

16. Help the resident to use bedpan or commode, or to get to the bathroom. Raise the head of the bed if resident is using the bedpan. If the

resident uses a commode or toilet, put on the robe and nonskid footwear. Lower the bed to its lowest position before the resident gets up.

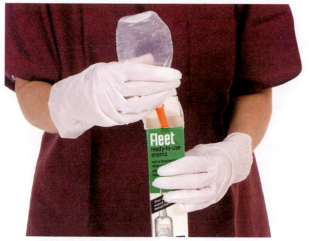

Fig. 17-7. Place enema bottle upside down in the box.

17. Remove and discard gloves. Wash your hands.

18. Place toilet paper and wipes within the resident's reach. Ask the resident to clean his hands with a hand wipe when finished if he is able. If the resident is using the toilet, ask him not to flush it when finished.

19. Place the call light within resident's reach. Ask resident to signal when done. Leave the room and close the door.

20. When called by the resident, return and wash your hands. Put on clean gloves.

21. Lower the head of the bed if raised. Make sure the resident is still covered.

22. Remove the bedpan carefully and cover it with a bedpan cover or towel.

23. Give perineal care if help is needed. Wipe from front to back. Dry the perineal area with a towel. Help the resident put on his undergarment. Cover the resident and remove the bath blanket.

24. Remove and discard the bed protector. Place the towel and bath blanket in a hamper or bag, and discard disposable supplies.

25. Take bedpan to the bathroom. Call the nurse to observe the enema results. Empty the contents of bedpan carefully into the toilet.

26. Turn the faucet on with a paper towel. Rinse the bedpan with cold water and empty it into the toilet. Flush the toilet. Place bedpan in the proper area for cleaning or clean it according to facility policy.

27. Remove and discard gloves.

28. Wash your hands.

29. Make resident comfortable.

30. Return bed to lowest position. Remove privacy measures.

31. Place call light within resident's reach.

32. Report any changes in resident to the nurse.

33. Document procedure using facility guidelines.

5. Demonstrate how to collect a stool specimen

Stool (feces) specimens are collected so that the stool can be tested for blood, pathogens, and other things, such as worms or amoebas. Worms and amoebas can be detected with an ova and parasites test. If the specimen is to be examined for ova and parasites, it must be taken to the lab immediately. This examination must be made while the stool is still warm.

If the resident uses a bedpan or portable commode for elimination, that is where the nursing assistant will collect the stool specimen. If the resident uses the toilet, a hat (collection container) will be used.

The NA should ask the resident to let her know when he needs to have a bowel movement, and she should be ready to collect the specimen. The NA should explain that urine or toilet paper should not be included in the sample because they can ruin the sample and create the need for a new specimen.

Collecting a stool specimen

Equipment: specimen container and lid, completed label (labeled with resident's name, date of birth, room number, date, and time), specimen bag, 2 pairs of gloves, 2 tongue blades, bedpan (if resident cannot use portable commode or toilet), hat for toilet (if resident uses portable commode or toilet), plastic bag, toilet paper, disposable wipes, paper towels, supplies for perineal care, lab slip

1. Identify yourself by name. Identify the resident by name.

2. Wash your hands.

3. Explain procedure to the resident. Speak clearly, slowly, and directly. Maintain face-to-face contact whenever possible.

4. Provide for resident's privacy with curtain, screen, or door.

5. Put on gloves.

6. When the resident is ready to move bowels, ask him not to urinate at the same time and not to put toilet paper in with the sample. Provide a plastic bag to discard toilet paper and wipes separately.

7. Fit hat to toilet or commode, or provide resident with bedpan.

8. Place toilet paper and disposable wipes within resident's reach. Ask resident to clean his hands with a wipe when finished if he is able.

9. Remove and discard gloves. Wash your hands.

10. Place the call light within resident's reach. Ask resident to signal when done. Leave the room and close the door.

11. When called by the resident, return and wash your hands. Put on clean gloves. Give perineal care if help is needed.

12. Using the two tongue blades, take about two tablespoons of stool and put it in the container. Without touching the inside of the

container, cover it tightly. Apply the label and place the container in a clean specimen bag. Seal the bag.

13. Wrap the tongue blades in toilet paper and put them in plastic bag with used toilet paper and wipes. Discard bag in proper container.

14. Empty the bedpan or container into the toilet. Turn the faucet on with a paper towel. Rinse the bedpan with cold water and empty it into the toilet. Flush the toilet. Place equipment in the proper area for cleaning or clean it according to facility policy.

15. Remove and discard gloves.

16. Wash your hands.

17. Remove privacy measures.

18. Place call light within resident's reach.

19. Report any changes in resident to the nurse.

20. Take specimen and lab slip to proper area. Document procedure using facility guidelines. Note amount and characteristics of stool.

6. Explain occult blood testing

Fecal occult blood testing (sometimes called the *stool guaiac* test) is performed to detect blood in stool. **Occult** means something that is hidden or difficult to see or observe. Hidden, or occult, blood in stool may be an indication of colorectal cancer or of other illnesses.

There are different types of tests to detect occult blood in stool. Stool specimens may be sent to the laboratory for this test; however, in some facilities, nursing assistants may be asked to perform this test if they are trained and allowed to do so.

Testing a stool specimen for occult blood

Equipment: labeled stool specimen, occult blood test kit (Fig. 17-8), 2 tongue blades, plastic bag, gloves

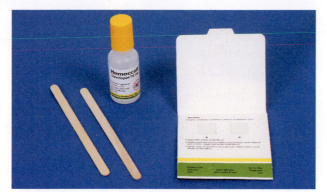

Fig. 17-8. This is one type of occult blood test kit.

1. Wash your hands.

2. Put on gloves.

3. Open the test card.

4. Pick up a tongue blade. Get a small amount of stool from the specimen container.

5. Using a tongue blade, smear a small amount of stool onto Box A of test card (Fig. 17-9).

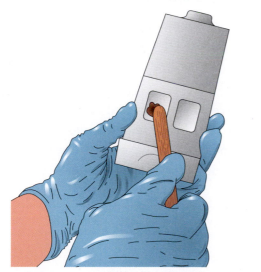

Fig. 17-9. Smear a small amount of stool onto Box A.

6. Flip the tongue blade (or use a new tongue blade). Get some stool from another part of the specimen. Smear a small amount of stool onto Box B of test card.

7. Close the test card. Turn over to other side.

8. Open the flap.

9. Open the developer. Apply developer to each box. Follow manufacturer's instructions.

10. Wait the amount of time listed in the instructions, usually between 10 and 60 seconds.

11. Watch the squares for any color changes. Record color changes. Follow instructions.

12. Place tongue blade and test packet in plastic bag, and dispose of plastic bag properly.

13. Remove and discard gloves.

14. Wash your hands.

15. Document procedure using facility guidelines.

7. Define *ostomy* and list care guidelines

An **ostomy** is the surgical creation of an opening from an area inside the body to the outside. The terms *colostomy* and *ileostomy* refer to the surgical removal of a portion of the intestines. In a resident with one of these ostomies, the end of the intestine is brought out of the body through an artificial opening in the abdomen. This opening is called a *stoma*. Stool, or feces, is eliminated through the ostomy rather than through the anus. (When a ureter is opened to the abdomen for urine to be eliminated, it is called a **ureterostomy**.) An ostomy may be necessary due to bowel disease, cancer, or trauma. It may be temporary or permanent.

The terms *colostomy* and *ileostomy* indicate what section of the intestine was removed and the type of stool that will be eliminated. A **colostomy** is a surgically-created opening into the large intestine to allow stool to be expelled. With a colostomy, stool will generally be semi-solid. An **ileostomy** is a surgically-created opening into the end of the small intestine to allow stool to be expelled. Stool will be liquid and may be irritating to the resident's skin.

Residents who have had an ostomy wear a disposable pouching system that fits over the stoma to collect the feces (Fig. 17-10). The pouching system is attached to the skin by adhesive, and a belt may also be used to secure it.

Many people manage the ostomy appliance by themselves. Nursing assistants should receive training before providing ostomy care. Because state and local guidelines vary, NAs should follow facility policy regarding ostomy care.

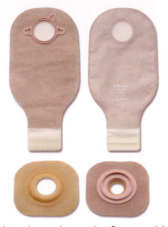

Fig. 17-10. *This photo shows the front and back of a two-piece system. The top is an ostomy drainage bag, and the bottom is a skin barrier.* (PHOTOS COURTESY OF HOLLISTER INCORPORATED, LIBERTYVILLE, ILLINOIS)

Guidelines: Ostomies

G Always wash hands carefully and wear gloves when providing ostomy care. Follow Standard Precautions.

G Help residents with ostomies to wash their hands properly.

G Make certain that the resident receives regular, careful skin care. Observe and report any changes in the skin to help prevent skin breakdown.

G Empty and clean or replace the ostomy pouch whenever stool is eliminated.

G Skin barriers protect the skin around the stoma from irritation from the waste products and/or the adhesive material that is used to secure the pouch to the body. Barriers may come in the form of a powder, gel, cream, ring, paste, wafer, or square.

G Residents who have an ileostomy may experience food blockage. A food blockage is a large amount of undigested food, usually high-fiber

food, that collects in the small intestine and blocks the passage of stool. Food blockages can occur if the resident eats large amounts of foods that are high-fiber and/or if the resident does not chew the food well. Follow the diet instructions in the care plan and the nurse's instructions for assisting with feeding.

G Encourage fluids and proper diet. Residents with ileostomies need to drink plenty of fluids because they lose extra liquid in their stools. They may also be on high-potassium diets due to rapid elimination.

G Many residents with ostomies feel they have lost control of a basic bodily function. They may be embarrassed or angry about the ostomy. Be sensitive and supportive when working with these residents. Always provide privacy for ostomy care. Behave professionally and do not act uncomfortable with any aspect of ostomy care.

G Ostomy pouches are made to be odor resistant. If odors are present, they may be due to a leak or improper cleaning. Report odors to the nurse.

G Observe how the resident is reacting to the ostomy and his general attitude. Report any emotional or physical problems with adjusting to the ostomy to the nurse.

Observing and Reporting: Ostomies

Report any of the following to the nurse:

O/R Changes in color, amount, frequency, or odor of stool

O/R Any skin changes at the stoma site, such as sores, excessive redness, or swelling

O/R Leaking stool

O/R Absence of stool

O/R Watery stool with green, stringy material

O/R Abdominal cramps

O/R Vomiting

Caring for an ostomy

Equipment: disposable bed protector, bath blanket, clean ostomy pouching system, belt (if needed), disposable wipes (made for ostomy care), basin of warm water, washcloth, 2 towels, plastic bag, gloves

1. Identify yourself by name. Identify the resident by name.

2. Wash your hands.

3. Explain procedure to the resident. Speak clearly, slowly, and directly. Maintain face-to-face contact whenever possible.

4. Provide for resident's privacy with curtain, screen, or door.

5. Adjust bed to a safe level, usually waist high. Lock bed wheels.

6. Put on gloves.

7. Place the bed protector under resident. Cover resident with a bath blanket. Pull down the top sheet and blankets. Expose only the ostomy site. Offer resident a towel to keep clothing dry.

8. Undo the ostomy belt if used. Remove the ostomy pouch carefully. Place it in the plastic bag. Note the color, odor, consistency, and amount of stool in the pouch.

9. Wipe the area around the stoma with disposable wipes for ostomy care. Discard wipes in plastic bag.

10. Using a washcloth and warm water, wash the area in one direction, away from the stoma (Fig. 17-11). Rinse. Pat dry with another towel.

11. Place the clean ostomy drainage pouch on the resident. Hold in place and seal securely. Make sure the bottom of the pouch is clamped.

12. Remove the bed protector and discard. Place soiled linens in proper container. Discard plastic bag properly.

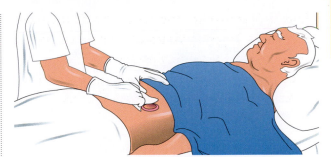

Fig. 17-11. Wash area gently, moving away from the stoma.

13. Remove and discard gloves.

14. Wash your hands.

15. Make resident comfortable.

16. Return bed to lowest position. Remove privacy measures.

17. Place call light within resident's reach.

18. Report any changes in resident to the nurse. Note any changes to the stoma and surrounding area. A normal stoma is red and moist, and looks like the lining of the mouth. Call the nurse if the stoma appears very red or blue or if swelling or bleeding is present. Report any signs of skin breakdown around the stoma.

19. Document procedure using facility guidelines.

8. Explain guidelines for assisting with bowel retraining

Residents who have had a disruption in their bowel routines from illness, injury, or inactivity may need help to reestablish a regular routine and normal function. To assist with bowel retraining, the doctor may order suppositories, laxatives, stool softeners, or enemas. Bowel elimination issues may be difficult for residents to discuss. Nursing assistants should be sensitive to this and should remain professional when assisting residents with bowel retraining.

Residents' Rights

Bowel Retraining

Residents who have problems controlling their bowels need to be treated with dignity. The nursing assistant should think about how he might feel in the same situation. For example, if a resident has a bowel movement in her bed, she probably feels extremely embarrassed about this and the fact that an NA has to clean her and change the sheets. The NA can help the resident maintain her dignity by being kind and supportive. He should promote the resident's right to privacy by keeping his voice low and not discussing her accident in a public area.

Guidelines: Bowel Retraining

G　Follow Standard Precautions. Wear gloves when handling body wastes.

G　Explain the bowel training schedule to the resident. Follow the schedule carefully.

G　Keep a record of the resident's bowel habits. When you see a pattern of elimination, you can predict when the resident will need a bedpan or a trip to the bathroom.

G　Encourage the resident to drink plenty of fluids.

G　Encourage the resident to eat foods that are high in fiber. Encourage residents to follow special diets as ordered. Chapter 15 has more information on diet and nutrition.

G　Answer call lights promptly. Leave call lights within reach.

G　Provide privacy for elimination—both in the bed and in the bathroom.

G　Do not rush the resident during elimination.

G　Help residents with careful perineal care. This prevents skin breakdown and promotes proper hygiene. Carefully observe for skin changes.

G　Discard wastes according to your facility's policies.

G　Discard clothing protectors and incontinence briefs properly. Double-bag these items if ordered.

G　Some facilities use washable bed pads or briefs. Follow Standard Precautions when placing these items in the laundry.

G　Keep an accurate record of elimination.

G　Praise successes or attempts to control bowels. However, do not talk to residents as if they were children. Keep your voice low and do not draw attention to any aspect of bowel retraining.

G　Never show frustration or anger toward residents who are incontinent. Remember that the problem is out of their control. Be positive and professional.

Chapter Review

1. How does stool normally appear?

2. List five things to observe and report to the nurse about stool.

3. What is the best position for bowel elimination? What should be done if a person cannot get out of bed for elimination?

4. What may need to be increased in a resident's diet if she is prone to constipation?

5. List three signs of a fecal impaction.

6. List three causes of diarrhea.

7. What is gastroesophageal reflux disease (GERD)?

8. What are two things that people with peptic ulcers should avoid?

9. What are three symptoms of colorectal cancer?

10. In what position must the resident be placed for an enema?

11. What should the nursing assistant do if a resident feels pain or if the nursing assistant feels resistance while giving an enema?

12. What two things should not be included in a stool specimen?

13. If a stool specimen needs to be tested for ova and parasites, what should be done immediately and why?

14. What may occult blood in stool indicate?

15. What are three reasons that a resident may need a colostomy or ileostomy?

16. How often should an ostomy pouch be emptied?

17. What kinds of foods may need to be eaten when a resident is going through bowel retraining?

18
Common Chronic and Acute Conditions

Diseases and conditions are either acute or chronic. An **acute illness** means that the illness has a rapid onset; this type of illness is usually short-term and is treated immediately. A **chronic illness** is long-term or long-lasting, even lasting over a lifetime. The symptoms are managed. Chronic conditions may have short periods of severity. The person may be hospitalized to stabilize the disease.

This chapter organizes diseases or conditions under the body system in which they are located. Common diseases of the urinary and gastrointestinal systems are located in Chapters 16 and 17.

1. Describe common diseases and disorders of the integumentary system

Pressure injuries, a common disorder of the integumentary system, are covered in Chapter 13. Burns are covered in Chapter 7.

Scabies

Scabies is a skin infection caused by a tiny mite called *Sarcoptes scabiei*. The mite burrows into the skin, where it lays eggs, which causes intense itching and a skin rash that may look like thin burrow tracks. These tracks typically appear in the folds of the skin.

Scabies is contagious and is spread through direct contact with an infected person. It can spread quickly in crowded places, such as long-term care facilities and child care facilities. Treatment of scabies involves medications, often in the form of prescription creams and lotions (Chapter 13 has information on applying lotions). Oral medications may be used if the person does not respond to the creams and/or lotions.

Shingles

Shingles, also called *herpes zoster*, is a skin rash caused by the varicella-zoster virus (VZV), which is the same virus that causes chickenpox. (Herpes zoster is not the same virus that causes the sexually transmitted infection.) Any person who has had chickenpox is at risk for developing shingles. After having chickenpox, the virus remains in the body, where it usually does not cause problems. However, it can reappear later in life and cause shingles.

Initial signs and symptoms of shingles include pain, tingling, or itching in an area, which later develops into a rash of fluid-filled blisters that is similar to chickenpox (Fig. 18-1). The rash usually goes away within two to four weeks.

Shingles cannot be transmitted to other people. However, if a person has never had chickenpox, he may acquire chickenpox from a person who has active shingles (when the rash is in the blister phase). The risk of getting shingles increases as a person ages. People with immune systems weakened by diseases such as cancer and HIV are at greater risk of getting shingles.

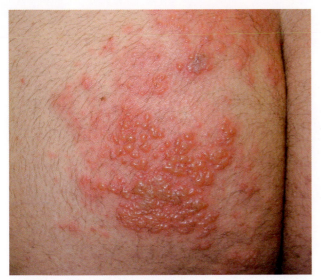

Fig. 18-1. Shingles in blister form. (PHOTO COURTESY OF DR. JERE MAMMINO, DO)

Keeping the rash covered, especially while it is in blister form, is important. Infected people should wash their hands often and should not scratch or touch the rash.

Shingles is treated with medication, which should be started as soon as possible. Starting medication immediately can help reduce the severity of the disease and can shorten the length of the illness. There is a vaccine for shingles that is often recommended for people 60 years or older who have had chickenpox. The vaccine can help reduce the risk of contracting shingles.

Wounds

A **wound** is a type of injury to the skin. Wounds are classified as either open or closed. An open wound has skin that is not intact. An open wound can be categorized in the following ways: incision, laceration, abrasion, and puncture wound. An incision is caused by a sharp-edged object, such as a knife or razor. An example of this type of open wound is a cut made during surgery with a surgical instrument. A laceration is an irregular wound caused by ripping or blunt trauma, such as tearing of skin during childbirth. An abrasion is a wound in which the top layer of skin is scraped or worn off, often by coming into moving contact with a rough surface. A puncture wound is a break in the skin caused by a sharp object such as a nail or a needle.

In a closed wound, the skin's surface has not been broken. Closed wounds can be contusions (bruises) or hematomas. A contusion is caused by blunt force trauma that damages tissue under the skin. A hematoma is caused by damage to a blood vessel that causes blood to collect under the skin.

Wounds are examined and cleaned with various liquids, such as tap water, sterile saline, or antiseptic solution. Bleeding may need to be stopped. Dressings, bandages, sutures, staples, or special strips or glue may need to be applied.

Dermatitis

Dermatitis is a general term that refers to an **inflammation**, or swelling, of the skin. There are different types of dermatitis, including atopic dermatitis, also known as *eczema*, and stasis dermatitis. Dermatitis usually involves swollen, reddened, irritated, and itchy skin.

Atopic dermatitis commonly occurs along with allergies, including asthma or chronic hay fever. Physical and mental stressors are causes, or it may be hereditary. This condition usually begins in childhood and may not be as severe later in life. Symptoms include dry, itchy, and inflamed skin, usually on the cheeks, arms, and legs, although it can cover other parts of the body. Symptoms improve and worsen at various times. Atopic dermatitis is not contagious. Special lotions are used to treat this condition. Further measures to help cracked skin may be prescribed, such as wet dressings. Antihistamines may help intense itching.

Stasis dermatitis is a skin condition that commonly affects the lower legs and ankles. The condition occurs due to a buildup of fluid under the skin. This buildup causes problems with circulation, and poor circulation results in skin that is fragile and poorly nourished. Stasis dermatitis can also lead to severe skin problems such as open ulcers and wounds.

Early signs of stasis dermatitis include a rash, a scaly, red area, or itching. Other signs are swelling of the legs, ankles, or other areas; thin, tissue-like skin; darkening skin at ankles or legs; thickening skin at ankles or legs; signs of skin irritation; and leg pain. Nursing assistants should report any of these signs to the nurse.

Ways to treat stasis dermatitis include surgery for varicose veins and medications, such as diuretics, to reduce fluid in the body. The resident should wear stockings and shoes that fit properly and are not too tight. Elevating the feet may be ordered, and the legs should not be crossed. NAs may need to apply elastic (anti-embolic) stockings to help promote circulation and should be gentle when handling or cleaning the skin. The resident may be on a low-sodium diet.

Fungal Infections

Mushrooms, mold, and yeasts (*Candida*) are all examples of fungi. Some types of fungi, such as *Candida*, normally live in and on the body, in such places as the skin and in the vagina and intestines. However, sometimes normal balances of fungi can change, resulting in fungal infections, such as *tinea pedis* (athlete's foot), *tinea cruris* (jock itch), or vaginal yeast infections. *Tinea*, often called *ringworm*, is another example of a fungal infection (Fig. 18-2). These imbalances that result in infections can be caused by a weakened immune system or by taking antibiotics.

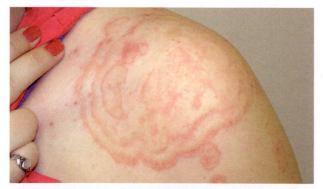

Fig. 18-2. *Tinea is a fungal infection that causes red, ring-like patches to appear on the upper body, hands, and/or feet.* (PHOTO COURTESY OF DR. JERE MAMMINO, DO)

Fungi can be difficult to kill. Treatment generally consists of applying antifungal drugs directly on the infection, such as on the skin, inside the mouth, or in the vagina. Medication may also need to be taken orally or injected if the infection is more serious.

> **Residents' Rights**
>
> **Diseases and Disorders**
>
> Nursing assistants must respect the privacy of residents who are ill. Residents' conditions should not be discussed in public areas. NAs should not make negative comments or show negative facial reactions to unpleasant symptoms, such as vomiting, or to conditions like skin disorders.

2. Describe common diseases and disorders of the musculoskeletal system

Arthritis

Arthritis is a general term that refers to inflammation, or swelling, of the joints. It causes stiffness, pain, and decreased mobility. Arthritis may be the result of aging, injury, or an **autoimmune illness**. An autoimmune illness causes the body's immune system to attack normal tissue in the body. Two common types of arthritis are osteoarthritis and rheumatoid arthritis.

Osteoarthritis, also called *degenerative arthritis* or *degenerative joint disease (DJD)*, is a common type of arthritis that affects the elderly. It may occur with aging or as the result of joint injury. Hips and knees, which are weight-bearing joints, are usually affected. Joints in the fingers, thumbs, and spine can also be affected. Pain and stiffness seem to increase in cold, damp weather.

Rheumatoid arthritis can affect people of any age. Joints become red, swollen, and very painful (Fig. 18-3). Deformities can result and may be severe and disabling. Movement is eventually restricted. Fever, fatigue, and weight loss are also symptoms. Rheumatoid arthritis usually affects the smaller joints first, then progresses to larger ones. Other parts of the body that may be affected are the heart, lungs, eyes, kidneys, and skin. Rheumatoid arthritis is considered an auto-immune disease.

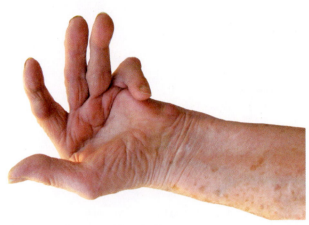

Fig. 18-3. Rheumatoid arthritis.

Arthritis is generally treated with the following:

- Anti-inflammatory medication such as aspirin or ibuprofen, as well as other medication

- Local applications of heat to reduce swelling and pain

- Range of motion exercises (Chapter 21)

- Regular exercise and/or activity routine

- Diet to reduce weight or maintain strength

Guidelines: Arthritis

G Watch for stomach irritation or heartburn caused by anti-inflammatory medications. Some residents cannot take these medications. Report signs of stomach irritation or heartburn immediately.

G Encourage activity. Gentle activity can help reduce the effects of arthritis. Follow care plan instructions carefully. Use canes or other walking aids as needed.

G Adapt activities of daily living (ADLs) to allow independence. Many assistive devices are available to help residents bathe, dress, and feed themselves even when they have arthritis (Chapter 21) (Fig. 18-4).

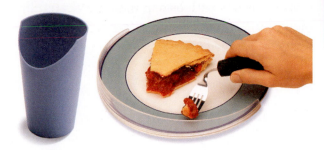

Fig. 18-4. Special equipment, such as this plate, fork, and cup, can help a person with arthritis remain independent.
(PHOTO COURTESY OF NORTH COAST MEDICAL, INC., WWW.NCMEDICAL.COM, 800-821-9319)

G Choose clothing that is easy to put on and fasten. Encourage the use of handrails and safety bars in the bathroom.

G Promote person-centered care by treating each resident as an individual. Arthritis is very common among elderly residents. Do not assume that each resident has the same symptoms and needs the same care.

G Help maintain the resident's self-esteem by encouraging self-care. Maintain a positive attitude. Listen to the resident's feelings. You can help him remain independent as long as possible.

Osteoporosis

Osteoporosis is a condition in which bones lose density, which causes them to become porous and brittle. Brittle bones can break easily. Osteoporosis is caused by any one or a combination of the following: a lack of calcium in the diet, the loss of estrogen, a lack of regular exercise or reduced mobility, or age. Osteoporosis is more common in women, especially after menopause (the end of menstruation; occurs when a woman has not had a menstrual period for 12 months). Signs and symptoms of osteoporosis include low back pain, stooped posture, becoming shorter over time, and fractures.

To prevent or slow osteoporosis, nursing assistants should encourage residents to walk and do other light exercise as ordered. Exercise can strengthen bones as well as muscles. NAs must move residents with osteoporosis very carefully. Medication and supplements are also used to treat osteoporosis.

Fractures

A fracture is a broken bone caused by an accident or by osteoporosis. A **closed fracture** is a broken bone that does not break the skin. An **open fracture**, also known as a compound fracture, is a broken bone that penetrates the skin. An open fracture carries a high risk of infection and usually requires immediate surgery.

Preventing falls, which can lead to fractures, is very important. Fractures of arms, wrists, elbows, legs, and hips are the most common. Signs and symptoms of a fracture are pain, swelling, bruising, changes in skin color at the site, and limited movement.

When bones are fractured, the sections of broken bone must be placed back into alignment so the body can heal. The body can grow new bone tissue and fuse the sections of fractured bone together. The bone must be unable to move to allow this healing to occur. This is often, although not always, accomplished by the use of a cast.

Casts are generally made of fiberglass. A fiberglass cast is lightweight and dries quickly after it is made. A cast must be completely dry before a person can bear weight on it.

Guidelines: Cast Care

G   Elevate the extremity that is in a cast. This helps stop swelling (Fig. 18-5). Use pillows to assist with elevation. If the resident is in bed, elevate the arm or leg slightly above the level of the heart.

G   Observe the affected extremity for swelling, skin discoloration, cast tightness or pressure, sores, skin that feels hot or cold, pain, burning, numbness or tingling, drainage, bleeding, or odor. Compare to the extremity that does

not have a cast. Report any of these signs or symptoms to the nurse, along with any signs of infection, such as fever or chills.

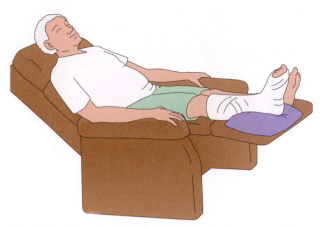

Fig. 18-5. *Elevating the extremity can help stop swelling.*

G   Protect the resident's skin from the rough edges of the cast. The stocking that lines the inside of the cast can be pulled up and over the edges and secured with tape. Tell the nurse if cast edges irritate the resident's skin.

G   Keep the cast dry at all times. Although fiberglass is waterproof, the padding inside the cast is not. Some fiberglass casts may have a waterproof lining, but unless instructed otherwise, keep the cast dry. Keep the cast clean.

G   Do not insert or allow the resident to insert anything inside the cast, even when the skin itches. Pointed or blunt objects may injure the skin, which is already dry and fragile. Skin can become infected under the cast.

G   Tell the nurse prior to moving the resident or before the resident exercises if pain medication is needed. Help with range of motion exercises as ordered. Allow plenty of time for movement. Assist the resident with cane, walker, or crutches as needed.

G   Use bed cradles as needed to reduce pressure from bed linens.

Hip Fractures

Weakened bones make hip fractures more common. A sudden fall can result in a fractured hip that takes months to heal. Preventing falls is very important. Hip fractures can also occur because of weakened bones that fracture and then cause a fall. A hip fracture is a serious condition. The elderly heal slowly, and they are at risk for secondary illnesses and disabilities.

Most fractured hips require surgery. Total hip replacement (THR) is the surgical replacement of the head of the long bone of the leg (femur) where it joins the hip. This surgery is often performed for the following reasons:

- Fractured hip from an injury or fall that does not heal properly

- Weakened hip due to aging

- Hip is painful and stiff because the joint is weak and the bones are no longer strong enough to bear the person's weight

After the surgery, the person may not be able to bear full weight on that leg while the hip heals. A physical therapist will assist after surgery. The goals of care include surgical incision healing, slowly strengthening the hip muscles, mobility and gait improvement, and increased endurance.

The resident's care plan will state when the resident may begin putting weight on the hip. It will also give instructions on how much the resident is able to do. It is important for nursing assistants to help with personal care and using assistive devices, such as walkers or canes.

Guidelines: Hip Replacement

G Keep often-used items, such as medications, phone, tissues, call lights, and water within easy reach. Avoid placing items in high places.

G Dress the affected (weaker) side first.

G Never rush the resident. Use praise and encouragement often. Do this even for small tasks.

G Ask the nurse to give pain medication prior to moving and positioning if needed.

G Have the resident sit to do tasks in order to save energy.

G Follow the care plan exactly, even if the resident wants to do more than is ordered. Follow orders for weight-bearing. After surgery, the doctor's order will be written as *partial weight-bearing* (PWB) or *non-weight-bearing* (NWB). **Partial weight-bearing** means the resident is able to support some body weight on one or both legs. **Non-weight-bearing** means the resident is unable to touch the floor or support any weight on one or both legs. Once the resident can bear full weight again, the doctor's order will be written for *full weight-bearing* (FWB). **Full weight-bearing** means that both legs can bear 100 percent of the body weight on a step. Help as needed with cane, walker, or crutches.

G Never perform range of motion exercises on the operative leg unless directed by the nurse.

G Caution the resident not to sit with his legs crossed in bed or in a chair or turn his toes inward or outward. The hip cannot be bent or flexed more than 90 degrees. It also cannot be turned inward or outward (Fig. 18-6).

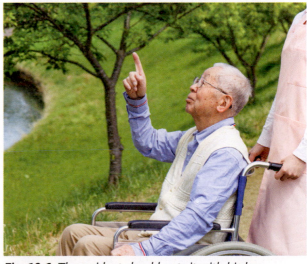

Fig. 18-6. *The resident should not sit with his legs crossed.*

G An abduction pillow may be used for six to 12 weeks after surgery while the resident is sleeping in bed. The abduction pillow immobilizes and positions the hips and lower extremities. The pillow is placed in between the legs. The legs are secured to the sides of the pillow using straps (Fig. 18-7). Follow the nurse's and the care plan's instructions for application and positioning.

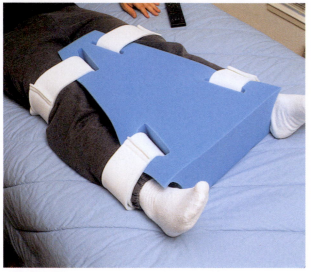

Fig. 18-7. *An abduction pillow is placed in between the legs to immobilize and position the hips and lower extremities.* (PHOTO COURTESY OF NORTH COAST MEDICAL, INC., WWW.NCMEDICAL.COM, 800-821-9319)

G   When transferring from the bed, use a pillow between the thighs to keep the legs separated. Raise the head of the bed to allow the resident to move her legs over the side of the bed with the thighs still separated. Stand on the side of the unaffected hip so that the strong side leads in standing, pivoting, and sitting.

G   With chair or toilet transfers, the operative leg should be straightened. The stronger leg should stand first (with a walker or crutches) before bringing the foot of the affected leg back to the walking position.

Observing and Reporting: Hip Replacement

Report any of these to the nurse:

O/R   Redness, drainage, bleeding, or warmth in the incision area

O/R   An increase in pain

O/R   Numbness or tingling

O/R   Tenderness or swelling in the calf of the affected leg

O/R   Shortening and/or external rotation of the affected leg

O/R   Abnormal vital signs, especially a change in temperature

O/R   Resident cannot use equipment properly and safely

O/R   Resident is not following doctor's orders for activity and exercise

O/R   Any problems with appetite

O/R   Any improvements, such as increased strength and improved ability to walk

A cast or traction may also be used to immobilize the hip. Traction helps to immobilize a fractured bone, relieve pressure, and lessen muscle spasms due to injury. A resident in traction will require special care that will be included in the care plan. The traction assembly must never be disconnected, and nursing assistants should keep the weights off the floor and not add or remove weights. Proper skin care and repositioning are essential for all residents who are immobilized. Skin will rapidly deteriorate over pressure points. Range of motion exercises should be performed as directed. Nursing assistants should report complaints of pain, numbness or tingling, or burning, as well as the presence of swelling, redness, bleeding, or sores.

Knee Replacement

Total knee replacement (TKR) is the surgical replacement of the knee with a prosthetic knee. A **prosthesis** is a device that replaces a body part that is missing or deformed because of an accident, injury, illness, or birth defect. It is used to improve a person's ability to function and/or to improve appearance. Total knee replacement surgery is performed to relieve pain and to restore motion to a knee damaged by injury or arthritis. It can help stabilize a knee that buckles or gives out repeatedly. After the surgery, care is similar to that for the hip replacement, but the recovery time is much shorter. These residents have a greater ability to care for themselves.

Guidelines: Knee Replacement

G   To prevent blood clots, apply special stockings as ordered. One type is a compression stocking. It is a plastic, air-filled, sleeve-like device that is applied to the legs and hooked to a machine. This machine inflates and deflates on its own. It acts in the same way that the muscles usually do during normal circumstances. The sleeves are normally applied after surgery while the resident is in bed. Anti-embolic stockings are another type of special stocking. They aid circulation. See later in the chapter for more information on this type of stocking.

G   Perform ankle pumps as ordered. These are simple exercises that promote circulation to the legs. Ankle pumps are done by raising the toes and feet toward the ceiling and lowering them again.

G   Encourage fluids, especially cranberry and orange juices, which contain vitamin C, to prevent urinary tract infections (UTIs).

G   Assist with deep breathing exercises as ordered.

G   A continuous passive motion (CPM) machine may be used after a knee replacement. This machine constantly moves the knee through its normal range of motion (Fig. 18-8). The person does not have to actively help; the machine does the work. Using a CPM machine can help speed recovery. The goal is to decrease stiffness, increase range of motion, and promote healing. The nurse or physical therapist will set the rate and posi-

tion the resident. You may be asked to stay with the resident while the machine is on.

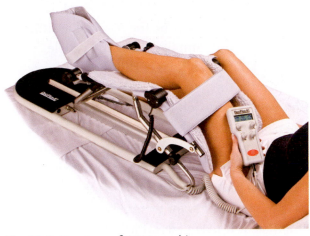

Fig. 18-8. *One type of CPM machine.* (PHOTO COURTESY OF THE MEDCOM GROUP, LTD., 800-231-4276, WWW.MEDCOMGROUP.COM)

G   Ask the nurse to give pain medication prior to moving and positioning if needed.

G   Report to the nurse if you notice redness, swelling, heat, or deep tenderness in one or both calves.

Muscular Dystrophy (MD)

Muscular dystrophy (MD) refers to a number of progressive diseases that cause a variety of physical disabilities due to muscle weakness. Progressive means the disease gets worse with time. MD is an inherited disease; it causes a gradual wasting away of muscle, weakness, and deformity. The muscles of the hands are impaired, and there may be twitching of the hand and arm muscles. Legs may be weak and stiff. The person may be in a wheelchair.

Most forms of MD are present at birth or become apparent during childhood. Many forms of MD are very slow to progress. Often people with MD can live to middle or even late adulthood.

In the early stages of this disease, nursing assistants should help with activities of daily living (ADLs) or range of motion (ROM) exercises. In the more advanced stages, assistance with skin care and positioning may be necessary, as well as performing activities of daily living for the resident.

Amputation

Amputation is the surgical removal of some or all of a body part, usually an arm, hand, leg, or foot. Amputation may be the result of an injury or disease. After amputation, some people feel that the amputated limb is still there, or they feel pain in the part that has been amputated. **Phantom sensation** is the term used when a person feels that the body part is still there. The person may experience warmth, tingling, or itching in the area where the limb existed. **Phantom limb pain** occurs when the person feels pain in a limb (or extremity) that has been amputated. It may persist for a short time or for several years. The pain or sensation, which has various possible causes, including remaining damaged nerve endings, is real. It should not be ignored. Medication or physical therapy may be used to treat these conditions.

Guidelines: Amputation

G Residents who have had a body part amputated must make many physical, psychological, social, and occupational adjustments due to their disability. Be supportive during the continuing process of adjustment. When a body part has been amputated, day-to-day activities may be limited. A resident will need special care to help him adjust to these changes. When the condition is new, a physical and/or occupational therapist may work with the resident.

G Assist residents in performing their ADLs.

G Assist with changes of position as ordered to prevent pressure injuries.

G Perform range of motion exercises as instructed. These exercises will help prevent contractures and other complications.

G Phantom limb pain is real pain and should be treated that way. Report complaints of pain to the nurse.

G Follow the care plan for care of the prosthesis and the stump. See Chapter 21 for more information on prosthetics and related care.

Complementary or Alternative Health Practices

Many people use complementary or alternative health practices. **Complementary medicine** refers to treatments that are used in addition to the conventional treatments prescribed by a doctor. **Alternative medicine** refers to practices and treatments used instead of conventional methods. Residents may use any of the following:

• Chiropractic medicine concentrates on the spine and musculoskeletal system. Chiropractors believe that a misaligned spine can interfere with the body's proper function. Chiropractors do not use drugs or surgery; they use hands-on manipulations, also called *adjustments*, of the spine or other joints. They also teach exercises and provide nutrition and other health counseling.

  Heat, cold, and muscle stimulation are used to improve function. Chiropractors are frequently consulted for back, neck, and joint pain, as well as for headaches.

• Massage therapy manipulates soft body tissues with touch and pressure and is used to reduce stress and to promote relaxation, healing, and pain relief.

• Acupuncture is a very old Chinese healing technique. Very fine needles are inserted into specific points on the body in order to restore health, relieve pain, or treat other conditions.

• Homeopathy involves giving small doses of a substance to stimulate the body's ability to heal itself.

• Herbs and other dietary supplements may be taken for prevention as well as treatment of diseases or conditions. If an NA knows that a resident is taking herbs or supplements, she should report this to the nurse, as some can cause serious problems if taken with certain medications.

If residents are using complementary or alternative medicine, the NA should not make judgments about their treatment or discuss her opinions. She should not make recommendations about these methods or offer suggestions. Any concerns should be reported to the nurse.

3. Describe common diseases and disorders of the nervous system

Chapter 19 has information on dementia and Alzheimer's disease. Dementia and Alzheimer's disease are common disorders of the nervous system.

CVA or Stroke

The medical term for a stroke is a cerebrovascular accident (CVA). CVA, or stroke (sometimes called *brain attack*), occurs when the blood supply to a part of the brain is blocked or a blood vessel leaks or ruptures within the brain. A stroke can be mild or severe. Afterward, a resident may experience paralysis, weakness, inability to speak or understand words, trouble swallowing, and loss of bowel or bladder control. Chapter 4 has a more comprehensive list of how a CVA may affect a person.

Strokes occur on either the right or left side of the brain. Symptoms resulting from a stroke differ; they depend on which side of the brain is affected. Strokes that occur on the right side of the brain affect functioning on the left side of the body. Strokes that occur on the left side of the brain affect functioning on the right side of the body.

If the stroke was mild, the resident may experience few, if any, complications. Physical therapy may help restore physical abilities. Speech and occupational therapy can also help with communication and performing activities of daily living.

Guidelines: CVA/Stroke

G   Residents with paralysis, weakness, or loss of movement will usually receive physical or occupational therapy. Range of motion exercises will help strengthen muscles and keep joints mobile. Residents may also need to perform leg exercises to improve circulation. Safety is important when residents are exercising. Assist carefully with exercises as ordered.

G   Never refer to the weaker side as the "bad side," or talk about the "bad" leg or arm. Use the terms *weaker* or *involved* to refer to the side with paralysis.

G   Residents with speech loss or communication problems may receive speech therapy. You may be asked to help. This includes helping residents recognize written or spoken words. Speech-language pathologists will also evaluate a resident's swallowing ability. They will decide if swallowing therapy or thickened liquids are needed.

G   Use verbal and nonverbal communication to express your positive attitude. Let the resident know you have confidence in his abilities through smiles, touches, and gestures. Gestures and pointing can also help give information or allow the resident to communicate with you. More ideas for communicating with residents recovering from stroke are listed in Chapter 4.

G   Experiencing confusion or memory loss is upsetting. People often cry for no apparent reason after suffering a stroke. Be patient and understanding. Your positive attitude will be important. Keeping a routine may help residents feel more secure.

G   Encourage independence and self-esteem. Let the resident do things for himself whenever possible, even if you could do a better or faster job. Make tasks less difficult for the resident to do. Appreciate and acknowledge residents' efforts to do things for themselves, even when they are unsuccessful. Praise even the smallest successes to build confidence.

G   Always check on the resident's body alignment. Sometimes an arm or leg can be caught on something and the resident is unaware.

G   Pay special attention to skin care and observe for changes in the skin if a resident is unable to move.

G   If residents have a loss of touch or sensation, check for potentially harmful situations. Diminished sensation or paralysis causes a lack of awareness about such things as water temperature and sharpness of razors. If residents are unable to sense or move a part of the body, check and change positioning often to prevent pressure injuries.

G   Adapt procedures when caring for residents with one-sided paralysis or weakness. Carefully assist with shaving, grooming, and bathing.

G   When assisting with transfers or walking, always use a gait belt for safety. Stand on the weaker side. Support the weaker side. Lead with the stronger side (Fig. 18-9).

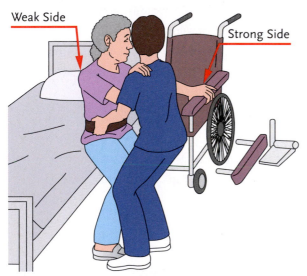

Weak Side

Strong Side

Fig. 18-9. *When helping a resident transfer, support the weaker side while leading with the stronger side.*

When assisting with dressing, remember to

G   Dress the weaker side first. Place the weaker arm or leg into the clothing first. This prevents unnecessary bending and stretching of the limb. Undress the stronger side first, then remove the weaker arm or leg from clothing to prevent the limb from being stretched and twisted.

G   Use assistive equipment to help the resident dress himself (see Chapters 13 and 21). Encourage self-care.

When assisting with eating, remember to

G   Place food in the resident's field of vision. The nurse will determine a resident's field of vision.

G   Use assistive devices such as silverware with built-up handle grips, plate guards, and drinking cups.

G   Watch for signs of choking. Report any difficulty with swallowing. Soft foods may be ordered in the care plan if swallowing is difficult. Straws should not be used for someone who has a swallowing problem.

G   Always place food in the unaffected, or stronger, side of the mouth. Make sure food is swallowed before offering more bites.

Home Care Focus

Monitoring the home safety of clients who have had a stroke is essential. Clients who are unsteady, weak, or confused are at risk of falling. Clients with loss of sensation are at risk of burning themselves in the bathroom or at the stove. Here are some safety tips for the home health aide to remember:

•   Report any safety hazards, such as unnecessary clutter or throw rugs, to the supervisor.

•   Unplug appliances like toasters and coffee makers when not in use.

•   Check the refrigerator and cabinets for spoiled food. A stroke may impair a person's sense of smell and taste.

Chapters 4 and 7 contain more information about cerebrovascular accidents.

Parkinson's Disease

Parkinson's disease is a progressive, incurable disease that causes a section of the brain to degenerate. Parkinson's disease affects the muscles, causing them to become stiff. In addition, it causes stooped posture and a shuffling gait, or walk. It can also cause pill-rolling. Pill-rolling is a circular movement of the tips of the thumb and the index finger when brought together, which looks like rolling a pill. Tremors or shaking make it very difficult for a person to perform

ADLs such as eating and bathing. A person with Parkinson's disease may have a mask-like facial expression. Medications are commonly used to treat this disease. Surgery may be an option for some people.

Guidelines: Parkinson's Disease

G Residents are at a high risk for falls. Visual and spatial impairments may occur, causing problems with bumping into doorways and navigating areas. Protect residents from any unsafe areas and conditions. Assist with ambulation as necessary.

G Help with ADLs as needed.

G Assist with range of motion exercises exactly as ordered to prevent contractures and to help strengthen muscles (Fig. 18-10).

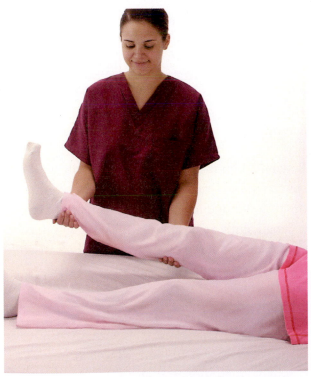

Fig. 18-10. Range of motion exercises help prevent contractures, strengthen muscles, and increase circulation.

G Observe for any swallowing problems and report them to the nurse.

G Encourage self-care. Be patient with self-care and communication.

Multiple Sclerosis (MS)

Multiple sclerosis (MS) is a progressive disease that affects the central nervous system. When a person has MS, the myelin sheath that covers the nerves, spinal cord, and white matter of the brain breaks down over time. Without this covering, or sheath, nerves cannot send messages to and from the brain in a normal way.

MS progresses slowly and unpredictably. Residents who have this disease will have widely varying abilities. Symptoms will vary as well and may include blurred vision, fatigue, tremors, poor balance, and trouble walking. Weakness, numbness, tingling, incontinence, and behavior changes are also symptoms. MS can eventually cause blindness, contractures, and loss of function in the arms and legs (Fig. 18-11).

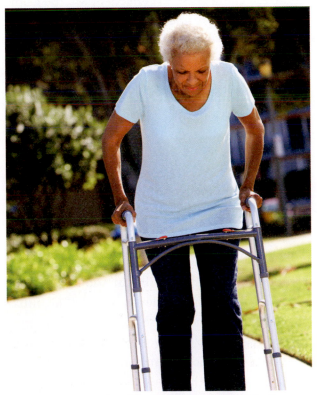

Fig. 18-11. Multiple sclerosis is an unpredictable disease that causes varying symptoms and abilities. MS can cause a range of problems, including fatigue, poor balance, and trouble walking.

Multiple sclerosis is often diagnosed in early adulthood. The exact cause is not known, but it may be an autoimmune disease. There is no cure for this disease; it is mostly treated with medication. Some people who have MS use complementary treatments.

Guidelines: Multiple Sclerosis

G Assist with activities of daily living as needed. Be patient with self-care and movement. Allow enough time to perform tasks. Offer rest periods as necessary.

G Give the resident plenty of time to communicate. People with MS may have trouble forming their thoughts. Be patient. Do not rush them.

G Prevent falls, which may be due to a lack of coordination, fatigue, or vision problems.

G Stress can worsen the effects of MS. Be calm and listen to residents when they want to talk.

G Symptoms of MS can sometimes change daily; offer support and encouragement, and adapt care to the symptoms reported.

G Encourage a healthy diet with plenty of fluids.

G Give regular skin care to prevent pressure injuries.

G Assist with range of motion exercises to prevent contractures and strengthen muscles.

Head and Spinal Cord Injuries

Diving, sports injuries, falls, car and motorcycle accidents, industrial accidents, war, and criminal violence are common causes of head and spinal cord injuries. Problems from these injuries range from mild confusion or memory loss to coma, paralysis, and death.

Head injuries can cause permanent brain damage. Residents who have had a head injury may have the following problems: intellectual disabilities, personality changes, breathing problems, seizures, coma, memory loss, loss of consciousness, paresis, and paralysis. *Paresis* is paralysis, or loss of muscle function, that affects only part of the

body. Often, paresis is used to mean a weakness or loss of ability on one side of the body.

The effects of spinal cord injuries depend on the force of impact and the location of the injury. The higher the injury on the spinal cord, the greater the loss of function. People with head and spinal cord injuries may have **paraplegia**, or loss of function of the lower body and legs. These injuries may also cause **quadriplegia**, which is loss of function in the legs, trunk, and arms (Fig. 18-12).

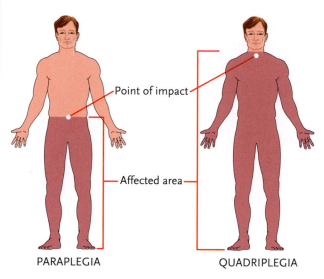

PARAPLEGIA   QUADRIPLEGIA

Fig. 18-12. *Loss of function depends on where the spine is injured.*

Rehabilitation is necessary for residents with spinal cord injuries. It will help them maintain the muscle function that remains and to live as independently as possible. Residents will need emotional support as they adjust to their disability. Their specific needs will vary.

Guidelines: Head or Spinal Cord Injury

G Give emotional support, as well as physical help. Frustration and anger may surface as residents attempt to deal with the reality of their lives. Try not to take it personally.

G Safety is very important. Be very careful that residents do not fall or burn themselves. Because residents who are paralyzed have no sensation, they are unable to feel a burn.

G Be patient with self-care. Allow as much inde-pendence as possible with ADLs.

G Give careful skin care. It is essential to pre-vent pressure injuries when mobility is limited.

G Assist residents to change positions at least every two hours to prevent pressure injuries. Be gentle when repositioning.

G Perform range of motion exercises exactly as ordered to prevent contractures and strength-en muscles.

G Immobility leads to constipation. Encourage fluids and a high-fiber diet if ordered in the care plan.

G Loss of ability to empty the bladder may lead to the need for a urinary catheter. Urinary tract infections are common. Encourage high intake of fluids. Juices high in vitamin C, such as orange juice and cranberry juice, help prevent UTIs. Give extra catheter care as needed.

G Lack of activity leads to poor circulation and fatigue. Offer rest periods as necessary. Special stockings to help increase circulation may be ordered.

G Difficulty coughing and shallow breathing can lead to pneumonia. Encourage deep breath-ing exercises as ordered.

G Male residents may have involuntary erec-tions. Provide for privacy and be sensitive if this happens. Behaving professionally helps put residents at ease.

G Assist with bowel and bladder training as directed.

Epilepsy

Epilepsy is a brain disorder that results from a disruption in normal electrical impulses in the brain, which causes repeated seizures. However, not all seizures are due to epilepsy. Epileptic seizures can range from mild tremors or brief blackouts to violent convulsions lasting several minutes. Epilepsy may be due to illness or in-jury that affects the brain, or the cause may be unknown. It is diagnosed by various medical tests, including an electroencephalogram (EEG) to check the electrical activity in the brain. Treatment for epilepsy includes medication or surgery. Chapter 7 contains information on re-sponding to seizures.

Vision Impairment

Vision impairment can affect people of all ages. Some vision impairment causes people to wear corrective lenses, such as eyeglasses or contact lenses. Some people need to wear eyeglasses all the time. Others only need them to read or for activities that require seeing distant objects, such as driving (Fig. 18-13).

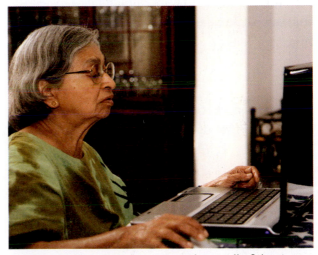

Fig. 18-13. Some people wear eyeglasses all of the time, while others only need them for certain activities that re-quire seeing distant objects.

People over the age of 40 are at risk for develop-ing certain serious vision problems. These in-clude cataracts, glaucoma, and blindness. When a **cataract** develops, the lens of the eye, which is normally clear, becomes cloudy. This prevents light from entering the eye. Vision blurs and dims initially. Vision is eventually lost entirely. This disease process can occur in one or both eyes. It is corrected with surgery, in which a per-manent lens implant is usually performed.

Glaucoma is a disease that is the leading cause of blindness in the United States. With glaucoma, the pressure in the eye (intraocular pressure) increases. This eventually damages the retina and the optic nerve. It causes loss of vision and blindness. Glaucoma can occur suddenly, causing severe pain, nausea, and vomiting. It can also occur gradually, with symptoms that include blurred vision, tunnel vision, and blue-green halos around lights. Glaucoma is treated with eye drops and other medications and sometimes surgery.

Diabetic retinopathy is a complication of diabetes caused by damage to the retina. Symptoms include seeing spots, blurred vision, and difficulty seeing well at night. Diabetic retinopathy can lead to blindness. The longer a person has diabetes, the greater the risk for developing this condition. Other risk factors include diabetes that is not managed well, high blood pressure, high cholesterol, and tobacco use. Diabetic retinopathy is treated with laser treatment, surgery, or injection of medication into the eye.

Age-related macular degeneration (AMD) is a condition that usually affects older adults (50 and over). It occurs when the macula, which is part of the retina, gradually deteriorates, eventually causing vision loss and such problems as the inability to recognize faces, drive, read, and write. Peripheral (side) vision is not affected.

This condition may evolve slowly, and symptoms may not be apparent in the early stages. A person may experience dark or blurred areas in the center of vision, or objects may appear less bright. The two forms of this condition are wet and dry age-related macular degeneration. The dry form is more common.

Risk factors include age, smoking, gender, race (Caucasians are more likely to develop it), and family history of the disease. There is no cure for AMD, but dry AMD may be treated with zinc and antioxidants to slow its progression. Wet AMD may be treated with injections and laser

surgery. Chapter 4 has more information on vision and hearing impairments.

4. Describe common diseases and disorders of the circulatory system

Hypertension (HTN) or High Blood Pressure

When blood pressure consistently measures 140/90 or higher, a person is diagnosed as having **hypertension (HTN)**, or high blood pressure. The major cause of hypertension is **atherosclerosis**, or a hardening and narrowing of the blood vessels (Fig. 18-14). It can also result from kidney disease, tumors of the adrenal gland, pregnancy, and certain medications.

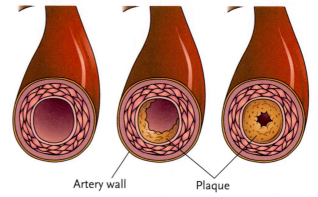

Artery wall   Plaque

Fig. 18-14. Arteries may harden or narrow because of a buildup of plaque. Hardened arteries are one cause of high blood pressure.

Hypertension can develop in people of any age. Signs and symptoms of hypertension are not always obvious, especially in the early stages. Often it is only discovered when a blood pressure measurement is taken by a healthcare provider. People with the disease may complain of headaches, blurred vision, and dizziness.

Guidelines: Hypertension

G   Because it can lead to serious conditions such as CVA, heart attack, kidney disease, and blindness, treatment to control hypertension is vital. Residents may take medication that lowers blood pressure. They may take diuretics. Diuretics are medication that reduce fluid in the body. Offer trips to the bathroom regularly. Answer call lights promptly.

G Residents may have prescribed exercise programs and special diets, such as low-fat or low-sodium diets. Reducing the amount of sodium in the diet can help reduce extra fluid in the body. You may be required to measure blood pressure frequently. You can also help by encouraging residents to follow their diet and exercise programs.

Coronary Artery Disease (CAD)

Coronary artery disease occurs when the blood vessels in the coronary arteries narrow. This reduces the supply of blood to the heart muscle and deprives it of oxygen and nutrients. Over time, as fatty deposits block the arteries, the muscles that are supplied by the blood vessels die. CAD can lead to heart attack or stroke.

The heart muscle that is not getting enough oxygen causes chest pain, pressure, or discomfort, called **angina pectoris**. The heart needs more oxygen during exercise, stress, and excitement, as well as to digest a heavy meal. In CAD, narrow blood vessels prevent the extra blood with oxygen from getting to the heart (Fig. 18-15).

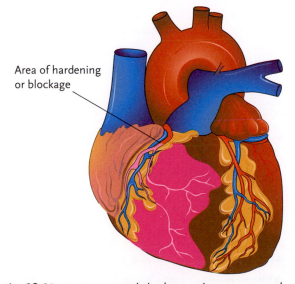

Area of hardening or blockage

Fig. 18-15. Angina pectoris is chest pain or pressure that results from the heart not getting enough oxygen.

The pain of angina pectoris is usually described as pressure or tightness in the left side or the center of the chest, behind the sternum or breastbone. Some people have pain moving down the inside of the left arm or to the neck and left side of the jaw. A person suffering from angina pectoris may sweat or appear pale. The person may feel dizzy and have trouble breathing.

Risk factors for coronary artery disease include aging, gender (men are more likely to get CAD than women), family history of heart disease, tobacco use, high cholesterol, hypertension, lack of activity, obesity, and diabetes.

Guidelines: Angina Pectoris

G Encourage residents to rest. Rest is extremely important. Rest reduces the heart's need for extra oxygen. It helps the blood flow return to normal, often within three to 15 minutes.

G Medication is also needed to relax the walls of the coronary arteries. This allows them to open and get more blood to the heart. This medication, **nitroglycerin**, is a small tablet that the resident places under the tongue. There it dissolves and is rapidly absorbed. Residents who have angina pectoris may keep nitroglycerin on hand to use as symptoms arise. To maintain potency, the nitroglycerin bottle should be kept tightly closed. Nursing assistants are not allowed to give any medication unless they have had special training. Tell the nurse if a resident needs help taking the medication.

Nitroglycerin is also available as a patch. Do not remove the patch. Tell the nurse immediately if the patch comes off. Nitroglycerin may also come in the form of a spray that the resident sprays on or under the tongue.

G Residents may also need to avoid heavy meals, overeating, intense exercise, and exposure to cold or hot and humid weather.

Myocardial Infarction (MI) or Heart Attack

When all or part of the blood flow to the heart muscle is blocked, oxygen and nutrients fail to reach the cells in that area (Fig. 18-16). Waste products are not removed, and the muscle cell dies. This is called a **myocardial infarction (MI)**, or a heart attack. The area of dead tissue may be large or small, depending on the artery involved. Someone having a myocardial infarction must receive emergency treatment from medical personnel. This helps minimize damage and may prevent further illness or death. Chapter 7 has a list of warning signs of an MI.

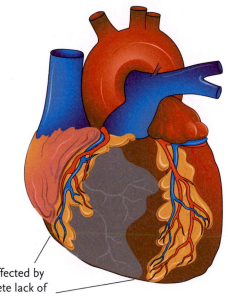

Area affected by complete lack of blood flow

Fig. 18-16. *A heart attack occurs when all or part of the blood flow to the heart is blocked.*

Guidelines: Myocardial Infarction

G   After a myocardial infarction, cardiac rehabilitation is usually ordered. This ongoing program is comprehensive and consists of a variety of components:

- Low-cholesterol, low-fat, and low-sodium diet

- Regular exercise program

- Medications to regulate the heart rate and blood pressure, to lower cholesterol, and to lower triglycerides

- Regular blood testing

- Stopping smoking

- Avoiding cold temperatures

- Stress management program

G   Encourage residents to follow their special diets and to follow their exercise programs.

G   Be encouraging if residents have quit or are trying to quit smoking.

G   Reduce stress as much as possible. Listen when residents want to talk, and report signs of and complaints of stress to the nurse.

Congestive Heart Failure (CHF)

Coronary artery disease, myocardial infarction, hypertension, or other disorders may all damage the heart. When the heart muscle has been severely damaged, the heart fails to pump effectively. When the left side of the heart is affected, blood backs up into the lungs. When the right side of the heart is affected, blood backs up into the legs, feet, or abdomen. When one or both sides of the heart stop pumping blood effectively, it is called **congestive heart failure (CHF)**.

Signs and symptoms of congestive heart failure include the following:

- Fatigue

- Rapid or irregular heartbeat

- Shortness of breath

- Dizziness

- Weakness

- Swelling of the feet and ankles (edema)

- Increased urination at night

- Weight gain

Guidelines: Congestive Heart Failure

G   Although congestive heart failure is a serious illness, it can be treated and controlled.

Medications can strengthen the heart muscle and improve its pumping.

G Assist the resident as needed with getting to the toilet or commode. Because medications help eliminate excess fluids, the resident will need more frequent trips to the bathroom. Answer call lights promptly. Keep a portable commode nearby if the resident is weak and has trouble getting out of bed and walking to the bathroom.

G Encourage residents to follow special diet orders or restrictions. A low-sodium diet or fluid restrictions may be ordered.

G A weakened heart may make it hard for residents to walk, carry items, or climb stairs. Limited activity or bedrest may be prescribed. Allow for a period of rest after an activity.

G Measure intake of fluids and output of urine as ordered (Chapter 15).

G Weigh residents as instructed. Resident may need to weigh daily at the same time to note weight gain from fluid retention.

G Apply elastic leg stockings as ordered to reduce swelling in feet and ankles.

G Assist with range of motion (ROM) exercises as ordered. These exercises improve muscle tone when activity and exercise are limited.

G Extra pillows may help residents who have trouble breathing. Keeping the head of the bed elevated may also help with breathing.

G Assist with personal care and activities of daily living (ADLs) as needed.

G A common side effect of medications for congestive heart failure is dizziness. This may result from a lack of potassium, although not all medications for CHF deplete potassium. Check with the nurse to see if high-potassium foods and drinks such as winter squash, baked sweet or regular potatoes, beans, raisins, apricots, prunes, bananas, prune juice, and orange juice can help.

Peripheral Vascular Disease (PVD)

Peripheral vascular disease (PVD) is a disease in which the legs, feet, arms, or hands do not have enough blood circulation. This is due to fatty deposits in the blood vessels that harden over time. The legs, feet, arms, and hands feel cool or cold. Nail beds and/or feet become ashen or blue. Swelling occurs in the hands and feet. Ulcers of the legs and feet may develop and can become infected. Pain may be very severe when walking; however, it is usually relieved with rest.

Risk factors for peripheral vascular disease include smoking, diabetes, high cholesterol, hypertension, inactivity, and obesity. Treatment includes quitting smoking, medications, exercise, and surgery.

For some cases of poor circulation to legs and feet, elastic stockings are ordered. These special stockings help prevent swelling and blood clots. They promote blood circulation by gently squeezing the legs to increase blood flow. Elastic stockings are also known as *anti-embolic* stockings or *TED hose*. They are referred to as anti-embolic because they help prevent embolisms. An *embolism* is an obstruction of a blood vessel, usually by a blood clot. The embolism can travel from where it was formed to another part of the body, blocking blood flow. It can cause serious damage and even death.

Elastic stockings may either be knee-high or thigh-high. They need to be put on in the morning, before the resident gets out of bed. Legs are at their smallest size then. They are usually removed in the evening. Nursing assistants should follow the manufacturer's instructions for how to put on stockings.

Putting elastic stockings on a resident

Equipment: elastic stockings

1. Identify yourself by name. Identify resident by name.

2. Wash your hands.

3. Explain procedure to resident. Speak clearly, slowly, and directly. Maintain face-to-face contact whenever possible.

4. Provide for resident's privacy with curtain, screen, or door.

5. The resident should be in the supine position (on her back) in bed. With the resident lying down, remove her socks, shoes, or slippers, and expose one leg. Expose no more than one leg at a time.

6. Take one stocking and turn it inside out at least to heel area (Fig. 18-17).

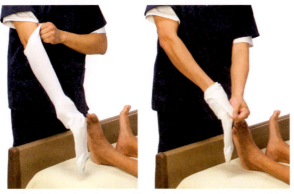

Fig. 18-17. *Turning the stocking inside out allows stocking to roll on gently.*

7. Gently place the foot of the stocking over the toes, foot, and heel (Fig. 18-18). Make sure the heel is in the right place (heel of foot should be in heel of stocking).

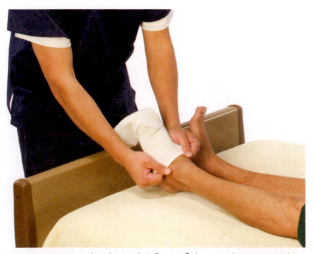

Fig. 18-18. *Gently place the foot of the stocking over the toes, foot, and heel. Promote the resident's comfort and safety. Avoid force and overextension of joints.*

8. Gently pull the top of stocking over the foot, heel, and leg.

9. Make sure there are no twists or wrinkles in the stocking after it is on the leg. It must fit smoothly (Fig. 18-19). Make sure the heel of the stocking is over the heel of the foot. If the stocking has an opening in the toe area, make sure the opening is either over or under the toe area, depending upon the manufacturer's instructions.

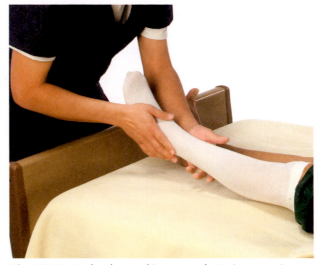

Fig. 18-19. *Make the stocking smooth. Twists or wrinkles cause the stocking to be too tight, which reduces circulation.*

10. Repeat steps 6 through 9 for the other leg.

11. Place call light within resident's reach.

12. Wash your hands.

13. Report any changes in resident to nurse.

14. Document procedure using facility guidelines.

Elastic stockings should be removed at least once a day as directed in the care plan. The stockings must be washed regularly. After removing them, the NA should bathe the skin underneath, dry the skin, and reapply them. The skin should be observed for changes in color, temperature, and swelling or sores. The NA should report any changes.

5. Describe common diseases and disorders of the respiratory system

Chronic Obstructive Pulmonary Disease (COPD)

Chronic obstructive pulmonary disease (COPD) is a chronic, progressive disease. This means a person may live for years with it but never be cured. Residents with COPD have trouble breathing, especially with getting air out of their lungs. There are two chronic lung diseases that are grouped under COPD: chronic bronchitis and emphysema.

Bronchitis is an irritation and inflammation of the lining of the bronchi. Chronic bronchitis is a form of bronchitis that is usually caused by cigarette smoking. Symptoms include coughing that brings up sputum (phlegm) and mucus. Breathlessness and wheezing may be present. Treatment includes stopping smoking and possibly medications.

Emphysema is a chronic disease of the lungs that usually results from chronic bronchitis and cigarette smoking. People with emphysema have trouble breathing. Other symptoms are coughing, breathlessness, and a rapid heartbeat. There is no cure for emphysema. Treatment includes managing symptoms and pain. Oxygen therapy, as well as medications, may be ordered. Quitting smoking is very important.

Over time, a resident with either of these lung disorders becomes chronically ill and weakened. There is a high risk of acute lung infections, such as pneumonia. **Pneumonia** is an illness that can be caused by a bacterial, viral, or fungal infection. Acute inflammation occurs in lung tissue. The affected person develops a high fever, chills, cough, greenish or yellow sputum, chest pains, and rapid pulse. Treatment includes antibiotics, along with plenty of fluids. Recovery from pneumonia may take longer for older adults and people with chronic illnesses.

When the lungs and brain do not get enough oxygen, all body systems are affected. Residents may live with a constant fear of not being able to breathe. This can cause them to sit upright in an attempt to improve their ability to expand the lungs. These residents can have poor appetites. They usually do not get enough sleep. All of this can add to feelings of weakness and poor health. They may feel they have lost control of their bodies, and particularly their breathing. They may fear suffocation.

Residents with COPD may experience the following symptoms:

- Chronic cough or wheeze

- Difficulty breathing, especially when inhaling and exhaling deeply

- Shortness of breath, especially during physical effort

- Pale, cyanotic, reddish-purple skin

- Confusion

- General state of weakness

- Difficulty completing meals due to shortness of breath

- Fear and anxiety

Guidelines: Chronic Obstructive Pulmonary Disease

G Colds or viruses can make COPD worse. Always observe and report signs and symptoms of colds or illness.

G Help residents sit upright or lean forward. Offer pillows for support (Fig. 18-20).

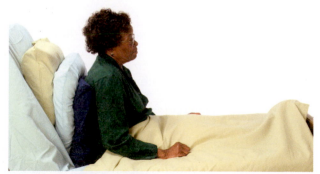

Fig. 18-20. It helps residents with COPD to sit upright and lean forward slightly.

G   Offer plenty of fluids and small, frequent meals.

G   Encourage a well-balanced diet.

G   Keep oxygen supply available as ordered.

G   Being unable to breathe or fearing suffocation can be very frightening. Be calm and supportive.

G   Use proper infection prevention practices. Wash your hands often and encourage the resident to do the same. Dispose of used tissues promptly.

G   Encourage as much independence with activities of daily living as possible.

G   Remind residents to avoid situations where they may be exposed to infections, especially colds and the flu.

G   Encourage pursed-lip breathing. Pursed-lip breathing involves inhaling slowly through the nose and exhaling slowly through pursed lips (as if about to whistle). A nurse should teach residents how to do this.

G   Encourage residents to save energy for important tasks. Encourage residents to rest.

Observing and Reporting: COPD

Report any of the following to the nurse:

O/R   Temperature over 101°F

O/R   Changes in breathing patterns, including shortness of breath

O/R   Changes in color or consistency of lung secretions

O/R   Changes in mental state or personality

O/R   Refusal to take medications as ordered

O/R   Excessive weight loss

O/R   Increasing dependence upon caregivers and family

Asthma

Asthma is a chronic inflammatory disease. It occurs when the respiratory system is hyper-reactive (that is, reacts quickly and strongly) to irritants, infection, cold air, or allergens such as pollen and dust. Exercise and stress can also worsen asthma. When the bronchi become irritated due to any one of these conditions, they constrict, making it difficult to breathe. As a response to irritation and inflammation, the mucous membrane produces thick mucus. This further inhibits respiration. As a result, air is trapped in the lungs, causing coughing and wheezing.

The exact cause of asthma is unknown. It may be caused by a combination of factors, such as family history and certain environmental exposures. Treatment for asthma includes medications that are delivered directly into the lungs by sprays or inhalers (Fig. 18-21). Residents with asthma should avoid triggers that bring on asthma attacks, such as allergens, smoke, strong odors, and strenuous exercise.

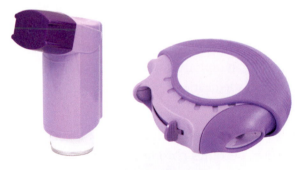

Fig. 18-21. *Two different types of asthma inhalers.*

Bronchiectasis

Bronchiectasis is a condition in which the bronchial tubes are abnormally enlarged. A person may have it in childhood or may acquire it later in life as a result of chronic infections and inflammation. Cystic fibrosis is a common cause of bronchiectasis. This abnormal state of the bronchial tubes is permanent. Bronchiectasis causes chronic coughing, which produces thick white or green sputum. A person with this disorder may have recurrent pneumonia and weight loss.

Treatment of bronchiectasis includes controlling infections and preventing complications. Antibiotics may be prescribed. Postural drainage may be ordered to eliminate fluid from the lungs. Postural drainage involves using different body positions to drain mucus from the lungs or to loosen it so that it can be coughed up.

Upper Respiratory Infection (URI)

Upper respiratory infection (URI) is commonly called *a cold*. It is the result of a viral infection or bacterial infection of the nose, sinuses, and throat. Symptoms usually include nasal discharge, sneezing, sore throat, fever, and fatigue. For most people, a cold can be dealt with by the body's immune system and by rest and fluids. If the infection is bacterial, antibiotics may be prescribed. People who have upper respiratory conditions should not be exposed to cigarette smoke or other irritants. Residents may be more comfortable sitting up, rather than lying down.

Lung Cancer

Lung cancer is the growth of abnormal cells or tumors in the lungs. Symptoms of lung cancer include chronic cough, shortness of breath, and bloody sputum. More information about cancer is located later in the chapter.

Tuberculosis (TB)

Tuberculosis (TB) is a highly contagious lung disease. Symptoms include fatigue, loss of appetite, slight fever, prolonged coughing, and shortness of breath. Chapter 5 includes more information about tuberculosis, care guidelines, and treatment.

Nursing assistants may need to collect a sputum specimen from residents who have tuberculosis.

Sputum is thick mucus coughed up from the lungs. It is not the same as saliva, which comes from the mouth. People with colds or respiratory illnesses may cough up large amounts of sputum. Sputum specimens may help diagnose respiratory problems, illness, or evaluate the effects of medication.

Early morning is the best time to collect sputum. The resident should cough up the sputum and spit it directly into the specimen container. Because sputum may be infectious, the NA should not let the resident cough on him. Standing behind the resident during the collection process may prevent sputum from coming into contact with the NA. Proper personal protective equipment (PPE) must be worn when collecting sputum. The required PPE are gloves and a special mask. It is important that the NA's hands and the specimen container are clean before beginning this procedure.

Collecting a sputum specimen

Equipment: specimen container and lid, completed label (labeled with resident's name, date of birth, room number, date, and time), specimen bag, tissues, gloves, N95 or other ordered mask, laboratory slip

1. Identify yourself by name. Identify resident by name.

2. Wash your hands.

3. Explain procedure to resident. Speak clearly, slowly, and directly. Maintain face-to-face contact whenever possible.

4. Provide for resident's privacy with curtain, screen, or door.

5. Put on mask and gloves. Coughing is one way that TB bacilli can enter the air. Stand behind the resident if the resident can hold the specimen container by himself.

6. Ask the resident to cough deeply, so that sputum comes up from the lungs. To prevent the spread of infectious material, give the resi-

dent tissues to cover his mouth while coughing. Ask the resident to spit the sputum into the specimen container.

7. When you have obtained a good sample (about two tablespoons of sputum), cover the container tightly. Wipe any sputum off the outside of the container with tissues. Discard the tissues. Apply label, place the container in a clean specimen bag, and seal the bag.

8. Remove and discard gloves and mask.

9. Wash your hands.

10. Place call light within resident's reach.

11. Report any changes in resident to the nurse.

12. Take specimen and lab slip to proper area. Document procedure using facility guidelines.

6. Describe common diseases and disorders of the endocrine system

Diabetes

Diabetes mellitus, commonly called **diabetes**, occurs when the pancreas produces too little insulin or does not properly use insulin. **Insulin** is a hormone that works to move **glucose**, or natural sugar, from the blood and into the cells for energy for the body. Without insulin to process glucose, these sugars collect in the blood and cannot get to the cells. This causes problems with circulation and can damage vital organs.

Diabetes is common in people with a family history of the illness, in the elderly, and in people who are obese. Diabetes is a chronic disease that has two major types: type 1 and type 2.

Type 1 diabetes is usually diagnosed in children and young adults. In type 1 diabetes, the pancreas does not produce any insulin. The condition will continue throughout a person's life.

Type 1 diabetes is managed with daily injections of insulin or an insulin pump and a special diet. Regular blood glucose testing must be done.

Type 2 diabetes is the most common form of diabetes. In type 2 diabetes, either the body does not produce enough insulin, or the body fails to properly use insulin. This is known as *insulin resistance*. Type 2 diabetes usually develops slowly and is the milder form of diabetes. It typically develops after age 35; the risk of getting this type increases with age. However, the number of children with type 2 diabetes is growing rapidly.

Type 2 diabetes often occurs in obese people or those with a family history of the disease. Type 2 diabetes can usually be controlled with diet and/or oral medications. Blood glucose levels should be tested regularly.

Pre-diabetes occurs when a person's blood glucose levels are above normal but not high enough for a diagnosis of type 2 diabetes. Research indicates that some damage to the body, especially to the heart and circulatory system, may already be occurring during pre-diabetes.

Pregnant women who have never had diabetes before but who have high blood sugar (glucose) levels during pregnancy are said to have **gestational diabetes**.

People with diabetes may have these signs and symptoms:

- Excessive thirst
- Extreme hunger
- Frequent urination
- Weight loss
- Elevated blood sugar levels
- Glucose (sugar) in the urine
- Sudden vision changes
- Tingling or numbness in hands or feet
- Feeling very tired much of the time
- Very dry skin

- Sores that are slow to heal

- More infections than usual

Diabetes can lead to further complications:

- Changes in the circulatory system can cause heart attack and stroke, reduced circulation to the extremities, poor wound healing, and kidney and nerve damage.

- Damage to the eyes can cause vision loss and blindness.

- Poor circulation and impaired wound healing may cause leg and foot ulcers, infected wounds, and gangrene. Gangrene can lead to amputation.

- Insulin reaction and diabetic ketoacidosis can be serious complications of diabetes. Chapter 7 has signs and symptoms of each.

Diabetes must be carefully controlled to prevent complications and severe illness. When working with people with diabetes, nursing assistants must follow care plan instructions carefully.

Guidelines: Diabetes

G Follow diet instructions exactly. The intake of carbohydrates, including breads, potatoes, grains, pastas, and sugars, must be regulated. Meals must be eaten at the same time each day. The resident must eat all that is served. If a resident will not eat what is served, or if you suspect that he is not following the diet, tell the nurse. More information on diabetic diets is found in Chapter 15.

G Encourage the resident to follow his exercise program. A regular exercise program is important. Exercise affects how quickly bodies use food. Exercise also helps improve circulation. Exercise may include walking or other active exercise (Fig. 18-22). It may also include passive range of motion exercises. Help with exercises as necessary. Be positive and try to make it fun. A walk can be a chore or it can be the highlight of the day.

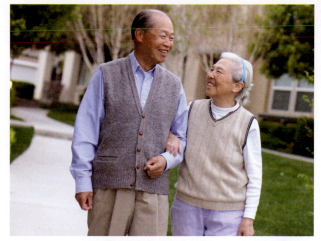

Fig. 18-22. Exercise is very important for residents who have diabetes. Exercise helps to increase circulation and maintain a healthy weight.

G Observe the resident's management of insulin. Doses are calculated exactly. They are given at the same time each day. Nursing assistants are not permitted to inject insulin, but it is important to know when residents take insulin and when their meals should be served. There must be a balance between the insulin level and food intake.

G Perform urine and blood tests as directed. A fingerstick blood glucose test is one type of blood test that may be used to check blood sugar. This is a simple test that is performed by quickly piercing the fingertip, then placing the blood on a chemically active disposable strip. The strip will indicate the result. Another type of test involves using strips, along with a blood glucose meter, a special glucose monitoring machine (Fig. 18-23). Sometimes the care plan will specify a daily blood or urine test for insulin levels. Not all states allow nursing assistants to do this. Know your state's rules. If allowed to assist with this procedure, your facility will provide training for it. Always wear gloves when helping with glucose monitoring. Follow facility policy and the manufacturer's instructions if you are responsible for disinfecting the blood glucose meter. Perform tests only as directed and allowed.

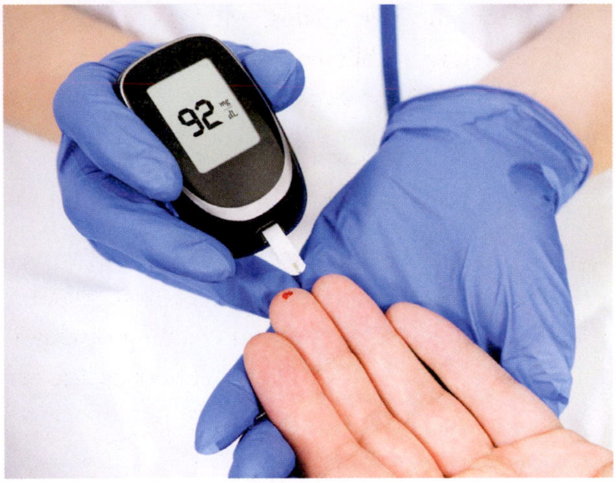

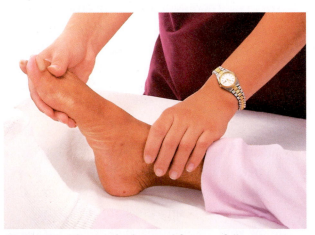

Fig. 18-23. *There are different types of equipment to measure glucose levels in the blood.*

G Proper foot care is vitally important for people with diabetes. Give foot care as directed. Because diabetes causes poor circulation, even a small sore on the leg or foot can grow into a large wound that may not heal. This can result in amputation. Careful foot care, including regular inspection, is very important (Fig. 18-24). The goals of diabetic foot care are to check for signs of irritation or sores, to promote blood circulation, and to prevent infection.

Fig. 18-24. *Observe the legs and feet carefully. Poor circulation can increase the risk of infection and the loss of toes, feet, or legs to gangrene.*

G Encourage residents to wear comfortable, supportive, well-fitting shoes that do not hurt their feet. Shoes made of material that breathes, such as leather, cotton, or canvas,

help prevent buildup of moisture. To avoid injuries to the feet, residents with diabetes should not go barefoot. Socks made of natural fibers such as cotton or wool are best because they absorb sweat. Socks should not be too tight. Nursing assistants should never trim or clip a resident's toenails. Only a nurse or doctor should do this.

Observing and Reporting: Diabetes

Report any of these to the nurse:

- Any sign of skin breakdown, especially on the feet and toes
- Change in appetite (resident overeating or not eating enough)
- Weight changes
- Change in mental status
- Increased thirst
- Increase or decrease in urine output
- Nausea or vomiting
- Irritability
- Nervousness or anxiety
- Feeling faint or dizzy
- Visual changes, especially blurred vision
- Change in mobility
- Change in sensation
- Sweet or fruity breath
- Numbness or tingling in arms or legs

Providing foot care for a resident with diabetes

Equipment: basin of warm water, bath thermometer, mild soap, washcloth, 2 towels, lotion, clean cotton socks, shoes or slippers, gloves

1. Identify yourself by name. Identify resident by name.

2. Wash your hands.

3. Explain procedure to resident. Speak clearly, slowly, and directly. Maintain face-to-face contact whenever possible.

4. Provide for resident's privacy with curtain, screen, or door.

5. Fill the basin halfway with warm water. Test water temperature with thermometer or against the inside of your wrist. Ensure it is safe. Water temperature should be no higher than 105°F. Have resident check water temperature. Adjust if necessary.

6. Place the basin on a bath towel on the floor (if the resident is sitting in a chair) or on a towel at the foot of the bed (if the resident is in bed). Make sure the basin is in a position that is comfortable for the resident. Support the foot and ankle throughout the procedure.

7. Put on gloves.

8. Remove the resident's socks and completely submerge the resident's feet in the water. Soak the feet for 10 to 20 minutes.

9. Put soap on a wet washcloth. Remove one foot from the water. Wash the entire foot gently, including between the toes and around the nail beds.

10. Rinse the entire foot, including between the toes.

11. Using a towel, pat the foot dry gently, including between the toes.

12. Repeat steps 9 through 11 for the other foot.

13. Starting at the toes and working up to the ankles, gently rub lotion into the feet with circular strokes. Your goal is to increase circulation, so take several minutes on each foot. **Do not put lotion between the toes.** Remove excess lotion (if any) with a towel. Make sure lotion has been absorbed and feet are completely dry.

14. Observe the feet, ankles, and legs for dry skin, irritation, blisters, redness, sores, corns, discoloration, or swelling.

15. Help the resident put on clean socks and shoes or slippers.

16. Put soiled linens in appropriate container. Pour water into the toilet and flush it. Place the basin in proper area for cleaning or clean and store it according to facility policy. Store supplies.

17. Remove and discard gloves.

18. Wash your hands.

19. Place call light within resident's reach.

20. Report any changes in resident to the nurse.

21. Document procedure using facility guidelines.

Hyperthyroidism (Overactive Thyroid Gland)

Hyperthyroidism is a condition in which the thyroid produces too much thyroid hormone. Body processes speed up, and metabolism increases, causing weight loss, a rapid heartbeat, sweating, and nervousness. Graves' disease, an autoimmune disorder, often causes hyperthyroidism. Hyperthyroidism is usually treated with medication. Occasionally, part of the thyroid is surgically removed.

Hypothyroidism (Underactive Thyroid Gland)

Hypothyroidism is a condition in which the body lacks thyroid hormone. This causes body processes to slow down. It is an autoimmune disorder in which the body produces antibodies that attack the thyroid, interfering with the production of thyroid hormone. Hypothyroidism is often caused by Hashimoto's thyroiditis, a type of autoimmune disorder. Symptoms of hypothyroidism include fatigue, weight gain, constipation, and intolerance to cold. Dry skin, hair loss, slow heart rate, and low blood pressure are other symptoms. Hypothyroidism is treated with thyroid hormone replacement therapy.

7. Describe common diseases and disorders of the reproductive system

Sexually Transmitted Infections

Sexually transmitted infections (STIs), or sexually transmitted diseases (STDs), are caused by sexual contact with an infected person. Sexually transmitted infections do not always have apparent signs and symptoms.

These infections are mostly transmitted through sexual contact, which includes sexual intercourse (vaginal and anal), contact of the mouth with the genitals or anus, and contact of the hands with the genital area. Some STIs can also be transmitted during pregnancy or childbirth. The human immunodeficiency virus (HIV) and some kinds of hepatitis can be transmitted via needles, as well as through sexual contact. (HIV and AIDS are discussed in detail in the next learning objective.)

Sexually transmitted infections cause a variety of signs and symptoms and health problems, which are detailed below. The transmission of some STIs can be reduced or stopped by using latex or polyurethane condoms (Fig. 18-25).

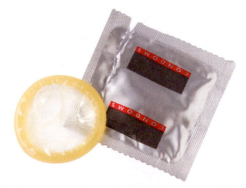

Fig. 18-25. Latex or polyurethane condoms can reduce or stop the transmission of some sexually transmitted infections.

Residents may be unaware of or embarrassed by symptoms of this type of infection. The nursing assistant should remain professional when discussing sexually transmitted infections and should report signs and symptoms to the nurse.

Chlamydia is an infection is caused by organisms introduced into the mucous membranes of the reproductive tract. Chlamydia can cause serious infection, including pelvic inflammatory disease (PID) in women. PID can lead to sterility. Signs and symptoms of chlamydia include yellow or white discharge from the penis or vagina, burning during urination, swelling of the testes, painful intercourse, and abdominal and low back pain. Chlamydia is treated with antibiotics.

Syphilis is caused by bacteria. It can be treated effectively in the early stages, but if left untreated, it can cause brain damage, mental illness, and even death. Babies born to mothers infected with syphilis may be born blind or with other serious birth defects. Syphilis is easier to detect in men than in women. This is due to open sores called **chancres** that develop on the penis soon after infection. In women, these sores may form inside the vagina. The chancres are painless and can go unnoticed. If untreated, the infection progresses to rashes, headache, fever, weight loss, and muscle aches. Then, over time, if the infection is still not treated with penicillin or other antibiotics, it spreads to the heart, brain, and other vital organs. Untreated syphilis will eventually be fatal. The sooner the disease is treated, the better the person's chances of preventing long-term damage and avoiding infection of others.

Gonorrhea is caused by bacteria. Like syphilis, it is easier to detect in men than in women because many women with gonorrhea show no early symptoms. Men infected with gonorrhea will typically have a white, yellow, or green discharge from the penis. Painful or swollen testes and burning during urination are other common symptoms in men. Symptoms in women include cloudy vaginal discharge, along with vaginal bleeding between periods. Rectal itching, soreness, bleeding, or painful elimination of stool can occur in both men and women. If untreated, gonorrhea can cause blindness, joint infection, sterility, and pelvic inflammatory disease. Gonorrhea is treated with antibiotics.

Genital herpes, unlike the STIs discussed previously, is caused by a virus—herpes simplex type 1 (HSV-1) or type 2 (HSV-2). HSV-2 is generally the cause of genital herpes. Genital herpes cannot be treated with antibiotics, nor can it be cured. Once infected with genital herpes, a person may suffer repeated outbreaks of the disease for the rest of his or her life. A herpes outbreak includes burning, painful, red sores on the genitals that may take weeks to heal. The sores are infectious, but a person with genital herpes can spread the infection even when sores are not present.

Some people infected with genital herpes never experience repeated outbreaks. The later episodes may not be as painful as the initial outbreak. Treatment with antiviral medication can help people stay symptom-free for longer periods of time. The medication can also help lessen the duration and intensity of the episodes. Babies born to women infected with genital herpes can be infected during birth. Pregnant women experiencing an outbreak are usually delivered by Cesarean section, or C-section.

Genital HPV infection is a sexually transmitted infection caused by human papillomavirus (HPV). HPV is a different virus than HIV and HSV (herpes). Genital HPV infection is spread primarily through genital contact and can infect the genital area of both men and women. This includes the penis, vulva, lining of the vagina, cervix, rectum, or anus. Many people have no signs or symptoms of HPV. Some HPV infections cause women to have an abnormal pap test. Genital warts may appear. They may also lead to the development of cervical cancer. Treatment to remove warts is done in a doctor's office or through the use of medication. There is no cure for HPV. However, an HPV vaccine, licensed by the Food and Drug Administration (FDA), is available and is recommended for young women through age 26 and young men through age 21. It may help prevent genital warts and anal, vaginal, and vulvar cancers in women, and genital warts and anal cancer in men.

The human immunodeficiency virus (HIV) can be transmitted sexually as well and is discussed in the next learning objective.

Benign Prostatic Hypertrophy

Benign prostatic hypertrophy (BPH) is a disorder that is common in men over the age of 60. The prostate becomes enlarged and causes pressure on the urethra. This pressure leads to frequent urination, dribbling of urine, and difficulty in starting the flow of urine. Urinary retention (urine remaining in the bladder) may also occur, causing urinary tract infection. Urine can also back up into the ureters and kidneys, causing damage to these organs. The cause of benign prostatic hypertrophy is unknown. Medications and/or surgery are used to treat this disorder. A test is also available to screen for cancer of the prostate. As men age, they are at increased risk for prostate cancer. Prostate cancer is usually slow-growing and responsive to treatment if detected early.

Vaginitis

Vaginitis is an inflammation of the vagina. It may be caused by a bacteria, protozoa (one-celled animals), or fungus (yeast). Bacterial vaginosis occurs when there is an overgrowth of normal bacteria inside the vagina. Yeast infections are caused by an overproduction of a fungus called *Candida albicans*. Vaginitis may also be the result of hormonal changes after menopause. Women who have vaginitis have a white vaginal discharge, accompanied by itching and burning. Treatment of vaginitis includes oral medications, as well as vaginal creams or suppositories.

8. Describe common diseases and disorders of the immune and lymphatic systems

Acquired Immune Deficiency Syndrome (AIDS)

Acquired immune deficiency syndrome (AIDS) is a disease caused by the human immunodeficiency virus (HIV). HIV attacks the body's immune system and gradually weakens and disables it. AIDS is caused by acquiring the HIV virus through blood or body fluids from an infected person. AIDS is the final stage of HIV infection in which infections, tumors, and central nervous system symptoms appear due to a weakened immune system that is unable to fight infection. It can take years for HIV to develop into AIDS.

HIV is a sexually transmitted disease. It can also be spread through the blood and from infected needles.

In general, HIV affects the body in stages. The first stage involves symptoms similar to the flu, with fever, muscle aches, cough, fatigue, and swollen lymph glands. These are symptoms of the body's immune system fighting the infection. As the infection worsens, the immune system overreacts and attacks not only the virus, but also normal tissue.

When the virus weakens the immune system in later stages, a group of problems may appear. These include opportunistic infections, tumors, and central nervous system symptoms that would not occur if the immune system were healthy. This stage of the disease is known as AIDS. The diagnosis of AIDS is made when a person's CD4+ lymphocyte (a type of white blood cell) count falls to 200 or below.

In the late stages of AIDS, damage to the central nervous system may cause memory loss, poor coordination, paralysis, and confusion. These symptoms together are known as **AIDS dementia complex**.

The following are signs and symptoms of HIV infection and AIDS:

- Flu-like symptoms, including fever, cough, weakness, and severe or constant fatigue

- Appetite loss

- Weight loss

- Night sweats

- Swollen lymph nodes in the neck, underarms, or groin

- Severe diarrhea

- Dry cough

- Skin rashes

- Painful white spots in the mouth or on the tongue

- Cold sores or fever blisters on the lips and flat, white ulcers in the mouth

- Cauliflower-like warts on the skin and in the mouth

- Inflamed and bleeding gums

- Bruising that does not go away

- Low resistance to infection, particularly pneumonia, but also tuberculosis, herpes, bacterial infections, and hepatitis

- **Kaposi's sarcoma**, a rare form of skin cancer that appears as purple, red, or brown skin lesions

- *Pneumocystis jiroveci pneumonia*, a lung infection

- AIDS dementia complex

Opportunistic infections, such as pneumonia or tuberculosis, invade the body because the immune system is weak and cannot defend itself. These illnesses complicate AIDS. They further weaken the immune system. It is difficult to treat these infections because generally, over time, a person with AIDS develops resistance to some antibiotics. These infections can cause death in people with AIDS.

There is no cure for this disease, and there is no vaccine to prevent the disease. People who are infected with HIV are treated with drugs that slow the progress of the disease. Without medication, however, the HIV-infected person's weakened resistance to infections may lead to AIDS and eventually to death.

Common Chronic and Acute Conditions

Many people are living longer with HIV by taking combinations of medications every day. HAART, or highly active antiretroviral therapy, has been shown to control the HIV virus. Three or more medications are used for this therapy. Medicines must be taken at precise times. They have many unpleasant side effects. Gastrointestinal symptoms like nausea, vomiting, and diarrhea, as well as fever and skin rashes, are some of the side effects. For some people, the medications are less effective than for others. Other aspects of HIV treatment include relief of symptoms and prevention and treatment of infection.

Specific behaviors put people at high risk for acquiring HIV. HIV is most commonly transmitted by the following:

- Having unprotected or poorly protected anal sex with an infected person
- Having unprotected or poorly protected vaginal sex with an infected person
- Having sexual contact with many partners
- Sharing drug needles or syringes

In the healthcare setting, infections can be spread through accidental contact with contaminated blood or body fluids, needles or other sharp objects, or contaminated supplies or equipment.

Ways to protect against the spread of HIV and AIDS include the following:

- Following Standard Precautions at work
- Never sharing needles or syringes
- Not having unprotected sex (always using condoms when having sex)
- Staying in a monogamous relationship (being monogamous means having only one sexual partner)
- Practicing abstinence (abstinence means not having sexual contact with anyone)
- Getting tested for HIV and retested if necessary (HIV is able to be detected in most people within three to eight weeks after exposure. However, it can take up to three months for HIV to be able to be detected and up to six months in rare cases.)

Residents' Rights

The Facts about HIV and AIDS

A handshake or a hug cannot spread the HIV virus. The disease cannot be transmitted by telephones, doorknobs, tables, chairs, toilets, mosquitoes, or by breathing the same air as an infected person. Nursing assistants should spend time with residents who have HIV or AIDS. These residents need the same thoughtful, personal attention that NAs give to all residents.

Guidelines: HIV and AIDS

G Follow Standard Precautions. Follow Transmission-Based Precautions in addition to Standard Precautions if ordered.

G People with poor immune system function are more sensitive to infections. Wash your hands often and keep everything clean.

G Involuntary weight loss occurs in almost all people who develop AIDS. High-protein, high-calorie, and high-nutrient meals can help maintain a healthy weight.

G Some people with HIV/AIDS lose their appetites and have difficulty eating. These residents should be encouraged to relax before meals and to eat in a pleasant setting. Familiar and favorite foods should be served. Report appetite loss or difficulty eating to the nurse. If appetite loss continues to be a problem, the doctor may prescribe an appetite stimulant.

G Residents who have infections of the mouth and esophagus may need food that is low in acid and neither cold nor hot. Spicy seasonings should be removed. Soft or pureed foods may be easier to swallow. Drinking liquid meals and fortified drinks, such as milkshakes, may ease the pain of chewing. Warm rinses may help painful sores of the mouth. Careful mouth care is vital.

G A person who has nausea or vomiting should eat small, frequent meals and should eat slowly. The person should avoid high-fat and spicy foods and eat a soft, bland diet. Cool foods that have little odor are usually easier to eat than hot foods. When nausea and vomiting persist, liquids and salty foods should be encouraged. Residents should drink fluids in between meals. Care must be taken to maintain proper intake of fluids to balance lost fluids.

G Residents who have mild diarrhea may have small, frequent meals that are low in fat, fiber, and dairy products. The doctor may order a BRAT (bananas, rice, applesauce, and toast) diet. This diet is helpful for short-term use.

G Diarrhea rapidly depletes the body of fluids. Fluid replacement is necessary. Good re-hydration fluids include water, juice, caffeine-free soda, and broth. Caffeinated drinks should be avoided.

G **Neuropathy**, or numbness, tingling, and pain in the feet and legs is usually treated with pain medications. Wearing loose, soft slippers may be helpful. If blankets and sheets cause pain, a bed cradle can keep sheets and blankets from resting on legs and feet (Fig. 18-26).

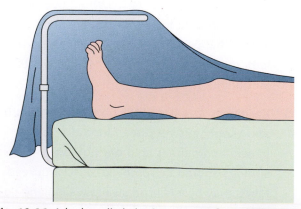

Fig. 18-26. A bed cradle helps keep covers from resting on the feet.

G Give emotional support as well as physical care. Residents with HIV/AIDS may suffer from anxiety and depression. In addition, they are often judged by family, friends, and society. Some people avoid a person with AIDS due to homophobia, which is a fear of lesbians and gay men. Some people blame them for their illness. People with HIV/AIDS may have tremendous stress. They may feel uncertainty about their illness, health care, and finances. They may also have lost friends who have died from AIDS. Listen closely to residents to understand their individual needs and concerns. This is part of providing person-centered care. Treat them with respect, and help provide needed emotional support.

Residents with this disease need support from others. This support may come from family, friends, religious and community groups, and support groups, as well as the care team. Report to the nurse if you feel that residents need more resources and services.

G Withdrawal, apathy, avoidance of tasks, and mental slowness are early symptoms of HIV infection. Medications may also cause side effects of this type. AIDS dementia complex may develop, causing further mental prob-lems. There may also be muscle weakness and loss of muscle control, making falls a risk. Residents in this stage of the disease will need a safe environment and close super-vision in their activities of daily living.

The right to confidentiality may be especially important to a person who has HIV or AIDS. Others may pass judgment on people with this disease. HIV testing requires consent; a per-son cannot be tested for HIV unless he agrees. HIV test results are confidential and cannot be shared with a person's family, friends, or em-ployer without his consent. A person with HIV or AIDS cannot be fired from a job because of the disease. However, a healthcare worker with HIV or AIDS may be reassigned to duties that have a lower risk of transmitting the disease.

Home Care Focus

When working in the home, it is very important for home health aides to carefully follow guidelines for safe food preparation and storage when working with a client who has HIV or AIDS. Foodborne illnesses caused by improperly cooking or storing food can cause death for someone with HIV or AIDS. (Chapter 28 has information about safe food handling practices.) The HHA should wash her hands frequently. She should keep everything clean, especially countertops, cutting boards, and knives after they have been used to cut meat. Food should be thawed in the refrigerator, and it should be washed and cooked thoroughly. When storing food, cold foods should be kept cold and hot foods should be kept hot. Small containers that seal tightly are best. The HHA should check expiration dates and remember "When in doubt, throw it out."

Cancer

Cancer is a general term used to describe a disease in which abnormal cells grow in an uncontrolled way. Cancer usually occurs in the form of a tumor or tumors growing on or within the body. A **tumor** is a cluster of abnormally growing cells. **Benign tumors** are considered noncancerous. They usually grow slowly in local areas. **Malignant tumors** are cancerous. They grow rapidly and invade surrounding tissues.

Cancer invades local tissue, and can spread to other parts of the body. When cancer spreads from the site where it first appeared (metastasizes), it can affect other body systems. In general, treatment is more difficult, and cancer is more deadly after this has occurred. Cancer often appears first in the breast, colon, rectum, uterus, prostate, lungs, or skin. There is no known cure for cancer. However, some treatments are effective. They are discussed later in the chapter.

Known causes of cancer include the following:

- Genetic factors
- Tobacco use
- Alcohol use
- Poor diet/obesity
- Lack of physical activity
- Certain infections
- Environmental exposure, such as radiation
- Sun exposure (Fig. 18-27)

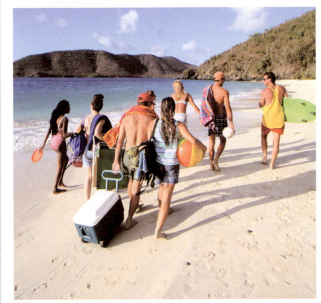

Fig. 18-27. *Prolonged sun exposure puts a person at risk for skin cancer.*

When diagnosed and treated early, cancer can often be controlled. The American Cancer Society (cancer.org) has identified some warning signs of cancer:

- Unexplained weight loss
- Fever
- Fatigue
- Pain
- Skin changes, such as change in skin color (e.g., reddened skin)
- Change in bowel or bladder function
- Sores that do not heal
- Unusual bleeding or discharge
- Thickening or lump in the breast, testicle, or other parts of the body
- Indigestion or difficulty swallowing
- New mole or recent change in appearance of a mole, wart, or spot
- Nagging cough or hoarseness

People with cancer can live longer and sometimes recover when treated using the following methods. These treatments are most effective when tumors are discovered early. Often these treatments are combined.

Surgery is the front line of defense for most forms of cancer. It is the key treatment for malignant tumors of the skin, breast, bladder, colon, rectum, stomach, and muscle. Surgeons attempt to remove as much of the tumor as possible to prevent cancer from spreading.

Chemotherapy refers to medications given, usually intravenously, to fight cancer. Certain drugs destroy cancer cells and limit the rate of cell growth. However, many of these drugs are toxic to the body. They destroy healthy cells as well as cancer cells. Chemotherapy can have severe side effects, including nausea, vomiting, diarrhea, oral sores, hair loss, fatigue, and decreased resistance to infection.

Radiation therapy (radiotherapy) directs radiation to a limited area to kill cancer cells. However, normal or healthy cells in the radiation's path are also destroyed (Fig. 18-28). By controlling cell growth, radiation can reduce pain. Radiation can cause the same side effects as chemotherapy. The skin of the area exposed to radiation may become sore, irritated, and sometimes burned.

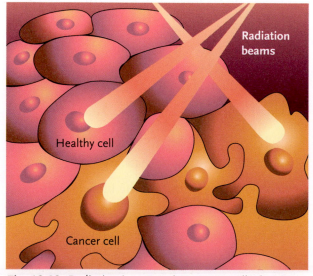

Fig. 18-28. Radiation is targeted at cancer cells, but it also destroys some healthy cells in its path.

Targeted therapy is a specific type of chemotherapy. Traditional chemotherapy typically destroys healthy cells as well as cancer cells. Scientists have developed targeted chemotherapy drugs using the differences between cancer cells and normal cells. These drugs can attack cancer cells and the cells that help cancer grow. Side effects of these drugs can be similar to those associated with other chemotherapy drugs, and can also include high blood pressure, rashes or other skin changes, bleeding and clotting problems, and more.

Immunotherapy is a general term for treatment that uses a person's own immune system to fight disease. Immunotherapy can be helpful in treating some forms of cancer. It can work by making the immune system work harder to fight the cancer or by adding something to the immune system, like man-made proteins, to change how it works. Immunotherapy for cancer includes cancer vaccines, which make the immune system attack specific types of cancer cells. These may be used to help treat cancer or to stop cancer from coming back after other treatments. Different immunotherapy drugs have different side effects, but in general they have fewer side effects than chemotherapy drugs.

Guidelines: Cancer

G   Each case is different. Cancer is a general term and refers to many individual situations. Residents may live many years or only several months. Treatment affects each person differently. Do not make assumptions about a resident's condition.

G   Residents may want to talk or may avoid talking. Respect each resident's needs. Listen if a resident wants to share feelings or experiences with you. However, never push a resident to talk. Be honest. Never tell a resident, "Everything will be okay." Be sensitive. Remember that cancer is a disease, and its cause is unknown. Maintain a positive attitude and focus on concrete details. For example, comment if a resident seems stronger, or mention that the sun is shining outside.

G Proper nutrition is important for residents with cancer. Follow the care plan carefully. Residents frequently have poor appetites. Encourage a variety of food and small portions. Liquid nutrition supplements may be used in addition to, not in place of, meals. If nausea or swallowing is a problem, foods such as soups, gelatins, or starches may appeal to the resident. Use plastic utensils for a resident receiving chemotherapy. It makes food taste better. Metal utensils cause a bitter taste.

G Cancer can cause great pain, especially in the late stages. It can affect the ability to sleep, eat, and move. Be alert for signs of pain. Report them to the nurse. Help with comfort measures, such as repositioning, and providing distractions, such as conversation, music, or reading materials (Fig. 18-29). Report to the nurse if pain seems to be uncontrolled.

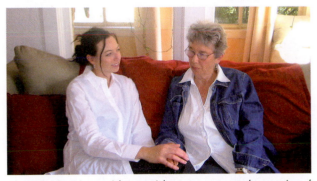

Fig. 18-29. *Give residents with cancer as much emotional support as possible. Distractions such as conversation can help a person deal with pain.*

G Offer back rubs to provide comfort and increase circulation. For residents who spend many hours in bed, special pads or other positioning devices may make them more comfortable. Moving to a chair for some period of time may improve comfort as well. Residents who are very weak or immobile need to be repositioned at least every two hours.

G Check the skin often to help prevent pressure injuries. Keep the skin clean and dry.

Use lotion regularly on dry or delicate skin. Do not apply lotion to areas receiving radiation therapy. Do not remove markings that are used in radiation therapy. Follow any skin care orders (for example, no hot or cold packs, no soap, lotion, or cosmetics, or no tight stockings).

G Help residents brush teeth regularly. Chemotherapy medications, nausea, vomiting, or mouth infections may cause pain and a bad taste in the mouth. You can help ease discomfort by using a soft-bristled toothbrush, rinsing with baking soda and water, or using a prescribed rinse. Do not use a commercial mouthwash. The alcohol in mouthwash can further irritate a resident's mouth. For residents with mouth sores, using oral swabs rather than toothbrushes may be preferable. The swabs can be dipped in a rinse and gently wiped across the gums. Mouth sores can make oral care very painful; be very gentle when giving residents oral care.

G People with cancer may suffer from poor self-image because they are weak and their appearance has changed. For example, hair loss is a common side effect of chemotherapy. Assist with grooming if desired. Your concern and interest can help improve self-image.

G If visitors help cheer your resident, encourage them and do not intrude. If some times of day are better than others, suggest this to visitors. Support groups exist for people with cancer and their families. Check with the nurse for groups in your area. It may help a person with cancer to think of something besides cancer and treatment for a while. Pursue other topics. Get to know what interests your residents have. As always, report any signs of depression immediately.

G Having a family member with cancer can be very difficult. Be alert to needs that are not being met or stresses created by the illness. Report observations.

Observing and Reporting: Cancer

Report any of these to the nurse:

O/R Increased weakness or fatigue

O/R Weight loss

O/R Nausea, vomiting, or diarrhea

O/R Changes in appetite

O/R Fainting

O/R Signs of depression (see Chapter 20)

O/R Confusion

O/R Blood in stool or urine

O/R Change in mental status

O/R Changes in skin

O/R New lumps, sores, or rashes

O/R Increase in pain, or unrelieved pain

O/R Blood in the mouth

Care after a Mastectomy

A **mastectomy** is the surgical removal of all or part of the breast and sometimes other surrounding tissue. This operation is usually performed because of a tumor.

After a mastectomy, the care plan may include arm exercises for the side of the body on which the surgery was performed. The goal of arm exercises is to strengthen the arm and chest muscles and reduce swelling in the arm and underarm. Exercises may include raising the arm, opening and closing the hand, and bending and straightening the elbow. The resident should wear loose, comfortable clothing while doing arm exercises.

The care plan's instructions may include keeping the arm on the affected side raised on pillows to decrease swelling. The resident may use a sling to keep the arm elevated. In addition, deep breathing exercises may be ordered. Blood pressure should not be measured on the arm on the affected side.

9. Identify community resources for residents who are ill

Numerous services and support groups are available for people who are ill and their families

or caregivers. These resources can help them through difficult times and help solve problems. Social service agencies, hospitals, hospice programs, churches, and synagogues offer many resources. These include meal services, transportation to doctors' offices or hospitals, counseling, and support groups.

Here are a few of the many community resources available to help residents meet different needs:

- Eldercare Locator, a public service of the U.S. Administration on Aging (eldercare.gov or 800-677-1116)

- National Association of Agencies on Aging (n4a.org or 202-872-0888)

- National Resource Center on LGBT Aging (lgbtagingcenter.org or 212-741-2247)

- Alzheimer's Association (alz.org or 800-272-3900)

- American Cancer Society (cancer.org or 800-227-2345)

- AIDSinfo, a service of the U.S. Department of Health and Human Services (aidsinfo.nih.gov or 800-448-0440)

- American Association on Intellectual and Developmental Disabilities (AAIDD, aaidd.org or 202-387-1968)

- National Institute of Mental Health (NIMH, nimh.nih.gov or 866-615-6464)

Chapter Review

1. What is an acute illness? What is a chronic illness?

2. What are signs and symptoms of scabies? How is scabies spread?

3. What causes shingles?

4. What is an open wound? What is a closed wound?

5. What is dermatitis and how does it generally look?

6. What can cause fungal infections?

7. What causes arthritis?

8. What health problems can anti-inflammatory medications cause?

9. What can happen to bones when they are brittle?

10. What can a nursing assistant do to prevent or slow osteoporosis?

11. Why should extremities in casts be elevated?

12. When dressing a person who has just had a hip replacement, which side should be dressed first: the affected/weaker side or the unaffected/stronger side?

13. What is the difference between partial weight-bearing (PWB) and non-weight-bearing (NWB)?

14. List reasons that knee replacements are necessary.

15. List three physical problems that muscular dystrophy can cause.

16. What is phantom limb pain? What is phantom sensation?

17. What causes a CVA (stroke)?

18. What terms should an NA use to refer to the weaker side of a person who has had a stroke?

19. When helping a resident who has had a stroke with transfers or walking, on which side should an NA stand—the weaker or stronger?

20. When dressing a resident with a one-sided weakness, which side should an NA dress first?

21. In which side of the mouth should food be placed if a resident has a one-sided weakness?

22. Why may people with Parkinson's disease have trouble eating and bathing themselves?

23. When a person has multiple sclerosis, what covering breaks down over time?

24. What is paraplegia? What is quadriplegia?

25. What consistent blood pressure measurement is classified as hypertension?

26. What is the medical term for chest pain, pressure, or discomfort?

27. What are some components of a cardiac rehabilitation plan?

28. List seven care guidelines for a resident who has congestive heart failure.

29. What time of day should elastic stockings be put on?

30. What position might a resident with chronic obstructive pulmonary disease (COPD) prefer to be in?

31. What are two causes of emphysema?

32. How is asthma treated?

33. How is bronchiectasis treated?

34. When is the best time of day to collect a sputum specimen?

35. Why is proper foot care especially important for a resident with diabetes?

36. Why is it important for an NA to follow diet instructions exactly for a resident with diabetes?

37. What is a sexually transmitted infection?

38. How is human immunodeficiency virus (HIV) spread?

39. Which stage of HIV infection is classified as acquired immune deficiency syndrome (AIDS)?

40. Because people who have HIV/AIDS are sensitive to infections, what steps should the nursing assistant follow?

41. What are the side effects of chemotherapy and radiation?

19

Confusion, Dementia, and Alzheimer's Disease

1. Describe normal changes of aging in the brain

As a person ages, some of the ability to think logically and clearly may be lost. This ability is called **cognition**. When some of this ability is lost, a person is said to have **cognitive impairment**. How much cognition is lost depends on the individual. Cognitive impairment affects concentration and memory. Elderly residents may lose their memories of recent events, which can be frustrating for them. Nursing assistants can help by encouraging them to make lists of things to remember and writing down names, events, and phone numbers. Other normal changes of aging in the brain include slower reaction time, difficulty finding or using the right words, and sleeping less.

2. Discuss confusion and delirium

Confusion is the inability to think clearly and logically. A confused person has trouble focusing his attention and may feel disoriented. Confusion interferes with the ability to make decisions. The person's personality may change. He may not know his name, the date, other people, or where he is. A confused person may be angry, depressed, or irritable.

Confusion may come on suddenly or gradually. It can be temporary or permanent. Confusion is more common in the elderly. It may occur when a person is in the hospital. Some common causes of confusion include the following:

- Urinary tract infection (UTI)
- Low blood sugar
- Head trauma or head injury
- Dehydration
- Nutritional problems
- Fever
- Sudden drop in body temperature
- Lack of oxygen
- Medications
- Infections
- Brain tumor
- Diseases or illnesses
- Loss of sleep
- Seizures

Guidelines: Confusion

G Do not leave a confused resident alone.

G Stay calm. Provide a quiet environment.

G Speak in a lower tone of voice. Speak clearly and slowly.

G Introduce yourself each time you see the resident. Remind the resident of his or her location and name, as well as the date. A calendar can help.

G   Explain what you are going to do, using simple instructions.

G   Be patient. Do not rush the resident.

G   Talk to confused residents about plans for the day. Keeping a routine may help.

G   Encourage the use of eyeglasses and hearing aids. Make sure they are clean and are not damaged.

G   Promote self-care and independence.

G   Do not leave cleaning agents, such as liquid soap, or personal care products, such as lotions or toothpaste, where the resident can access them. A person who is confused may try to eat or drink these products.

G   Report observations to the nurse.

Delirium is a state of severe confusion that occurs suddenly; it is usually temporary. Some causes are infections, disease, fluid imbalances, and poor nutrition. Drugs and alcohol may also cause delirium. Signs and symptoms of delirium include the following:

*   Agitation

*   Anger

*   Depression

*   Irritability

*   Disorientation

*   Trouble focusing

*   Problems with speech

*   Changes in sensation and perception

*   Changes in consciousness

*   Decrease in short-term memory

Nursing assistants should report these signs and symptoms to the nurse. The goal of treatment is to control or reverse the cause. Emergency care may be needed, as well as a stay in a hospital.

Confusion and Delirium

When communicating with a person who is confused or disoriented, the nursing assistant should

*   Not raise her voice or shout

*   Use the person's name, and speak clearly in simple sentences

*   Use facial expressions and body language to aid in understanding

*   Take action to reduce distractions in the environment, such as turning down the TV

*   Be gentle and try to decrease fears

3. Describe dementia and define related terms

Dementia is a general term that refers to a serious loss of mental abilities such as thinking, remembering, reasoning, and communicating. As dementia advances, these losses make it difficult to perform activities of daily living such as eating, bathing, dressing, and eliminating. Dementia is not a normal part of aging (Fig. 19-1).

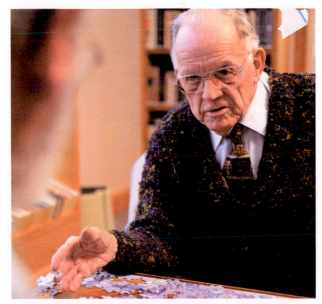

Fig. 19-1. *Some loss of cognitive ability is normal; however, dementia is not a normal part of aging.*

Here are some terms that are related to dementia:

Progressive: Once it begins, a progressive disease advances. It tends to spread to other parts of the body and affects many body functions.

Degenerative: A degenerative disease gets continually worse. It eventually causes a breakdown of body systems. It causes a greater and greater loss of mental and physical health and abilities. A degenerative disease can cause death.

Onset: The onset of a disease is the time the signs and symptoms begin.

Irreversible: An irreversible disease or condition cannot be cured. Someone with irreversible dementia (like Alzheimer's disease) will either die from the disease or die with the disease.

The following are a few of the common causes of dementia:

- Alzheimer's disease

- Multi-infarct or vascular dementia (a series of strokes causing damage to the brain)

- Lewy body dementia (abnormal structures, called *Lewy bodies*, develop in areas of the brain, causing a variety of symptoms)

- Parkinson's disease

- Huntington's disease (an inherited disease that causes certain nerve cells in the brain to waste away)

A diagnosis of dementia involves getting a patient's medical history and having a physical, as well as neurological, exam. Blood tests and imaging tests (a CT or MRI scan, for example) may be ordered. An electroencephalogram (EEG), a test using electrodes on the scalp to trace brain wave activity, may be performed. Diagnosis is a process of ruling out other possible diseases that mimic symptoms of dementia.

4. Describe Alzheimer's disease and identify its stages

Alzheimer's disease (AD) is the most common cause of dementia in the elderly. The Alzheimer's Association (alz.org/facts) estimates that 5.5 million Americans are living with Alzheimer's disease. One in 10 people age 65 and older has Alzheimer's disease. Women are more likely than men to have Alzheimer's disease and dementia. African-Americans are about two times as likely to get Alzheimer's disease as older whites, while Hispanics are about 1.5 times as likely. Although the risk of getting AD increases with age, it is not a normal part of aging.

Alzheimer's disease is a progressive, degenerative, and irreversible disease. AD causes tangled nerve fibers and protein deposits to form in the brain, eventually causing dementia. There is no known cause of AD, and there is no cure. Diagnosis is difficult, involving many physical and mental tests to rule out other causes. However, the only sure way to determine AD at this time is by autopsy. The length of time it takes AD to progress from onset to death varies greatly. According to the Alzheimer's Association, on average a person with Alzheimer's disease lives four to eight years after diagnosis. However, the person can live as long as 20 years, depending on other factors.

Symptoms of AD appear gradually. It generally begins with memory loss. As the disease progresses, it causes greater and greater loss of health and abilities. People with AD may get disoriented. They may be confused about time and place. Communication problems are common. They may lose their ability to read, write, speak, or understand. Mood and behavior changes. Aggressiveness, wandering, and withdrawal are all part of AD. Alzheimer's disease generally progresses in stages. In each stage, the symptoms become progressively worse. The majority of victims are eventually completely dependent on others for care.

Each person with Alzheimer's disease will show different symptoms at different times. For example, one resident may continue to read, but not be able to recognize a family member. Another person may be able to play a musical instrument, but may not know how to use the phone. Skills that a person has used often over a lifetime are usually kept longer (Fig. 19-2).

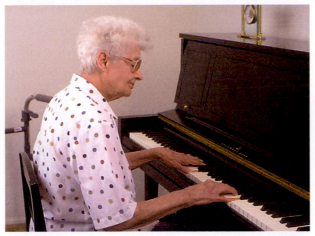

Fig. 19-2. A person with AD may continue to have skills she has used her whole life.

The Alzheimer's Association identifies three general stages of Alzheimer's disease:

Mild Alzheimer's disease (early-stage)

At this stage, the person may show some problems, such as memory loss and forgetting some words and the location of familiar objects. The person's medical examination may show problems with memory and concentration. However, the person may still be independent and able to work, drive, and do other activities.

Moderate Alzheimer's disease (middle-stage)

Generally speaking, this stage has the longest duration. At this stage, the person may show signs and symptoms such as forgetting recent events, forgetting some of one's own past experiences and background, changes in personality and behavior, and being moody or withdrawn. Other changes include changes in sleep patterns, confusion about time and place, and needing help with some activities of daily living, such as choosing appropriate clothing.

Severe Alzheimer's disease (late-stage)

During this final stage, a person may be unable to communicate with others, control movement, or respond to his surroundings. The person needs significant help with activities of daily living, including eating and eliminating. The ability to walk, sit, and swallow may be affected.

It is important for nursing assistants to encourage independence, regardless of what signs and symptoms a resident with Alzheimer's disease shows. The resident should be encouraged to do whatever he is able to do. This helps keep the resident's mind and body as active as possible. Working, socializing, reading, problem solving, and exercising should all be encouraged (Fig. 19-3). Tasks should be challenging but not frustrating. Nursing assistants can help residents succeed in doing these tasks.

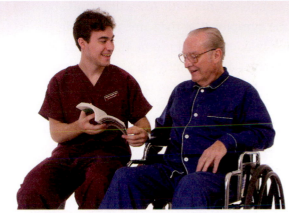

Fig. 19-3. Nursing assistants should encourage reading and other activities.

5. Identify personal attitudes helpful in caring for residents with Alzheimer's disease

These attitudes will help nursing assistants give the best possible care to residents with AD:

Do not take things personally. Alzheimer's disease is a devastating mental and physical disorder. It affects everyone who surrounds and cares for the person with AD. People with Alzheimer's disease do not have control over their words and actions. They may often be unaware of what they say or do. A resident with AD may not recognize a caregiver or do what he is supposed to do. He may ignore, accuse, or insult staff members. When this happens, it is important to remember that the behavior is due to the disease.

Be empathetic. It is helpful if the NA thinks about what it would be like to have Alzheimer's disease. She can imagine being unable to do activities of daily living and being dependent on others for care. It would be very frustrating to have no memory of recent events or to be unable to find words for what one wants to say. Nursing assistants should assume that people with AD have insight and are aware of the changes in their abilities. They should treat residents with AD with dignity and respect.

Work with the symptoms and behaviors noted. Each person with Alzheimer's disease is an individual. Residents with AD will not all show the same symptoms at the same times (Fig. 19-4). Each resident will do some things that others will never do. The best plan is to work with the behaviors that are seen on any particular day. For example, a resident with Alzheimer's disease may want to go for a walk one day, when the day before he did not want to go to the bathroom without help. If allowed by the care plan, the NA should try to go for a walk with him. Nursing assistants should notice and report changes in behavior, mood, and independence.

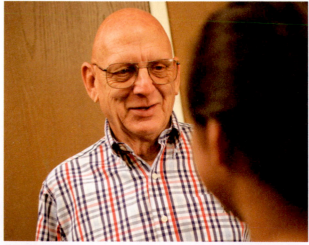

Fig. 19-4. *Each resident with AD should be treated as an individual. The NA should work with the symptoms that she sees.*

Work as a team. Symptoms and behaviors change daily. When nursing assistants observe and report carefully, as well as listen to others' reports, the care team may be better able to develop solutions. For example, a resident with AD may refuse to eat her meals. An NA might

discover that if he sits next to the resident and eats something while she has food in front of her, the resident will also eat. The NA may also notice that the resident always eats her bite-sized sandwiches or some other specific food. This is important to report to the team and can help the team provide better nutrition for the resident. Nursing assistants are in a great position to give details about residents. Being with residents often allows them to be experts on each case. NAs should make the most of this opportunity. Residents with AD may not be able to recognize or distinguish between aides, nurses, or administrators. All staff members should be prepared to help when needed.

Be aware of the difficulties associated with caregiving. Caring for someone with dementia can be physically and emotionally exhausting, as well as incredibly stressful. NAs should take care of themselves so they can continue to provide the best care (Fig. 19-5). Being aware of the body's signals to slow down, rest, or eat better is important. Each NA's feelings are real; they have a right to them. Mistakes should be viewed as learning experiences. Unmanaged stress can cause physical and emotional problems. When stress feels overwhelming, an NA can talk to her supervisor. Chapter 31 has more information on handling stress.

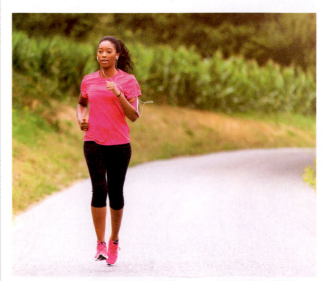

Fig. 19-5. *Regular exercise is an important part of taking care of oneself.*

Work with family members. Family members can be a wonderful resource. They can help a nursing assistant learn more about a resident. They also give stability and comfort to the person with Alzheimer's disease. NAs should build relationships with family members and keep the lines of communication open.

In addition, NAs should be reassuring to family members. It is very difficult for families to see a loved one's health and abilities decline. When residents with AD exhibit problem behaviors, it can be stressful for the family. NAs can help by reassuring family members that they understand that this behavior is part of the disease.

Remember the goals of the care plan. Along with the practical tasks that nursing assistants perform, the care plan will also call for maintaining residents' dignity and self-esteem. NAs should help residents be as independent as possible.

6. List strategies for better communication with residents with Alzheimer's disease

Many things can be done to improve communication with residents who have Alzheimer's disease. Providing person-centered care for residents with AD means responding to each resident as an individual. The guidelines below can help with communication:

Guidelines: Communicating with Residents Who Have Alzheimer's Disease

G   Always approach from the front, and do not startle the resident.

G   Smile and look happy to see the resident. Be friendly.

G   Determine how close the resident wants you to be.

G   Communicate in a calm area with little background noise and distraction.

G   Always identify yourself and use the resi-

dent's name. Continue to use the resident's name during the conversation.

G   Speak slowly, using a lower tone of voice than normal. This is calming and easier to understand.

G   Repeat yourself, using the same words and phrases, as often as needed.

G   Use signs, pictures, gestures, or written words to help communicate.

G   Break complex tasks into smaller, simpler ones. Give simple, step-by-step instructions as necessary.

In addition, communication with residents with AD can be helped by using these techniques for specific situations:

If the resident is frightened or anxious:

G   Speak slowly in a low, calm voice. Speak in a quiet area with few distractions (Fig. 19-6).

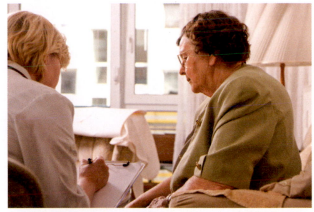

Fig. 19-6. Nursing assistants should try to find a room with little background noise and distraction when communicating with a resident with AD.

G   Try to see and hear yourself as they might. Always describe what you are going to do.

G   Use simple words and short sentences. If helping with care, list steps one at a time.

G   Check your body language; make sure you are not tense or hurried.

If the resident forgets or shows memory loss:

G   Repeat yourself, using the same words if you need to repeat an instruction or question. However, you may be using a word the resident does not understand, such as *tired*. Try other words like *nap*, *lie down*, or *rest*. Repetition can be soothing for a resident with Alzheimer's disease. Many people with AD will repeat words, phrases, questions, or actions. This is called **perseveration**. Do not try to stop a resident who is perseverating. Answer the questions, using the same words each time, until he stops. Even though responding over and over may frustrate you, it communicates comfort and security.

G   Keep messages simple. Break complex tasks into smaller, simpler ones.

If the resident has trouble finding words or names:

G   Suggest a word that sounds correct. If this upsets the resident, learn from it. Try not to correct a resident who uses an incorrect word. As words (written and spoken) become more difficult, smiling, touching, and hugging can help show care and concern (Fig. 19-7). Remember, however, that some people find touch frightening or unwelcome.

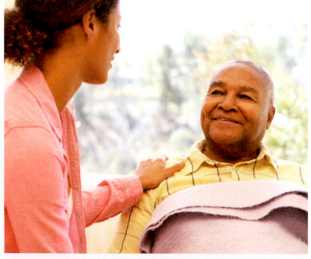

Fig. 19-7. Touch, smiles, and laughter will be understood longer, even after speaking abilities decline.

If the resident seems not to understand basic instructions or questions:

G   Ask the resident to repeat your words. Use short words and sentences, allowing time to answer.

G   Note the communication methods that are effective and use them.

G   Watch for nonverbal cues as the ability to talk lessens. Observe body language—eyes, hands, and face.

G   Use signs, pictures, gestures, or written words. For example, a picture of a toilet on the bathroom door can help remind a resident where the bathroom is. Combining verbal and nonverbal communication is helpful. For example, you can say, "Let's get dressed now," while holding up clothes.

If the resident wants to say something but cannot:

G   Encourage the resident to point, gesture, or act it out.

G   If the resident is obviously upset but cannot explain why, offer comfort with a smile, or try to distract him. Verbal communication may be frustrating.

If the resident does not remember how to perform basic tasks:

G   Break each activity into simple steps. For instance, "Let's go for a walk. Stand up. Put on your sweater. First the right arm..." Always encourage residents to do what they can.

If the resident insists on doing something that is unsafe or not allowed:

G   Redirect activities toward something else. Try to limit the times you say "Don't."

If the resident hallucinates (sees or hears things that are not really happening) or is paranoid or accusing:

G   Try not to take it personally.

G   Try to redirect behavior or ignore it. People with AD often have a limited attention span. This behavior usually passes quickly.

If the resident is depressed or lonely:

G   Take time, one-on-one, to ask how he is feeling and really listen to the response.

G Try to involve the resident in activities. Always report signs of depression to the nurse (Chapter 20).

If the resident repeatedly asks to go home:

G Ask the resident to tell you what his home was like and how he felt being there.

G Redirect or guide the conversation and/or the resident's activities to something he enjoys.

G Expect that the resident may continue to ask to go home and be patient and gentle in your response.

If the resident is verbally abusive or uses bad language:

G Remember it is the dementia speaking, not the person. Try to ignore the language, and redirect attention to something else.

If the resident has lost most verbal skills:

G Use nonverbal skills. As speaking abilities decline, people with AD will still understand touch, smiles, and laughter for much longer. Remember that some people do not like to be touched. Approach touching slowly and be gentle. Softly touch the hand or place your arm around the resident. A smile can show affection and caring and say you want to help (Fig. 19-8).

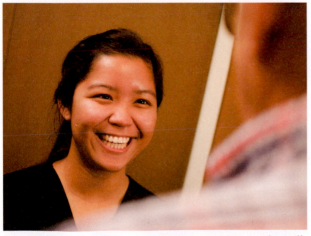

Fig. 19-8. Smiling can communicate positivity and a willingness to help.

G Even after verbal skills are lost, signs, labels, and gestures can reach people with dementia.

G Assume people with AD can understand more than they can express. Do not talk about them as though they were not there or treat them like children.

7. Explain general principles that will help assist residents with personal care

Nursing assistants should use the same procedures for personal care and activities of daily living for residents with Alzheimer's disease as they would with other residents. However, here are some general principles that will help NAs give the best care:

1. **Develop a routine and stick to it.** Being consistent is important for residents who are confused and easily upset.

2. **Promote self-care.** Helping residents care for themselves as much as possible will help them cope with this difficult disease.

3. **Take care of yourself, both mentally and physically.** This will help give the best care.

8. List and describe interventions for problems with common activities of daily living (ADLs)

As Alzheimer's disease worsens, residents will have trouble doing their activities of daily living. Below are interventions to help residents with these problems. An **intervention** means a way to change an action or development.

Guidelines: Assisting with ADLs for Residents Who Have Alzheimer's Disease

If the resident has problems with bathing:

G Schedule bathing when the resident is least agitated. Be organized so the bath can be quick. Give sponge baths if the resident resists a shower or tub bath.

G Prepare the resident before bathing. Hand him the supplies (washcloth, soap, shampoo, towels). This serves as a visual aid.

G   Take a walk with the resident down the hall, stopping at the tub or shower room, rather than talking directly about the bath.

G   Make sure the bathroom is well lit and is at a comfortable temperature.

G   Provide privacy during the bath.

G   Be calm and quiet when bathing a resident and keep the process simple.

G   Be sensitive when talking to a resident about bathing.

G   Give the resident a washcloth to hold. This can distract him while you finish the bath.

G   Always follow safety precautions. Ensure safety by using nonslip mats, tub seats, and handholds.

G   Be flexible about when to bathe a resident. A resident may not always be in the mood. Also, be aware that not everyone bathes with the same frequency. Understand if a resident does not want to bathe.

G   Be relaxed and allow the resident to enjoy the bath. Offer encouragement and praise.

G   Let the resident do as much as possible during the bath.

G   Check the skin regularly for signs of irritation or breakdown during the bath.

If the resident has problems with grooming and dressing:

G   Help with grooming to help residents feel attractive and dignified (Fig. 19-9).

G   Avoid delays or interruptions while dressing.

G   Provide privacy by closing doors and curtains. The resident should be dressed in the resident's room.

G   Show the resident some of her clothing. This brings up the idea of dressing.

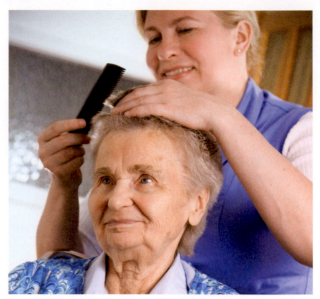

Fig. 19-9. *Assist residents with grooming to promote dignity and self-esteem.*

G   Encourage the resident to pick clothes to wear. Simplify this by giving just a few choices. Make sure the clothing is clean and appropriate. Lay out clothes in the order in which they are put on (Fig. 19-10). Choose clothes that are simple to put on, such as slip-on instead of lace-up shoes and pants or skirts instead of dresses. Some people with Alzheimer's disease make a habit of layering clothing regardless of the weather.

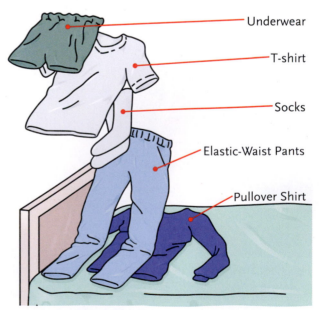

Underwear

T-shirt

Socks

Elastic-Waist Pants

Pullover Shirt

Fig. 19-10. *Clothes should be laid out in the order in which they should be put on.*

G   Break the task down into simple steps. Introduce one step at a time. Do not rush the resident.

G   Use a friendly, calm voice when speaking. Praise and encourage the resident at each step.

Residents' Rights

Rights with Alzheimer's Disease

Residents with AD may not be aware when their bodies are exposed. Nursing assistants can protect residents' legal rights to privacy by keeping them dressed or covered when in bed. Residents with AD should be encouraged to make the decisions they are able to make, such as what shirt to wear or where to sit to eat.

If the resident has problems with elimination:

G   Encourage fluids. Never withhold or discourage fluids because a resident has problems with urinary incontinence. Report to the nurse if the resident is not drinking fluids. Follow the schedule in the care plan for drinking fluids.

G   Mark the bathroom with a sign or a picture as a reminder of where it is and to use the toilet.

G   Make sure there is enough light in the bathroom and on the way there.

G   Note when the resident is incontinent over two to three days. Check her every 30 minutes. This can help determine "bathroom times." Take the resident to the bathroom just before her bathroom time.

G   Observe toilet patterns for two to three nights for incontinence in order to try to determine nighttime bathroom times.

G   Take the resident to the bathroom after drinking fluids. Take the resident to the bathroom before and after meals and before bedtime. Make sure the resident actually urinates before getting off the toilet.

G   Put lids on trash cans, wastebaskets, or other containers if the resident urinates or defecates in them.

G   Family or friends may be upset by their loved one's incontinence. Be professional when cleaning after episodes of incontinence. Do not show disgust or irritation.

If the resident has problems with nutrition:

G   Encourage nutritious food. Food may not interest a resident with Alzheimer's disease, or he may forget to eat. It may be of great interest, but he may only want to eat a few types of food. A resident with AD is at risk for malnutrition.

G   Have meals at regular, consistent times each day. You may need to remind the resident that it is mealtime. Familiar foods should be served and should look and smell appetizing.

G   Make sure there is adequate lighting.

G   Keep noise and distractions to a minimum during meals.

G   Keep the task of eating simple. If the resident is restless, try smaller, more frequent meals. Finger foods (foods that are easy to pick up with the fingers) work best. They allow residents to choose the food they want to eat. Examples of finger foods that may be good to serve are sandwiches cut into fourths, chicken nuggets or small pieces of cooked boneless chicken, fish sticks, cheese cubes, halved hard-boiled eggs, and fresh fruit and soft vegetables cut into bite-sized pieces.

G   Do not serve steaming or very hot foods or drinks.

G   Use a simple place setting with a single eating utensil. Remove other items from the table (Fig. 19-11). Plain plates without patterns or colors work best.

G   Put only one item of food on the plate at a time. Multiple kinds of food on a plate or a tray may be overwhelming.

G   Give simple, clear instructions. Residents with AD may not understand how to eat or use utensils. Help the resident taste a sample of the meal first. Place a spoon to the lips. This will encourage the resident to open her mouth. Ask the resident to open her mouth.

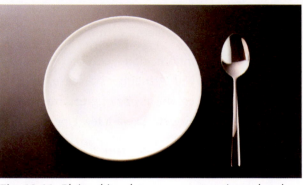

Fig. 19-11. Plain white plates on a contrasting-colored surface may help avoid confusion and distraction.

G   Guide the resident through the meal, providing simple instructions. Offer regular drinks of water, juice, and other fluids to prevent dehydration.

G   Use adaptive equipment for eating, such as special spoons and bowls, as needed.

G   If the resident needs to be fed, do so slowly. Offer small pieces of food.

G   Make mealtimes simple and relaxed, not rushed. Give the resident time to swallow before the next bite or drink.

G   Seat the resident with others at small tables. This encourages socializing.

G   Observe and report eating or swallowing problems, as well as changes in eating habits. Monitor weight accurately and frequently.

To promote the resident's physical health:

G   Prevent infections and follow Standard Precautions.

G   Observe the resident's physical health and report any potential problems. People with dementia may not notice their own health problems.

G   Help residents wash their hands frequently.

G   Give careful skin care to prevent pressure injuries.

G   Watch for signs of pain. A person who has Alzheimer's disease may not be able to express that he is in pain. Nonverbal signs that a resident may be in pain include grimacing or clenching fists (Fig. 19-12). A resident may be agitated or have an angry outburst. Report possible signs of pain to the nurse.

G   Maintain a daily exercise routine.

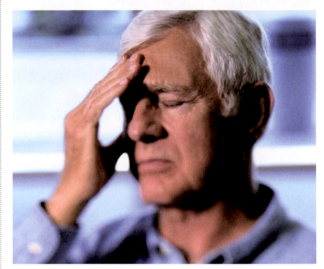

Fig. 19-12. Be aware of nonverbal signs of pain, such as holding or rubbing a body part. Report these signs to the nurse.

To promote the resident's mental and emotional health:

•   Maintain self-esteem by encouraging independence in activities of daily living.

•   Share in enjoyable activities, such as looking at pictures, talking, and reminiscing.

•   Reward positive and independent behavior with smiles and warm touches.

9. List and describe interventions for common difficult behaviors related to Alzheimer's disease

Below are some common difficult behaviors that nursing assistants may face when working with residents who have Alzheimer's disease. Each resident is different, and NAs should work with each person as an individual. Details of behavior should be reported to the nurse.

Agitation: A resident who is excited, restless, or troubled is said to be **agitated**. Feeling insecure or frustrated, encountering new people or places, and changing a routine can all trigger this behavior. A **trigger** is a situation that leads to agitation. Even watching television can cause agitation, as a person with AD may lose his ability to distinguish fiction from reality. If a resident is agitated, the NA should

* Try to remove triggers, keep a routine, and avoid frustration. Redirecting the resident's attention may help.

* Reduce noise and distractions. Focusing on a familiar activity, such as sorting things or looking at pictures, may help.

* Stay calm and use a low, soothing voice to speak to and reassure the resident.

Sundowning: When a person with AD gets restless and agitated in the late afternoon, evening, or night, it is called **sundowning**. Sundowning may be caused by hunger or fatigue, a change in routine or caregiver, or any new or frustrating situation. If a resident experiences sundowning, the NA should

* Avoid stressful situations during this time. Limit activities, appointments, trips, and visits.

* Play soft music.

* Set a bedtime routine and keep it.

* Recognize when sundowning occurs and plan a calming activity just before.

* Remove caffeine from the diet.

* Provide snacks.

* Give a soothing back massage.

* Distract the resident with a simple, calm activity like looking at a magazine.

* Maintain a daily exercise routine.

Catastrophic Reactions: When a person with AD overreacts to something, it is called a **cata-**

strophic reaction. It may be triggered by any of the following:

* Fatigue

* Change of routine, environment, or caregiver

* Overstimulation (too much noise or activity)

* Difficult choices or tasks

* Physical pain or discomfort, including hunger or a need to use the toilet

An NA can respond to catastrophic reactions as she would to agitation or sundowning. For example, she can remove triggers and help the resident focus on a soothing activity.

Violent Behavior. A resident who attacks, hits, or threatens someone is using violence. Violence may be triggered by many situations. These include frustration, overstimulation, or a change in routine, environment, or caregiver. If a resident is violent, the NA should

* Call for help if needed.

* Block blows but never hit back.

* Step out of reach and stay calm.

* Avoid leaving residents alone.

* Try to remove triggers.

* Use the same techniques to calm residents as for agitation.

Pacing and Wandering: A resident who walks back and forth in the same area is **pacing**. A resident who walks aimlessly around the facility or the facility grounds is **wandering** (Fig. 19-13). Pacing and wandering may have some of the following causes:

* Restlessness

* Hunger

* Disorientation

* Incontinence or the need to use the bathroom

* Constipation

- Pain

- Forgetting how or where to sit down

- Too much daytime napping

- Need for exercise

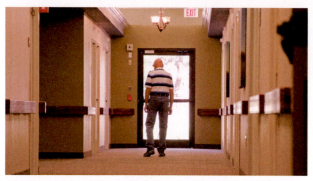

Fig. 19-13. A resident with AD who is walking aimlessly around the facility is wandering.

If a resident paces or wanders, the NA should

- Remove causes when possible. For example, give nutritious snacks, encourage an exercise routine, and maintain a toileting schedule.

- Let residents pace or wander in a safe and secure (locked) area where staff can keep an eye on them (Fig. 19-14).

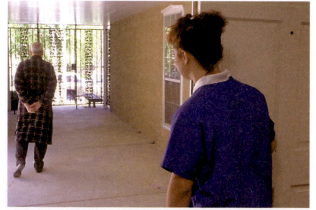

Fig. 19-14. Residents should be in a safe, secured area if they pace or wander.

- Redirect attention to something the resident enjoys, such as suggesting going on a walk together.

- Mark rooms with signs or pictures, such as stop signs or "closed" signs, as this may prevent residents from wandering into areas where they should not go.

- Report to the nurse immediately if a resident wanders away from a protected area and does not return, or **elopes**.

Elopement

Residents with Alzheimer's disease or other forms of dementia might try to elope, or leave a facility unsupervised and unnoticed. It is very important that residents who elope are located and returned to the facility as quickly as possible. The longer a resident is gone, the greater danger he or she might encounter. If an NA believes a resident might have eloped, she must alert her supervisor immediately. Residents who elope are often found near where they were last seen, and the earlier a search is begun, the more likely the resident is to be found nearby and safe.

Hallucinations or Delusions: A resident who sees, hears, smells, tastes, or feels things that are not there is having **hallucinations**. A resident who believes things that are not true is having **delusions**. If a resident is experiencing hallucinations and/or delusions, the NA should

- Ignore harmless hallucinations and delusions.

- Reassure a resident who seems agitated or worried.

- Not argue with a resident who is imagining things. Challenging the resident serves no purpose and can make matters worse. The feelings are real to the resident. The NA should not tell the resident that she sees or hears his hallucinations. She should redirect the resident to other activities or thoughts.

- Be calm and reassure the resident that she is there to help.

Depression: People who become withdrawn, isolated, lack energy, and stop eating or doing things they used to enjoy may be depressed. Depression may have many causes, including the following:

- Loss of independence

- Inability to cope

- Feelings of failure or fear

- Reality of facing a progressive, degenerative illness

- Chemical imbalance

Chapter 20 contains more information about depression and its symptoms. If a resident is depressed, the NA should

- Report signs of depression to the nurse immediately. It is an illness that can be treated with medication.

- Observe for triggers that cause changes in mood.

- Encourage independence, self-care, and activity.

- Listen to residents if they want to share their feelings or talk about their moods.

- Find ways to encourage social interaction.

Perseveration or Repetitive Phrasing: Residents who have dementia may repeat words, phrases, questions, or activities over and over again. This is called *perseverating* or **repetitive phrasing**. Such behavior may be caused by several factors, including disorientation or confusion. The NA should be patient with this behavior and not try to silence or stop the resident. She should answer questions each time they are asked, using the same words each time.

Disruptiveness: Disruptive behavior is anything that disturbs others, such as yelling, banging on furniture, and slamming doors. Often this behavior is triggered by pain, constipation, frustration, or a wish for attention. To prevent or respond to disruptive behavior, the NA should

- Be calm and friendly, and try to find out why the behavior is occurring. There may be a physical reason, such as pain or discomfort.

- Gently try to direct the resident to a private area.

- Notice and praise improvements in the

resident's behavior, being sensitive to avoid treating the resident like a child.

- Tell the resident about any changes in schedules, routines, or the environment in advance. Involving the resident in developing routine activities and schedules may help.

- Encourage the resident to join in independent activities that are safe (for example, folding towels). This helps the resident feel in charge and can prevent feelings of powerlessness. Independence is power.

- Help the resident find ways to cope. Focusing on activities the resident may still be able to do, such as knitting or crafts, can provide a diversion.

Inappropriate Social Behavior: Inappropriate social behavior may include cursing, name-calling, or yelling. As with violent or disruptive behavior, there may be many reasons why a resident is behaving in this way. The NA should try not to take it personally. The resident may only be reacting to frustration or other stress. The NA should remain calm and be reassuring. She can try to find out what caused the behavior. Possible causes include too much noise, too many people, and too much stress, pain, or discomfort. If the resident is disturbing others, the NA should gently direct him to a private area if possible. Any physical abuse or serious verbal abuse should be reported to the nurse.

Inappropriate Sexual Behavior: Inappropriate sexual behavior, such as removing clothing, touching one's own genitals in public, or trying to touch others can disturb or embarrass those who see it. It is helpful to stay calm and be professional when this behavior occurs. The NA should not overreact, as this may reinforce the behavior. Trying to determine the cause of the problem may help. Is the behavior actually intentional? Is it consistent? If distracting the resident does not work, the NA can gently direct him to a private area and inform the nurse. A resident may be reacting to a need for physical stimulation or affection. Ways to provide physical stimulation include giving backrubs, offering a soft stuffed animal to cuddle, providing comforting blankets, or giving physical touch that is appropriate.

Hoarding and Rummaging: Rummaging is going through drawers, closets, or personal items that belong to oneself or to other people. **Hoarding** is collecting and putting things away in a guarded way. These behaviors are not within the control of a person with Alzheimer's disease. Rummaging and hoarding should not be considered stealing. Stealing is planned and requires a conscious effort. In most cases, the person with AD is only collecting something that catches his attention. It is common for those with AD to wander and collect things. They may carry these objects around for a while, and then leave them in other places. This is not intentional. People with AD will often take their own things and leave them in another room, not knowing what they are doing. If the resident hoards or rummages, the NA should

- Label all personal belongings with the resident's name and room number. This way there is no confusion about what belongs to whom.

- Place a label, symbol, or object on the resident's door. This helps the resident find his own room.

- Not tell the family that their loved one is stealing from others.

- Prepare the family so they are not upset when they find items that do not belong to their family member.

- Ask the family to tell staff if they notice unfamiliar items in the room.

- Regularly check areas where residents store items. They may store uneaten food in these places. Providing a rummage drawer—a drawer with items that are safe for the resident to take with him—can help.

Sleep Disturbances: Residents with AD may experience a number of sleep disturbances. If a resident experiences sleep problems, the NA should

- Make sure that the resident gets moderate exercise throughout the day, appropriate to his condition. The NA can encourage him to participate in activities he enjoys.

- Allow the resident to spend some time each day in natural sunlight if possible. Exposure to light and dark at appropriate times can help establish restful sleep patterns.

- Reduce light and noise as much as possible during nighttime hours.

- Discourage sleeping during the day if possible.

Suspicion: A person with Alzheimer's disease often becomes suspicious as the disease progresses. Residents may accuse staff or family members of lying to them or stealing from them. Suspicion may escalate to paranoia (having intense feelings of distrust and believing others are "out to get them"). When a resident is acting suspicious, the NA should not argue with him. Arguing just increases defensiveness. Instead, the NA should offer reassurance and be understanding and supportive.

Safety in the Home for a Client with AD

A nurse should assess a home's safety before the home health aide (HHA) visits a client with Alzheimer's disease. She will suggest changes that need to be made. Examples include using gates on stairways, putting locks on certain doors, and removing clutter. When the client's condition changes, the HHA should report it to her supervisor. Another visit will be made to reassess the home and make further changes. In general, the HHA can follow these safety guidelines:

For disoriented clients:

- Use signs to mark rooms, including stop signs on rooms that should not be entered.

- Use calendars and other reminders of day, date, and location.

- Put bells on the door to indicate when someone is coming or going.

- Keep pictures and familiar objects around.

- Put stickers or brightly colored tape on glass doors, large windows, or glass furniture.

For clients who wander:

- Use locks on doors. These can be installed lower or higher than usual, so the client will not see them.

- Install alarms that sound when exit doors are opened.

- Have clients wear identification. Sew labels into clothes.

- Alert neighbors that the client may wander. Show them a recent photo of the client. Keep a recent photo handy, as well as a piece of clothing the client has worn. These can help police and police dogs track a client who has wandered away.

For clients who pace:

- Remove clutter and throw rugs.

- Do not rearrange furniture.

- Do not wax floors.

- Be sure shoes and slippers fit and have nonslip soles.

For clients who have difficulty walking:

- Keep areas well lit, even at night.

- Block access to stairs with a gate.

- Clear walkways of electrical cords and clutter.

General tips include the following:

- Keep medications and other chemicals out of reach.

- Display emergency numbers, including Poison Control, and the client's home address somewhere they can be easily seen.

- Use red tape around radiators or heating vents to prevent burns.

- Check refrigerator and hiding places for spoiled food.

- Prevent kitchen accidents by removing knobs on stoves, unplugging toasters and other small appliances, and supervising kitchen visits.

Residents' Rights

Abuse and Alzheimer's Disease

People with Alzheimer's disease may be at a higher risk for abuse. One reason for this is that caring for someone with Alzheimer's disease is very difficult. There are many psychological and physical demands placed on caregivers.

To help manage the stress of caring for people with AD, nursing assistants should take care of themselves, both mentally and physically. This will help them give the best care. If needed, a supervisor can provide more resources to help an NA cope.

Nursing assistants must never abuse residents in any way. If an NA notices someone else abusing a resident, he is legally required to report it. All nursing assistants are responsible for residents' safety and should take this responsibility seriously.

10. Describe creative therapies for residents with Alzheimer's disease

Although Alzheimer's disease cannot be cured, there are techniques to improve the quality of life for residents with AD, including the following.

Validation therapy means letting residents believe they live in the past or in imaginary circumstances. **Validating** means giving value to or approving. When using validation therapy, the NA should make no attempt to reorient the resident to actual circumstances. She can explore the resident's beliefs and should not argue with or correct him. Validating can give comfort and reduce agitation. Validation therapy is useful in cases of severe dementia.

Example: Mr. Baldwin tells the NA that he does not want to eat lunch today because he is going out to a restaurant with his wife. The NA knows his wife has been dead for many years and that Mr. Baldwin can no longer eat out in restaurants. Instead of telling him that he is not going out to eat, the NA asks what restaurant he is going to and what he will order. She suggests that he eat a good lunch now because sometimes the service is slow in restaurants (Fig. 19-15).

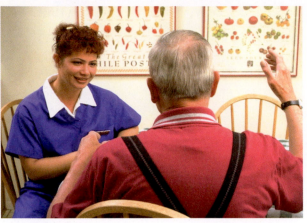

Fig. 19-15. Validation therapy accepts a resident's fantasies without attempting to reorient him to reality.

Benefits: By playing along with Mr. Baldwin's fantasy, the NA lets him know that she takes him seriously. She does not think of him as a crazy person or a child who does not know what is happening in his own life. She also learns more about the resident. He used to enjoy eating in restaurants and liked certain dishes. Eating out is something he probably associates with being with his wife. This knowledge can help the NA give better care in the future.

Reminiscence therapy involves encouraging residents to remember and talk about the past. The NA can explore memories by asking about details. Reminiscence therapy can help elderly people remember pleasant times in their past and allow caregivers to increase their understanding of clients. It is useful in many stages of Alzheimer's disease, but especially with moderate to severe dementia.

Example: Mr. Benton, an 86-year-old man with Alzheimer's disease, fought in the Korean War. In his room are many mementos of the war—pictures of his war buddies, a medal he was given, and more. The NA asks him to tell him where he was sent in the war. The NA asks him more detailed questions about his experiences. Eventually the resident shares a lot: the friends he made in the service, why he was given the medal, times when he was scared, and how much he missed his family (Fig. 19-16).

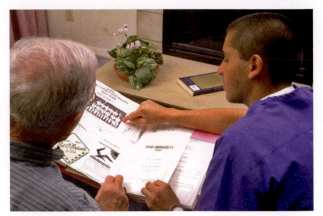

Fig. 19-16. Reminiscence therapy encourages a resident to remember and talk about his past.

Benefits: By asking questions about Mr. Benton's experiences in the war, the NA shows an interest in him as a person, not just as a resident. This lets the resident show that he is a person who was competent, social, responsible, and brave. This boosts his self-esteem. The NA also learns that Mr. Benton cared very much for his wife and daughter.

Activity therapy uses activities that the resident enjoys to prevent boredom and frustration. These activities also promote self-esteem. The NA can help the resident take walks, do puzzles, listen to music, read, or do other things she enjoys (Fig. 19-17). Activities may be done in groups or one-on-one. Activity therapy is useful in most stages of AD.

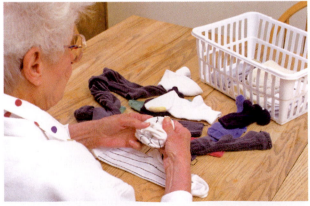

Fig. 19-17. Activities that are not frustrating can be helpful for residents with AD. They promote mental exercise.

Example: Mrs. Hoebel, a 70-year-old woman with AD, was a librarian for almost 45 years. She loves books and reading, but she cannot read much anymore. The NA obtains books from the facility that are filled with pictures. Mrs. Hoebel sits with the books, sorting them, turning pages, and looking at pictures.

Benefits: Mrs. Hoebel can enjoy an activity that always brought her pleasure. She feels competent, because she is sorting books and looking at books, which are tasks she can handle. The NA shows her that she cares about her by taking the time to show an interest in her past. This may lead the resident to associate positive feelings with the NA.

Music Therapy

Music therapy involves using music to accomplish specific goals, such as managing stress and improving mood and cognition. This type of therapy has been used successfully with people who have Alzheimer's disease. Music is a form of sensory stimulation. Hearing familiar songs can cause a response in people with dementia who do not respond well or at all to other treatments. Music & Memory is a nonprofit organization that brings personalized music into the lives of the elderly. Their website, musicandmemory.org, provides more information.

11. Discuss how Alzheimer's disease may affect the family

Alzheimer's disease requires the person's family to make adjustments, which may be difficult. The disease progresses at different rates, and people with AD will need more care as it progresses. Eventually most people with AD need constant care. How well the family is able to cope with the effects of the disease depends, in part, on the family's emotional and financial resources.

A person with AD may be living alone, which can cause the family to worry about her health and safety. Financial resources may be limited, which adds to stress levels. Finding money needed to pay expenses of home care or adult day services can be difficult. Families do not

know what goes on when no one is in the home. They may be afraid that the person is not caring for herself, may not take medications properly, could wander away, or could cause a fire.

A person with AD may be living with her family, which can cause stress and other emotional difficulties for all involved. The household schedule has to change; family members will lose the freedom to come and go as they please. Family members must monitor the loved one's activities and provide constant care. They may lose sleep, as well as lose time to do their own activities and relax.

Alzheimer's disease introduces other stressors, too. It is very difficult to watch a loved one's personality change and her health and abilities deteriorate. It is also hard to switch roles—to go from being a child who was once cared for by the parent to being the one caring for the parent.

Families may make the decision to place a loved one with AD into a long-term care facility for any number of reasons. They may have safety concerns or may not be able to care for the person at home. The family may not be able to handle the issues that AD causes, such as the problem behaviors or the inability to perform personal care. The person with AD may not want her family to do the needed personal care. There may be no available family caregiver.

After making the decision to place a person with AD in a long-term care facility, family members usually feel guilty, even if they know that placement is necessary. The person with AD may be angry and unable to understand the decision. Families worry about mistreatment and are sensitive to being judged by others. They also feel loss and a change in the relationship with their family member.

Family members are making emotional adjustments, just as residents are. They may be experiencing frustration, fear, sadness, anger, loneliness, and depression. It is important for families to be able to express their feelings. Chapter 8 contains more information about how to respond to emotional needs of families. Nursing assistants should be sensitive to the big adjustments that residents and their families are making. If help is needed, the NA can refer them to her supervisor.

12. Identify community resources available to people with Alzheimer's disease and their families

There are many resources, such as organizations, books, counseling, and support groups, available for people with Alzheimer's disease and their families. The Alzheimer's Association has a helpline that is available 24 hours a day, seven days a week for information, referral, and support. The number is 800-272-3900, and the website is alz.org. The National Institute on Aging has information available by calling 800-438-4380 or on their Alzheimer's Disease Education and Referral (ADEAR) Center website, nia.nih.gov/alzheimers. Healthcare professionals can also be of assistance. Support groups are often helpful because many people in the group are experiencing the same kinds of emotions and problems. People often find it is helpful to know that they are not alone in what they are going through. People in support groups often share tips and ideas for care and interventions for problems, which can be beneficial. NAs should inform the nurse if they think residents and/or their families could benefit from a list of community resources.

Chapter Review

1. What does cognitive impairment affect?

2. How can confusion affect a person?

3. Define *delirium* and list five possible causes.

4. What is dementia?

5. Alzheimer's disease is a progressive, degenerative, and irreversible disease. What does this mean?

6. What type of skills does a person with Alzheimer's disease usually retain?

7. What can a nursing assistant encourage residents to do that may help slow the progression of Alzheimer's disease?

8. Why should an NA work with the symptoms and behaviors she observes in a resident who has Alzheimer's disease?

9. What is the best way for an NA to respond to a resident who is perseverating (repeating words, phrases, questions, or actions)?

10. Why may developing a routine be helpful for a resident who has Alzheimer's disease?

11. How many items of food should be put on a plate or tray at a time?

12. How might the NA remind a resident who has Alzheimer's disease where the bathroom is?

13. What are six ways that an NA can respond to a resident who is experiencing sundowning (becoming restless and agitated in the late afternoon, evening, or night)?

14. Describe these creative therapies for Alzheimer's disease: validation therapy, reminiscence therapy, and activity therapy.

15. What difficulties might families of people who have Alzheimer's disease face?

16. List two community resources that may help a person who has Alzheimer's disease.

20 Mental Health and Mental Illness

1. Identify seven characteristics of mental health

Mental health is the normal functioning of emotional and intellectual abilities. A person who is mentally healthy is able to:

- Get along with others (Fig. 20-1)
- Adapt to change
- Care for self and others
- Give and accept love
- Deal with situations that cause anxiety, disappointment, and frustration
- Take responsibility for decisions, feelings, and actions
- Control and fulfill desires and impulses appropriately

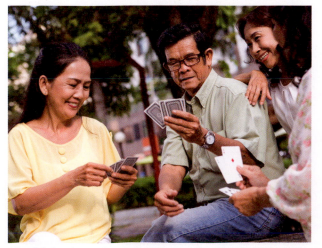

Fig. 20-1. The ability to interact well with other people is a characteristic of mental health.

2. Identify four causes of mental illness

Although it involves the emotions and mental functions, **mental illness** is a disorder like any physical disorder. It produces signs and symptoms and affects the body's ability to function. It responds to proper treatment and care. Mental illness disrupts a person's ability to function at a normal level in the family, home, or community. It often causes inappropriate behavior. Some signs and symptoms of mental illness are confusion, disorientation, agitation, and anxiety.

However, signs and symptoms like those of mental illness can also occur when mental illness is not present. A personal crisis, temporary physical changes in the brain, side effects from medications, or a severe change in the environment may cause a **situation response**. In a situation response, the signs and symptoms are temporary.

Mental illness can be caused or made worse by chronic stress from any of these conditions:

1. **Physical factors**: Illness, disability, or aging can cause stress that may lead to mental illness. Substance abuse or a chemical imbalance can also lead to mental illness. Self-respect and self-worth are the building blocks of mental health. They are challenged when people who are ill or disabled have difficulty with their activities of daily living (ADLs). They may become fearful of the future. They may be concerned about their dependence on others.

2. **Environmental factors**: Weak interpersonal or family relationships or traumatic early life experiences (such as suffering abuse as a child) can lead to mental illness.

3. **Heredity**: Mental illness can occur repeatedly in some families. This may be due to inherited traits or family influence.

4. **Stress**: People can tolerate different levels of stress. People have different ways of coping with stress. When the amount of stress becomes too great, a person may not be able to cope with it, and mental illness may arise.

3. Distinguish between fact and fallacy concerning mental illness

A **fallacy** is a false belief. The greatest fallacy about mental illness is that people who are mentally ill can control it. People who are mentally ill cannot simply choose to be well. Mental illness is a disorder like any physical disorder. People who are mentally healthy are usually able to control their emotions and responses. People who are mentally ill may not have this control.

Fact and Fallacy

Fact: Mental illness is a disorder like any physical illness. People with mental illness cannot control their illness through sheer force of will.

Fallacy: People with mental illness can control their illness or choose to be well.

Intellectual Disability and Mental Illness

Sometimes people confuse the meaning of the terms *intellectual disability* and *mental illness*. They are not the same. Intellectual disability is a developmental disability that causes below-average mental functioning. It may affect a person's ability to care for himself, as well as to live independently. It is not a type of mental illness. Here are some ways that it differs from mental illness:

- Intellectual disability is a permanent condition; mental illness can be temporary.

- Intellectual disability is present at birth or emerges in childhood. Mental illness may occur at any time during a person's life.

- Intellectual disability affects mental ability. Mental illness may or may not affect mental ability.

- There is no cure for an intellectual disability, although persons who are intellectually disabled can be helped. Many mental illnesses can be cured with treatment, such as medications and therapy.

Although they are different conditions, persons who have either condition need emotional support, as well as care and treatment.

4. Explain the connection between mental and physical wellness

Mental health is important to physical health. Reducing stress can help prevent some physical illnesses (Fig. 20-2). It can help people cope if illness or disability occurs. Mental health can help protect and improve physical health. The reverse is also true. Physical illness or disability can cause or worsen mental illness. The stress these conditions create takes a toll on mental health.

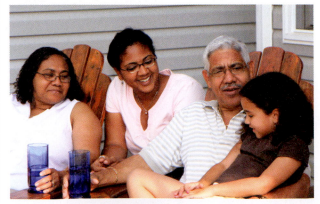

Fig. 20-2. *Social interaction can promote mental and physical health.*

5. List guidelines for communicating with residents who are mentally ill

Different types of mental illness will affect how well residents communicate. Nursing assistants should treat each resident as an individual. They should tailor their approach to the situation.

Guidelines: Communication and Mental Illness

G   Do not talk to adults as if they were children.

G   Use simple, clear statements and a normal tone of voice.

G   Be sure that what you say and how you say it show respect and concern.

G   Sit or stand at a normal distance from the resident. Be aware of your body language.

G   Be honest and direct, as you would with any resident.

G   Avoid arguments.

G   Maintain eye contact and listen carefully (Fig. 20-3).

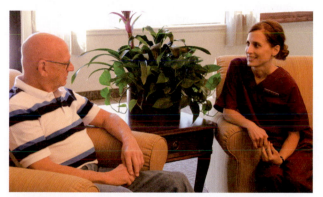

Fig. 20-3. *Maintain eye contact and sit a normal distance when communicating with residents who have a mental illness.*

6. Identify and define common defense mechanisms

Defense mechanisms are unconscious behaviors used to release tension or cope with stress. They help to block uncomfortable or threatening feelings. All people use defense mechanisms at times. However, people who are mentally ill use them to a greater degree. An overuse of these mechanisms prevents a person from understanding his emotional problems and behaviors. If a person is unable to recognize problems, he will not address them. The problems may get worse. Common defense mechanisms include the following:

Denial: Completely rejecting the thought or feeling—"I'm not upset with you!"

Projection: Seeing feelings in others that are really one's own—"My teacher hates me."

Displacement: Transferring a strong negative feeling to a safer situation—for example, an unhappy employee cannot yell at his boss for fear of losing his job. He later yells at his wife.

Rationalization: Making excuses to justify a situation—for example, after stealing something, saying, "Everybody does it."

Repression: Blocking unacceptable thoughts or painful feelings from the mind—for example, not remembering a traumatic experience.

Regression: Going back to an old, usually immature behavior—for example, throwing a temper tantrum as an adult.

7. Describe anxiety, depression, and schizophrenia

There are many degrees of mental illness, from mild to severe. A person with severe mental illness may lose touch with reality and become unable to communicate or make decisions. Some people with mild mental illness, however, seem to function normally. They may sometimes become overwhelmed by stress or overly emotional. Many signs of mental illness are simply extreme behaviors most people occasionally experience. Being able to recognize such behaviors may make it easier to understand residents who are mentally ill.

Anxiety Disorders: Anxiety is uneasiness, worry, or fear, often about a situation or condition. When a person who is mentally healthy feels anxiety, he can usually identify the cause. The anxiety fades once the cause is removed. A person who is mentally ill may feel anxiety all the time. She may not know the reason for feeling anxious. Anxiety causes physical symptoms, such as shaking, muscle aches, sweating, cold and clammy hands, dizziness, chest pain, rapid heartbeat, cold or hot flashes, a choking or smothering sensation, and a dry mouth.

Some types of anxiety disorders include the following:

Generalized anxiety disorder (GAD) is characterized by chronic anxiety and worry, even when there is no reason for concern. A person with GAD may be excessively worried about health, finances, work, or other issues.

A panic attack is an episode of intense fear that occurs along with physical symptoms, such as rapid heartbeat, chest pain, dizziness, and shortness of breath. A person having a panic attack may think he is having a heart attack or dying. Having regular panic attacks or living with constant anxiety about having another attack is classified as **panic disorder**.

Obsessive-compulsive disorder (OCD) is an anxiety disorder characterized by obsessive behavior or thoughts, which may cause the person to repeatedly perform a behavior or routine. For example, a person may wash his hands over and over again or repeatedly check to make sure the door is locked as a way to ease anxiety.

Posttraumatic stress disorder (PTSD) is an anxiety disorder brought on by experiencing or witnessing a traumatic event, such as being a victim of a violent crime or being involved in combat while in the military.

A **phobia** is an intense, irrational fear of or anxiety about an object, place, or situation. Many people are very afraid of certain things or situations. Examples include fear of dogs or fear of flying. A phobia can be long-lasting and can prevent a person from participating in normal activities. For example, the fear of being in a confined space, **claustrophobia**, may make using an elevator a terrifying experience.

Mood Disorders: Mood disorders are marked by changes in mood. **Depression** (often called **major depressive disorder** or *clinical depres-*

sion) is a type of mood disorder. Depression is characterized by a loss of interest in everything a person once cared about, and may interfere with the person's ability to work, sleep, and eat. It may cause intense mental, emotional, and physical pain and disability. Depression also makes other illnesses worse. If left untreated, it may result in suicide. The National Institute of Mental Health (NIMH, nimh.nih.gov) lists depression as one of the most common conditions associated with suicide in older adults.

Clinical depression is not a normal reaction to stress. Sadness is only one sign of this illness. Not all people who have depression complain of sadness or appear sad. Other common symptoms of clinical depression include the following:

- Pain, including headaches, abdominal pain, and other body aches

- Low energy or fatigue

- **Apathy**, or lack of interest in activities

- Irritability

- Anxiety

- Loss of appetite or overeating

- Problems with sexual functioning and desire

- Sleeplessness, difficulty sleeping, or excessive sleeping

- Lack of attention to basic personal care tasks (e.g., bathing, combing hair, changing clothes)

- Intense feelings of despair

- Guilt

- Difficulty concentrating

- Withdrawal and isolation

- Repeated thoughts of suicide and death

Depression is very common in the elderly population. It can occur in conjunction with other illnesses. Cancer, AIDS, Alzheimer's disease, diabetes, and heart attack may be associated with increased rates of depression. It can happen after the death of a loved one. Depression may be caused by abnormal levels of chemicals in the brain.

Clinical depression is an illness and must be treated as such. A person cannot simply overcome depression through sheer will. It can be treated successfully. People who suffer from depression need compassion and support. A nursing assistant needs to know the symptoms so that she can recognize the beginning or worsening of depression. Any suicide threat should be taken seriously and reported immediately. It should not be dismissed as an attempt to get attention.

Bipolar disorder causes a person to have mood swings and changes in energy levels and the ability to function. A person may swing from periods of extreme activity or excitement (a manic episode) to periods of deep depression or sadness (a depressive episode). Characteristics of manic episodes include high energy, little sleep, big speeches, rapidly changing thoughts and moods, inflated self-esteem, overspending, and poor judgment.

Psychotic Disorders: Psychotic disorders are severe mental disorders marked by abnormal thinking and problems with understanding reality. Schizophrenia is one type of psychotic disorder. **Schizophrenia** affects a person's ability to think and communicate clearly. It also affects the ability to manage emotions, make decisions, and understand reality. It affects a person's ability to interact with other people. Treatment makes it possible for many people to lead relatively normal lives.

Hallucinations and delusions are two symptoms of schizophrenia. **Hallucinations** are false or distorted sensory perceptions. A person may see someone or something that is not really there, or hear a conversation that is not real. **Delusions** are persistent false beliefs. For example, a per-

son may believe that other people are controlling his thoughts.

Other symptoms of schizophrenia include disorganized thinking and speech. This makes a person unable to express logical thoughts. Disorganized behavior means a person moves slowly, repeating gestures or movements. People with schizophrenia may also show less emotion. They may seem to have less interest in things around them and lack energy.

8. Explain how mental illness is treated

It is extremely important to remember that mental illness can be treated. Medication and psychotherapy are common treatment methods. Medication is widely used for several diseases and can have a very positive effect. These medications affect the brain and have been successful in treating the symptoms and behaviors of many people with mental disorders. Medication may allow people who are mentally ill to function more completely. Medication used to treat mental illness must be taken properly to promote benefits and reduce side effects. NAs may be assigned to observe residents taking their medications.

Psychotherapy is a method of treating mental illness that involves talking about one's problems with mental health professionals. Individuals, groups, couples, or families meet with trained, licensed professionals to work on their problems. Therapists work with their clients to identify problems and causes. They use different techniques to help clients learn more about themselves and to teach them new ways to handle problems and be more in control of their lives.

Cognitive behavioral therapy (CBT) is a type of psychotherapy that is often used to treat anxiety disorders and depression. This type of therapy is usually short-term and focuses on skills and solutions that a person can use to modify negative thinking and behavior patterns.

Residents' Rights

Residents' Rights

Mental Illness

Residents have the right to participate in the planning of their care. They also have the right to have their medical and personal records handled confidentially. A resident with a history of mental illness has the right to go to his care plan meetings and state his preferences for care and treatment. He also has the right to refuse care and treatment. The fact that the resident has a mental illness is confidential information. This information should not be shared with anyone.

9. Explain the nursing assistant's role in caring for residents who are mentally ill

Personal care of residents who are mentally ill is similar to care of any resident. As with any resident, care should be provided in a way that is respectful of and responsive to each resident as an individual. This is part of providing person-centered care. The care plan will contain instructions for what care to perform. The NA will also have some special responsibilities, including the following:

Home Care Focus

A stable home environment is important in managing many forms of mental illness. By assisting the family with meeting their basic needs, the home health aide helps the recovery process. Even if not caring directly for the person who is mentally ill, the HHA's role is important. For example, knowing that their children are being well cared for can greatly assist people being treated for depression. The HHA may be assigned to provide these services:

- Food shopping, meal planning, and food preparation

- Housecleaning and laundry

- Assistance with activities of daily living and personal care, such as bathing

- Caring for children and other family members

If assisting in a client's home, the HHA should help preserve the client's role and authority in the family. The HHA is not replacing the client. He or she is only filling in until the client is well enough to resume his role in the family.

Guidelines: Residents Who Are Mentally Ill

G Observe residents carefully for changes in condition or abilities. Document and report your observations.

G Support the resident and his family and friends. Coping with mental illness can be very frustrating. Your positive, professional attitude encourages the resident and the family. If you need help coping with stress of caring for someone who is mentally ill, speak to the nurse.

G Encourage residents to do as much as possible for themselves. Progress may be very slow. Be patient, supportive, and positive.

10. Identify important observations that should be made and reported

Nursing assistants should carefully observe residents. They should not draw conclusions about the cause of the behavior they see; they should only report the facts of their observations, including what they saw or heard, how long the behavior lasted, and how frequently it occurred.

Observing and Reporting: Residents Who Are Mentally Ill

O/R Changes in ability

O/R Positive or negative mood changes, especially withdrawal (Fig. 20-4)

O/R Behavior changes, including changes in personality, extreme behavior, and behavior that is not appropriate to the situation

O/R Comments, even jokes, about hurting oneself or others

O/R Failure to take medicine or improper use of medicine

O/R Real or imagined physical symptoms

O/R Events, situations, or people that upset or excite residents

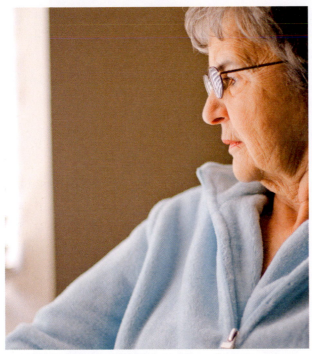

Fig. 20-4. Withdrawal is an important change to report.

11. List the signs of substance abuse

Substance abuse is the repeated use of legal or illegal substances in a way that is harmful to oneself or others. Many types of substances are abused, including alcohol, tobacco, legal and illegal drugs, glue, and paint.

It is not necessary for a substance to be illegal for it to be abused (Fig. 20-5). Alcohol and cigarettes are legal for adults, but are often abused. Over-the-counter medications, including diet aids and decongestants, can be addictive and harmful. Even household substances such as paint or glue can be abused, causing injury and death.

The harm caused by substance abuse may come in many forms: damage to the person's health, legal problems, and damage to the person's relationships with family and friends. Chemical dependency is more severe; it may involve needing greater amounts of the drug and having symptoms even when not using it. Chemical dependency is a disease. It affects a person physically, mentally, and emotionally. Like many other diseases, chemical dependency can develop at

any age. It is treatable but frequently requires diagnosis and care by specialists. Treatment is not as simple as just stopping the drug.

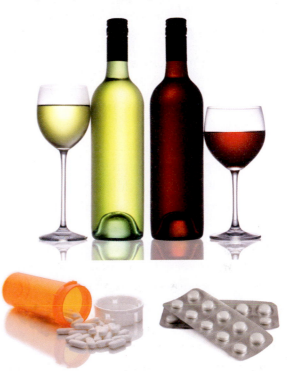

Fig. 20-5. Prescription drugs, cigarettes, and alcohol are examples of legal substances that may be abused.

A nursing assistant may be in a position to observe signs of substance abuse in residents. These signs should be reported to the nurse. Observations can be made without accusing anyone of abuse. The NA should simply report what she sees, not what she thinks the cause may be.

Observing and Reporting: Substance Abuse

- °/ᵣ Changes in physical appearance (red eyes, dilated pupils, weight loss)
- °/ᵣ Changes in personality (moodiness, strange behavior, disruption of routines, lying)
- °/ᵣ Irritability
- °/ᵣ Smell of alcohol, cigarettes, or other substances on breath or on clothing
- °/ᵣ Diminished sense of smell
- °/ᵣ Unexplained changes in vital signs

%R Loss of appetite

%R Inability to function normally

%R Need for money

%R Confusion or forgetfulness

%R Blackouts or memory loss

%R Frequent accidents

%R Problems with family or friends

Some of the same signs listed above may also indicate other problems. Depression, dementia, medication issues, or medical conditions can also produce many of these same symptoms.

Residents' Rights

Rights with Alcohol

Most residents in long-term care facilities are adults and have the legal right to drink alcohol. However, there are instances when alcohol is not allowed. A doctor may have issued an order for a resident not to drink alcohol. A facility may have policies against any alcohol being consumed, which would have been known and agreed to by potential residents before admission.

If a doctor has not issued an order stating that a resident may not have alcohol and the facility has no rules against it, a resident may drink alcohol. If a resident is allowed to do so and enjoys having an alcoholic beverage, nursing assistants should not make judgments. They should not gossip about it with other residents or staff members. However, if an NA knows that a resident should not be drinking alcohol, he should report it to the nurse.

Chapter Review

1. For each of the seven characteristics of mental health in Learning Objective 1, give one example of a behavior that demonstrates the characteristic.

2. What are four possible causes of mental illness?

3. What is the most common fallacy about mental illness?

4. Why might a physical illness cause or make a mental illness worse?

5. At what distance should a nursing assistant be when communicating with a resident who has a mental illness?

6. What are defense mechanisms?

7. What is anxiety?

8. When a resident makes a suicide threat, what should the nursing assistant do?

9. What are the most common treatments for mental illness?

10. List three care guidelines for residents who are mentally ill.

11. List five important observations to make about a resident who is mentally ill.

12. List four legal substances that can be abused.

13. List ten signs and symptoms of substance abuse.

21

Rehabilitation and Restorative Care

1. Discuss rehabilitation and restorative care

When a resident loses some ability to function due to an illness or injury, rehabilitation may be ordered. **Rehabilitation** is care that is managed by professionals to help restore a person to his or her highest possible level of functioning. It involves helping residents move from illness, disability, and dependence toward health, ability, and independence. Rehabilitation involves all parts of the person's disability, including physical needs (e.g., eating, elimination) and psychosocial needs (e.g., independence, self-esteem). Goals of a rehabilitative program include the following:

- To help a resident regain function or recover from illness

- To develop and promote a resident's independence

- To allow a resident to feel in control of his life

- To help a resident accept or adapt to the limitations of a disability

Rehabilitation will be used for many residents, particularly those who have suffered a stroke, accident, joint replacement, or trauma.

When the goals of rehabilitation have been met, **restorative care** may be ordered. The goal of restorative care is to keep the resident at the level achieved by rehabilitative services. Restorative care works to maintain a resident's functioning, to improve his quality of life, and to increase independence.

With both rehabilitation and restorative care, the care team uses a holistic, person-centered approach. The physician and nurses will establish goals of care (Fig. 21-1). These include promoting independence in activities of daily living (ADLs) and restoring health to optimal condition. The physical therapist, occupational therapist, and/or speech-language pathologist will work with the resident to help restore or adapt specific abilities. Social workers or other counselors may see the resident to help promote attitudes of independence and acceptance. The effects of the illness or injury cannot always be reversed. Social workers and counselors help people adjust to trauma and loss.

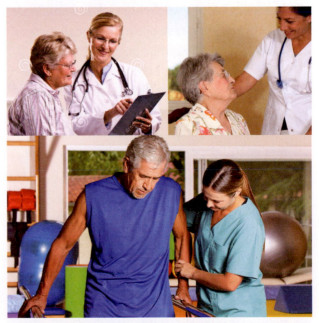

Fig. 21-1. *A team of specialists, including doctors, nurses, physical therapists, and other kinds of therapists, helps residents with rehabilitation.*

Because nursing assistants spend many hours with these residents, they are a very important part of the team. NAs play an important role in helping residents recover and regain independence. When assisting with restorative care, these guidelines are critical to residents' progress:

Guidelines: Restorative Care

G   Be patient. Progress may be slow, and it will seem slower to you and the residents if you are impatient. Residents must do as much as possible for themselves. Encourage independence and self-care, regardless of how long it takes or how poorly they are able to do it. The more patient you are, the easier it will be for them to regain abilities and confidence.

G   Be positive and supportive. A positive attitude can set the tone for success. Family members and residents will take cues from you as to how they should behave. If you are encouraging and positive, you help create a supportive atmosphere for rehabilitation.

G   Focus on small tasks and small accomplishments. For example, dressing themselves may seem like an overwhelming task to some residents. Break the task down into smaller steps. Today the goal might be putting on a shirt without buttoning it. Next week the goal could be buttoning the shirt if that seems manageable. When the resident can put the shirt on without help, congratulate him on reaching this goal. Take everything one step at a time.

G   Recognize that setbacks occur. Progress occurs at different rates. Sometimes a resident can do something one day that he cannot do the next. Reassure residents that setbacks are normal. Focus on the things that the resident can do and not on what he cannot do. However, document any decline in a resident's abilities.

G   Be sensitive to the resident's needs. Some residents may need more encouragement than others. Some may feel embarrassed by certain kinds of encouragement. Get to know your residents. Understand what motivates them. Adapt your encouragement to fit each person's personality.

G   Encourage independence. A resident's independence may help his ability to be active in the process of rehabilitation. Independence improves self-image and attitude. It also helps speed recovery.

G   Provide privacy. Ensure residents' privacy when they are trying to do skills or activities of daily living. Doing this promotes dignity and maintains residents' legal rights.

G   Involve residents in their care. Residents who feel involved and valued may be more motivated to work hard in rehabilitation. Fears may be eased by including family and friends in the rehabilitation program (Fig. 21-2). A team approach is inspiring.

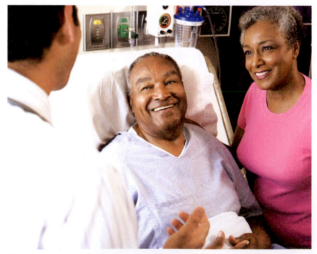

Fig. 21-2. Involving family and friends in rehabilitation may help the resident be motivated and successful.

Residents' Rights

Call Lights

Residents may need help often while going through rehabilitation. No matter how often a resident uses his call light or how demanding he is, it is never acceptable for a nursing assistant to unplug a resident's call light. Call lights should always be left within reach of the resident's unaffected/stronger hand. Staff must respond kindly and promptly to call lights every time they are used.

Observing and Reporting: Restorative Care

O/R Any increase or decrease in abilities (For example, note, "Yesterday Mr. Martinez used the bedside commode without help. Today he asked for the bedpan.")

O/R Any change in attitude or motivation, positive or negative

O/R Any change in general health, such as changes in skin condition, appetite, energy level, or general appearance

O/R Signs of depression or mood changes

Working with residents going through rehabilitation and restorative care can be a very rewarding part of caregiving. Nursing assistants should take pride in their contributions to residents' improving health and independence.

Residents' Rights

Rehabilitation

Residents receiving rehabilitation and restorative care services have been ill or injured and are likely to feel tired, afraid, and depressed, or to be in pain. NAs can help them feel safe and secure by being kind, patient, and helpful. For example, if a therapy schedule interferes with mealtimes, the NA can collect the resident's meal when the resident is ready. A resident who is frightened may benefit from an unrushed conversation. If a resident says she is in pain, the NA should talk to the nurse. She should take action to help the resident. Comfort measures, such as a back rub, can be offered.

2. Describe the importance of promoting independence and list ways that exercise improves health

Maintaining independence is vital during and after rehabilitation and restorative services. When an active and independent person is dependent, physical and mental problems may result. The body becomes less mobile, and the mind is less focused. Studies show that the more active a person is, the better the mind and body work.

Exercise is important for improving and maintaining physical and mental health. Inactivity and immobility can result in loss of self-esteem, depression, pneumonia, urinary tract infections, constipation, blood clots, and dulling of the senses. People who are in bed for long periods of time are more likely to develop muscle atrophy or contractures. When atrophy occurs, the muscle wastes away, decreases in size, and becomes weak. A contracture is the permanent and often painful shortening of a muscle, tendon, or ligament.

A lack of mobility may cause other problems as well. Immobility reduces the amount of blood that circulates to the skin. Residents who have restricted mobility have an increased risk for pressure injuries. In addition, a lack of mobility can also cause problems with independence and self-esteem.

The staff's job is to keep residents as active as possible—whether they are bedbound or are able to get out of bed and walk (ambulate). Regular ambulation and exercise help improve the following:

- Quality and health of the skin
- Circulation
- Strength
- Sleep and relaxation
- Mood
- Self-esteem
- Appetite
- Elimination
- Blood flow
- Oxygen level

Promoting social interactions and thinking abilities is important, too. Most facilities have activities geared to residents' ages and abilities. Social involvement should be encouraged. When possible, nursing assistants should join in activities with residents (Fig. 21-3). This promotes independence. It also gives NAs a chance to observe residents' abilities.

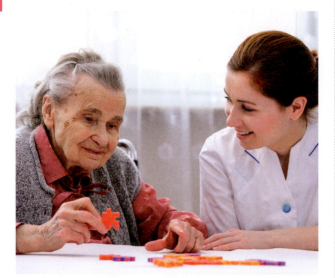

Fig. 21-3. *Promoting mental and physical activity is important. When possible, NAs should join in activities with residents.*

Basic Exercise Principles

It is important to get a doctor's approval before starting a new exercise or activity program. It is not safe to exercise with certain heart conditions. Exercising with high blood pressure can be risky. Caution must be used after surgery. It is also necessary to limit exercise if a person has unstable bones, fractures, osteoporosis, or extreme breathing problems.

Warming up should be done before doing any other exercises. This consists of light exercise, such as walking. The warm-up begins to increase heart rate and breathing. It helps prevent injury. Some people like to stretch at the beginning of their workout. Stretching should not be done until the muscles are warm.

Cool-down exercises are done to slowly lower the heart rate. They return other body functions to normal. Suddenly ending an exercise session without cooling down can cause blood to pool in the large leg muscles. This may cause dizziness or even fainting. It is a good idea to stretch after the cool-down, while the muscles are still warm. Stretching keeps muscles flexible and helps them relax.

3. Describe assistive devices and equipment

Many devices are available to help people who are recovering from or adapting to a physical condition. Assistive or adaptive equipment was first explained in Chapter 2. This equipment helps residents perform their activities of daily living. Each device is made to support a particular disability. Raised seating, for example, makes it easier for a resident with weak legs to stand.

Personal care equipment includes long-handled brushes and combs. Plate guards prevent food from being pushed off the plate and make it easier to scoop food onto utensils. Reachers can help with putting on underwear or pants. A sock aid can pull on socks, and a long-handled shoehorn assists in putting shoes on without bending. Long-handled sponges help with bathing.

Supportive devices, such as canes, walkers, and crutches, are used to assist residents with ambulation (Chapter 10). Safety devices, such as shower chairs and gait or transfer belts, help prevent accidents. Safety bars/grab bars are often installed in and near the tub and toilet to give the resident something to hold on to while changing position. The items shown in Fig. 21-4 can be useful as residents relearn old skills or adapt to new limitations.

Residents' Rights

Walking Aids

Residents using new ambulatory aids, such as canes, walkers, boots, crutches, etc., are likely to be off-balance. The nursing assistant should stay close by to be sure they are using these devices safely. She should observe residents for signs of dizziness. Residents should not be rushed while they are using these aids. The NA should let residents set the pace. To avoid falls, pathways should remain clear and spills should be wiped up immediately.

Trapeze

A trapeze is a triangular piece of equipment that hangs over the head of the bed. It may be mounted to the bed or freestanding. People in bed can grasp the trapeze with their hands, which enables them to lift themselves. The trapeze assists with repositioning and exercise activities.

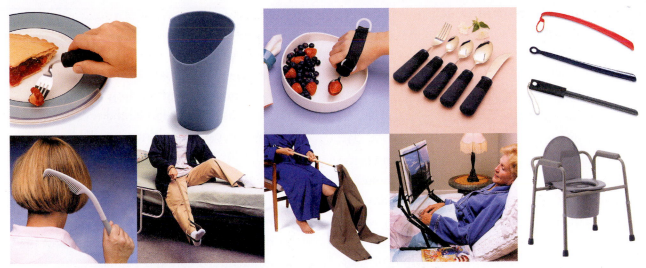

Fig. 21-4. *Many assistive items are available to help residents adapt to physical changes.* (PHOTOS COURTESY OF NORTH COAST MEDICAL, INC., WWW.NCMEDICAL.COM, 800-821-9319)

4. Explain guidelines for maintaining proper body alignment

Residents who are confined to bed need to maintain proper body alignment. This aids recovery and prevents injury to muscles and joints. Chapter 10 includes specific instructions for positioning residents. These guidelines help residents maintain proper alignment and make progress when they are able to get out of bed:

Guidelines: Alignment and Positioning

G Observe principles of alignment. Remember that proper alignment is based on straight lines. The spine should lie in a straight line. Pillows or rolled or folded blankets can support the small of the back and raise the knees or head in the supine position. They can support the head and one leg in the lateral position (Fig. 21-5).

G Keep body parts in natural positions. In a natural hand position, the fingers are slightly curled. Use a rolled washcloth, gauze bandage, or rubber ball inside the palm to support the fingers in this position. Use bed cradles to keep covers from resting on feet if the resident is in the supine position.

G Prevent external rotation of hips. When legs and hips turn outward during long periods of bedrest, hip contractures can result. A rolled blanket or towel tucked alongside the hip and thigh can keep the leg from turning outward.

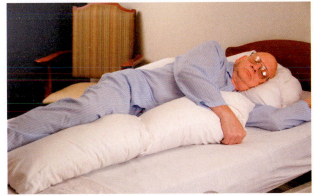

Fig. 21-5. *Pillows or rolled or folded blankets help provide extra support.*

G Change positions often to prevent muscle stiffness and pressure injuries. This should be done at least every two hours. Which position the resident uses will depend on the resident's condition and preference. Check the skin every time you reposition the resident.

G Give backrubs as ordered for comfort and relaxation.

5. Explain care guidelines for prosthetic devices

A prosthesis is a device that replaces a body part that is missing or deformed because of an accident, injury, illness, or birth defect. It is used to improve a person's ability to function and/or to improve appearance. Examples of prostheses include the following:

- Artificial limbs, such as artificial hands, arms, feet, and legs, are made to resemble the body part that they are replacing (Fig. 21-6). Many advances have been made and continue to be made in the field of prosthetic limbs. Today's artificial limbs are usually made of strong and lightweight plastics and other materials, such as carbon fiber. Most artificial limbs are attached by belts, cuffs, or suction. Direct bone attachment is a newer method of attaching the limb to the body.

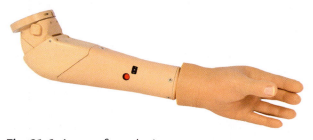

Fig. 21-6. *A type of prosthetic arm.* (MOTION CONTROL UTAH ARM. PHOTO BY KEVIN TWOMEY.)

- An artificial breast is made of a lightweight, soft, spongy material. It usually fits into a regular bra or in the pocket of a special bra, called a *mastectomy bra.*

- A hearing aid is a small device that amplifies sound for persons with hearing loss. Many elderly residents have hearing aids. Chapter 4 has more information on hearing aids.

- An artificial eye, or ocular prosthetic, replaces an eye that has been lost to disease or injury. It is usually made of plastic. It is held in place by suction. An ocular prosthetic does not provide vision; it can, however, improve appearance.

- Dentures are artificial teeth. They may be necessary when a tooth or teeth have been damaged, lost, or must be removed. Many elderly residents have dentures. Chapter 13 has more information about denture care.

Guidelines: Prosthetic Devices

G Because prostheses are specially fitted, expensive pieces of equipment (some cost tens of thousands of dollars), only care for them as assigned. Handle them carefully. Follow the care plan. Know exactly how to care for the equipment before you begin. If you have any questions, talk to the nurse.

G A therapist or nurse will demonstrate application of a prosthesis. Follow instructions to apply and remove the prosthesis. Follow the manufacturer's care directions.

G Respect a resident's decision not to wear a prosthetic limb. Some residents may find the limb uncomfortable and only wish to wear it for special occasions.

G Keep the prosthesis and the skin under it dry and clean. The socket of the prosthesis must be cleaned at least daily. Follow the care plan and the nurse's instructions.

G If ordered, apply a stump sock before putting on the prosthesis.

G Observe the skin on the stump. Watch for signs of skin breakdown caused by pressure and abrasion. Report redness or open areas.

G Never try to fix a prosthesis. Report any problems to the nurse.

G Do not show negative feelings about a resident's stump during care.

G If instructed to care for an artificial eye, review the care plan with the nurse. Always wash your hands and don gloves before handling an artificial eye. Provide privacy for the resident. Put on gloves before beginning care. Artificial eyes are held in place by suction. They will come out quickly when pressure is applied below the lower eyelid. Some artificial eyes do not require frequent removal. Others need daily removal and cleaning.

G If the artificial eye is removed, wash the eye with solution and rinse in warm water. Never clean or soak the eye in rubbing alcohol. It will crack the plastic and destroy it.

G   When the artificial eye is removed, wash the eye socket with warm water or saline. Use a clean gauze square to clean it. Clean the eyelid with a clean cotton ball. Wipe gently from inner corner (canthus) outward.

G   If the artificial eye is to be removed and not reinserted, line an eye cup or basin with a soft cloth or a piece of 4x4 gauze. This prevents scratches and damage. Fill with water or saline solution. Place the artificial eye in the container and close the container. Make sure the container is labeled with the resident's name and room number.

G   To reinsert the eye, moisten it and place it far under the upper eyelid. Pull down on the lower eyelid; the eye should slide into place.

6. Describe how to assist with range of motion exercises

Range of motion (ROM) exercises put a particular joint through its full arc of motion. The goals of range of motion exercises are to decrease or prevent contractures or atrophy, improve strength, and increase circulation. Types of range of motion exercises are as follows:

Active range of motion (AROM) exercises are performed by a resident himself, without help. The nursing assistant's role in AROM exercises is to encourage the resident.

Active assisted range of motion (AAROM) exercises are done by the resident with some assistance and support from the nursing assistant or other caregiver.

Passive range of motion (PROM) exercises are used when residents are not able to move on their own. PROM exercises are performed by the caregiver, without the resident's help. When assisting with these type of range of motion exercises, the NA should support the resident's joints while moving them through the range of motion.

Range of motion exercises are specific for each body area. They include the following movements (Fig. 21-7):

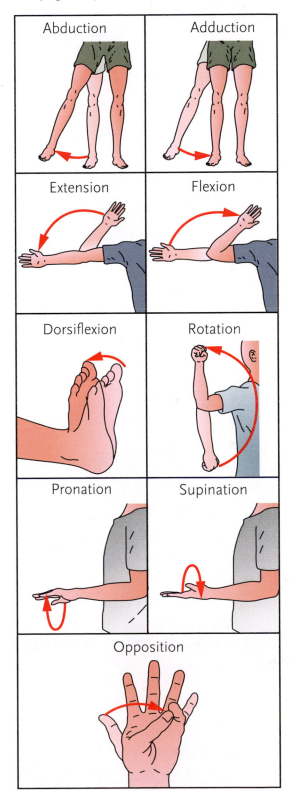

Fig. 21-7. *The different range of motion body movements.*

- **Abduction**: moving a body part away from the midline of the body

- **Adduction**: moving a body part toward the midline of the body

- **Extension**: straightening a body part

- **Flexion**: bending a body part

- **Dorsiflexion**: bending backward

- **Rotation**: turning the joint

- **Pronation**: turning downward

- **Supination**: turning upward

- **Opposition**: touching the thumb to any other finger

Range of motion exercises are not performed without a specific order from a doctor, nurse, or physical therapist. Depending on the care plan, the NA will repeat each exercise three to five times, once or twice a day, working on both sides of the body. When performing ROM exercises, the NA should begin at the resident's shoulders and work down the body. The upper extremities (arms) should be exercised before the lower extremities (legs). The NA should give support above and below the joints. The joints should be moved gently, slowly, and smoothly through the range of motion to the point of resistance. The NA should ask the resident to let her know if the resident experiences pain. She should watch for nonverbal signs that the resident is in pain during the procedure. It is important to stop the exercises if the resident complains of pain and to report the pain to the nurse.

Assisting with passive range of motion exercises

1. Identify yourself by name. Identify the resident by name.

2. Wash your hands.

3. Explain procedure to resident. Speak clearly, slowly, and directly. Maintain face-to-face contact whenever possible.

4. Provide for resident's privacy with curtain, screen, or door.

5. Adjust bed to a safe level, usually waist high. Lock bed wheels.

6. Position the resident lying supine—flat on her back—on the bed. Use proper alignment.

7. While supporting the limbs, move all joints gently, slowly, and smoothly through the range of motion to the point of resistance. Repeat each exercise at least three times. Watch for signs of pain and stop performing exercises if resident appears to be in pain or complains of pain. Report pain to the nurse.

8. **Shoulder**. Support the resident's arm at the elbow and wrist while performing ROM for the shoulder. Place one hand under the elbow and the other hand under the wrist. Raise the straightened arm from the side position upward toward the head to ear level and return the arm down to side of the body (extension/flexion) (Fig. 21-8).

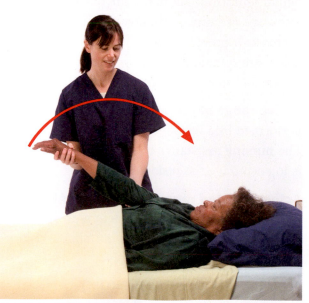

Fig. 21-8. Raise the straightened arm upward toward head to ear level, and return it to the side of the body.

Move straightened arm away from side of body to shoulder level and return arm to side of body (abduction/adduction) (Fig. 21-9).

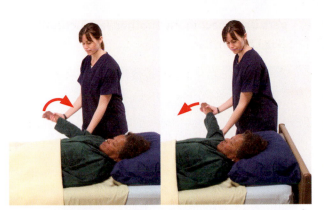

Fig. 21-9. Move the straightened arm away from side of body to shoulder level and return the arm to side.

9. **Elbow**. Hold the resident's wrist with one hand and the elbow with the other hand. Bend the elbow so that the hand touches the shoulder on that same side (flexion). Straighten the arm (extension) (Fig. 21-10).

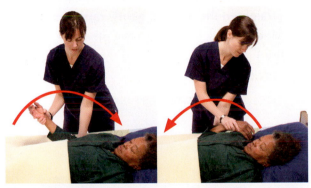

Fig. 21-10. Bend the elbow so that the hand touches the shoulder on the same side, and then straighten the arm.

Exercise the forearm by moving it so the palm is facing downward (pronation) and then the palm is facing upward (supination) (Fig. 21-11).

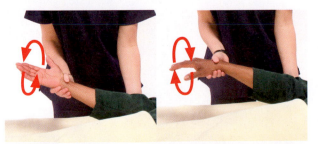

Fig. 21-11. Exercise the forearm so that the palm is facing downward and then upward.

10. **Wrist**. Hold the wrist with one hand and use the fingers of your other hand to help move

the joint through the motions. Bend the hand down (flexion). Bend the hand backward (dorsiflexion) (Fig. 21-12).

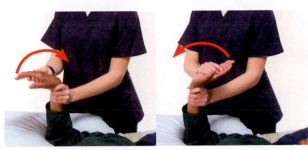

Fig. 21-12. While supporting the wrist, gently bend the hand down and then backward.

Turn the hand in the direction of the thumb (radial flexion). Then turn the hand in the direction of the little finger (ulnar flexion) (Fig. 21-13).

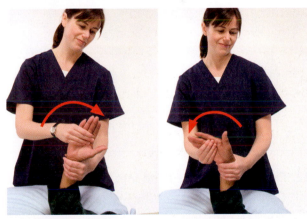

Fig. 21-13. Turn the hand in the direction of the thumb, then turn it in the direction of the little finger.

11. **Thumb**. Move the thumb away from the index finger (abduction). Move the thumb back next to the index finger (adduction) (Fig. 21-14).

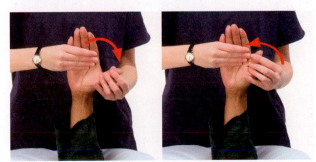

Fig. 21-14. Move the thumb away from the index finger and then back to the index finger.

Touch each fingertip with the thumb (opposition) (Fig. 21-15).

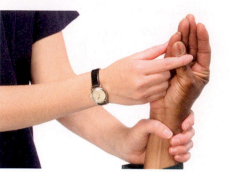

Fig. 21-15. *Touch each fingertip with the thumb.*

Bend the thumb into the palm (flexion) and out to the side (extension) (Fig. 21-16).

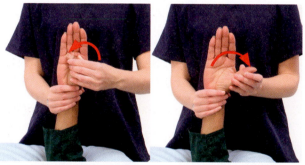

Fig. 21-16. *Bend the thumb into the palm and then out to the side.*

12. **Fingers**. Make the hand into a fist (flexion). Gently straighten out the fist (extension) (Fig. 21-17).

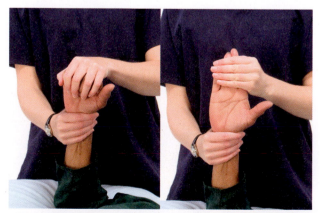

Fig. 21-17. *Make the fingers into a fist and then gently straighten out the fist.*

Spread the fingers and the thumb far apart from each other (abduction). Bring the fin-

gers back next to each other (adduction) (Fig. 21-18).

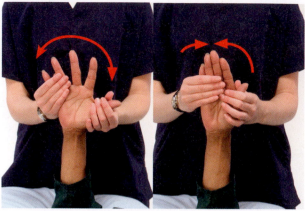

Fig. 21-18. *Spread the fingers and thumb far apart from each other and then bring them back next to each other.*

13. **Hip**. Support the leg by placing one hand under the knee and one under the ankle. Straighten the leg and gently raise it upward. Move the leg away from the other leg (abduction). Move the leg toward the other leg (adduction) (Fig. 21-19).

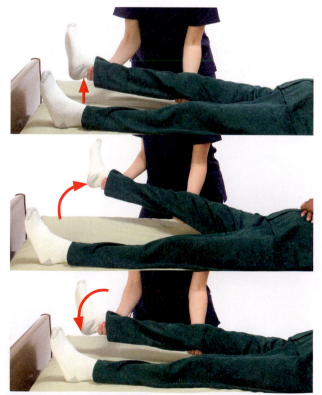

Fig. 21-19. *Straighten the leg and gently raise it. Move the leg away from the other leg and then back toward the other leg.*

Gently turn the leg inward (internal rotation), then turn the leg outward (external rotation) (Fig. 21-20).

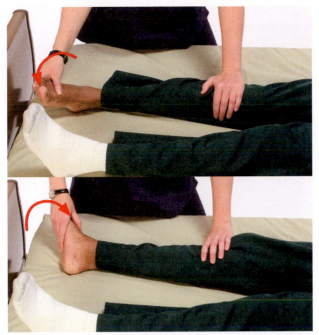

Fig. 21-20. Gently turn the leg inward and then outward.

14. **Knee**. Support the leg under the knee and under the ankle while performing ROM for the knee. Bend the knee to the point of resistance (flexion). Return the leg to resident's normal position (extension) (Fig. 21-21).

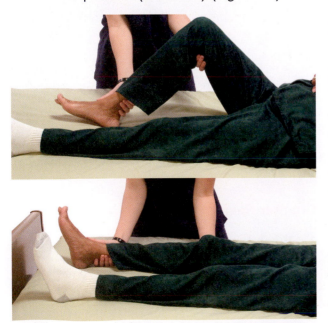

Fig. 21-21. Gently bend the knee to the point of resistance and return the leg to its normal position.

15. **Ankle**. Support the foot and ankle close to the bed while performing ROM for the ankle. Push/pull foot up toward the head (dorsiflexion). Push/pull foot down, with the toes pointed down (plantar flexion) (Fig. 21-22).

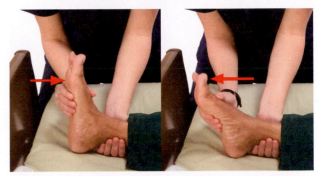

Fig. 21-22. Push the foot up toward the head and then push it back down.

Turn the inside of the foot inward toward the body (supination). Bend the sole of the foot away from the body (pronation) (Fig. 21-23).

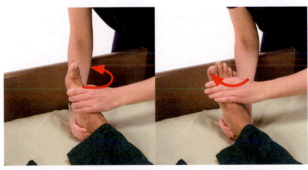

Fig. 21-23. Turn the inside of foot inward, toward the body, and then bend it to face away from the body.

16. **Toes**. Curl and straighten the toes (flexion and extension) (Fig. 21-24).

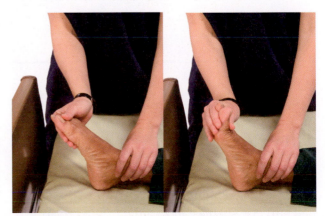

Fig. 21-24. Curl and straighten the toes.

Gently spread the toes apart (abduction) (Fig. 21-25).

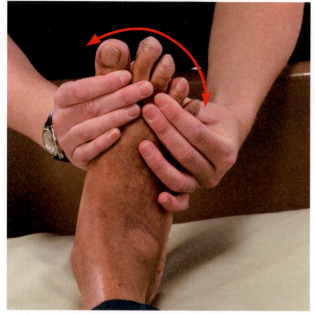

Fig. 21-25. *Gently spread the toes apart.*

17. Return resident to a comfortable position. Return bed to lowest position. Remove privacy measures.

18. Place call light within resident's reach.

19. Wash your hands.

20. Report any changes in resident to nurse.

21. Document procedure using facility guidelines. Note any decrease in range of motion or any pain experienced by the resident. Notify the nurse or the physical therapist if you find increased stiffness or physical resistance. Resistance may be a sign that a contracture is developing.

7. Describe the benefits of deep breathing exercises

Deep breathing exercises help expand the lungs, clearing them of mucus and preventing infections such as pneumonia. Residents who have had surgery, such as abdominal or hip replacement surgery, or who are paralyzed are often in-

structed to do deep breathing exercises regularly to expand the lungs. The care plan may include using a deep breathing device called an *incentive spirometer* (Fig. 21-26). Incentive spirometry helps the resident to take long, slow, deep breaths. Nursing assistants should not assist with these exercises if they have not been trained; they must ask the nurse for instructions.

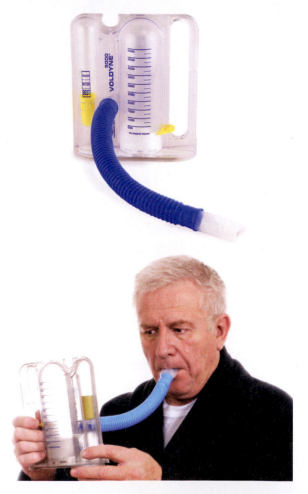

Fig. 21-26. *Incentive spirometers are used for deep breathing exercises.*

Chapter Review

1. What does rehabilitation involve?

2. What attitudes should the nursing assistant adopt to assist residents in rehabilitation and restorative care?

3. List 10 problems that a lack of mobility can cause.

4. What are some benefits of regular exercise?

5. Look at the adaptive devices in Figure 21-4. Choose one and briefly describe how it might help a resident who is recovering from or adapting to a physical condition.

6. List three guidelines an NA should follow to help residents maintain proper alignment.

7. What is a prosthesis?

8. What should be observed about the skin on the stump of an amputated body part?

9. Why should alcohol not be used to clean an artificial eye?

10. What is the purpose of range of motion (ROM) exercises?

11. When performing ROM exercises, where should the NA begin? Which parts of the body should be exercised first?

12. Describe the difference between passive, active, and active assisted range of motion exercises.

13. Why are deep breathing exercises performed?

22

Special Care Skills

1. Understand the types of residents who are in a subacute setting

Subacute care is a kind of specialized care that falls between acute care and long-term care. This type of care can be given in hospitals or in skilled nursing facilities. People in subacute settings require more treatment, monitoring, and services than regular long-term care provides.

Recent surgery, injuries, or chronic illnesses, such as AIDS or cancer, may require subacute care (Fig. 22-1). Complex wound care, specialized infusion therapy, dialysis, and mechanical ventilation are other reasons subacute care may be needed. Dialysis cleans the body of waste that the kidneys cannot remove due to chronic renal failure (Fig. 22-2). A mechanical ventilator is a machine that assists with or replaces breathing when a person cannot breathe on his own.

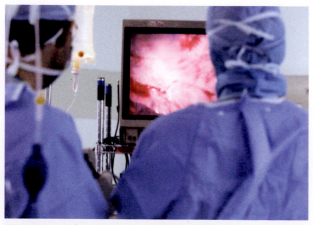

Fig. 22-1. *Subacute care provides a higher level of care; it may be necessary due to surgery, illness, serious wounds, dialysis, or mechanical ventilation.*

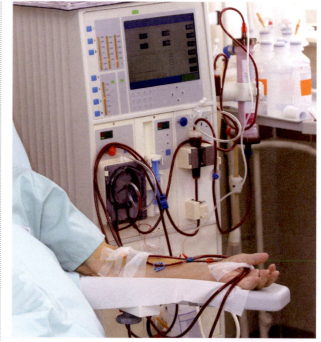

Fig. 22-2. *A patient hooked up to a dialysis machine.*

2. Discuss reasons for and types of surgery

There are many reasons why surgery is performed, including the following:

- To relieve symptoms of a disease

- To repair or remove problem tissues and structures

- To improve the appearance or correct function of damaged tissues

- To diagnose disease

- To cure a disease

Surgeries generally fall into three categories: elective, urgent, and emergency. Elective surgery is surgery that is chosen by the patient and is planned in advance. Generally, the surgery is not absolutely necessary. Plastic surgery, such as having a facelift, is an example of an elective surgery.

Urgent surgery is surgery that must be performed for health reasons, but is not an emergency. Urgent surgery may even be planned and scheduled in advance, as with heart surgery such as coronary artery bypass surgery.

Emergency surgery is unexpected and unscheduled surgery that is performed immediately to save a patient's life or a limb. A gunshot wound, car accident, or ruptured appendix are examples of situations that can require emergency surgery.

When a person has surgery, anesthesia will usually be given. **Anesthesia** involves the use of medication to block pain during surgery and other medical procedures. Local anesthesia involves the injection of an anesthetic directly into the surgical site or area to block pain. It is used for minor surgical procedures, and the person may remain awake during the surgery. Regional anesthesia involves injection of an anesthetic into a nerve or group of nerves to block sensation in a particular region of the body. It is limited to an area, but to a larger area than for a local anesthetic. One example of a regional anesthetic is an epidural, which is used during childbirth to block pain in the lower half of the body, from the waist down. General anesthesia is inhaled or injected directly into a vein and affects the brain and the entire body. The person is unaware of his surroundings and does not feel any pain. It blocks any memory of the procedure. This type of anesthesia is stopped when the surgery has been completed.

3. Discuss preoperative care

Depending on where a nursing assistant works, his duties may include giving **preoperative**, or before-surgery, care. Preoperative care includes both physical and psychological preparation. Before a person has surgery, a doctor will explain the procedure, the risks and benefits, and what to expect after surgery. The person will be encouraged to ask questions and give opinions. This is part of informed consent (Chapter 3), a process in which a person, with the help of a doctor, makes informed decisions about her health care. The person must sign a written consent form for surgery or have one signed by a guardian or someone with medical power of attorney.

People who are going to have surgery often experience anxiety, fear, worry, sadness, and other emotions (Fig. 22-3). It is often helpful to express these concerns to members of the healthcare team. Being prepared psychologically may help the resident cope better after surgery. Part of a nursing assistant's role in assisting with this preparation is listening to a resident's concerns. The NA should report any concerns or questions, including requests for a visit from clergy, to the nurse.

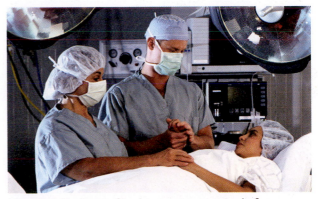

Fig. 22-3. *Patients often have many worries before surgery. A compassionate response by staff may help alleviate concerns.*

A person who is having surgery will require preoperative physical preparation as well. These general guidelines explain physical preparation for surgery:

Guidelines: Preoperative Care

G　Before surgery, there will be an order for the resident to receive nothing by mouth (NPO). This time usually ranges anywhere from two to eight hours. Having this medical order means that nothing is allowed by mouth, including water, ice chips, food, etc. Remove the water pitcher, glass, and any other food and fluids from the immediate area. Explain to the resident why you are doing this. Report any concerns to the nurse.

G   Assist the resident with urinating before surgery.

G   For some residents having surgery of the gastrointestinal tract, the bowels may need to be cleared. An enema or rectal suppository may be ordered. Assist as trained, ordered, and allowed. Be ready to bring the bedpan or portable commode when needed. Provide plenty of privacy.

G   Assist with bathing as needed. Dressing the person in loose-fitting clothes may make it easier to change into a gown later.

G   Make sure call light is within reach every time you leave the room.

G   Measure and record vital signs as ordered.

G   Remove dentures, eyeglasses, contact lenses, hearing aids, jewelry, hairpieces, hairpins, and any other personal items. Store these safely according to policy. For local or regional anesthetic, the doctor may want the person to wear hearing aids and dentures, so that communication will be easier.

G   Help the resident to change into a gown if required.

G   Transfer to a stretcher/gurney if necessary.

G   Make sure the resident's identification bracelet is accurate and on the wrist or ankle prior to transport. You may need to verify if the resident has any known allergies by asking this question or verifying what is written on an allergy bracelet.

4. Describe postoperative care

Postoperative, or after-surgery, care begins immediately following surgery. The goal of

postoperative care is to prevent infections, promote healing, and return the person to a state of health. Immediate postoperative concerns are problems with breathing, mental status, pain, and wound healing. Complications of surgery can also include urinary retention or infections, constipation, blood pressure variances, and blood clots. Careful postoperative monitoring is critical.

After surgery, the resident is taken to the recovery room and may remain there for some time. This depends on the type of surgery that the resident had, as well as how long the surgery was, what type and how much anesthetic was used, and the resident's level of consciousness.

While the resident is in recovery, the nursing assistant's duties will include changing bed linens and gathering equipment. Equipment needed may include the following:

*   Bed protector

*   Towels and washcloths

*   Vital signs equipment

*   Emesis basin

*   Pillows and other positioning devices

*   Warming blankets

*   IV pole

*   Oxygen and suction equipment

When the resident returns to the room, the following guidelines are used in providing postoperative care:

Guidelines: Postoperative Care

G   Move furniture as needed to allow for the transfer back into bed from the stretcher.

G   Assist with transferring the resident back into bed. (Chapter 10 has information on stretcher transfers.)

G   Return dentures, eyeglasses, contact lenses, and hearing aids to the resident. Remember that without these items, residents may not be able to talk, eat, see, or hear.

G   Measure and record vital signs often after surgery as directed. The schedule may look like this: every 15 minutes for the first hour, every 30 minutes for the next hour to two hours, every hour for the next four hours, and then every four hours. Report any changes immediately.

G   Reposition the resident every one to two hours, or as ordered. Elevate the extremities as ordered.

G   Assist with deep breathing and coughing exercises (Chapter 21).

G   Anti-embolic hose and sequential compression devices (SCDs) may be ordered to increase circulation and reduce the risk of blood clots. A sequential compression device is a plastic, air-filled sleeve that is put on the leg and hooked up to a machine. When turned on, the machine inflates and deflates the sleeve, creating pressure and promoting blood flow. Assist with anti-embolic hose, SCDs, and leg exercises as instructed.

G   Binders are stretchable pieces of fabric that can be fastened. They hold dressings in place and give support to surgical wounds. Binders can also reduce swelling and ease discomfort. Apply binders as ordered.

G   Surgical drains may be placed near the incision (Fig. 22-4). These drains help prevent fluid buildup, which can lead to infection. Surgical drains are connected to a collection device such as a bulb, which is emptied regularly. Observe the amount and appearance of the drainage as directed. Sometimes nursing assistants are also responsible for measuring the amount of drainage. If this is part of your responsibilities, the nurse will train you how to do it.

G   Encourage the resident to follow diet orders. A postoperative resident may have a nothing by mouth (NPO) order or an order for a clear liquid diet. The resident may be on a high-protein diet to promote wound healing. Following diet orders can help speed the recovery process.

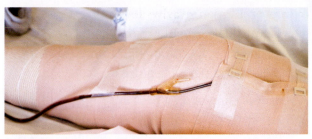

Fig. 22-4. *This photo shows a postoperative knee with a drainage tube in it.*

G   Assist with elimination. Always provide plenty of privacy for elimination.

G   Help with bathing and grooming as requested and as ordered.

G   Assist with ambulation as needed and as ordered. Be encouraging and positive.

Observing and Reporting: Postoperative Care

Report the following signs and symptoms of complications to the nurse immediately:

O/R   Changes in vital signs

O/R   Difficulty breathing

O/R   Mental changes, such as confusion or disorientation

O/R   Changes in consciousness

O/R   Pale or cyanotic (bluish) skin

O/R   Skin that is cold or clammy

O/R   Increase in amount of drainage

O/R   Swelling at IV site

O/R   IV that is not dripping

O/R   Nausea or vomiting

O/R   Numbness or tingling

O/R   Resident complaints of pain

5. List care guidelines for pulse oximetry

When residents have had surgery, are on oxygen, are in intensive care, or have cardiac or respiratory problems, a pulse oximeter may be used. A **pulse**

oximeter is a noninvasive device that uses a light to determine the amount of oxygen in the blood (also called *oxygen saturation*). A pulse oximeter also measures a person's pulse rate.

A sensor is clipped on a person's finger, earlobe, or toe (Fig. 22-5). A light passes through the skin, and the percentage of oxygen in the blood and the pulse rate are displayed. An alarm will sound if the oxygen level becomes less than optimal.

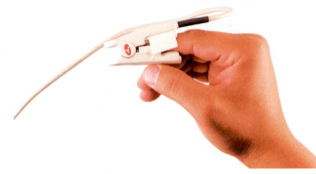

Fig. 22-5. *A pulse oximeter sensor is usually clipped on a person's finger.*

Normal blood oxygen level usually measures between 95% and 100%. However, normal ranges may differ from person to person. Nursing assistants should report any increase or decrease in oxygen levels to the nurse.

Guidelines: Pulse Oximetry

G   Report to the nurse immediately if the alarm on the pulse oximeter sounds.

G   Tell the nurse if the pulse oximeter falls off or if the resident requests that you remove it.

G   Check the skin around the device often. Report any of the following:

- Swelling
- Cyanotic skin
- Shiny, tight skin
- Skin that is cold to the touch
- Sores, redness, or irritation
- Numbness or tingling
- Pain or discomfort

G   Check vital signs as ordered. Report changes to the nurse.

6. Describe telemetry and list care guidelines

Telemetry is used to measure the heart rhythm and rate on a continuous basis. Wires are attached to the chest with sticky pads or patches (also called *leads* or *electrodes*) (Fig. 22-6). The wires are connected to a battery-powered portable unit, which sends data to computer screens at a monitoring station (Figs. 22-7 and 22-8). This data is monitored and assessed at all times by specially trained staff.

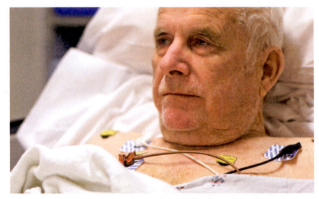

Fig. 22-6. *Pads, or leads, are attached to the person's chest.*

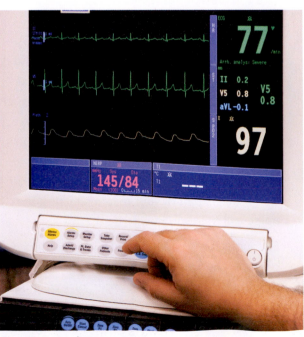

Fig. 22-7. *A telemetry monitoring unit.*

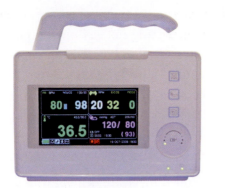

Fig. 22-8. A smaller portable telemetry monitoring unit that can be carried by the person.

Telemetry may be necessary due to chest pain, heart or lung disease, heart or lung surgery, irregular heartbeats, or certain medications that affect heart rhythm or rate.

Guidelines: Telemetry

G   Report to the nurse if the pads become wet or soiled. Report if pads appear loose or fall off.

G   Report if the alarm sounds. The alarm may sound if the pads disconnect or if the battery is low.

G   Check the skin around the pads often. Report any of the following:

   • Swelling

   • Sores, redness, or irritation

   • Fluid or blood draining from skin

   • Broken skin

G   Report resident complaints of chest pain or discomfort, as well as any difficulty breathing.

G   Check vital signs as ordered. Report changes to the nurse.

7. Explain artificial airways and list care guidelines

An **artificial airway** is any tube inserted into the respiratory tract to maintain or promote breathing. Artificial airways keep the airway open. This is necessary when the airway is ob-structed due to illness, injury, secretions, or aspiration. Some residents who are unconscious will need an artificial airway.

The artificial airway is inserted using a method called **intubation**. Intubation involves the passage of a plastic tube through the mouth, nose, or an opening in the neck and into the trachea (windpipe). There are different types of artificial airways (Fig. 22-9). One common type is a **tracheostomy**, which is a surgically-created opening through the neck into the trachea. A hollow tube, called a *tracheostomy tube* or *trach tube*, is inserted through this opening into the trachea. More information on this type of artificial airway may be found in the next learning objective.

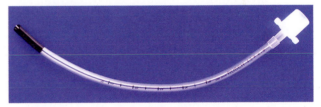

Fig. 22-9. An endotracheal tube is a type of artificial airway that is inserted through the mouth and then into the trachea. (PHOTO COURTESY OF TELEFLEX)

Guidelines: Artificial Airways

G   Check the resident regularly. If the tubing falls out, tell the nurse immediately.

G   Monitor vital signs as ordered. Report changes to the nurse.

G   Perform oral care often, as directed.

G   Watch for biting and tugging on tube. If a resident is doing this, tell the nurse.

G   Use other methods of communication if the resident cannot speak. Try writing notes, drawing pictures, and using communication boards. Watch for hand and eye signals.

G   Be supportive and reassuring. It can be frightening and uncomfortable to have an artificial airway. Some residents may choke or gag. Be empathetic. Imagine how it might feel to have a tube in your nose, mouth, or throat.

8. Discuss care for a resident with a tracheostomy

A tracheostomy is a type of artificial airway commonly seen in long-term care facilities (Fig. 22-10). Tracheostomies may be necessary for many reasons, including the following:

- Tumors/cancer

- Infection

- Severe neck or mouth injuries

- Facial surgery and facial burns

- Long-term unconsciousness or coma

- Obstruction in the airway

- Paralysis of muscles related to breathing

- Aspiration as a result of muscle or sensory problems in the throat

- Severe allergic reaction

- Gunshot wound

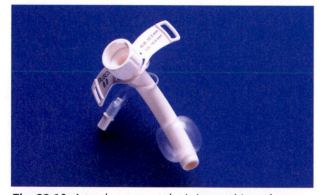

Fig. 22-10. A tracheostomy tube is inserted into the trachea through a surgically-created opening in the neck.
(PHOTO COURTESY OF TELEFLEX)

This procedure is usually temporary, but it can be permanent. It is easier to suction and attach respiratory equipment with a tracheostomy than with other artificial airways.

When the tracheostomy is first placed, it may be difficult for the resident to adapt to breathing through the tube. This can cause anxiety and frustration. It may be impossible for the resident to talk or make sounds at first, which also causes fear. During this time, nursing assistants should be especially supportive and encourag-

ing. They can use other methods of communication, such as writing notes, drawing pictures, using communication boards, and using hand and eye signals. Checking on the resident often and answering call lights immediately may help lessen anxiety. People can usually learn to talk through a trach tube.

General tracheostomy care includes keeping skin around the opening clean, helping with dressing changes, and cleaning the device. Suctioning may be required. Nursing assistants do not perform suctioning or tracheostomy care. Their responsibilities will mostly involve observing and reporting.

Observing and Reporting: Tracheostomies

Report any of the following to the nurse:

O/R Shortness of breath

O/R Trouble breathing

O/R Gurgling sounds

O/R Any signs of skin breakdown around the opening, such as irritation, rash, cracks, breaks, sores, or bleeding on the skin

O/R The type and amount of discharge that the resident coughs up through the tracheostomy (normal discharge looks like white mucus or saliva)

O/R Any increase in the amount of discharge

O/R Discharge that is thick, yellow, green, bloody, or has an odor (this may indicate an infection or other problem in the lungs)

O/R Mouth sores or discomfort

O/R Disconnected tubing

It is very important to prevent infection when caring for residents with tracheostomies. They are prone to respiratory infections. Nursing assistants must wash their hands often and wear gloves when indicated. NAs should wear masks if residents are coughing. It is vital that equipment be kept clean. Anything that is dropped on the floor must be sterilized before it can come in contact with the tubes. Great care must be taken so that nothing gets into the tube, which can cause an infection in the lungs.

9. List care guidelines for residents requiring mechanical ventilation

Residents in a subacute unit may be on a mechanical ventilator. **Mechanical ventilation** is using a machine to inflate and deflate the lungs when a person is unable to breathe on his own. A person may require mechanical ventilation due to cardiac or respiratory arrest, lung injuries and diseases, or head and spinal cord injuries.

Residents will not be able to speak while on the mechanical ventilator. This is because air will no longer reach the larynx (vocal cords). Not being able to speak may increase anxiety. The resident may think that no one will know if he is having trouble breathing. Being on a ventilator has been compared to breathing through a straw. Nursing assistants should be empathetic and think about how that might feel. Residents will need a lot of support while connected to the ventilator. NAs should enter the room often so that residents on ventilators can see them. This helps to reassure residents that they are being carefully observed. Clipboards, notepads, and communication boards will help with communication.

Residents on ventilators are often heavily sedated. A **sedative** is an agent or drug that helps calm and soothe a person and may cause sleep. Being sedated helps prevent people on ventilators from feeling discomfort and anxiety. Even if a resident seems unaware of what is happening, the NA must continue to speak to him and explain what she is doing.

Guidelines: Mechanical Ventilator

G Ventilators cause an increased risk for a special type of pneumonia. Wash your hands often when working with residents on mechanical ventilators.

G Report to the nurse if the alarm sounds.

G If you notice tubing that is disconnected or loose, report it immediately.

G Answer the call light promptly.

G Follow the care plan for repositioning instructions. The head of the bed may need to remain elevated.

G Give regular, careful skin care to prevent pressure injuries. Check the skin around the intubation site often, as well as on the rest of the body. Report any of the following:

- Swelling
- Sores, redness, irritation
- Fluid or blood draining from skin
- Broken skin

G Report if the resident is pulling on or biting the tube. Report if the resident is anxious, fearful, or upset.

G Be patient during communication. Observe body language. Watch for hand or eye signals.

G Check on the resident often, so that the resident can see that you are there. Be supportive, kind, and empathetic.

10. Describe suctioning and list signs of respiratory distress

Subacute care units include residents who require suctioning by nurses or respiratory therapists. Suctioning removes mucus and secretions from the lungs when a person cannot do this on his own. A person who has a tracheostomy may require suctioning. Suctioning can be performed through the nose, mouth, or throat.

Suctioning is normally a sterile procedure. Nursing assistants do not perform suctioning; nurses or respiratory therapists will perform the suctioning. Suction comes from a wall hook-up or a portable pump, operated on battery power or electrical power (Fig. 22-11). A canister or bottle on the pump collects the mucus and secretions.

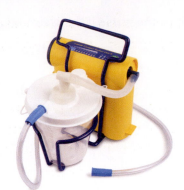

Fig. 22-11. This is one type of suctioning pump. Nursing assistants do not perform suctioning. They help by reporting signs of respiratory distress and monitoring vital signs. (PHOTO COURTESY OF LAERDAL MEDICAL)

A resident who needs frequent suctioning may show signs of respiratory distress. Signs of respiratory distress include the following:

- Gurgling sounds
- Difficulty breathing
- Elevated respiratory rate
- Pale, cyanotic, or gray skin around the eyes, mouth, fingernails, or toenails
- Nostrils flaring (nostrils opening wider when breathing in may show that a person is having to work harder to breathe)
- Retracting (chest appears to sink in below the neck with each breath)
- Sweating
- Wheezing

Guidelines: Suctioning

G Report signs of respiratory distress to the nurse immediately.

G Monitor vital signs closely, especially respiratory rate. Report changes.

G Follow Standard Precautions. Don gloves, gown, mask, or goggles as directed.

G Assist the nurse with suctioning as needed. You may be asked to have a towel or washcloth ready to clean the resident after suctioning. Give oral care as ordered.

G Report resident complaints of pain or difficulty breathing.

11. Describe chest tubes and explain related care

Chest tubes are hollow drainage tubes that are inserted into the chest during a sterile procedure (Fig. 22-12). They can be inserted at the bedside or during surgery. Chest tubes drain air, blood or other fluid, or pus that has collected inside the pleural cavity or space. The *pleural cavity* is the space between the layers of the pleura, the thin membrane that covers and protects the lungs. Chest tubes are also inserted to allow a full expansion of the lungs. Some conditions that require chest tube insertion include the following:

- Air or gas in the pleural space (pneumothorax)
- Blood in the pleural space (hemothorax)
- Pus in the pleural space (empyema)
- Certain types of surgery
- Chest trauma or injuries

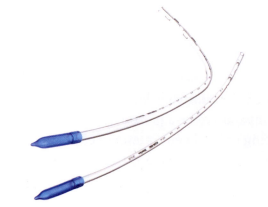

Fig. 22-12. A chest tube is inserted into the chest to drain air, fluid, or pus. (PHOTO COURTESY OF TELEFLEX)

A doctor normally inserts chest tubes. The chest tube is connected to a drainage system. Suction is sometimes attached to the system to encourage drainage. This system must be sealed so that air cannot enter the pleural cavity. The system must be airtight.

When X-rays show that the air, blood, or fluid has been drained, the tube is removed. Medications may be used to prevent or treat infection.

Guidelines: Chest Tubes

G Be aware of the number and location of chest tubes. Tubes may be in the front, back, or on the side of the body.

G Check vital signs as directed. Report any changes immediately to the nurse.

G Report signs of respiratory distress to the nurse immediately. Report complaints of pain.

G Keep the drainage system below the level of the resident's chest.

G Make sure drainage containers remain upright and level at all times.

G Make sure that tubing is not kinked. If tubing becomes kinked, report to the nurse right away.

G Watch for disconnected tubing. If this happens, report it immediately.

G Certain equipment is kept nearby in case tubes are pulled out. Do not remove these items from the area.

G Observe chest drainage for color and amount. Report any changes in color or amount immediately.

G Report if there is an increase or decrease in bubbling in the drainage system. Report if there are clots in the tubing.

G Follow the repositioning schedule. Be very gentle with turning and repositioning. You must move the resident and the tubes at the same time to prevent tubes from coming out. Always get enough help.

G Report odor in the chest tube area.

G Provide rest periods as needed.

G Follow fluid intake orders. Measure intake and output carefully, as ordered.

G If asked to help with coughing and deep breathing exercises, be encouraging and patient.

Other residents who require more direct care and close observation by staff include residents who have intravenous therapy (Chapter 14) and residents who have tube feedings (Chapter 15).

Chapter Review

1. What kinds of conditions require subacute care?

2. Briefly describe three types of surgeries.

3. Which type of anesthesia is inhaled or injected directly into a vein and affects the brain and entire body?

4. List eight guidelines for assisting with pre-operative care.

5. List eight guidelines for assisting with post-operative care.

6. List 10 signs and symptoms to report about a resident after surgery.

7. What does a pulse oximeter measure?

8. What is important to report about the skin when a resident is using a telemetry unit?

9. What are alternate methods of communication that nursing assistants can use with residents who have artificial airways?

10. What are a nursing assistant's responsibilities with tracheostomy care?

11. In what ways can a nursing assistant show support for a resident who is on a ventilator?

12. Why might a resident be anxious while on a ventilator?

13. List five signs of respiratory distress.

14. What types of fluids are drained by chest tubes?

15. List 12 guidelines for caring for residents with chest tubes.

Dying, Death, and Hospice

23
Dying, Death, and Hospice

1. Discuss the stages of grief

Death can occur suddenly without warning, or it can be expected. Older people or people with terminal illnesses may have time to prepare for death. A **terminal illness** is a disease or condition that will eventually cause death. Preparing for death is a process that affects the dying person's emotions and behavior.

Grief is deep distress or sorrow over a loss. It is an adaptive, or changing process, and usually involves healing. Dr. Elisabeth Kübler-Ross studied and wrote about the grief process. She theorized that dying people share a common grief process. Her book, *On Death and Dying*, describes five stages that dying people and their families or friends may experience before death. These five stages are described below. Not all residents go through all the stages. Some may stay in one stage until death occurs. Others may move back and forth between stages during the process.

Denial: People in the denial stage may refuse to believe they are dying. They often believe that a mistake has been made. They may demand lab work be repeated. They may talk about the future and avoid discussion about their illnesses. They may simply act like it is not happening. This is the "No, not me" stage.

Anger: Once people start to face the possibility of their death, they may become angry. They may be angry because they think they are too young to die. They may be angry because they feel they have always lived a healthy lifestyle and have always taken care of themselves. This anger may be directed at staff, visitors, roommates, family, or friends. Anger is a normal and healthy reaction. Even though it may be upsetting, the caregiver must try not to not take anger personally. This is the "Why me?" stage.

Bargaining: Once people have begun to believe that they really are dying, they may make promises to God or a higher power or somehow try to bargain for their recovery. This is the "Yes me, but..." stage.

Depression: As dying people become weaker and their symptoms get worse, they may become deeply sad or depressed (Fig. 23-1). They may cry or withdraw. They may be unable to perform simple activities. They need additional physical and emotional support. It is important for caregivers to listen and be understanding.

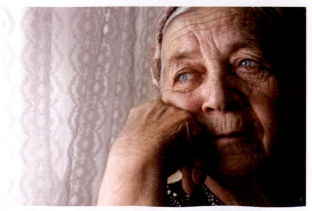

Fig. 23-1. *A person who is dying may become depressed and withdrawn. The nursing assistant should give extra emotional support to these residents.*

Acceptance: Peace or acceptance may or may not come before death. Some people who are dying are eventually able to accept death and prepare for it. They may make arrangements with attorneys and accountants. They may arrange with loved ones for the care of important people or things. They may make plans for their last days or for the ceremonies that may follow their death. At this stage, people who are dying may seem emotionally detached.

These stages may not be possible for someone who dies suddenly, unexpectedly, or quickly. Nobody can force anyone to move from stage to stage. Nursing assistants can help by listening and being ready to offer their help.

2. Describe the grief process

Dealing with grief after the death of a loved one is a process as well. Grieving is an individual process. No two people will grieve in exactly the same way. Clergy, counselors, and social workers can provide help for people who are grieving. Family members or friends may have any of the following reactions to the death of a loved one:

Shock: Even when death is expected, family members and friends may still be shocked after death occurs. Many people do not know what to expect after the death of a loved one and may be surprised by their feelings.

Denial: It is easy to want to believe that everything will quickly return to normal after a death. Denying or refusing to believe they are grieving can help people deal with the initial hours or days after a death. But eventually it is important to face feelings. Grief can be so overwhelming that some people may take years to face their feelings. Professional help can be very valuable.

Anger: Although it is hard to admit it, many people feel angry after a death. They may be angry with themselves, at God, at the doctors, or even at the person who died. There is nothing wrong with feeling anger as a part of grief.

Guilt: It is very common for families, friends, and caregivers to feel guilty after a death. They may wish they had done more for the dying person. They may simply feel that he or she did not deserve to die. They may feel guilty that they are still living or that they feel relieved.

Regret: Often people regret what they did or did not do for the dying person. They may regret things they said or did not say to the person who has died. Many people have regrets for years.

Relief: People may feel relieved that the person who has died is no longer suffering. They may be relieved that they no longer have a responsibility (emotional, physical, or financial) regarding care.

Sadness: It is very common to feel depressed or emotionally unstable after a death. People may suffer headaches or insomnia when they cannot express their sadness.

Loneliness: Missing someone who has died is very normal. It can bring up other feelings, such as sadness or regret. Many things may remind people of the person who died. The memories may be painful at first. With time, those who survive usually feel less lonely, and memories are less painful.

3. Discuss how feelings and attitudes about death differ

Death is a very sensitive topic. Many people find it hard to discuss death. Feelings and attitudes about death can be formed by many factors:

Experience with death: Someone who has been through other deaths may have a different understanding of death than someone who has not.

Personality type: Open, expressive people may have an easier time talking about and coping with death than those who are very reserved or quiet. Sharing feelings is one way of working through fears and concerns.

Religious beliefs: Religious practices and beliefs affect a person's experience with death. These include the process of dying, rituals at the time of death, burial or cremation practices, services held after death, and mourning customs (Fig. 23-2). For example, some Catholics do not believe in cremation. Orthodox Jews may not believe in viewing the body after death. Beliefs about what happens after death can also influence grieving. People who believe in an afterlife, such as heaven, may be comforted by this belief.

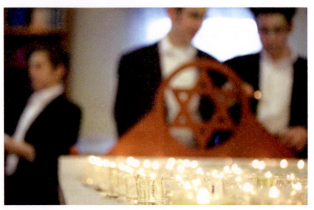

Fig. 23-2. *Religious beliefs and practices influence a person's feelings about death.*

Cultural background: The practices people grow up with affect how they deal with death. Cultural groups may have different practices to deal with death and grieving. Some groups have meals and other services but say very little about a person's death. In other groups, talking about and remembering the person who has died may be a comfort to family and friends (Fig. 23-3).

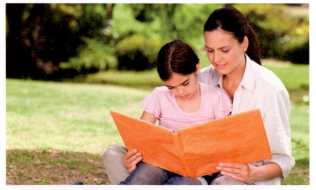

Fig. 23-3. *Looking at photos and sharing stories about a person who is dying or who has died is one way that family and friends may grieve.*

Learning Objective 10 in this chapter contains more information about different practices relating to death.

4. Discuss how to care for a resident who is dying

Care for a resident who is dying should focus on meeting physical needs, as well as providing comfort and emotional support. Promoting independence is important.

Guidelines: Resident Who Is Dying

G **Diminished senses**: Vision may begin to fail. Reduce glare and keep room lighting low (Fig. 23-4). Hearing is usually the last sense to leave the body, so speak in a normal tone. Tell the resident about care that is being done or what is happening in the room. Do not expect an answer. Ask few questions. Encourage the family to speak to the resident, but to avoid subjects that are disturbing. Observe body language to anticipate a resident's needs.

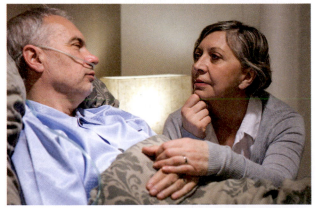

Fig. 23-4. *Keep a dying resident's room softly lit without glare.*

G **Care of the mouth and nose**: Give mouth care often. If the resident is unconscious, give mouth care every two hours. The lips and nostrils may be dry and cracked. Apply lubricant, such as lip balm, to lips and nose.

G **Skin care**: Give bed baths and incontinence care as needed. Bathe perspiring residents often. Skin should be kept clean and dry. Change sheets and clothes for comfort. Keep sheets wrinkle-free. Giving regular skin care and repositioning the resident often is important to help prevent pressure injuries.

G **Pain control and comfort**: Residents who are dying may be in pain. Pain relief is critical. Observe and report signs of pain to the nurse immediately. Residents may be connected to a patient-controlled analgesia (PCA) device. A PCA device is a method of pain control that allows patients to administer pain medication to themselves. They press a button to give themselves a dose of pain medication. Report any complaints of pain or discomfort to the nurse immediately. Because some residents may not be able to communicate that they are in pain, observe body language and watch for other signs.

Frequent changes of position, back massage, skin care, mouth care, and proper body alignment may help. Body temperature usually rises. Many residents are more comfortable with light covers. However, fever may cause chills. Use extra blankets if residents need more warmth.

G **Environment**: Display favorite objects and photographs where the resident can easily see them. They may provide comfort. Play music if the resident requests it. Make sure the room is comfortable, appropriately lit, and well ventilated. When leaving the room, place the call light within reach, even if the resident is unaware of his surroundings.

G **Emotional and spiritual support**: Residents who are dying may be afraid of what is happening and of death. Listening may be one of the most important things you can do for a resident who is dying. Pay attention to these conversations. Report any comments about fear to the nurse.

People who are dying may also need the quiet, reassuring, and loving presence of another person. Touch can be very important. Holding the resident's hand as you sit quietly can be very comforting.

Do not avoid the dying person or his family. Do not deny that death is approaching, and do not tell the resident that anyone knows how or when it will happen. Do give accurate information in a reassuring way. No one can take away a person's fear of death. However, your supportive and reassuring presence can help.

Some residents who are dying may also seek spiritual comfort from clergy. Tell the nurse immediately if resident requests a clergyperson. Provide privacy for visits from clergy and others. Do not discuss your religious or spiritual beliefs with residents or their families or make recommendations.

Take the time to sort out your own feelings about death. If you are not comfortable with the topic, residents will feel it. Speak to the nurse if you need resources to help you deal with your feelings.

Advance Directives and Related Medical Orders

Advance directives and medical orders were first introduced in Chapter 3. Advance directives allow people to choose what medical care they want or do not want if they cannot make those decisions themselves. A DNR order tells medical professionals not to perform CPR. DNR orders may be issued for a person who has a terminal illness, someone who almost certainly will not be saved by CPR, a person who is not expected to live long, and/or a person who simply wants to let nature take its course.

If a resident has an advance directive in place, the NA may be asked to continue to monitor vital signs, such as temperature, pulse, respirations, and blood pressure, and to report the readings to the nurse. Comfort measures, such as pain medication, will continue to be used. However, depending on what the advance directive states, performing CPR or any extraordinary measures may be prohibited, no matter how the vital signs have changed or declined. Extraordinary measures are measures used to prolong life when there is no reasonable expectation of recovery. When a person with a DNR order stops breathing or the heart stops, he or she will die unless the heart or breathing restarts on its own. This is not likely to happen. By law, advance directives and DNR orders must be honored. Nursing assistants must respect each resident's decisions about advance directives.

5. Describe ways to treat dying residents and their families with dignity and how to honor their rights

Nursing assistants can treat residents with dignity when they are approaching death by respecting their rights and their preferences. These are some legal rights to remember when caring for people who are dying:

The right to refuse treatment. Nursing assistants must remember that whether they agree or disagree with a resident's decisions, the choice is not theirs. It belongs to the person involved and/or his or her family. NAs should be supportive of family members and not judge them. The family is most likely following the resident's wishes.

The right to have visitors. When death is close, it is an emotional time for all those involved. Saying goodbye can be a very important part of dealing with a loved one's death. It may also be very reassuring to the person who is dying to have someone in the room, even if the person does not seem to be aware of his surroundings.

The right to privacy. Privacy is a basic right, but privacy for visiting, or even when the person is alone, may be even more important now.

Other rights of a dying person are listed below in *The Dying Person's Bill of Rights*. This was created at a workshop, *The Terminally Ill Patient and the Helping Person*, sponsored by Southwestern Michigan In-Service Education Council, and appeared in the *American Journal of Nursing*, Vol. 75, January 1975, p. 99.

I have the right to:

- Be treated as a living human being until I die.
- Maintain a sense of hopefulness, however changing its focus may be.
- Be cared for by those who can maintain a sense of hopefulness, however changing this might be.
- Express my feelings and emotions about my approaching death in my own way.

- Participate in decisions concerning my care.
- Expect continuing medical and nursing attentions even though "cure" goals must be changed to "comfort" goals.
- Not die alone.
- Be free from pain.
- Have my questions answered honestly.
- Not be deceived.
- Have help from and for my family in accepting my death.
- Die in peace and dignity.
- Retain my individuality and not be judged for my decisions, which may be contrary to the beliefs of others.
- Discuss and enlarge my religious and/or spiritual experiences, whatever these may mean to others.
- Expect that the sanctity of the human body will be respected after death.
- Be cared for by caring, sensitive, knowledgeable people who will attempt to understand my needs and will be able to gain some satisfaction in helping me face my death.

Guidelines: Treating Residents Who Are Dying with Dignity

G   Respect the resident's wishes in all possible ways. Communication is extremely important at this time so that everyone understands what the resident's wishes are. Listen carefully for ideas on how to provide simple gestures that may be special and appreciated.

G   Do not isolate or avoid a resident who is dying. Enter his room regularly.

G   Be careful not to make promises that cannot or should not be kept.

G   Continue to involve the resident in his care and in any facility activities. Be person-centered. Do not talk with other staff members about your personal life when caring for a resident.

G Listen if a resident wants to talk but do not offer advice. Do not make judgmental comments.

G Do not babble or act especially cheerful or sad. Be professional.

G Keep the resident as comfortable as possible. The nurse needs to know immediately if pain medication is requested. Keep the resident clean and dry.

G Assure privacy when it is desired.

G Respect the privacy of the family and other visitors. They may be upset and not want to be social at this time. They may welcome a friendly smile, however, and should not be isolated either.

G Help with the family's physical comfort. If requested, get them coffee, water, chairs, blankets, etc.

Residents' Rights

Life Support Measures

Life support measures are used when vital body systems are not working well enough to support life on their own. These measures include feeding tubes, mechanical ventilation, dialysis, etc. The decision to remain on life support or to discontinue life support is often part of a person's advance directives. When the decision is made to discontinue life support and the body is not able to function without these supports, the person will die. This may happen immediately, or the person may live for a short time. As with any advance directive and personal decision regarding treatment, nursing assistants should not judge a resident's (or a family member's) choice to remain on or discontinue life support. This is a private and personal decision. NAs should respect the resident's wishes and not make comments about his or her choices to anyone, including family members, other residents, or other staff members.

6. Define the goals of a hospice program

Hospice care is the term for the special care that a dying person needs. It is a compassionate way to care for people who are dying and their families. Hospice care emphasizes a holistic, person-centered approach. It treats the dying person's physical, emotional, spiritual, and social needs.

Hospice care can be given seven days a week, 24 hours a day. It is available with a doctor's order. There is always a nurse on call to answer questions, make a visit, or solve a problem. Hospice care may be given in a hospital, at a care facility, or in the home. A hospice can be any location where a person who is dying is treated with dignity by caregivers.

Any caregiver may provide hospice care, but often specially trained nurses, social workers, and volunteers provide hospice care. The hospice team may include doctors, nurses, social workers, counselors, nursing assistants, home health aides, therapists, clergy, dietitians, and volunteers.

Hospice care helps meet all needs of the resident who is dying. The resident, as well as family and friends, is directly involved in care decisions. The resident is encouraged to participate in family life and decision-making as long as possible.

In long-term care, goals focus on the resident's recovery or on the resident's ability to care for herself as much as possible. In hospice care, however, the goals are the comfort and dignity of the resident. This type of care is called **palliative care**. Palliative care is a type of care given to people who are dying that emphasizes relieving pain, controlling symptoms, and preventing side effects and complications. Palliative care is also given to people who have serious, chronic diseases, such as cancer, congestive heart failure, and AIDS.

Focusing on pain relief, comfort, and managing symptoms is different than providing regular care. NAs will need to adjust their mindset when caring for residents in hospice.

Residents who are dying need to feel independent for as long as possible. Caregivers should allow residents to have as much control over their lives as possible. Eventually, caregivers may have to meet all of the resident's basic needs.

Nursing assistants should remember the following guidelines when working in hospice care:

Guidelines: Hospice Care

G Be a good listener. It is hard to know what to say to someone who is dying or to his relatives or friends. Most often, people need someone to listen to them (Fig. 23-5). A good listener can be a great comfort. Some people, however, will not want to confide in their caregivers, and you should never push someone to talk.

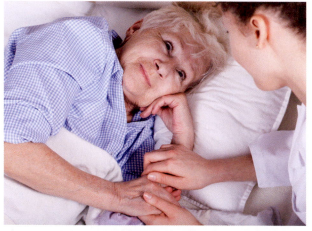

Fig. 23-5. Being a good listener can be a great help to a resident who is dying.

G Respect privacy and independence. Relatives, friends, clergy, and others may visit a resident who is dying. Make it easy for these difficult visits to take place. Stay out of the way when you can. Do not join in the conversation unless asked to do so. Understand that some people wish to be alone with their dying loved ones. Dying residents can have some independence even when they need total care. Let the resident make choices when possible, such as when to bathe, whether to eat or not, or what to eat or drink.

G Be sensitive to individual needs. Different residents and families will have different needs. The more you know what is needed, the more you can help. Some residents need a quiet and calm atmosphere. Others appre-

ciate a cheery presence and might like you to talk or stay close by. Ask family members or friends how you can help.

G Be aware of your own feelings. Caring for people who are dying can be draining. Know your limits and respect them. Discuss feelings of frustration or grief with another care team member.

G Recognize the stress. Just realizing how stressful it is to work with residents who are dying is a first step toward caring for yourself. Talking with a counselor about your experiences at work can help you understand and work through your feelings. Remember, however, that specific information must be kept confidential. A supervisor may be able to make a referral to a counselor or support group.

G Take care of yourself. Eating right, exercising, and getting enough rest are ways of taking care of yourself. Remember that caring for your emotional health is important too. Talk about and acknowledge your feelings. Take time to do things for yourself, such as reading a book, taking a bubble bath, or another activity that you enjoy. If you are a religious or spiritual person, these needs may be met by attending religious services, reading, praying, meditating, or just taking a quiet walk (Fig. 23-6). Meeting your needs allows you to best meet other people's needs.

G Take a break when you need to. Find ten minutes to sit down and relax or stand up and stretch. This may be enough of a break in some situations.

Hospice Volunteers

According to the National Hospice and Palliative Care Organization, an estimated 430,000 hospice volunteers provided 19 million hours of service to an estimated 1.6 to 1.7 million patients in 2014. Hospice volunteers go through a training program to prepare them for hospice work. The volunteers provide a variety of services. This includes caring for the home or family of a dying person, driving or doing errands, and providing emotional support. Their website, nhpco.org, has more information.

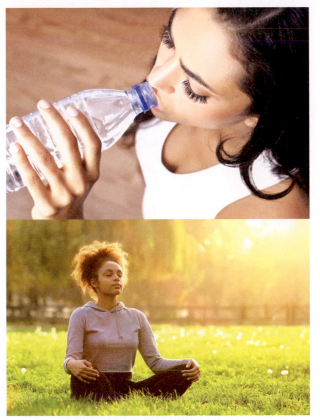

Fig. 23-6. *Taking care of yourself, including eating right, drinking plenty of water, and relaxing, is a way to help you tend to your needs while caring for people who are dying. Exercise, meditation, prayer, or reading are also ways to meet your needs.*

7. Explain common signs of approaching death

Death can be sudden or gradual. Certain physical changes occur that can be signs and symptoms of approaching death. Vital signs and skin color are often affected. Disorientation, confusion, and reduced responsiveness may occur. Vision, taste, and touch usually diminish. However, it is generally acknowledged that hearing is often present until death occurs.

Common signs of approaching death include the following:

* Blurred and failing vision
* Unfocused eyes
* Impaired speech
* Diminished sense of touch

* Loss of movement, muscle tone, and feeling
* A rising or below-normal body temperature
* Decreasing blood pressure
* Weak pulse that is abnormally slow or rapid
* Alternating periods of slow, irregular respirations and rapid, shallow respirations, along with short periods of apnea, called **Cheyne-Stokes** respirations
* A rattling or gurgling sound as the person breathes (which does not cause discomfort for the dying person)
* Cold, pale skin
* Mottling (bruised appearance), spotting, or blotching of skin caused by poor circulation
* Perspiration
* Incontinence (both urine and stool)
* Disorientation or confusion

8. List changes that may occur in the human body after death

When death occurs, the body will not have a heartbeat, pulse, respiration, or blood pressure. The eyelids may remain open or partially open with the eyes in a fixed stare. The mouth may remain open. The body may be incontinent of urine and stool. Between two to six hours after death, the muscles in the body become stiff and rigid. This is a temporary condition called ***rigor mortis***, which is Latin for *stiffness of death*. Though these things are a normal part of death, they can be frightening. The nursing assistant should inform the nurse immediately to help confirm the death.

9. Describe postmortem care

Postmortem care is care of the body after death. It takes place after the resident has been declared dead by a nurse or doctor. It is important for nursing assistants to be sensitive to the needs of the family and friends after death.

Family members may wish to sit by the bed to say goodbye. They may wish to stay with the body for a while. They should be allowed to do these things. NAs should be aware of religious and cultural practices that the family wants to observe. Facilities have different policies about postmortem care. NAs should follow their facility's policies and only perform assigned tasks.

Guidelines: Postmortem Care

G   After death, the muscles in the body become stiff and rigid. This may make the body difficult to move. Talk to the nurse if you need help performing postmortem care.

G   Bathe the body. Be very gentle to avoid bruising. Place drainage pads where needed, most often under the head and/or under the perineum (the genital and anal area). Be sure to follow Standard Precautions.

G   Do not remove any tubes or other equipment. A nurse or someone at the funeral home will do this.

G   If instructed to do so, put dentures back in the mouth and close the mouth. You may need to place a rolled towel under the chin to support the closed mouth position. If this is not possible, place dentures in a denture cup near the resident's head.

G   Close the eyes carefully.

G   Position the body on the back with legs straight and arms folded across the abdomen. Place a small pillow under the head.

G   Follow facility policy about personal items. Check to see if you should remove jewelry. Always have a witness if personal items are removed or given to a family member. Document what was given and to whom.

G   Once the body has been removed, strip the bed.

G   Open windows to air the room as needed and straighten up.

G   Document according to your facility's policy.

Organ Donation

Organ donation is the removal of organs and tissues for the purpose of transplanting into someone who needs them. Organ donors can be people who have recently died or living people. If a resident has designated himself an organ donor after death, specific policies and procedures will need be followed. Some organs must be taken from the body very soon after a person dies. NAs should follow the nurse's instructions regarding special preparations or transport.

Residents' Rights

Comforting Others

After a loved one has died, the nursing assistant should show family and friends to a comfortable place to sit and talk privately. She should ask if she can contact anyone for them. She should provide water or another beverage. If family members want to be left alone with the deceased, the NA can provide privacy by leaving the room and closing the door. Family and friends should not feel they are being rushed out of the facility.

It is natural to feel upset and not know what to say when someone has died. Many people talk a lot when feeling stressed. NAs can show support without talking very much. They should listen patiently and not interrupt (Fig. 23-7). The family may want to repeat what happened and how it occurred. It is helpful for them to repeat this story.

What an NA says is not as important as is being sincere. Simply saying, "I am so sorry," is fine. She should avoid clichés such as, "It is for the better." If the NA can say it honestly, saying something like, "Your mother will be missed here," is supportive and kind.

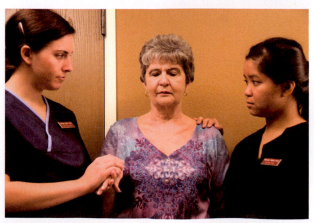

Fig. 23-7. Nursing assistants should be available for family and friends if they want to talk and should allow them to express their feelings.

10. Understand and respect different postmortem practices

When caring for those who are dying, nursing assistants will also interact with families and will witness many different responses to the death of a loved one. Dealing with the loss of a loved one is a monumental task that people face in different ways. It is a process that may begin with the diagnosis of a terminal illness and may not end until years after the loved one's death.

There is no right or wrong way to grieve. A person's initial response to the death of a loved one may be due in part to her cultural or religious background, or it may simply be how that person deals with death. When people respond differently than a nursing assistant would, it is important that the NA remember her professional duty and respect their responses.

When a death has occurred, some people may respond quietly, with very little obvious emotion, while others may be very vocal. Depending on the preferences of the family, the body may be removed very quickly or the family may wish for the body to remain for some time while people say goodbye, pray, or perform necessary religious rituals. Many cultures forbid leaving the body of the deceased alone. In some cultures and religious traditions, the body must be buried promptly, either on the day of death or within a certain period immediately after. An NA should not be alarmed if this happens or judge the practices of the resident's family.

A nursing assistant may be invited to attend a funeral or other ceremony following the death of a resident. As someone who has cared for the deceased person, the NA may be grieving as well (Fig. 23-8). If she wants to attend the service, she should check with her supervisor first to make sure it is appropriate. It is important to respect professional boundaries.

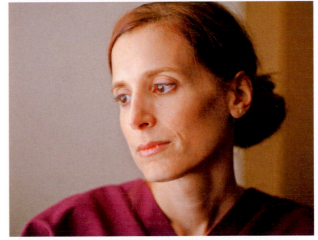

Fig. 23-8. *Nursing assistants should allow themselves to grieve. They will develop close relationships with some residents. It is normal for them to feel sad, angry, or lonely when residents die.*

Just as responses to death vary widely, funeral and burial practices vary from culture to culture and region to region. In some cultures, the family and friends of the deceased person hold a *wake*, or a watch over the body before burial. Traditionally the wake was held in the deceased person's home, and the body was present. Modern wakes may take place at a funeral home. There may be singing, eating, drinking, and storytelling at a wake. The mood is not necessarily sad or somber. A *viewing* is a period of time during which a deceased person's body may be visited by mourners. Viewings may be combined with a celebration of the person's life (as in a wake) or may simply be a time for mourners to pay their quiet respects.

Funerals or memorial services may also involve the display of the dead person's body. This is typically called an *open casket* funeral. The body will have been preserved for burial (embalmed) by a mortician (a person whose job it is to arrange for the burial or cremation of the dead) and may be dressed formally or in clothing dictated by the person's family, culture, or faith. Some cultures or religious traditions forbid the display of a dead body, and for some it is simply a preference that the body not be displayed. At a closed casket service, the casket, or coffin, is present, but is closed so that the body is not visible.

When a body is not buried in a casket, it may be cremated. Cremation is the burning of a body until it is reduced to ashes. Being cremated may be what the deceased person wanted for personal reasons, or it may be dictated by some religious traditions. An urn, or container for the ashes, may be displayed at a funeral or memorial service rather than a casket.

Natural burial (sometimes called *green burial*) is another option. The body is wrapped in a shroud (cloth) or put in a **biodegradeable** casket. The body is not embalmed and is placed in the ground to allow for natural decomposition.

Funerals and memorial services may be held in a place of worship or at a funeral home. They may be held in a family home, at a park, in a restaurant, or at any location that has personal significance. Services may involve readings either of religious scripture and prayers or philosophical excerpts. Many include eulogies, or speeches made in honor of the deceased. Friends and family members may share moving, memorable, or humorous stories about the person who has died. Spiritual leaders may offer words of comfort or remembrance. Some funerals are followed by a procession to the place of burial. Often only those closest to the deceased take part in the burial. In some cases, memorial services are entirely separate from the burial, and the deceased person's body is not present at all. A luncheon or reception often follows the service.

Services may incorporate elements of the dead person's religious faith and culture. If an NA is attending a service for a resident who practiced a faith different from her own or who came from a culture different from her own, she should be respectful of the resident's traditions.

The same is true of attending a service for a resident who was an atheist (a person who does not believe in any higher power). Such services will not involve prayers, hymns, or any religious rituals.

No matter what rituals or services take place after a person has died, nursing assistants should not be judgmental or make critical comments. They should be respectful and professional.

Chapter Review

1. Describe one behavior that a nursing assistant might see at each stage of grief.

2. Describe five possible feelings/responses in the grief process.

3. How would you describe your personality type? What helps you work through difficult feelings like those associated with grief?

4. Which sense is usually present until death occurs?

5. What are some of the ways that an NA might provide emotional and spiritual support for a dying resident?

6. What measures may help a dying resident who is in pain?

7. List three legal rights to remember when caring for the terminally ill.

8. What is the focus in palliative care? How does it differ from the usual care NAs provide?

9. List 10 common signs of approaching death.

10. List five changes that may occur in the human body after death.

11. What is postmortem care?

12. Where are drainage pads most often needed during postmortem care?

13. What is a wake?

14. What is cremation?

24

Introduction to Home Care

1. Explain the purpose of and need for home health care

Health care delivered in hospitals and long-term care facilities is expensive. To reduce costs, hospitals discharge patients earlier. Many people who are discharged have not recovered their strength and stamina. Many require skilled assistance or monitoring. Others need only short-term assistance at home. Most insurance companies are willing to pay for a part of this care because it is less expensive than a long stay at a hospital or extended care facility.

The growing numbers of older people and chronically ill people are also creating a demand for home care services. Family members who in the past would care for aging or ill relatives frequently live in distant areas. In addition, they often have other responsibilities that interfere with their ability to provide care. For example, family members who work may be unable to look after aging relatives as they become frail and less functional.

Most people who need some medical care prefer the familiar surroundings of home to an institution. They choose to live alone or receive care from a relative or friend. Home health aides (HHAs) can provide assistance to the chronically ill, the elderly, and family caregivers who need relief from the physical and emotional stress of caregiving. Many home health aides also work in assisted living facilities. Assisted living facilities allow independent living in a home-like environment, with professional care available as needed. Home

health aides may be former nursing assistants who decided to make a change from working in facilities or hospitals to working in the home.

As advances in medicine and technology extend the lives of people with chronic illnesses, the number of people needing health care will increase. Home services will be needed to provide continued care and assistance as chronic illnesses progress. Healthcare professionals are becoming more and more aware of the importance of providing person-centered care (Chapter 1). This means providing care that takes each client's individual preferences, choices, dignity, interests, and capabilities into consideration. One of the most important reasons for health care in the home is that most people who are ill or disabled feel more comfortable at home (Fig. 24-1). Home health care lends itself very well to person-centered care. Health care in familiar surroundings improves mental and physical well-being. It has proven to be a major factor in the healing process.

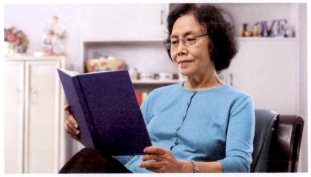

Fig. 24-1. *People who are ill or disabled often feel more comfortable being cared for in their own homes, where everything is familiar.*

2. Describe a typical home health agency

Many home health aides are employed by home health agencies. **Home health agencies** are businesses that arrange for health care and personal services to be provided in the home. Healthcare services provided by home health agencies may include nursing care, specialized therapy, specific medical equipment, pharmacy and intravenous (IV) products, and personal care. Personal care services may include helping with activities of daily living (ADLs), housekeeping, shopping, and cooking.

Clients who need home care are referred to a home health agency by their doctors. They can also be referred by a hospital discharge planner, a social services agency, the state or local department of public health, a local agency on aging, or a senior center. Clients and family members may also choose an agency that meets their needs.

Once an agency is chosen and the doctor has made a referral, a staff member performs an assessment of the client. This determines how the care needs can best be met. The home environment will also be evaluated to determine whether it is safe for the client.

The services home health agencies provide depend on the size of the agency. Small agencies may provide basic nursing care, personal care, and housekeeping services. Larger agencies may provide speech, physical, and occupational therapies and medical social work. Some common services include the following:

- Physical, occupational, and speech therapy

- Medical-surgical nursing care, including medication management; wound care; care of different types of tubes; catheterization; and management of clients with HIV, diabetes, chronic obstructive pulmonary disease (COPD), and congestive heart failure (CHF)

- Intravenous infusion therapy

- Maternal, pediatric, and newborn nursing care

- Nutrition therapy/dietary counseling

- Medical social work

- Personal care, including bathing; measuring vital signs; skin, nail and hair care; meal preparation; light housekeeping; ambulation; and range of motion exercises

- Homemaker/companion services

- Medical equipment rental and service

- Pharmacy services

- Hospice services

All home health agencies have professional staff who make decisions about what services are needed. These professionals, who may be doctors, nurses, or other licensed professionals, also reassess clients' need for services, write care plans, and schedule services.

Once staff members determine the amount and types of care needed, assignments are given. A home health aide may be assigned to spend a certain number of hours each day or week with a client providing care and services. While the care plan and the assignments are developed by the supervisor or case manager, input from all members of the care team is needed. All home health aides are under the supervision of a skilled professional. It may be a nurse, a physical therapist, a speech-language pathologist, or an occupational therapist. Figure 24-2 shows a typical home health agency organization chart.

3. Explain how working for a home health agency is different from working in other types of facilities

In some ways, working as a home health aide is similar to working as a nursing assistant. Most of the basic medical procedures and many of the personal care procedures will be the same. However, some aspects of working in the home are very different from working in care facilities.

Housekeeping: An HHA may have light housekeeping responsibilities, including cooking, cleaning, laundry, and grocery shopping, for at least some clients.

Family contact: An HHA may have a lot more contact with clients' families in the home than in a facility.

Independence: An HHA will work independently. A supervisor will monitor her work, but most hours working with clients will be spent without direct supervision. Thus, the HHA must be a responsible and independent worker.

Communication: Careful written and verbal communication skills are important. An HHA must stay informed of changes in the client care plan. She must keep others informed of changes observed in the client and the client's environment.

Transportation: Traveling from one client's home to another is a necessity. An HHA needs to have a dependable car or know how to use public transportation. She may face bad weather conditions, but clients need care, regardless of rain, sleet, or snow.

Safety: An HHA needs to be aware of personal safety when traveling alone to visit clients. She may be visiting clients in areas where crime is a problem. It is important that she remain aware of her surroundings, walk confidently, and avoid dangerous situations. She should make sure others know her travel plans/schedule for the day.

Flexibility: Each client's home will be different. An HHA will need to adapt to the changes in the environment. In a care facility, certain supplies will be available, and working conditions will be clean and organized. In home care, an

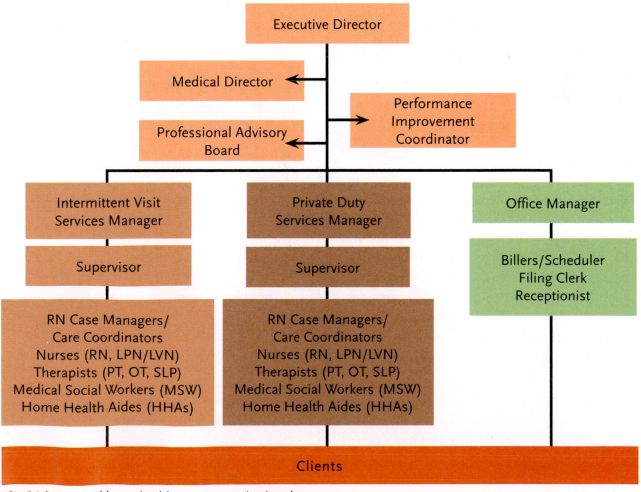

Fig. 24-2. A typical home health agency organization chart.

HHA may not know what will be available at a client's home until she gets there.

Working environment: Long-term care facilities are built to make caregiving easier and safer. They have wide doors, large bathing facilities, and special equipment for transferring residents. If needed, other caregivers are close by and can help move a resident or answer questions. In home care, lack of equipment, stairs, cramped bathrooms, rugs, clutter, the layout of rooms, and even pets can complicate caregiving.

Client's home: In a client's home, the HHA is a guest (Fig. 24-3). She needs to be respectful of the client's property and customs. The client is in control most of the time. If there are any customs that seem unsafe, the HHA should talk to her supervisor.

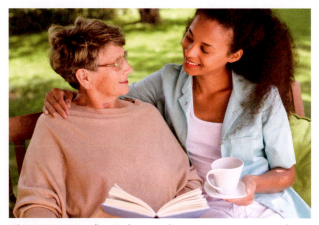

Fig. 24-3. In a client's home, the HHA is a guest and must respect the client's personal items and customs.

Clients' comfort: One of the best things about home care is that it allows clients to stay in the familiar and comfortable surroundings of their own homes. This can help most clients recover or adapt to their condition more quickly.

4. Discuss the client care plan and explain how team members contribute to the care plan

Just as a resident in long-term care has a personal care plan, so does a client in home health care. The care plan is individualized for each client. It is developed to help achieve the goals of care. It lists tasks that team members, including home health aides, must perform. It states how often these tasks should be performed and how they should be carried out. For example, the care plan for a client who has had a stroke may list the following HHA responsibilities:

- Perform range of motion exercises daily

- Measure vital signs, such as temperature, pulse, and blood pressure, once a day or more

- Meet diet and fluid requirements

The care plan is a guide to help the client attain and maintain the best possible level of health. **Activities not listed on the care plan should not be performed**. The HHA care plan is part of this overall plan of care. It must be followed very carefully.

Care planning should involve input from the client and/or the family, as well as from health professionals. When the client is involved in care planning, he is more likely to participate in and continue treatment. In addition, the client has a legal right to participate in his own care. Person-centered care places special emphasis on the importance of the client's input. Professionals will assess the client's physical, financial, social, and psychological needs. After the doctor prescribes treatment, the supervisor, nurses, and other care team members create the care plan. Many factors are considered when creating a care plan. These include the following:

- The client's health and physical condition

- The client's diagnosis and treatment

- The client's goals, priorities, or expectations

- Whether additional services and resources, including transportation, equipment, or supplementary income, are needed (for example, a social worker may arrange transportation for the client to and from appointments with his or her doctor)

The psychological (mental and emotional) and socioeconomic (social and economic) status of the client and the family are other important considerations. The agency will assess how the client and family are reacting to the medical problems that the client is experiencing. Family members may be unavailable for some clients. For example, a client may have only elderly and ailing relatives to help with care. Family members may have jobs to go to or children to care for. Some families may have relatives who are unwilling to assist in care. For some families, problems like alcoholism and substance abuse can make it difficult to provide care. Housing and financial resources may also be lacking. A medical social worker may be sent to the home to assess the situation, make referrals, and assist with long-term care planning.

Input from all members of the care team is needed to develop the client care plan. For instance, a 250-pound, elderly client requests a tub bath. The supervisor assigns it. The home health aide finds that the client has no adaptive equipment and is unable to move to the tub. The assignment puts the HHA and the client at risk of injury. The home health aide must communicate this to his supervisor. The assignment needs to be changed to a bed bath or shower, or the client needs to obtain adaptive equipment. The supervisor is responsible for reassessing the assignment and making changes to the care plan.

Multiple care plans may be necessary for some clients. In these situations, the supervisor will coordinate the client's overall care. There will be one care plan for the home health aide to follow. There will be separate care plans for other providers, such as the physical therapist.

Care plans must be updated as the client's condition changes. Reporting changes and problems to the supervisor is a very important role of the home health aide. That is how the care team revises care plans to meet the client's changing needs (Fig. 24-4).

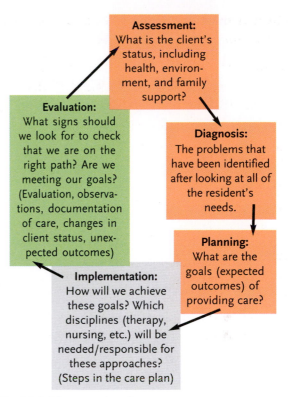

Fig. 24-4. *The care planning process.*

Clients' Rights

Care Team and Client

Just as the resident is an important team member in long-term care, the client is the focus in home health care. The client has the right to make decisions and choices about his or her own care. The client's family may also be involved in these decisions. The care team revolves around the client and his or her condition, treatment, and progress. Without the client, there is no care team. Chapter 2 contains more information.

5. Describe the role of the home health aide and explain typical tasks performed

The role of home health aides is to improve or maintain the independence, health, and well-being of clients. This is done by providing or assisting with personal care, assisting with activities of daily living (ADLs), and performing assigned tasks. It is also accomplished by promoting self-care. HHAs can reinforce the teachings of other team members and promote behavior that improves health, such as maintaining a healthy diet and exercising.

Home health aides provide services directly to their clients in several ways. HHAs provide care or assist with self-care, depending on the care plan. A care plan may include the following, depending on state regulations:

- Bathing
- Dressing
- Grooming
- Toileting
- Assisting with range of motion (ROM) exercises and ambulation (walking)
- Transferring from bed to chair or wheelchair
- Measuring vital signs (temperature, pulse rate, respiratory rate, blood pressure, and pain level)
- Feeding
- Reminding the client about medications
- Giving skin care
- Using medical supplies and equipment, such as walkers and wheelchairs
- Changing simple dressings
- Making and changing beds
- Light cleaning, including dusting, vacuuming, and washing dishes
- Teaching home management and safety

HHAs maintain a safe, secure, and comfortable home life for clients and their families. This may include light housekeeping, food shopping, meal preparation, and laundry.

Home health aides are also role models. They promote clients' independence by practicing proper housekeeping, nutrition, and healthcare skills. Encouraging clients to do tasks for themselves helps ensure that health will be maintained between visits.

In addition, home health aides teach by example. By performing procedures and giving help ef-

ficiently and cheerfully, they provide the family with a model for caregiving. Home health aides are not intended to replace a family member. Rather, HHAs support and strengthen the family.

In Chapter 2, scope of practice was introduced. A scope of practice defines the tasks that healthcare providers are legally allowed to do as permitted by state and federal law. Laws and regulations about what aides can and cannot do vary from state to state. However, some procedures are not performed by home health aides under any circumstances. Tasks that are said to be outside the scope of practice of a home health aide include the following:

- HHAs do not administer medications unless trained and assigned to do so. Only a few states allow home health aides to do this. However, additional training is always required. Home health aides may assist the clients with self-administered medications in certain situations.

- HHAs do not insert or remove tubes or objects (other than a thermometer) into or from a client's body. These procedures are called *invasive*, and are performed only by licensed professionals.

- HHAs do not honor a request to do something outside the scope of practice, not listed in the job description, or not on the assignment sheet. In this situation, an HHA should explain that he cannot do the task requested. The request should then be reported to a supervisor. This is true even if a nurse or doctor asks the HHA to perform the task. The HHA should refuse to perform the task and explain why. Refusing to do something that the HHA cannot legally do is the HHA's right and responsibility.

- HHAs do not perform procedures that require sterile technique. For example, changing a sterile dressing on a deep, open wound requires sterile technique.

- HHAs do not diagnose illnesses or prescribe treatments or medications.

- HHAs do not tell the client or the family the diagnosis or the medical treatment plan. This is the responsibility of the doctor or nurse.

Home health aides must know which tasks are outside their scope of practice and not perform them. Many of these specialized tasks require more training. HHAs must learn how to refuse a task for which they have not been trained or which is outside their scope of practice.

Maintaining Boundaries

In professional relationships, boundaries must be set. Boundaries are the limits to or within relationships. Home health aides, like other professionals, are guided by ethics and laws which set limits for their relationships with clients. These boundaries help support a healthy client-worker relationship. Working in clients' homes may make it more difficult to honor the boundaries of professional relationships. Clients may feel that home health aides are their friends because they are in their homes. If the worker and client become personally involved with each other, it makes it more difficult to enforce rules. For example, an HHA may want to give a client extra help or let her skip the exercise she dislikes. The client may expect the HHA to break the rules because she thinks they are friends.

Emotional attachments to clients are unprofessional and may weaken an HHA's judgment. HHAs should be friendly, warm, and caring with clients, but should remain professional and stay within the limits of set boundaries. Agency rules and the care plan's instructions should be followed. They are in place for everyone's protection. An HHA can ask her supervisor for help if a client asks her to do things she is not allowed to do.

6. Explain common policies and procedures for home health aides

All home health agencies have policies and procedures that all staff members are expected to follow. Common policies at home health agencies include the following:

- All client information must remain confidential. Keeping information confidential means not telling anyone about it. This is not only an agency rule, it is also the law. Chapter 3 contains more information on confidentiality, including the Health Insurance Portability and Accountability Act (HIPAA). All agency employees must keep all information about clients and their families confidential. The HHA must be careful about where she keeps her notes and assignment sheets. Keeping paperwork in the open where someone could read it, or losing notes or assignments, is a breach of confidentiality. Confidentiality also extends to the agency's personnel files and clinical records. This means an employer cannot give out information about any employee from job applications or other records.

- The client's care plan must always be followed. Home health aides should perform all tasks assigned by the care plan. Tasks that are listed in the care plan or approved by the supervisor should not be performed. If the client or family requests changes, the HHA should report the requests to the supervisor.

- Home health aides must report to the supervisor at regular, arranged times, and more often if needed. For example, HHAs must report the following to their supervisors: important events or changes in clients and their families; an accident on the job; and anything that delays or prevents them from going to or completing an assignment.

- Personal problems should not be discussed with the client or the client's family. Discussing personal problems is unprofessional. HHAs must act professionally. Clients should see an HHA as a care provider rather than as a friend.

- Home health aides must be punctual and dependable. Employers expect this of all employees.

- Home health aides need to follow deadlines for documentation and paperwork. Timely and accurate documentation is very important.

- All client care must be given in a pleasant, professional manner.

- Home health aides should not give or accept gifts. Gift-giving and receiving is not allowed because it is unprofessional. Gift-giving can cause other problems as well. For example, a client may forget that she gave an object as a gift and report it as stolen. Some clients who give gifts may believe they deserve special treatment.

Employers will have policies and procedures for every client care situation. These have been developed to give quality care and protect client safety. HHAs must always follow their employer's policies and procedures. More information on professionalism and professional behavior, including proper grooming, may be found in Chapter 2.

7. Demonstrate how to organize care assignments

To finish all assignments each day, home health aides have to work efficiently. To be efficient, they need to decide the order in which to do their tasks. For example, an HHA is assigned to work with an elderly client from 2:00 to 4:00 p.m. on Monday. The care plan states that the client needs some housekeeping, dinner preparation, and personal care. When the HHA arrives at the client's home, she sees what tasks need to be done. She makes a list of the tasks she will do and the order in which she will do them (Fig. 24-5).

Two hours is not a lot of time to do all those tasks. The HHA will have to work quickly. If she does not plan the tasks before she starts, she might spend too long cleaning the kitchen and never make dinner. Making a list of tasks

makes for more efficient work. It is also helpful to include the client in the planning. A client may not cooperate with a schedule if he has different priorities. It takes communication, and sometimes negotiation, to arrange a schedule that works.

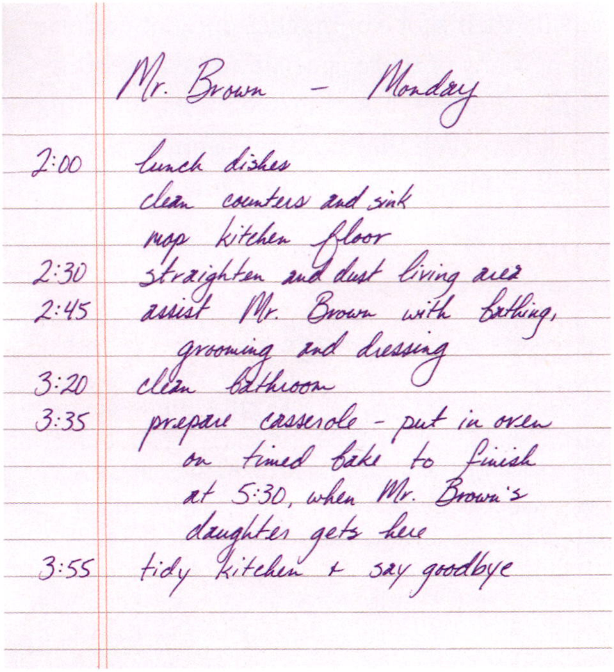

Fig. 24-5. *Making a list of tasks to be done will help an HHA perform them efficiently.*

If an HHA runs out of time with a client, she may have to leave some tasks uncompleted. This can negatively affect the client, and will put the HHA behind during her next visit. Completing assignments efficiently means not always trying to catch up. It means being able to complete necessary tasks in the time allowed.

8. Identify an employer's responsibilities

Agencies should teach home health aides about their policies and procedures. Agencies must make sure that HHAs are educated and are able to perform all assigned tasks. The employer's responsibilities include the following:

- Provide a written job description. The job description explains what the HHA is expected to do during work hours (Fig. 24-6).

Job Description

Home Health Aide I

The home health aide (HHA I) assists with environmental services such as housekeeping and homemaking services to preserve a safe, sanitary home and enhance family life. The HHA I should encourage the client and/or family to assume as much responsibility as possible for care and environment in accordance with the plan of care. The HHA I is not to provide any personal care.

Examples of duties: housekeeping; shopping; laundry; essential errands; basic meal preparation and meal planning (not for special diets); maintaining a safe environment; observing, monitoring and reporting on a client's condition; and teaching of those tasks to the client that will increase client independence and that the HHA I is qualified to teach.

Supervision: Supervision of the HHA I shall occur at least every 62 days in at least one home while the HHA I is on duty. Supervision may be performed by staff such as nurses, social workers, and home economists.

In-service: The HHA I shall be required to complete at least six hours of in-service training per year on topics relevant to appropriate clients and duties and meet applicable state laws.

Home Health Aide II

The home health aide II (HHA II) assists the client and/or family with home management activities and with non-medically-directed personal care. The HHA II is not to perform duties under a medically directed plan of care and is not to be assigned duties related to assistance with medications or wound care.

Examples of duties: All the duties of a HHA I plus: assistance with ambulation, bathing, hair care/grooming, dressing, toileting, transfer activities, special diets, activities of daily living, and appropriate client teaching consistent with training.

Training: The HHA II is to complete all the training units required of the HHA I (40 hours) prior to any assignment to a client involving the provision of care. The following additional units are to be completed within six months of the first assignment as HHA II. However, no HHA II shall be assigned to provide services for which the HHA II has not been trained and for which the HHA II has not demonstrated competency.

Additional Training (beyond HHA I requirement), 60 hrs. total training required within six months of first assignment.

Supervision: Supervision of the HHA II shall occur at least every 62 days in at least one home while the HHA II is on duty. Supervision must be performed by appropriate professionals.

Fig. 24-6. The employer should provide the home health aide with a job description.

- Provide testing and skills evaluation before sending HHAs to care for clients.

- Provide initial training and continuing in-service training. Initial training includes an explanation of the policies and procedures of the agency, including the agency's documentation system. In-service training is a federal requirement. It keeps skills fresh and helps the HHA do an even better job. OSHA regulations require employers to offer infection prevention education, among other topics.

- Provide appropriate preparation for each assignment. The agency should teach HHAs to properly care for each client's special needs and conditions. The HHA should be told why the client needs a service and what the goals of care are. If other team members are involved, their responsibilities should also be explained.

- Provide supervision. Supervisors support HHAs and teach them how to do new tasks. They help HHAs find solutions to problems and adjust to new situations. Supervisors check with clients to assure the goals of the care plan are being met. They will also check to see that clients are satisfied with the care they are receiving.

- Provide information about supervision. The employer should tell HHAs when and where they will meet with supervisors and what will be discussed in these meetings. The HHA should also be told how the supervisor can be reached for help and why the supervisor will visit clients' homes.

- Provide proper equipment and supplies for HHAs to safely do their work. For example, the agency should provide the gloves an HHA must sometimes wear to protect herself and her client from infection.

9. Identify the client's rights in home health care

Clients in home care have legal rights, just as residents in long-term care do. These rights relate to how clients must be treated. They provide an ethical code of conduct for healthcare workers. Home health agencies give clients a list of these rights and review each right with them. Chapter 3 has more information on legal rights.

Clients have the right to receive considerate, dignified, and respectful care. In addition, home health aides and nursing assistants are legally required to report abuse or suspected abuse. Two other basic clients' rights are the right to be fully informed of the goals of care and of the care itself, and the right to participate in care planning. The employer should develop an agreement with each client about the goals of care before service is provided. The employer should also make every effort to involve clients and their families in care planning (Fig. 24-7). Each person knows how his body works best and what makes him comfortable. People who feel in control of their bodies, lives, and health have greater self-esteem. They are more likely to continue a treatment plan and to cooperate with caregivers. Clients also have a right to know what results the agency expects to achieve from the care provided. These expected outcomes are sometimes called the goals of the care plan. Clients and the case manager should be informed of barriers to clients' care. For example, a client's failure to eat enough healthy food can be an obstacle to getting well.

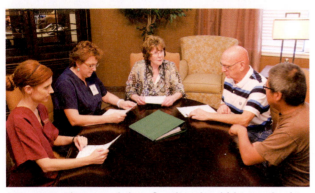

Fig. 24-7. *Clients and their families should be involved in care planning.*

Client's Bill of Rights

Home health clients and their formal caregivers have a right to not be discriminated against based on race, color, religion, national origin, age, gender, sexual orientation, or disability. Furthermore, clients and caregivers have a right to mutual respect and dignity, including respect for property. Caregivers are prohibited from accepting personal gifts and borrowing from clients.

Clients have the right

- To have relationships with home health providers that are based on honesty and ethical standards of conduct;

- To be informed of the procedure they can follow to lodge complaints with the home health provider about the care that is, or fails to be, furnished and about a lack of respect for property;

- To know about the disposition of such complaints;

- To voice their grievances without fear of discrimination or reprisal for having done so; and

- To be advised of the contact information for the state agency that handles questions and complaints about local home health agencies, including complaints about implementation of advance directive requirements.

Clients have the right

- To be notified in advance about the care that is to be furnished, the disciplines of the caregivers who will furnish the care, and the frequency of the proposed visits;

- To be advised of any change in the plan of care before the change is made;

- To participate in planning care and planning changes in care, and to be advised that they have the right to do so;

- To be informed in writing of rights under state law to make decisions concerning medical care, including the right to accept or refuse treatment and the right to formulate advance directives;

- To be notified of the expected outcomes of care and any obstacles or barriers to treatment*;

- To be informed in writing of policies and procedures for implementing advance directives, including any limitations if the provider cannot implement an advance directive on the basis of conscience;

- To have healthcare providers comply with advance directives in accordance with state law;

- To receive care without condition or discrimination based on the execution of advance directives; and

- To refuse services without fear of reprisal or discrimination.

* The home health provider or the client's physician may be forced to refer the client to another source of care if the client's refusal to comply with the plan of care threatens to compromise the provider's commitment to quality care.

Clients have the right

- To confidentiality of their medical record as well as information about their health, social, and financial circumstances, and about what takes place in the home; and

- To expect the home health provider to release information only as required by law or authorized by the client, and to be informed of procedures for disclosure.

Clients have the right

- To be informed of the extent to which payment may be expected from Medicare, Medicaid, or any other payer known to the home health provider;

- To be informed of the charges that will not be covered by Medicare;

- To be informed of the charges for which the client may be liable;

- To receive this information orally and in writing before care is initiated and within 30 calendar days of the date the home health provider becomes aware of any changes; and

- To have access, upon request, to all bills for service that the client has received, regardless of whether the bills are paid out-of-pocket or by another party.

Clients have the right

- To receive care of the highest quality;

- In general, to be admitted by a home health provider only if it has the resources needed to provide the care safely and at the required level of intensity, as determined by a professional assessment; a provider with less than optimal resources may nevertheless admit the client if a more appropriate provider is not available, but only after fully informing the client of the provider's limitations and the lack of suitable alternative arrangements; and

- To be told what to do in the case of an emergency.

The home health provider shall assure that

- All medically-related home care is provided in accordance with physicians' orders and that a plan of care specifies the services and their frequency and duration; and

- All medically-related personal care is provided by an appropriately trained home health aide who is supervised by a nurse or other qualified home health care professional.

Clients have the responsibility

- To notify the provider of changes in their condition (e.g., hospitalization, changes in the plan of care, symptoms to be reported);

- To follow the plan of care;

- To notify the provider if the visit schedule needs to be changed;

- To inform providers of the existence of any changes made to advance directives;

- To advise the provider of any problems or dissatisfaction with the services provided;

- To provide a safe environment for care to be provided; and

- To carry out mutually-agreed-upon responsibilities.

To satisfy Medicare certification requirements, the Centers for Medicare & Medicaid Services (CMS) requires that agencies

1. Give a copy of the Bill of Rights to each client in a language that they can understand during the admission process.

2. Explain the Bill of Rights to the client and document that this has been done.

Agencies may have clients sign a copy of the Client's Bill of Rights to acknowledge receipt.

Chapter Review

1. Name three reasons for the increase in demand for home health care.

2. Once a person is referred to home health care and a home health agency is chosen, what happens next?

3. How may the working environment differ in the home as opposed to a long-term care facility?

4. What are the factors considered when forming a client care plan?

5. How can home health aides be positive role models for clients and their families?

6. Should an HHA tell a client about his or her diagnosis or medical treatment plan? Why or why not?

7. What is one reason why a home health aide should not give or accept gifts?

8. Create a sample schedule for a two-hour morning visit to an elderly client named Mrs. Smith. Use tasks different from those listed in Figure 24-5.

9. What type of preparation should an employer provide before sending an HHA to care for clients?

10. How do supervisors help HHAs and clients?

11. If a home health aide sees or suspects that a client is being abused, what is her responsibility?

12. What is one important reason that clients should be involved in their care planning?

13. Pick five rights from the Client's Bill of Rights that are most important to you and explain why you chose those particular rights.

25

Infection Prevention and Safety in the Home

Chapter 5 contains most of the infection prevention and control material in this textbook. It includes information about Standard Precautions, Transmission-Based Precautions, hand hygiene, personal protective equipment (PPE), infectious diseases, handling spills, caring for equipment and linen, and much more. This chapter contains information on how infection prevention may need to be modified in the home. Chapter 6 contains most of the information on general safety guidelines. This chapter includes additional safety information for the home. It would be helpful to review both Chapters 5 and 6 before reading this chapter.

1. Discuss disinfection in the home

In health care, an object is called *clean* if it has not been contaminated with pathogens. An object that is *dirty* has been contaminated with pathogens. Here is a short list of some of the substances and objects that are considered dirty in the home:

- The floor

- Saliva and other discharges from the mouth and nose; this includes any objects that come into contact with these discharges, such as hands, toothbrushes, sinks, napkins, pillowcases, cigarettes, eating utensils, handkerchiefs, etc.

- Body wastes, such as stool (feces) and urine; this includes anything that comes into con-

tact with these wastes, such as toilet paper, underwear, bed linens, and toilets

- Drainage from wounds; this includes objects that come in contact with drainage, such as dressings, tissues, cloths, clothing, and bed linens

- Spoiled food; this includes objects that come into contact with this food, such as other food, dishes, cooking utensils, kitchen working areas, and surfaces

Measures like sterilization and disinfection are used to decrease the spread of pathogens that could cause disease. Disinfection is a process that kills pathogens but does not destroy all pathogens. It reduces the pathogen count to a level that is considered not infectious. Sterilization is a cleaning measure that destroys all microorganisms, including those that form spores.

Home health aides may disinfect items used by clients and will also disinfect some areas of the home while doing housekeeping tasks. The care plan and assignments will specify what disinfection needs to be done. General methods of disinfection are by wet and dry heat and by chemicals. Wet heat disinfection uses boiling water to disinfect. Dry heat disinfection means baking in the oven. Chapter 29 includes information about household chemical disinfecting solutions. The method used depends on the type of item that needs to be disinfected. Home health agencies have policies and procedures for disinfection in the home.

Disinfecting using wet heat

Equipment: items to be disinfected, clean pot with enough room to hold items, clean lid for pot, cold water, timer or clock, stove, potholders

1. Wash your hands.

2. Place items in the pot and fill it with water. Make sure water covers all items, leaving enough room at the top for steam to escape.

3. Place lid on pot and place covered pot on burner on stove.

4. Turn on heat and bring water to a boil. Do not open the lid at any time during boiling.

5. Set timer and boil for 20 minutes. You should see steam escaping from the sides of the pot.

6. Turn off heat. Allow items and water to cool.

7. After items have cooled, remove the cover with the potholders.

8. Remove the items. Place on a rack or a clean towel to air dry.

9. Wash and dry the disinfecting equipment. Return to proper storage.

10. Wash your hands.

11. Document the procedure.

Disinfecting using dry heat

Equipment: items to be disinfected, clean metal pan (cookie sheet, cake pan, etc.), timer or clock, oven, potholders

1. Wash your hands.

2. Place items in the pan.

3. Place sheet or cake pan in the oven.

4. Turn on oven to 350°F. Set timer and bake for one hour. Keep oven door closed while items are baking.

5. Turn off heat. Allow items to cool.

6. After items have cooled, remove with the potholders.

7. Store the items.

8. Wash and dry the disinfecting equipment. Return to proper storage.

9. Wash your hands.

10. Document the procedure.

2. Describe guidelines for assisting a client when isolation has been ordered

Transmission-Based Precautions are used when caring for persons who are infected or suspected of being infected with a disease. When ordered, these precautions are used in addition to Standard Precautions.

Guidelines: Isolation Procedures

G   Wash plates and utensils thoroughly in very hot water with antibacterial soap. Bleach may need to be added to the water. Follow agency policy. Encourage family members to use separate dishes and utensils.

G   Wear disposable gloves when handling soiled laundry. Bag laundry in the client's room and carry it to the laundry area in the bag. Wash the client's laundry separately. Use hot water and detergent.

G   The amount of non-disposable equipment brought into the home should be limited. Ideally, the client's care equipment should be left in the home until home health services are no longer needed. If some care equipment cannot remain in the home (for example, a stethoscope), clean and disinfect items before taking them from the home. Contaminated reusable items can also be placed in a plastic bag for transport.

G   A solution of bleach and water (one part bleach to nine parts water) should be mixed in a clearly-labeled plastic spray bottle and stored in a safe place. The bleach solution can be used to disinfect surfaces that may have been contaminated.

G Clean and disinfect frequently-touched surfaces and equipment, such as tables, bedside commodes, television remotes, canes, wheelchairs, and doorknobs at least daily. A client in contact or airborne isolation should use a separate bathroom if possible. If the client uses the same bathroom as others, disinfect it after each use by the client.

Clients in isolation may be fearful or concerned about what is happening to them. The home health aide should listen to what the client is saying and should allow time to talk with the client about his concerns. It is important to reassure clients that the disease is the reason for isolation. The HHA can explain why these steps are being taken. Any questions outside the HHA's scope of practice should be relayed to the supervisor.

Guidelines: Cleaning Spills in the Home

G When blood or body fluids are spilled, don gloves before starting. In some cases, industrial-strength gloves are best.

G If blood or body fluids are spilled on a hard surface such as a linoleum floor or countertop, clean immediately using a solution of one part household bleach to nine parts water. You can mix the solution in a bucket and, with gloves on, wipe up the spill with rags or paper towels dipped in the solution. Be careful not to spill bleach or bleach solution on clothes, carpets, or bedding. It can discolor and damage fabrics. Your employer may provide you with special products for cleaning spills.

G If blood or body fluids are spilled on fabrics such as carpets, bedding, or clothes, do not use bleach to clean the spill. Commercial disinfectants that do not contain bleach are available. When using these disinfectants, follow the manufacturer's directions for how to use the product. If you have no disinfectant, wear gloves and wipe up spills. Then use soap and water to clean the area. Clean carpet with regular carpet cleaner. Use gloves to load soiled bedding or clothes into the washing machine and add color-safe bleach to the washer with the laundry detergent.

3. List ways to adapt the home to principles of proper body mechanics

Chapters 6 and 10 contain more in-depth information on body mechanics. HHAs can use the following guidelines to help them practice proper body mechanics in the home:

Guidelines: Using Proper Body Mechanics in the Home

G Have the right tools for a job. For example, if you cannot reach an object on a high shelf, use a step stool rather than climbing on a counter or straining to reach.

G Have footrests and pillows available. Tasks that require standing for long periods can be more comfortable if you rest one foot on a footrest. This position flexes the muscles in the lower back and keeps the spine in alignment. When sitting, using a footrest allows for a more comfortable leg position. Crossing the legs disrupts alignment and should be avoided. Use pillows behind the back to keep the back straight.

G Keep tools, supplies, and clutter off the floor. Keep frequently-used items on shelves or counters where they can be easily reached without lifting. Keeping things organized will also help you find what you need without straining.

G Whenever you can sit to do a job, do so. Chopping vegetables, folding clothes, and other tasks can be done easily while sitting. For jobs like scouring the bathtub, kneel or use a low stool. Avoid bending at the waist.

G Use gait or transfer belts when assisting clients with ambulation or transfers, as described in Chapter 10.

G Make sure the homes you work in are safe for your clients, their family members, and you. Working in a home that is neglected puts you at risk for injury. Do remember, however, that you are a visitor in the client's home. Unless an immediate danger exists, check with your supervisor and the client before making any significant changes. A nurse or case manager will assess the safety of the homes in which you work. However, you will spend more time in the home than any other member of the care team. Look for safety hazards. Immediately report any hazards to your supervisor.

4. Identify common types of accidents in the home and describe prevention guidelines

There is information about these common types of accidents—falls, burns/scalds, poisoning, cuts, and choking—in Chapter 6. The HHA needs to be able to identify hazards and take action to remove them. This will include working with the client, the client's family, and/or other members of the care team. Prevention is the key to safety. Below are guidelines for preventing common types of accidents in the home:

Falls: Falls can be caused by an unsafe environment, loss of abilities, diseases, and medications. Falls are particularly common among the elderly. Older people are often more seriously injured by falls because their bones are more fragile. HHAs should be especially alert to the risk of falls with elderly clients. HHAs must report all falls to their supervisor.

Guidelines: Preventing Falls

G Clear all walkways of clutter, throw rugs, and cords (Figs. 25-1 and 25-2).

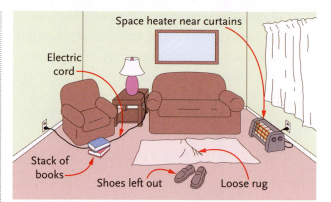

Fig. 25-1. Be aware of unsafe conditions in your clients' homes. This living room contains many hazards.

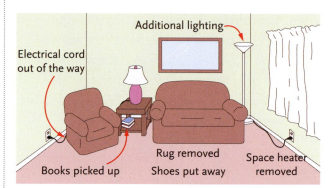

Fig. 25-2. You can help prevent accidents. The hazards shown in Figure 25-1 have been removed. Talk with your client about changes that need to be made to avoid hazards.

G Avoid waxing floors, and use mats or rugs with a nonslip backing where appropriate.

G Have clients wear nonskid, sturdy shoes. Make sure shoelaces are tied.

G Have clients wear clothing that is not too long and does not drag on the floor.

G Keep personal items that are used often close to clients.

G Immediately clean up spills on the floor.

G Mark uneven flooring or stairs with tape of a contrasting color to indicate a hazard.

G Improve lighting where needed.

G Lock wheels and move footrests out of the way before helping clients into or out of wheelchairs.

G Lock bed wheels before helping clients into and out of bed or when giving care.

G Before giving care, you will often need to raise adjustable beds to make your job easier and safer. After completing care, return beds to their lowest position.

G Offer help with toileting often. Respond to requests for help immediately.

G Leave furniture in the same place as you found it.

Burns/Scalds: Burns can be caused by dry heat (e.g., a hot iron, stove, other electrical appliances), wet heat (e.g., hot water or other liquids, steam), or chemicals (e.g., lye, acids). Small children, older adults, or people with loss of sensation (such as from paralysis or diabetes) are at the greatest risk of burns. Scalds are burns caused by hot liquids. It takes five seconds or less for a serious burn to occur when the temperature of a liquid is 140°F. Coffee, tea, and other hot drinks are usually served at 160°F to 180°F. These temperatures can cause almost instant burns that require surgery. Preventing burns and scalds is very important.

Guidelines: Preventing Burns and Scalds

G Roll up sleeves and avoid loose clothing when working at or near the stove (Figs. 25-3 and 25-4).

G Check that the stove and appliances are off when you leave.

G Suggest that the hot water heater be set lower than normal. It should be set at 120°F to 130°F to avoid burns from scalding tap water.

G Always check water temperature with a bath thermometer or on the inside of your wrist before using.

G Keep space heaters away from clients' beds, chairs, and draperies. Never allow space heaters to be used in the bathroom.

G Immediately report frayed electrical cords or appliances that look unsafe. Do not use these appliances.

G Let clients know when you are about to pour or set down a hot liquid.

G Pour hot drinks away from clients. Keep hot drinks and liquids away from edges of tables. Put a lid on them.

G Make sure clients are sitting down before serving hot drinks.

Poisoning: Homes contain many harmful substances that should not be swallowed. These include cleaning products, paints, medicines, toiletries, and glues. These products should be locked away from confused clients, clients with limited vision, and children. HHAs should check medication for expired dates. Clients who have a diminished sense of taste or smell due to stroke or head injury might eat spoiled food. HHAs should check the refrigerator and cabinets frequently for foods that are moldy, sour, or spoiled. They should investigate any odors they notice. Clients with dementia may hide food and let it spoil in closets, drawers, or other places. The number for the Poison Control Center should be kept handy (the website for the American Association of Poison Control Centers is aapcc.org).

Cuts: Cuts typically occur in the kitchen or bathrooms. Sharp objects, including knives, peelers, graters, food processor blades, scissors, nail clippers, and razors must be kept out of the reach of children. Sharp objects should also be locked away if there is a confused client in the home. When preparing food, an HHA should cut away from herself, use a cutting board, and keep her fingers out of the way. She must also know proper first aid for cuts (Chapter 7).

Choking: Choking can occur when eating, drinking, or swallowing medication. Babies and young children who put objects in their mouths are at great risk of choking. People who are weak, ill, or unconscious may choke on their own saliva. A person's tongue can also become swollen and obstruct the airway. Babies and small children should never have access to small

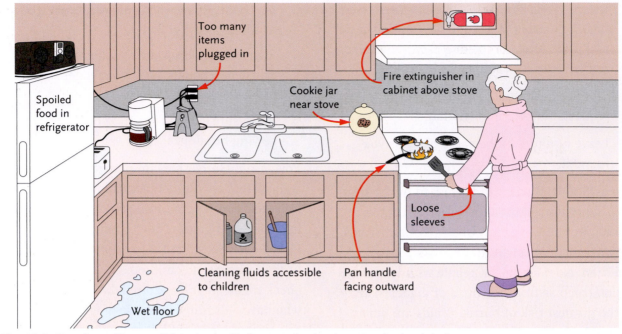

Fig. 25-3. *Unsafe working conditions in the kitchen can lead to burns and other injuries.*

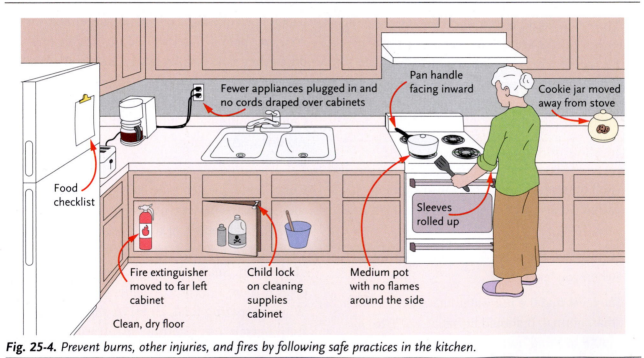

Fig. 25-4. *Prevent burns, other injuries, and fires by following safe practices in the kitchen.*

objects. HHAs should keep in mind that any object small enough to fit inside a toilet paper roll is small enough for a child to put in his mouth and could cause choking. Clients who have trouble with utensils and children who are too young to manage utensils on their own need their food cut into bite-sized pieces. Infants should sleep on their backs to reduce the risk of sudden infant death syndrome (SIDS). Pillows, small toys, and other objects should never be placed in a crib with an infant. Clients should eat in as upright a position as possible to avoid choking. Clients with swallowing problems may have a special diet with liquids thickened to the consistency of honey or syrup. Thickened liquids are easier to swallow.

Household Tips for Preventing Accidents

The majority of accidents occur in bathrooms and kitchens. Home health aides should be vigilant to prevent accidents.

Bathroom

Falls: Nonskid bathmats in tubs and showers can reduce the risk of falls. Grab bars for the tub, shower, and toilet are also helpful if the client is weak and unsteady (Figs. 25-5 and 25-6). A shower chair may be used for clients who are weak.

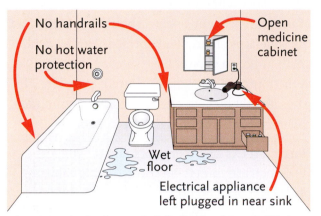

Fig. 25-5. *The bathroom is full of safety hazards if it is not properly maintained.*

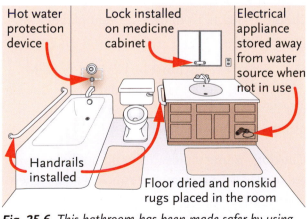

Fig. 25-6. *This bathroom has been made safer by using special devices and by cleaning and straightening.*

Burns: HHAs must always check water temperature with a bath thermometer or on the inside of the wrist. Electrical appliances should not be used near a water source and should be put away when not in use.

Drowning: Young children must never be left unattended near any water. This includes bathtubs, swimming pools, buckets or basins of water, puddles, ponds, drainage ditches, toilets, or sinks. An HHA should not leave anyone who is ill and weak alone in a tub. Clients who are dizzy or confused should not be alone in the tub or shower.

Poisoning: Home care providers can suggest that all medications be stored safely in containers with childproof caps and in locked cabinets. Children should never be told that medication is candy. Part of the HHA's job is to be sure that the client reads medicine labels carefully before taking a medication. If a medicine is not labeled, the HHA should report the situation to a supervisor. The client's medications should be stored separately from medications taken by other members of the family.

Cuts: Home health aides should put away razors and other sharp objects (such as nail scissors) when they are not in use.

Kitchen

Falls: If the HHA cares for an infant or small child who uses a high chair or booster seat, she should make sure safety belts are securely fastened.

Burns: It is important that pot handles be turned toward the back of the stove. Food should be stirred before serving, especially if cooked in a microwave. This ensures that the temperature is the same all the way through. Hot liquids can be cooled with an ice cube before serving.

Poisoning: Emergency numbers, including the Poison Control Center's number, should be kept handy. HHAs can suggest that all household cleaning products and other chemicals be locked away.

Cuts: Cutlery should be put away when not in use. If an HHA is using a knife and puts it down for a moment, she should place it away from the edge of the counter or table, making sure the blade is pointed away from the counter or table edge. Other sharp kitchen tools should also be stored in safe places, out of the reach of children and confused clients.

Choking: Popcorn, peanuts, hard candy, gum, and foods such as hot dogs or grapes are easily inhaled and pose a choking hazard to small children. HHAs should cut all foods into small, bite-sized pieces suitable for the age of the child. For elderly clients who have difficulty swallowing, the HHA can serve softer foods and foods cut into small pieces. When the HHA serves meals, she can encourage clients to take small bites of food, chew thoroughly, and eat slowly. Plastic storage bags should be kept out of reach, and dry-cleaning and other large plastic bags should be recycled or discarded.

Bedroom

Falls: A nightlight can illuminate pathways and reduce the risk of falls. It is very important that an HHA never leave children unattended on high surfaces. These surfaces include beds, changing tables, high chairs, and playpens. An HHA should not even turn his back when changing a child on a high surface. Movable crib rails are no longer considered safe, but some homes may still have cribs with rails that lower. If an HHA encounters a crib that has such rails, he should make sure they are raised before leaving a child's room.

Burns: Clients should not smoke in bed. It is especially important that clients and family members never smoke around oxygen tanks or equipment.

Cuts: Sharp objects should always be put away.

Choking: An HHA should report any cribs that have wide spaces between the slats. The infant's head could become wedged between them. Cribs should be positioned away from drapes and blinds, as infants and toddlers can become en-

tangled in the cords. Pillows and loose bedding in cribs can pose a risk of suffocation. HHAs should not prop up bottles for infants and toddlers, and they should examine toys for loose or removable parts.

Living Area

Falls: HHAs should request walkers or canes for clients who need support when walking. A supervisor can talk to a client or the client's family about having handrails installed where necessary. Floors should always be kept clear, and electrical and extension cords should be out of the way. A client's shoes should be sturdy and the shoelaces should be kept tied. Homes with small children should have safety gates installed at the tops and bottoms of stairs if possible. The gates should be kept closed. Hardware-mounted gates should be used at the tops of stairs.

Burns: HHAs or supervisors should suggest that electrical outlets be covered with baby-proof plugs. Nobody should smoke around children, and lighters and matches should be kept out of reach and out of sight.

Poisoning: Plants should be placed out of children's reach, as many common plants are poisonous.

Cuts: Sharp objects must be kept out of children's reach, and children should not be allowed to run, jump, or play roughly with any toy or object that could stab them.

Choking: Young children should not be permitted to play with balloons or rubber bands. These objects are easily inhaled. Children should not run or jump with food in their mouths.

Garage and Outdoors

An HHA should not leave children at home alone or alone in a vehicle. If an HHA transports children for any reason, she must make sure they are fastened into an appropriate car seat. Child car seats should be placed in the back seat of the automobile. Children under 12 should never sit in the front seat of a car. Airbags can kill children riding in the front seat. It is important that an HHA supervise children at play. Walkways should be kept clear of toys and other obstructions, and free of snow and ice.

Chapter 19 contains more information about safety in the home for clients with dementia.

5. List home fire hazards and describe fire safety guidelines

It is essential for home health aides to recognize and report fire hazards. Any of the following can be a fire hazard:

- Wood stoves and kerosene, gas, or electric heaters that appear old, damaged, or faulty

- Unvented heaters used in small, enclosed areas or sleeping areas

- Space heaters used near fabrics such as draperies, bedspreads, or towels, or used to dry clothing or towels

- Flammable materials such as gasoline, kerosene, or paint thinner stored near stoves, heaters, furnaces, hot water heaters, or other appliances

- Frayed or exposed electrical wires

- Matches or lighters left within reach of children or incapacitated adults

- Careless smoking; smoking in bed; cigarettes, pipes, or cigars left burning; or clients who are confused who are smoking

Guidelines: Reducing Fire Hazards

G Never work wearing loose or flowing clothing, especially around the stove. Roll up clients' sleeves and avoid loose clothing when clients are cooking or around the stove.

G Stay in or near the kitchen when anything is cooking or baking.

G Store potholders, dish towels, and other flammable kitchen items away from the stove.

G Never store cookies, candy, or other items that may attract children above or near the stove.

G Discourage careless smoking and smoking in bed. If clients must smoke, check to be sure that cigarettes are extinguished after use. Empty ashtrays frequently. Before emptying an ashtray, make sure there are no hot ashes, matches, or cigarette butts in the ashtray.

G Do not leave the clothes dryer on when you leave the house. Lint can catch fire. Empty lint traps each time you use the dryer.

G If you smell gas, report it immediately.

G Turn off space heaters when no one is home or everyone is asleep.

G Be sure there are working smoke alarms in the home. Check monthly to see that alarms are working. Replace batteries when needed.

G Have fire extinguishers on hand. Every home should have a fire extinguisher in the kitchen. Do not store the kitchen fire extinguisher near or above the stove, because you need to be able to get to it if the stove is on fire. Check that fire extinguishers have not expired. Know where the extinguisher is stored and how to operate it.

Chapter 6 contains more information on fire safety.

6. Identify ways to reduce the risk of automobile accidents

Since home health aides may be driving to and from clients' homes, they must be careful to protect themselves from possible dangers.

Guidelines: Traveling Safely

G Plan your route. Driving while trying to read a map or directions can be very dangerous.

Study the directions before beginning. If you are using a phone or other GPS device for navigation, listen to the voice instructions so you do not have to look at the device while you drive.

G Minimize distractions. Paying attention to the road can help avoid accidents. Drivers should keep their eyes on the road and hands on the wheel. If an HHA finds that music is distracting, she should not listen to it in the car. It is very dangerous to talk on a cell phone or to send or read text messages or e-mails while driving. An HHA should pull over in a safe location or wait until she reaches her destination before participating in any of these activities.

G Use turn signals. Using your turn signals lets other drivers know what you are planning to do. Always use turn signals when preparing to turn or change lanes.

G Use caution when backing up. Many accidents occur when drivers back up. Although rearview cameras are available in many cars, do not rely on them alone. When you back up, look around carefully. Turn your head to both sides and look behind your car.

G Drive at a safe speed. Follow speed limits to be sure you are not driving too fast. Road conditions such as ice or heavy rain may make it necessary to drive at a slower speed.

G Always wear your seat belt. Although it may not help you avoid an accident, it will certainly help protect you if an accident occurs. Always buckle up, no matter how short the distance you must drive. Require your passengers to wear their seat belts as well.

7. Identify guidelines for using a car on the job

The following guidelines apply to home health aides who use a car while working:

Guidelines: Using a Car on the Job

G Park in safe, well-lit areas.

G Lock car doors when you enter and exit your vehicle. Keep them locked while driving.

G Do not leave valuables in the car. If you must leave something in the car, put it out of sight.

G Have valid car insurance and carry the insurance card with you.

G Keep your proof of registration or registration card with you, not in the car. If your car is stolen, you do not want the thief to have this important document.

G Keep track of the miles you drive for work. Document them accurately. Lying about your mileage is the same as stealing from your employer.

G Keep your car in good working order. Get it serviced at the appropriate times. Make sure you have good tires. Keep a spare tire that is in good condition in the car in case you get a flat tire. Keep the gas tank full.

8. Identify guidelines for working in high-crime areas

If an assignment takes a home health aide to an area where crime is a problem, she should use caution. If using public transportation, she should be alert at all times. The following tips can help home health aides avoid trouble:

Guidelines: Staying Safe in High-Crime Areas

G Park in well-lit areas, as close as possible to the home you are visiting.

G Try to leave valuables at home when you must work in a dangerous area.

G Hold your home care bag tightly, close to your body. There are also special security and anti-theft bags available.

G   Lock your car and do not leave any valuables in it.

G   Walk confidently. Look as though you know where you are going (Fig. 25-7).

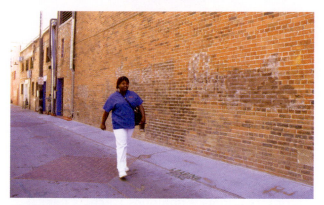

Fig. 25-7. *Look confident and be cautious if you enter a high-crime area.*

G   Carry a whistle so you can make a loud noise to startle any potential attacker and get help.

G   Carry your keys in your hand to unlock your car as soon as you arrive. If necessary, you can also use them as a weapon.

G   Do not sit in your car, even with the doors locked. Drive away as soon as you reach your car.

G   Try to avoid unsafe areas after dark.

G   If you are concerned about your safety in a particular area, leave the area immediately. Contact your supervisor.

G   Do not approach a home where strangers are hanging around. Go to your car and drive to a safe area. Use your cell phone or the nearest phone in a safe area, and call your supervisor.

G   Call your client before you visit so he or she knows approximately when to expect you.

G   Never enter a vacant home.

G   If necessary, ask your supervisor to arrange for an escort or another care provider to go with you.

G   Be sure someone knows your schedule. Call the office at the end of your work day.

Chapter Review

1. How would an HHA disinfect using wet heat? How would an HHA disinfect using dry heat?

2. List two items that are considered dirty in the home. Can you think of two examples of dirty items that are not listed in Learning Objective 1?

3. How should plates and utensils be washed when working with a client who has an infectious disease?

4. List five strategies for applying proper body mechanics in the home.

5. List eight tips to guard against falls in the home.

6. List eight tips to guard against burns in the home.

7. In what position should clients eat to avoid choking?

8. For each of the following rooms in a house, list one way to prevent accidents: bathroom, kitchen, bedroom, living area, garage, and outdoors.

9. List seven guidelines for reducing fire hazards.

10. Why is it a bad idea to talk on a cell phone when driving?

11. Why should car registration documents not be left in a person's car?

12. If an HHA approaches a house with strangers hanging around, what should he do?

13. Why should an HHA to carry her keys in her hand as she walks to her car?

26
Medications in Home Care

1. List four guidelines for safe and proper use of medications

People who need home care often need medications. Clients who have problems such as coronary artery disease, high blood pressure, and diabetes may take many drugs, all with different purposes and effects. Home health aides do not usually handle or give medications. However, HHAs need to understand the kinds of medicine that clients may be taking. They also need to know what to do if a client experiences side effects or refuses to take medication.

Guidelines: Safe and Proper Use of Medications

G Never handle or give medications unless you are specifically trained and assigned to do so. Do not touch the inside of a medicine bottle or the pills or other medicines themselves. Do not put any medication in a client's mouth. Handling or giving medication can have serious consequences. Only people who have had special training are allowed to give medications.

G Observe clients taking their medication. Although you cannot handle or give medication, you can remind clients to take their medications. You can also bring medication containers to clients, and provide water or food as needed to take with the medication. Always observe, report, and document as appropriate.

G Know the difference between prescription drugs and non-prescription (over-the-counter, or OTC) drugs. Antibiotics (such as penicillin), heart drugs (such as nitroglycerin), and potent pain medications (such as codeine) are examples of prescription drugs. Aspirin and cold medications, such as decongestants, are over-the-counter drugs (Fig. 26-1).

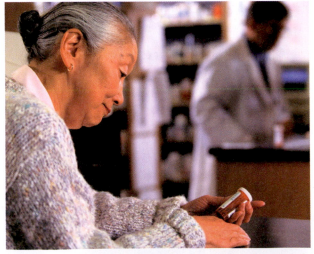

Fig. 26-1. Be aware of all medications that a client is taking. Know the difference between prescription and over-the-counter medications.

G Be aware of all medications that a client is taking. There are many possible side effects and interactions among medications. Watch for symptoms such as itching, trembling or shaking, anxiety, stomachache, diarrhea, confusion, vomiting, rash, hives, or headache. Any of these symptoms could indicate a side effect or interaction. Report any of these symptoms to your supervisor.

2. Identify the five "rights" of medications

Knowing and remembering the five "rights" of medications will help prevent mistakes.

1. **The Right Client**: Always check the label on the medication container to make sure the client's name is on it.

2. **The Right Medication**: Check the expiration date and the name of the medication before giving the container to the client. Make sure the medication name on the container matches the name listed in the care plan.

3. **The Right Time**: Make sure the instructions on the medication label about what time or how often to take the medication match the instructions in the care plan.

4. **The Right Route**: Check the label for instructions on how the medication is to be taken. Make sure the instructions on the label match those in the care plan.

5. **The Right Amount**: Make sure the instructions on the container label for how much medication to take match the instructions in the care plan.

An HHA should call her supervisor if the medication label and the care plan do not agree on any of the five rights. She should also call her supervisor if there is not enough information on the label or in the care plan, or if there is another problem with the medication (for example, the client's name is not on the container).

Dosages

Prescription medication comes from the pharmacy with the instructions printed on the label (Fig. 26-2). The information listed on the label includes the name of the medication, dosage instructions, how the medication should be taken, the quantity of medication included, the amount of refills allowed, the medication's expiration date, and any specific warnings. The patient's name and the pharmacy's name and contact information are also included.

When assisting a client to self-administer medication, the HHA should read the directions on the bottle before handing the bottle to the client. Dosage means how much medication should be taken each time (the right amount). A capsule, tablet, or pill will be ordered with both the strength of one pill and how many are to be taken each time. For example, the bottle may read *Zolpidem 10 mg tablets, take one tablet by mouth at bedtime as needed*.

The label will state how the medication should be taken (the right route). For example, the Zolpidem should be taken by mouth at bedtime. Sometimes the prescription states to *take as needed*. This means the client is not required to take the drug; the drug should be taken when the client has symptoms. The Zolpidem is to be taken as needed for sleep. However, medications that are ordered as needed will have a maximum daily dose/limit stated on the label.

Liquid oral medications may be ordered in teaspoons, tablespoons, or milliliters. The HHA should provide the client a measuring spoon or cup—not a spoon used at the table—to measure the dose. Medications which are to be put into the eyes or ears will be labeled with the number of drops per dose. A nasal spray label will state how many sprays are in one dose. Medications for inhalers may be premeasured into dose-sized packages.

The HHA should learn the abbreviations that are approved by his agency, and he should always call his supervisor if he has a concern or question.

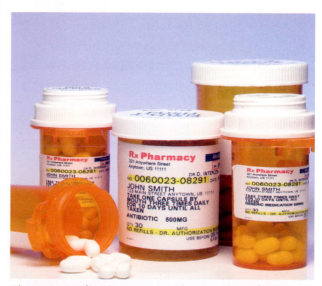

Fig. 26-2. *Medications come with instructions from the pharmacist. Instructions include the dosage and when and how to take the medication.*

3. Explain how to assist a client with self-administered medications

Some elderly people have a hard time remembering to take all their medications. In addition, there may be instructions to remember. Examples of instructions include taking pills with food or on an empty stomach, or drinking plenty of fluids. HHAs must pay close attention to the medication schedule. The nurse usually sets this schedule. HHAs should become familiar with all doctors' instructions on how and when to take medications and should use forms as ordered (Fig. 26-3). If the specified time for a dose passes, an HHA should remind the client to take the medicine. If a client does not take a medication that has been ordered, it should be reported to the supervisor.

Form 3481/2P
BRIGGS, Des Moines, IA 50306 (800) 247-2343
PRINTED IN U.S.A.

MEDICATION PROFILE

Patient Name ______ ID # ______
Pharmacy Name ______ Phone # ______ FAX # ______
Height ______ Weight ______ Type of venous access (if applicable) ______
Allergies: ❑ None known ❑ Yes (if yes, list and explain e.g. rash, hives, swelling) ______

Medications administered by: ❑ Self ❑ Caregiver/Family ❑ RN ❑ Other ______
Mediplanner filled: ❑ Yes ❑ No If yes, by whom ______ How often ______
Hospice staff orders medications: ❑ Yes ❑ No ❑ Other ______

MEDICATIONS (includes all prescription, O.T.C. and home remedies)
*medications are p.o. unless specified otherwise

Start Date	Stop Date	✓ If Hospice Pays	(N)ew (C)hanged (O)ngoing	Medication and Dose	Route *	Frequency	Instructed (Y)es (N)o	Pill Count If Applicable	
OXYGEN									
				Oxygen ______ ______ LPM	❑ N/C ❑ Trach ❑ Mask	❑ PRN ❑ Cont.			
INFUSION FLUSHES									
				Normal saline ______ ml/cc	IV				
				Heparin ____ u/ml ______ ml/cc	IV				
				Sterile water ______ ml/cc	IV				

Medication Device(s): Pump (type) ______
Nebulizer (type) ______
IV pole: ❑ Yes ❑ No

REVIEW/REVISE AREAS

Review/Revise dates	Date	Date	Date	Date	Date	Date
1. Potential adverse effects/ drug reactions	❑Y ❑N	❑Y ❑N	❑Y ❑N	❑Y ❑N	❑Y ❑N	❑Y ❑N
2. Significant side effects	❑Y ❑N	❑Y ❑N	❑Y ❑N	❑Y ❑N	❑Y ❑N	❑Y ❑N
3. Significant drug interactions	❑Y ❑N	❑Y ❑N	❑Y ❑N	❑Y ❑N	❑Y ❑N	❑Y ❑N
4. Duplicative drug therapy	❑Y ❑N	❑Y ❑N	❑Y ❑N	❑Y ❑N	❑Y ❑N	❑Y ❑N
5. Potential/actual ineffective therapy	❑Y ❑N	❑Y ❑N	❑Y ❑N	❑Y ❑N	❑Y ❑N	❑Y ❑N
6. Understands intructions	❑Y ❑N	❑Y ❑N	❑Y ❑N	❑Y ❑N	❑Y ❑N	❑Y ❑N
7. Needs further instructions	❑Y ❑N	❑Y ❑N	❑Y ❑N	❑Y ❑N	❑Y ❑N	❑Y ❑N
8. Potential noncompliance issues with drugs	❑Y ❑N	❑Y ❑N	❑Y ❑N	❑Y ❑N	❑Y ❑N	❑Y ❑N
Signature/Title						

Form 3481/2P © BRIGGS, Des Moines, IA 50306 (800) 247-2343 www.BriggsCorp.com PRINTED IN U.S.A. **MEDICATION PROFILE**
Part 1 – Clinical Record **Part 2 – Care Coordination**

Fig. 26-3. *Many home health agencies use medication forms to help the client or aide document the client's self-administered medication.* (REPRINTED WITH PERMISSION OF BRIGGS CORPORATION, 800-247-2343, WWW.BRIGGSCORP.COM)

If specified, HHAs may be instructed to help a client with self-medication in these ways:

- Remind the client when it is time for medication.
- Check for right person, medication, time, expiration date, route, and amount.
- Read the medication label for the client.
- Identify the container and bring the bottle or container of medication to the client.
- Bring client equipment needed to prepare and self-administer medication.
- Provide food or water to take with the medication as directed.
- Shake liquid medications if ordered by the care plan.
- Open and close containers.
- Position client for taking medication.
- Observe the client taking the medication.
- Document that the client took the medication, the time, and any other medications or food taken at the same time.
- Report any possible reactions to the supervisor. Call the supervisor if there are any problems or questions.
- Clean and store or dispose of special medication equipment after use.
- Return medication to storage.

Home health aides are NOT allowed to do any of the following:

- Break apart or crush capsules or tablets
- Mix medication with food or drink
- Pour or mix medication from one bottle into another, even if both contain the same medicine
- Touch medication directly with their hands
- Assist with self-administration of medication if the client's name is different from that on the label

- Assist with medication whose label has been removed or changed

- Assist with medicine if medication name does not match the name on the care plan

- Use appearance alone to identify a medication

- Assist client in taking more or less of a medication than is ordered

- Remove or change a medication label

- Assist client with medication at a time when it is not ordered

- Provide the wrong liquid for swallowing medications

- Put medication into the client's mouth

- Draw up solution for injections

- Give the client an injection

- Dispose of used injection needles/syringes

- Insert suppositories or other medication into the rectum

- Insert or apply vaginal medication

- Do special cleaning of the client's eyelids or eyelashes to prepare for eye medications

- Put drops into the eye, ear, or nose

- Apply prescription medications to the skin

Some clients have reactions to certain medications, and some medications may interact with others, causing problems. To avoid these problems, all medication that is taken must be documented. The HHA should report drugs, prescription or non-prescription, that the client takes that are not part of the care plan. Even a pill as common as aspirin should be noted. Reporting and documenting any reactions the client may have to medications is important.

Avoiding certain foods or substances can be important when taking certain medications. For example, drugs that have sedative effects should never be mixed with alcohol. If the client does not follow these restrictions, the HHA must notify her supervisor immediately. The doctor and pharmacist will inform the client and the family of any possible side effects from the medication. Common side effects include dizziness, drowsiness, headache, nausea and vomiting, and confusion. More serious side effects occur when there is an allergic reaction to the medication. Allergic reactions with symptoms like hives, fever, rash, or difficulty breathing can be life-threatening. They may require emergency help.

Medication Nebulizer

A medication nebulizer is a device that turns liquid medication into a fine mist so that it can be inhaled (Fig. 26-4). It is also known as an atomizer. This device helps clients who have lung problems to bring medication deep into the lungs. The medication loosens mucus in the lungs and helps the client cough it up.

Depending on an agency's and state's rules, an HHA may be allowed to assist the client with the use of the medication nebulizer. If allowed to assist, the HHA's duties may include the following:

- Gathering the necessary equipment and supplies

- Properly positioning the client

- Putting normal saline in the nebulizer

- Turning on the equipment

- Timing the treatment

- Checking to make sure the client is using the equipment properly

- Turning off the equipment

- Cleaning and storing the equipment properly

- Documenting observations and reporting to the supervisor

The HHA must be very careful to prevent infection when assisting with a nebulizer. If microorganisms get into the medicine or on the mouthpiece, they can go deep into the client's lungs when he uses the nebulizer. The HHA should always wash her hands before and after touching the air hose, medication container, or medication bottle.

If a client is using oxygen, it should be left on while using the medication nebulizer. Oxygen safety precautions must be observed. If the equipment is not working properly, the HHA should not try to repair the equipment and should contact her supervisor.

Any of the following signs might mean that the client is not getting enough oxygen while using the nebulizer:

- Rapid pulse and respirations
- Difficulty breathing
- Cold, clammy skin
- Blue or darkened lips, fingernails, or eyelids
- Inability to sit still
- Lack of response when you call his name

If a client shows any of these signs, the HHA should stop the procedure and immediately notify her supervisor.

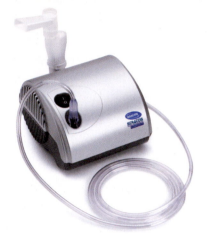

Fig. 26-4. *The mouthpiece, tubing, and compressor are all part of the nebulizing system.* (© INVACARE CORPORATION. USED WITH PERMISSION. WWW.INVACARE.COM)

4. Identify observations about medications that should be reported right away

If a client shows signs of a reaction to a medication or complains of side effects, the HHA must report it right away. Her supervisor can assess whether or not the symptom is caused by the medication. The HHA's responsibility is to report her observations.

Observing and Reporting: Medications

O/R Dizziness, fainting

O/R Nausea, vomiting

O/R Rash, hives, itching

O/R Difficulty breathing, swelling of the throat or eyes

O/R Drowsiness

O/R Headache, blurred vision

O/R Abdominal pain

O/R Diarrhea

O/R Any other unusual sign

In addition, report any of the following problems immediately:

O/R Client refuses to take medication as directed.

O/R Client takes the wrong dose (amount) of medication.

O/R Client takes medication at the wrong time.

O/R Client takes the wrong medication.

O/R A medication container is missing or empty.

5. Describe what to do in an emergency involving medications

If a client has a severe allergic reaction to a medication, takes the wrong dose, or takes medications together that cause complications, emergency medical treatment is necessary. An overdose, whether it was accidental or intentional, must be treated as a poisoning. The HHA must call the local Poison Control Center immediately and should follow their instructions. Poison Control will send paramedics if needed.

For severe drug reactions or interactions, the HHA should call 911 for emergency help. She should stay with the client and not give any liquids, food, or other medications unless instructed to do so by emergency personnel. The supervisor should be notified as soon as possible.

6. Identify methods of medication storage

When assisting with the proper storage of medications, the HHA should keep the following in mind:

- The client's medications should be kept in one place, separate from medicine used by other members of the household.

- If there are young children or a disoriented elderly person in the home, medications should be locked away.

- All medications should be kept in childproof containers if children are in the home. To avoid an accidental overdose, medications should be kept out of the reach of children.

- If medicine requires refrigeration, the bottle should be stored toward the back on an upper shelf, out of a child's reach (Fig. 26-5).

- All medications should be stored away from heat and light.

- The client or a family member should discard medications that have expired, are not labeled, or are discolored. Medications should not be discarded in the trash; children or animals may have access to them. Home care supervisors can provide specific disposal instructions. If the client or family will not dispose of expired medications, an HHA should inform her supervisor. She should not dispose of them herself.

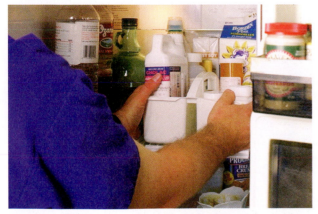

Fig. 26-5. *Medications should be stored properly and kept out of the reach of children.*

7. Identify signs of drug misuse and abuse and know how to report these

Drug misuse and abuse may be accidental or deliberate. It includes the following:

- Refusing to take medications

- Taking the wrong dose or taking it at the wrong time

- Mixing medication with alcohol

- Taking drugs that have not been prescribed

- Taking illegal drugs

- Sharing drugs with others

Misuse and abuse of drugs is extremely dangerous. It can even be fatal.

If a client refuses to take certain medications, an HHA can explain that recovery often depends on taking the right medication. If the client still refuses, he should notify his supervisor. The HHA should not push the client to take the medication, but he can try to find out what is making the client reluctant to take it. Getting the client to express uncertainties may help the HHA give information to the care team. A doctor or nurse can then either persuade the client to take the medication or adjust the treatment.

People may avoid taking prescribed medication because they cannot afford it or because they have difficulty obtaining it. Sometimes the client is confused about which drugs to take, at what hour, and in what quantities. Home health aides can help. If the client wants to know why he needs to be taking certain medications, an HHA can ask the nurse or doctor to provide an explanation. People who have conditions that affect mental function, such as dementia, will greatly benefit from friendly reminders. Other reasons people do not take medication are that they dislike the side effects and they have difficulty swallowing pills. These problems can be overcome once the supervisor is aware of them. HHAs should be alert to the signs of misuse or abuse of medications and report them immediately.

Observing and Reporting: Drug Misuse and Abuse

O/R Depression

O/R Anorexia

O/R Change in sleep patterns

O/R Withdrawn behavior or moodiness

O/R Secrecy

O/R Verbal abusiveness

O/R Poor relationships with family members

The drugs that pose the highest risk for causing drug dependency are pain medications, tranquilizers, muscle relaxers, and sleeping pills.

Chapter Review

1. What are the four guidelines for promoting safe and proper use of medications? Briefly describe why each guideline is important.

2. List the five "rights" of medications and explain what they mean.

3. What does dosage tell a person about medication?

4. What should an HHA do if she notices any problem with a client's medication?

5. List ten tasks an HHA may perform if she is instructed to help a client with self-administered medication.

6. List 18 tasks an HHA may NOT do with regard to medications.

7. Name five side effects of medications.

8. List seven signs an HHA should report immediately to her supervisor that might indicate a reaction to medication.

9. How should an HHA treat an overdose? Whom should she call?

10. What is the best place to keep medications if there are young children in the home?

11. List five signs of drug abuse and misuse.

12. What are two common reasons people avoid taking prescribed medications?

27

New Mothers, Infants, and Children

1. Explain the growth of home care for new mothers and infants

New mothers and their babies used to stay in the hospital for several days after delivery. Today, new restrictions by insurers and the popularity of natural childbirth techniques have changed that. Many new mothers and their babies are sent home as early as 24 hours after an uncomplicated delivery. Thus, new mothers today may return home more tired and uncomfortable. They may be less confident feeding and handling their babies than women were in the past.

Home care helps ease the transition from hospital to home. It allows the mother to rest and recover. Home health aides also assist with household management when an expectant mother is put on **bed rest** by her doctor. Bed rest is ordered if a woman shows signs of early labor, has a history of miscarriage or premature deliveries, or is extremely ill. Stopping all activity and staying in bed helps prevent the baby from being born prematurely. An expectant mother may have to stay mostly in bed for a period of a few weeks up to a few months.

2. Identify common neonatal disorders

Neonatal is the medical term for newborn. Doctors who specialize in caring for newborn babies are called **neonatologists**. A newborn baby is sometimes called a **neonate**. While most babies are born healthy, some babies are born with diseases or disorders that require special care. Babies born prematurely or at low birth weight, or who are injured during birth, will need special care. These are the most common neonatal disorders:

- Prematurity (birth more than three weeks before due date)

- Low birth weight

- Cerebral palsy

- Cystic fibrosis

- Down syndrome

- Viral or bacterial infections

- Susceptibility to sudden infant death syndrome (SIDS)

3. Explain how to provide postpartum care

Care for a new mother will be spelled out in the care plan. Each case will be different, and providing person-centered care means observing and responding to each new mother's particular situation. The care needed will depend on the mother's condition, the baby's condition, and the situation in the home. Care will depend on how much support the mother has from her spouse or partner, family, friends, and others. A new mother may need the following types of assistance:

- Basic care for the baby, such as feeding, diapering, and bathing

- Basic care for herself, such as rest, meal preparation, monitoring vital signs, and comfort measures, such as heat, ice, or sitz baths

- Light housekeeping and laundry

- Care of older children

- Meal planning and shopping for the family

The birth of a baby is a tremendous physical feat. Monitoring vital signs is important for understanding the stability of a mother during her initial recovery period. Temperature, pulse, respirations, blood pressure, and changes in pain level, if any, are vital measurements that track the successful physical transition from pregnancy to motherhood. After a woman has given birth, vital signs are usually checked often. A home health aide may be asked to monitor vital signs every 15 minutes, every 30 minutes, or every hour as ordered. HHAs should check with their supervisors if they have any questions.

An HHA may be required to monitor the amount and color of the new mother's lochia. The lochia is the vaginal flow that occurs after giving birth. This flow comes from the uterine wall where the placenta was attached. Similar to a monthly menses, the discharge is at first bright red in color. Over the next few days, the flow changes color to a duller red and then to pink. During the second week, the flow continues to change color from pink to a yellowish white and then finally disappears. The lochia may be quite heavy for a couple of days after birthing. It usually lessens gradually over the next seven to ten days. However, it can also last much longer, depending upon the person. The HHA should report the number of sanitary pads a new mother uses, and should also report any changes in flow or color to her supervisor. Increased amounts of lochia or a brightening in color are signs that should not be ignored.

In some cases, special care for the mother or baby may be needed. HHAs may be asked to assist the mother in caring for a Cesarean section incision or an episiotomy. A **Cesarean section**, or **C-section**, is a surgical procedure in which the baby is delivered through an incision in the mother's abdomen.

An **episiotomy** is an incision sometimes made in the perineal area during vaginal delivery that enlarges the vaginal opening for the baby's head. Self-dissolving stitches are generally used to repair this incision. An HHA's job duties regarding an episiotomy include careful observation and reporting. She should observe for signs of infection, including swelling at the site, redness, radiating heat, increased pain, and any wound changes such as discharge that is foul-smelling or yellow or green in color. An HHA may also assist with complete cleaning of the perineal area after voiding and bowel movements. It is common to use a squeeze bottle of warmed water to rinse the perineum, followed by drying from front to back. Other comfort measures HHAs may assist with are sitz baths and frequent sanitary pad changes.

If the baby is on a monitor (for pulse and respiration) or receiving oxygen, an HHA may be asked to monitor the equipment. Sometimes a new mother needs help with breastfeeding, and an HHA should report to her supervisor if a mother is having difficulties. She may need the assistance of a breastfeeding expert, called a *lactation consultant*.

Observing and Reporting: Postpartum Care

°/R Fever

°/R Change in amount of vaginal flow

°/R Odor in vaginal flow

°/R Changes in color of vaginal flow (e.g., bright red after it had been pink)

°/R Pain in the pelvic region

°/R Swelling, redness, or pain in the legs

°/R Changes in vital signs

°/R Swelling, redness, heat, pain, or discharge at surgical site or site of episiotomy

4. List important observations to report and document

A supervisor should instruct an HHA about observations to make. The HHA may be documenting the baby's or the mother's vital signs regularly. She may also be documenting how much and how often the baby eats, how long the baby nurses, the baby's sleeping patterns, and how many diapers are changed. The HHA should document any observations that seem important and should also check the following:

The home: Is it clean, healthy, and safe?

The family: Are older children maintaining their regular routines? Do the spouse or partner and other family members know how they can help?

The mother: Is she able to rest? Does she seem to be handling everything? Is she depressed, crying, or moody? An HHA should watch for signs of **postpartum** (after birth) **depression**, similar to signs of depression described in Chapter 20.

The baby: Is the baby eating regularly, wetting and soiling diapers, and sleeping well? Does the baby have good color?

The baby's room or space: Is there a safe place for the baby to sleep? Is the crib free of pillows, toys, or excess bedding that could cause suffocation? Is the room comfortably warm?

5. Explain guidelines for safely handling a baby

HHAs must wash their hands thoroughly before touching a baby or any baby supplies. It is extremely important to prevent the spread of bacteria around a newborn baby. All visitors and family members should also wash their hands often, especially before touching or holding the baby. People with colds or signs of illness should stay away from a newborn or wear a mask to prevent transmission of disease.

Babies must be lifted and held safely. Newborn babies cannot hold their heads up without assistance. Leaving the head unsupported can cause injury. All visitors and family members should hold the baby safely.

HHAs must be careful not to leave a baby in an unsafe location or position. **The only safe place to leave a baby is in a crib or in an adult's arms.** Babies should not be left in swings, carriers, seats, or on blankets on the floor unless they can be seen at all times. Baby seats, swings, or carriers must not be placed on tables, chairs, or countertops. Even during diaper changes, a baby should not be left on a table without one adult hand on the baby at all times. If the person lets go, even for one second, the baby can move and fall. A baby or small child should never be left alone in a bath, even for a short time.

Babies should be placed on their backs, not their abdomens. Crib mattresses should be firm, and infants should not be placed on blankets, comforters, pillows, or sheepskin to sleep. These items can cause suffocation and may contribute to SIDS, which occurs when a baby stops breathing and dies.

Older children and pets must be watched carefully around babies. Jealousy can cause even well-behaved children and pets to harm babies. Older children may not mean to hurt a baby, but may not know how to touch or handle a baby safely.

Picking up and holding a baby

1. Wash your hands.

2. Reach one hand under the baby and behind his head and neck. Cradle the head and neck in your hand. Support the head at all times when lifting or holding a newborn.

3. With the other hand, support the baby's back and bottom.

4. There are several ways to hold a baby safely: the cradle hold, the football hold, and upright against your chest (Figs. 27-1 through 27-3). Always be sure the baby's head and neck are supported.

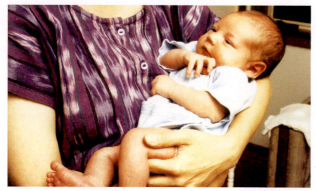

Fig. 27-1. The cradle hold has the baby's head and neck resting in the crook of one elbow and the legs in the other arm. You must support the baby's back with one or both hands.

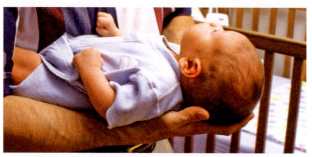

Fig. 27-2. The football hold is accomplished by holding the baby's head in one hand and supporting the baby's back with the arm on the same side of your body. The baby's body will lie along the side of your body.

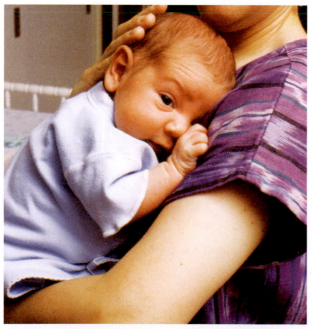

Fig. 27-3. When holding a baby upright against your chest, you must support the baby's head, neck, and back with one hand while keeping the other arm under the baby's bottom to support his weight.

Most infants love to be held. They are very sensitive to touch. HHAs should also talk to them while performing personal care; they respond well to stimulation. Although babies are helpless, they are sensitive to their environment. They can see, taste, hear, and smell.

6. Describe guidelines for assisting with feeding a baby

Assisting with Breastfeeding

Most pediatricians encourage mothers to breastfeed, or nurse, their babies. Breastfeeding provides the perfect nutrition for infants. The decision to breast- or bottle-feed is a personal one that each mother makes for herself. If a mother chooses breastfeeding, she may need support while learning how to breastfeed. Many professionals recommend that women try breastfeeding for at least two weeks before deciding whether to continue. The first two weeks may be challenging for the mother. An HHA's support can help her get off to a good start.

An HHA should discuss with the mother how much help she wants, asking questions to determine the mother's experience with and knowledge of breastfeeding: *Did you breastfeed your other children? If yes, for how long? If no, what made you decide to do so now? Did the nurses in the hospital teach you about breastfeeding? Did you take any newborn classes before delivery?* The mother may only want help getting into position, or she may want coaching throughout the process. The HHA can make sure the mother knows that lactation consultants can help solve breastfeeding problems. Help for nursing mothers is also available from La Leche League International, found online at llli.org. HHAs should report any problems observed or that the client shares with them.

Mothers nursing for the first time may experience embarrassment, fear of pain, and/or lack of self-confidence. An HHA can help the new mother by remaining calm, being supportive and confident in the mother's ability to nurse, and creating an atmosphere in which the mother can comfortably nurse without interruption.

Women have different breastfeeding styles. Some are very comfortable nursing in the presence of others. Others may want more privacy while nursing. HHAs should be sensitive to individual preferences. A calm setting where the mother can relax will help her body provide the most milk for the baby.

Guidelines: Helping a Mother with Breastfeeding

G Remind the mother to wash her hands. Help her get in position for breastfeeding, usually sitting upright in a comfortable chair or in bed supported by pillows. Provide a low foot-rest if possible and a pillow for the mother's lap (Fig. 27-4). Some mothers are able to breastfeed while lying down. Others, how-ever, find this more difficult, especially with a newborn baby.

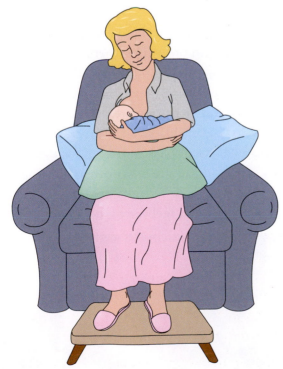

Fig. 27-4. *A new mother may prefer to nurse in an up-right sitting position. Provide support with pillows and a footrest.*

G Provide privacy. Close the door and occupy older children if necessary.

G Change the baby's diaper if needed before bringing him to the mother. If desired, use a towel or blanket to cover the mother's breast and baby's head after baby has latched on.

G If necessary, remind the mother how to hold the nipple and areola between thumb and forefinger to allow baby to latch on. If baby does not latch on right away, have the mother stroke his cheek with her nipple.

G Proper nutrition and plenty of fluids are important for nursing mothers. Offer snacks and frequent drinks of water, juice, or milk.

G Observe the nursing baby to be sure he stays latched on properly (Fig. 27-5). If needed, the mother can use one hand to hold the breast tissue away from the baby's nose.

There is no need to move the baby from one breast to the other until the baby stops nurs-ing on his own. The longer the baby nurses on one side, the more of the denser, fattier "hindmilk" he receives.

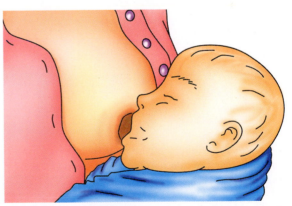

Fig. 27-5. *When the baby is properly latched on to the mother's nipple, his mouth covers much of the areola. The nipple is sucked straight out rather than at an angle. This ensures the best milk flow and prevents the nipples from becoming sore.*

G If the mother needs to reposition the baby or wishes to try for a better latch, she can break the suction by pressing down on the breast above the nipple or by gently putting her fin-ger in the baby's mouth.

G   Help the mother burp the baby when switching breasts and when finishing the feeding.

G   Change the baby's diaper after the feeding. Help the mother lay the baby down safely.

G   Many women find it helpful to tie a ribbon or place a pin on the side the baby last fed on. This helps them remember to start the baby's feeding on that side next time, so the breasts will be emptied more evenly.

Assisting with Bottle Feeding

Many women choose to bottle feed their babies some or all of the time. Bottle-fed newborns require special formula. Infant formula is commercially prepared and provides the nutrition babies need. Regular whole milk does not supply the proper nourishment for babies and would upset their digestive systems.

There are many brands and types of formula. The three most common types are ready-to-use formula, concentrated liquid formula, and powdered formula (Fig. 27-6).

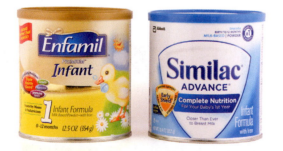

Fig. 27-6. Baby formula is available in three forms: powdered in cans, like the two options above, ready-to-use, and concentrated liquid.

Ready-to-use formula (sometimes called *ready-made*) is often sold in bottles. This formula is ready to use. It should not be diluted or mixed with water. If the formula comes in a bottle, an HHA can simply unscrew the cap and pour the formula into a clean bottle. Any formula remaining in the bottle after feeding should be discarded. Open containers of ready-to-use formula can usually be stored safely in the refrigerator, covered, for up to 48 hours. Ready-to-use for-

mula is the most convenient to use. It is also the most expensive.

Concentrated formula is sold in cans or bottles. It must be mixed with tap or bottled water before using. If the care plan's instructions state to use sterile water, it can be purchased in bottles or made by bringing water to a boil and then cooling it. The HHA should open the can and pour the amount indicated in the care plan into a clean bottle. An equal amount of water should be added to the bottle. After the nipple and ring have been screwed on, the HHA should shake the bottle to mix it well. Unused concentrate can be stored in the can, covered and refrigerated, for up to 48 hours.

Powdered formula is sold in cans of various sizes. It is carefully measured and mixed with tap or bottled water. A scoop is included in the can for measuring. The powder and water should be mixed in a clean bottle, following directions on the container. Any formula remaining in the bottle after a feeding should be discarded. Powdered formula is the most difficult to use, but is usually the cheapest to buy.

Before feeding, bottles should be warmed by immersing them in or holding them under warm tap water for several minutes (Fig. 27-7). Bottles of formula just out of the refrigerator will take longer to warm. A microwave oven should never be used to warm bottles. This can create hot spots in the liquid that can burn the baby. The HHA should shake the bottle after warming and shake a few drops of formula onto the inside of her wrist. It should feel warm, not hot or cold.

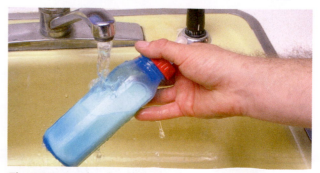

Fig. 27-7. Bottles should be warmed in warm tap water—not in the microwave.

Sterilizing bottles

Equipment: clean bottles, nipples, and rings to be sterilized (these should be washed in hot, soapy water using a bottle brush and allowed to drain), large pot filled halfway with water, tongs, clean dish or paper towels to set sterile bottles on

1. Wash your hands.

2. Bring water to a boil and put bottles, nipples, and rings in. Use tongs to push bottles under water.

3. Bring water to a boil again and boil for five minutes.

4. Using tongs, remove bottles, nipples, and rings, draining the water into the pot. Set everything on the clean towels. When dry, store in a clean, dry cabinet.

5. Discard water.

Assisting with bottle feeding

1. Wash your hands.

2. Prepare bottle and formula as directed.

3. Sit in a comfortable chair and hold the baby safely in either the cradle hold or football hold.

4. Stroke the baby's lips with the bottle nipple until he opens his mouth. Put the bottle nipple in the baby's mouth.

5. Be sure the baby's head is higher than his body during feeding. Also, make sure the nipple stays full of milk so that the baby does not swallow air (Fig. 27-8).

6. Talk or sing to the baby while feeding. Feedings are the high points of his days and should be special times.

7. When the baby is through or has stopped sucking, burp him (see procedure below). Resume feeding or, if finished, change the diaper (see procedure later in chapter). Put the baby down safely.

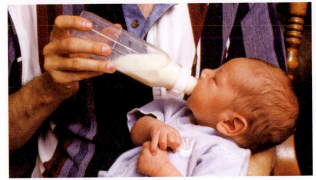

Fig. 27-8. *The baby's head should be higher than his body during feeding.*

8. Wash your hands and document the feeding, how much was consumed, and any other observations.

9. Discard unused formula left in bottle. Wash the bottle, nipple, and ring in hot soapy water with a bottle brush and allow to dry. Sterilize before using again.

Babies must be burped after each feeding to release air swallowed during feeding. Burping prevents babies from developing gas. Gas can be very uncomfortable for them. Burping in the middle of a feeding may allow a baby to eat more.

Burping a baby

Equipment: clean burp cloth, towel, or cloth diaper

1. Wash your hands.

2. Pick up the baby safely. There are two different positions to use for burping. Most people like to hold the baby against the shoulder to burp (Fig. 27-9). However, babies who are very small, who have breathing problems, or who tend to choke or spit up should be held on the lap with the head supported by holding the baby's chin with the thumb and forefinger (Fig. 27-10). This position allows you to watch the baby for signs of respiratory distress, especially color changes or spit-up. Whichever position you use, put the burp cloth under the baby's chin to catch any spit-up.

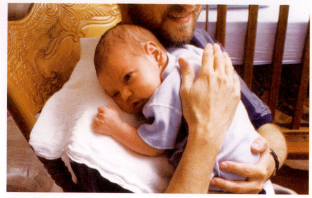

Fig. 27-9. *Holding a baby against the shoulder to burp is common.*

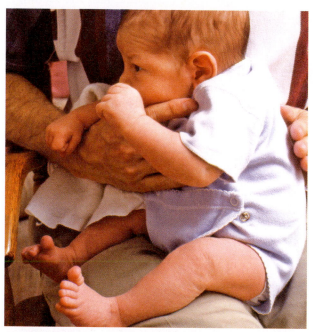

Fig. 27-10. *Babies who have breathing problems or who choke or spit up should be held on the lap with the head supported to burp.*

3. With the baby in a safe and comfortable position, pat the baby's back gently with your flat hand. Concentrate on the area between the shoulder blades. Some people like to pat up and down the baby's back. Others like to massage the back using an upward motion with the flat hand. Use any technique that works for you. The more relaxed and comfortable the baby is, the sooner the burp will come.

4. After the baby has burped, return him to a safe position or resume feeding.

Clients' Rights

Schedule and Feeding

The mother has the right to determine how to handle her new baby's schedule. For example, if a mother wants her baby to be fed whenever he cries, whether she is present or not, the HHA should respect her wishes. It is also the mother's decision what to feed her baby. The HHA should not make judgments or express opinions on whether the mother should breastfeed or use formula to feed her baby. If any behavior causes concern, it should be reported to the supervisor.

7. Explain guidelines for bathing and changing a baby

Keeping a baby clean is important to his health. These guidelines describe how to safely handle a baby:

Guidelines: Bathing and Changing a Baby

G Because you could come into contact with body fluids, wear disposable gloves when bathing or changing a baby. Remember, however, that gloves can make a wet baby slippery. Be very careful when handling a baby during a bath.

G Whether bathing or changing a baby, keep one hand on the infant at all times. Have all supplies ready so you **never** have to take both hands off the baby.

G Give baths in a warm place. Close doors and windows to prevent drafts. Dry the baby's head immediately after washing hair.

G Be very careful about bath temperature. Always test the temperature of the water (either on the inside of your wrist or with a bath thermometer).

G Keep the baby's bottom dry. Be sure the area is thoroughly dried after a bath. Moisture contributes to diaper rash. Dry the bottom after changing a diaper. Leaving the diaper off for a few moments when changing the baby allows air to circulate and helps prevent diaper rash.

G   Do not use powder unless directed to do so. Powder can cause breathing problems and lung damage if babies inhale the particles.

Giving an infant sponge bath

Equipment: clean basin, blanket or towel to pad surface, washcloth and towel, baby wash or baby shampoo, cotton hat, lotion, cotton balls, diaper ointment (if used), clean diaper, clean clothes or sleeper, clean receiving blanket, gloves

1.   Wash your hands.

2.   Put on gloves. Be careful—gloves make the baby slippery.

3.   Give the bath in a warm place. Use a blanket or towel to pad the surface that the baby will lie on. Have all your supplies within reach. You will need to keep one hand on the baby during the entire bath. Remove caps from wash or shampoo to make it easier.

4.   Fill the basin with warm water. Test the temperature on the inside of your wrist. Put the bottle of lotion in the warm water to warm it.

5.   With the baby still dressed, hold him in the football hold. Wet the washcloth or cotton ball and gently wipe the eyes, using a clean cotton ball or clean area of the washcloth for each wipe. Clean from the inner corner to the outer (Fig. 27-11). Then clean the rest of the face. Use only warm water—no soap.

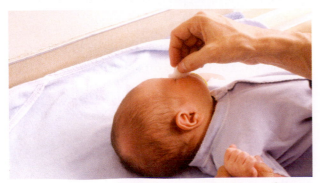

Fig. 27-11. *Using only warm water, wipe the eyes from the inner area to the outer area.*

6.   To wash hair, hold the baby in the football hold with the head over the basin. Use the washcloth to wet the hair. Using a small amount of baby wash, lather the hair (Fig. 27-12). Rinse with the washcloth. Pat the head dry immediately with the towel. Put a cotton hat over the baby's head. Body heat is lost through the head; keep the head warm.

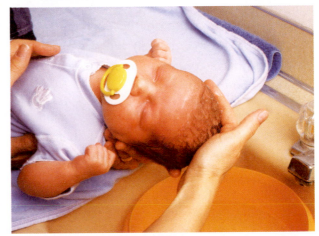

Fig. 27-12. *Lather the hair with a small amount of baby wash and immediately dry the head after rinsing.*

7.   Lay the baby down on the padded surface. Always keep at least one hand on the baby.

8.   Undress the upper body (Fig. 27-13). Wash the neck, chest, back, arms, and hands using the washcloth and small amounts of baby wash. Rinse using the washcloth and water from the basin. Pat dry. Cover the upper body with a towel.

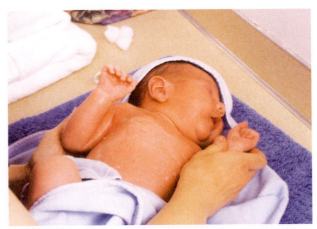

Fig. 27-13. *Uncover only the area that you are washing. Keep one hand on the baby at all times.*

9. Undress the lower body, removing the diaper. Wash the baby's abdomen and legs. Rinse. Pat dry.

10. Wash the perineal area last. For a girl, wipe the perineal area from front to back. For a boy who has recently been circumcised, do not wash the area of the circumcision. Follow instructions to care for the circumcision.

11. Wash the baby's bottom thoroughly, and dry the entire area completely with the towel. Moisture can contribute to diaper rash. Use diaper ointment if needed.

12. As gently and quickly as possible, rub lotion over the baby's body. Avoid the umbilical cord stump if it has not yet healed. Avoid using lotion on the baby's face unless ordered to do so. Keep the baby covered except for the part you are rubbing.

13. Diaper and dress the baby. Wrap baby in a clean blanket and put him down safely.

14. Put used towels and washcloth in the laundry. Discard water. Clean basin and store. Store other supplies. Discard gloves.

15. Wash your hands.

16. Document the bath, including any observations.

Giving an infant tub bath

In addition to the supplies listed in the procedure above for a sponge bath, you will need a large basin or baby bath tub. You may also bathe a baby in a clean sink. Follow the first six steps in the procedure for a sponge bath to prepare the bath and wash the baby's face and hair.

1. Lay the baby down on the padded surface and undress him completely. Immerse baby in basin. Support the head and neck above water with one hand at all times (Fig. 27-14).

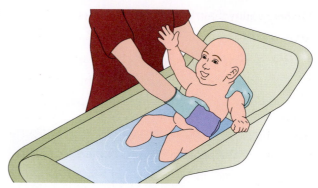

Fig. 27-14. *The baby's head and neck must be supported at all times.*

2. Using the washcloth and small amounts of baby wash, wash the baby from the neck down.

3. Remove the baby from the bath and lay him down on the padded surface. Keep one hand on the baby at all times. Cover baby with a towel and pat dry (Fig. 27-15).

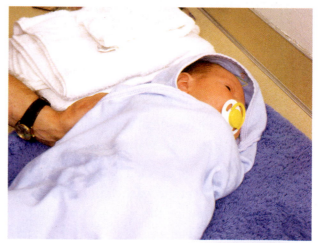

Fig. 27-15. *Immediately dry and cover the baby after the bath.*

4. Apply lotion, keeping the baby covered as much as possible.

5. Diaper, dress, and wrap the baby in a clean blanket. Put baby down safely.

6. Put used linens in the laundry. Discard bath water. Clean and store basin. Store all supplies. Discard gloves.

7. Wash your hands.

8. Document the bath, including any observations.

Diapers catch the baby's urine and feces. Children wear diapers until they are toilet trained—generally between two and three years of age. Diapers are either cloth or disposable. There are different types of cloth diapers with different types of closures, like Velcro, fasteners, snaps, or pins. Most cloth diapers are used with a special waterproof cover that needs to be secured.

A newborn will need between eight and 12 diaper changes in 24 hours. As babies get older, they use fewer diapers each day. The appearance, consistency, and smell of a baby's feces will depend on what he is fed. Some newborn babies have loose bowel movements with every feeding, as many as eight a day. Others have different schedules. Babies must be changed frequently to avoid diaper rash or irritation.

Changing cloth or disposable diapers

Equipment: clean disposable diaper or clean cloth diaper, diaper cover and closure (if needed for cloth diapers), wipes or a warm, wet washcloth, diaper ointment (if used), clean clothes if clothes are soiled or wet, gloves

1. Wash your hands.

2. Put on gloves.

3. Change the diaper in a warm place. You need a padded surface, which may be a special changing table or a countertop. Never turn your back on the baby. Keep one hand on baby at all times. Have supplies within reach.

4. Undress the baby as necessary and remove wet or soiled diaper. Set it aside for handling later.

5. Clean the perineal area with wipes or washcloth. Remove all traces of feces. Spread the legs to clean thoroughly. For girls, wipe from front to back and spread the labia to clean as needed.

6. Let air circulate on the bottom for a moment. Exposure to air prevents diaper rash. Apply ointment as directed.

7. **For disposable diapers**: Unfold the diaper and expose tapes. Place the diaper flat under the baby's bottom with the tapes in back. Bring the front of the diaper up between the baby's legs and bring the back sides around and over the front (Fig. 27-16). Peel tapes open, and tape the side of the diaper securely to the front.

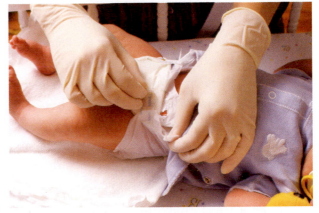

Fig. 27-16. *A disposable diaper is fastened with adhesive tapes that are located on the back sides of the diaper.*

For cloth diapers with a diaper cover: Fold the diaper in thirds lengthwise. Then open out the back corners about three inches (Fig. 27-17). Lay the back of the diaper inside the back of the diaper cover (the back of the diaper cover has the tabs extending from it). Place the diaper and cover underneath the baby's bottom. Bring the front of the diaper and cover up through the baby's legs. Bring the tabs around from the sides to the front of the diaper cover and use them to close the cover securely over the diaper. Check that all the edges of the diaper are tucked under the cover.

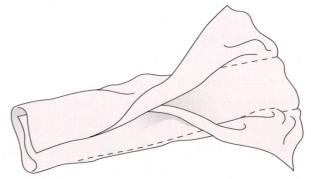

Fig. 27-17. *After folding the diaper in thirds, open out the back corners about three inches.*

For cloth diapers with fasteners and waterproof pants: Fold the diaper lengthwise in thirds, then open out the back corners about three inches. Place the diaper under the baby's bottom, and bring the front of the diaper up between the baby's legs. Fold down the front of the diaper to the inside (next to baby's skin) so that the diaper covers the genitals and lower abdomen. Bring the corners of the diaper around the baby's sides and fasten them to the front of the diaper. If using a stretchable fastener, hook it on the outside of the diaper, on the left, then stretch it across and hook it on the right. Stretch it down and hook the center. It should go from a "T" shape to a "Y" shape when stretched properly. When diaper is securely fastened, put waterproof pants over the diaper to keep urine from leaking.

8. Dress the baby in clean clothes and put him down safely.

9. Dispose of diaper properly. Disposable diapers can be rolled into a ball (dirty side in), sealed with tapes, and disposed of in a special trash bag in a sealed container to prevent odors. Cloth diapers may need to be soaked before washing or before a diaper service removes them. Check with the baby's mother or your supervisor for instructions.

10. Remove and discard gloves.

11. Wash your hands.

12. Clean changing area and store supplies.

13. Wash hands again as needed.

14. Document any observations, including unusual color, consistency, or odor.

8. Identify how to measure weight and length of a baby

As part of an HHA's duties, she may be asked to measure a new baby's weight and length. Measurement of a newborn is not normally difficult, but they do tend to squirm and wiggle when naked and on a hard, flat surface. The HHA should keep one hand on the baby at all times.

The infant may need to be naked for an accurate weight. The HHA should follow her supervisor's instructions and should use an infant scale when measuring the baby's weight.

Measuring a baby's weight

Equipment: infant scale, clean paper or pad

1. Wash your hands.

2. Place an infant scale on a firm surface.

3. Place a clean paper or pad on the scale.

4. Start with scale balanced at zero before weighing baby.

5. Undress the baby.

6. Place the baby on the scale, protecting the sides so he does not roll. Keep at least one hand on the baby at all times.

7. Read and remember the weight. If possible, lock the weight into place.

8. Remove the baby and dress him. Put baby in crib.

9. Wash your hands.

10. Document the weight, including any observations.

A baby's length measurement can be obtained with the baby dressed.

Measuring a baby's length

Equipment: paper with inch markings on it or plain paper, tape measure, pencil

1. Wash your hands.

2. Prepare a clean, firm surface with a clean sheet of paper that has inch markings on it.

3. Place the baby on the firm surface. Keep at least one hand on the baby at all times.

4. Place the baby's head at the beginning of the measured markings.

5. Straighten the baby's knee.

6. Make a pencil mark on the paper at the baby's heel.

7. Determine and remember length.

8. Remove the baby and put him in his crib.

9. Wash your hands.

10. Document the length, including any observations.

When a paper with inch markings is not available, follow these steps:

1. Wash your hands.

2. Prepare a clean, firm surface with a plain sheet of paper on it. The paper must be longer than the baby.

3. Place the baby on the firm surface. Keep at least one hand on the baby at all times.

4. Make a pencil mark on the paper at the top of the baby's head.

5. Straighten the baby's knee.

6. Make another mark at the baby's heel.

7. Remove the baby and put him in his crib.

8. With the tape measure, measure the distance between the marks. Remember length.

9. Wash your hands.

10. Document the length, including any observations.

9. Explain guidelines for special care

At birth, the **umbilical cord** that connected the baby to the placenta inside the mother's uterus is cut. The stump of the cord remains attached to a newborn's navel for up to three weeks

(Fig. 27-18). Proper care of the cord stump is necessary to prevent infection and allow healing.

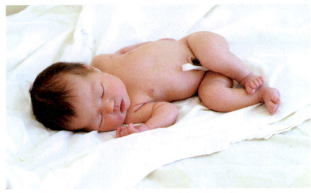

Fig. 27-18. The stump of an umbilical cord remains attached to the navel for up to three weeks. The stump needs to be kept clean and dry until it falls off.

Guidelines: Umbilical Cord Care

G Keep the stump clean. It used to be common to swab the stump with alcohol after every diaper change. However, research suggests that the stump may heal faster if left alone. If the stump becomes dirty, gently wash it with mild soap and water. Make sure the area is dry after cleaning it. Use a clean, dry cloth to gently absorb any moisture, or fan it dry using a piece of paper.

G Never pull on or handle the cord. It will fall off by itself. The baby will feel no pain when the cord falls off.

G Keep diapers folded down away from the cord to allow air to circulate and prevent irritation. Quickly change wet or soiled diapers.

G Do not give an infant a tub bath until the cord has fallen off. Until then, giving a sponge bath is best.

Measuring an infant's axillary, tympanic, or temporal artery temperature

Equipment: mercury-free thermometer, digital thermometer, tympanic thermometer, or temporal artery thermometer, disposable probe cover (if needed)

1. Wash your hands.

2. Be sure thermometer is clean. Put on disposable probe cover if used. For mercury-free thermometer, shake thermometer down to below the lowest number.

3. **For axillary temperature**: Undress the upper body on one side. Lay the baby on a padded surface. Place the tip of the thermometer under the arm, and hold the baby's arm close to his body so the thermometer tip touches skin on all sides (Fig. 27-19). Keep thermometer in place for three to five minutes for a mercury-free thermometer or until the digital thermometer blinks or beeps.

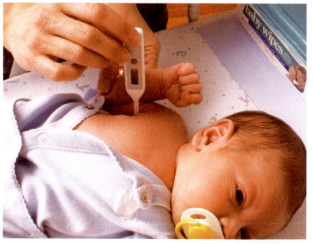

Fig. 27-19. *Leave the thermometer in place for three to five minutes or until it blinks or beeps.*

For tympanic temperature: Lay the baby on his side. Pull the outside of the ear gently toward the back of the head. Gently insert the thermometer tip into the ear, pointing toward the opposite eye. Be sure the ear is sealed by the thermometer. Press the button and hold the thermometer in place until thermometer blinks or beeps.

For temporal artery temperature: Turn on the thermometer. Place the thermometer flat on the forehead, usually midway between the eyebrow and the hairline. Press and hold the scan button. Gently sweep the thermometer across the baby's forehead, keeping the thermometer in contact with the skin. Release the scan button.

4. For all methods, remove the thermometer and read the temperature. Keep one hand on the baby at all times.

5. If you measured the axillary temperature, dress the baby. Put the baby down safely.

6. Clean and store thermometer and supplies.

7. Wash your hands.

8. Document temperature.

Circumcision is the removal of part of the foreskin of the penis. It is commonly performed on male babies. Some religions require circumcision. Parents may choose to have their baby circumcised for other reasons.

Circumcision is usually performed in the hospital or at the doctor's office when the baby is only days old. Afterwards, the circumcision site needs special care to heal. This usually includes covering the tip of the penis with a gauze pad rubbed with petroleum jelly to prevent the diaper from irritating the site. However, some types of circumcision require different care. The HHA's supervisor's instructions and the care plan will explain the care required.

Some babies who need special care will have medical equipment in the home. HHAs will probably not be responsible for operating or handling the equipment. However, it is helpful for them to be familiar with various items. HHAs should always follow their supervisor's instructions before touching any medical equipment.

Apnea monitor: Apnea is the state of not breathing. Some babies may stop breathing for periods of time due to immaturity of the lungs or other reasons. The apnea monitor alerts parents or caregivers if breathing stops. Many apnea monitors also monitor heart rate.

Ventilator or oxygen equipment: Some babies with breathing problems need to be given oxygen. Oxygen is considered a medication. In most states it cannot be given by a home health aide.

In addition, HHAs are not allowed to change the amount of oxygen being given. As always, HHAs should be careful when working around oxygen, as it is flammable, and should follow instructions carefully when working in a home where oxygen is in use. Chapter 14 has more information about oxygen and related care.

10. Identify special needs of children and describe how children respond to stress

Home health aides may have contact with children in several ways. They may be assigned to care for a client's children when the client is unable to care for them. The client may be absent or unable to care for them due to illness, injury, or disability. In this case the HHA is a substitute for the parent. In other cases, the client may be the child and may be suffering from a disease or disability that requires home care. In either case, it is important that HHAs understand some basic principles of caring for and working with children.

Children have the same basic physical and emotional needs as adults (Chapter 8). They also have some special physical, mental, and emotional needs. Children's growing bodies need adequate and nutritious food and fluids, exercise, fresh air, and plenty of sleep. Their developing minds need to be stimulated by age-appropriate activities, opportunities for learning, and chances for increasing independence. Emotionally, children need love and affection, reassurance, encouragement, security, and guidance. They also need consistent and constructive discipline. In addition, children need protection from injury and illness. Chapter 8 describes child development in more detail.

Children with disabilities have the same physical and emotional needs as other children. HHAs should remember to treat these children as children first. Disabilities may make normal social contact with other children difficult. However, it is important for children with disabilities to interact with others their own age (Fig. 27-20).

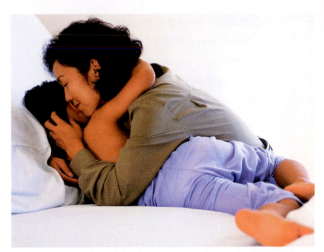

Fig. 27-20. *Children with disabilities have the same emotional needs as other children. They should be encouraged to interact with others their own age.*

Children may experience stress due to a variety of reasons, including unmet needs, problems at school or at home, unstable families, disability, illness, and unfamiliar caregivers in the home. Many factors influence how children respond to stress, such as the age of the child, what is causing the stress, how severe the stress is, how long it lasts, and how often the stress occurs.

School-age children may react to stress by rebelling, skipping school, daydreaming, lying, cheating, or stealing. They may also feel guilty and feel that they are to blame for the family's problems. Adolescents may react to stress in negative ways too, such as by staying out all night, dropping out of school, and abusing drugs or alcohol.

11. List symptoms of common childhood illnesses and the required care

Most childhood illnesses are caused by bacterial or viral infections. These include colds, flu, and various infections causing fever, diarrhea, vomiting, or coughing. Home health aides can help avoid illness by preventing the spread of infection in the home. Handwashing, cleaning, and disinfection are the best ways to prevent infection (Chapter 5). Treatments for some of the most common symptoms of childhood illnesses are described below.

Fever: Fever may indicate serious illness. An HHA should always report it to his supervisor. Rest and fluids are recommended for fevers. Treatment for a fever may also include acetaminophen or a lukewarm bath or sponging. Home health aides never give any medication, including over-the-counter medications, but they can assist by making sure the family caregiver follows a doctor's dosage instructions for all medications. The strength of over-the-counter drugs varies in infant, children, and adult formulas. It is especially important to follow dosage instructions. For example, giving too much acetaminophen can cause liver damage or failure. In general, children should not be given aspirin, as it has been associated with some serious disorders.

Diarrhea: Diarrhea, or frequent loose or watery bowel movements, can have many causes. In children, it is often caused by a virus. Cramps and abdominal pain may accompany diarrhea. Children with diarrhea should rest and drink plenty of clear liquids, including water, broth, and diluted juices. Doctors may recommend electrolyte-replacement drinks to prevent dehydration. Although it used to be common to recommend the BRAT (bananas, rice, applesauce, and toast) diet until diarrhea subsided, doctors now recommend that kids resume their normal, well-balanced diet within 24 hours of getting sick.

Vomiting: The treatment for vomiting is similar to the treatment for diarrhea, including rest and clear liquids.

An HHA should always call his supervisor if symptoms continue and should follow instructions in the care plan or his assignment sheet.

12. Identify guidelines for working with children

The following suggestions may help an HHA establish a trusting and honest relationship with the children in his care:

G   Introduce yourself. Treat children as important members of the family who are worthy of your notice. Be friendly, tell the children your name, and explain why you are there.

G   Maintain routine. As much as possible, stick with the family's regular schedule. The comfort of a routine can help ease the stress children may feel if someone in their household needs home care.

G   Give comfort. Children who are hurt, angry, or sad may need a hug, a pat, or soothing words to make them feel more secure (Fig. 27-21).

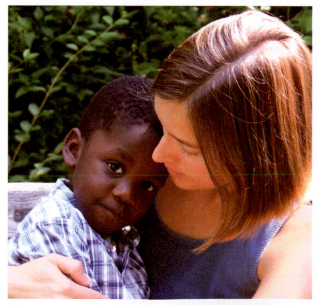

Fig. 27-21. *Comforting children can make them feel more secure.*

G   Offer encouragement and praise. Praise and encouragement contribute to the child's sense of self-worth and self-confidence. Word your praise so that it does not belittle other children.

G   Do not make comparisons. Children should not be compared to each other.

G   Use positive phrases. Children often respond better to guidance such as, "Let's try it this way..." rather than "no" or "don't."

G Listen. Pay attention when children attempt to communicate. Do not interrupt them or deny their feelings. Help them to express what they are feeling by using your communication skills.

G Answer. Respond to children's questions immediately, willingly, and clearly. If you do not know the answer or are not sure you are the right person to answer it, tell the child. Take the child's question to the appropriate person.

G Do not force children to eat. Like adults, children do not always feel like eating. Do not allow a meal to become a power struggle. Children are usually motivated to eat when meals are simple but attractive and contain their favorite foods.

G Involve children in household activities. Children feel capable and responsible when they are given household tasks to perform (Fig. 27-22). Like all people, they like to feel they are making a contribution to the family.

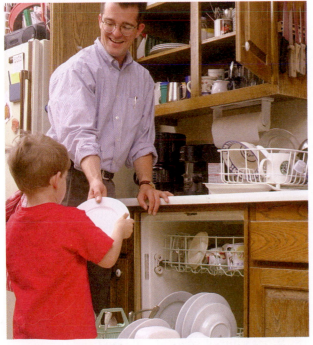

Fig. 27-22. Help children contribute.

G Encourage children to play. Children need to exercise and socialize with other children (Fig. 27-23). Playing helps children express themselves and be creative. Exercise is important for their growth and health. Socialization is especially important for children who are learning social skills.

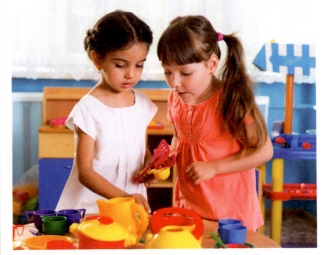

Fig. 27-23. Encourage children to play with others.

G Recognize individual needs. Not all children are the same. They have different needs for sleep, food, and exercise. They grow and develop at different paces.

G Be nonjudgmental. As with any client, treat a child with disabilities or problems with respect.

13. List the signs of child abuse and neglect and know how to report them

Child abuse is the physical, sexual, or psychological mistreatment of a child. Children who are abused can range in age from infant to adolescent. Sexual abuse of children includes inappropriate touching of a child's body, sexual contact, penetration, or sharing sexual stories or material with children. Psychological abuse includes verbal abuse, such as name-calling, social isolation, and seclusion. **Child neglect** is the purposeful or unintentional failure to provide for the needs of a child. Children who are neglected may not receive adequate food, water, medications, supervision, or shelter.

Children should never be harmed, threatened, or made fun of. They must be treated with respect and concern. Adults must talk to children calmly and quietly and give them positive comments, praise, and encouragement.

Child abuse or neglect can come from anyone who is responsible for a child's care. This includes parents, guardians, paid caregivers, teachers, friends, or relatives. The law requires that health professionals report suspected child abuse. **If a home health aide observes or suspects abuse or neglect, or if a child reports that someone has abused or neglected him or her, the HHA must immediately report this to the supervisor.** It not only is the right thing to do, but the HHA and her agency can get into trouble for not reporting suspected abuse or neglect. HHAs must follow their employer's procedures for reporting abuse or suspected abuse.

Observing and Reporting: Child Abuse

If you observe any of these signs of child abuse or neglect, or if you suspect abuse or neglect, speak to your supervisor immediately.

- O/R Child has burns, cuts, bruises, abrasions, or fractured bones

- O/R Child stares vacantly or watches intensely

- O/R Child is extremely quiet

- O/R Child avoids eye contact, although in some cultures, it is the norm to avoid eye contact

- O/R Child is afraid of adults

- O/R Child behaves aggressively

- O/R Child exhibits excessive activity or hyperactivity (some hyperactive children, however, have a chemical imbalance that produces this behavior)

- O/R Child tells you that someone is abusing him or her

Chapter Review

1. Why are new mothers often more tired and uncomfortable when they get home than women were in the past?

2. What kind of doctor specializes in working with newborns?

3. List five tasks an HHA may do to assist a new mother.

4. What is important to report about a new mother's lochia?

5. What types of information might an HHA be asked to routinely document in caring for a newborn and mother?

6. What should an HHA always do before touching or picking up a baby?

7. Where are the only safe places to leave a baby?

8. Why must a baby's head be supported when he is being held?

9. Why should a baby NOT be put to sleep on his stomach or on a blanket or comforter?

10. Why are women encouraged to breastfeed?

11. How should a bottle be warmed?

12. How is concentrated formula mixed?

13. For what length of time can ready-to-use formula be refrigerated?

14. How does burping help a baby?

15. Why must an HHA have all supplies ready before bathing or changing a baby?

16. How can an HHA test the temperature of a baby's bath water?

17. How many diaper changes will a newborn typically need within 24 hours?

18. What kind of scale should be used to measure an infant's weight?

19. Why should the umbilical cord stump be left alone unless it is dirty?

20. What does circumcision care generally require?

21. Why may an HHA be assigned to care for a client's children?

22. Why is it important to treat children with disabilities as children first?

23. List five factors that influence how children respond to stress.

24. Name each of the three symptoms of illness outlined in Learning Objective 11 and describe one common treatment for each.

25. If a child asks an HHA a question, and she does not know the answer, what should the HHA do?

26. Why is maintaining routine important for children?

27. List six common signs of child abuse.

28

Meal Planning, Shopping, Preparation, and Storage

1. Explain how to prepare a basic food plan and list food shopping guidelines

Home health aides should plan meals for a week or at least several days before shopping. When planning, the client's dietary restrictions, food preferences, the number of people present at meals, and the client's budget should be taken into account. On a large sheet of paper, the HHA should write the days for which she will shop, leaving space under each day for meals and snacks. She may end up serving the meals in a different order. However, by planning for each day, she will plan the right number of meals and buy the right amount of food (Fig. 28-1).

The HHA can fill in breakfasts, lunches, dinners, and snacks for each day. She can ask the client for ideas or look online (epicurious.com, allrecipes.com, and foodnetwork.com are a few options) or in cookbooks. A good plan will include leftovers that can be easily reheated on days the HHA will not be in the home. Nutritious snacks should be part of the plan; clients may need as many as three snacks a day. Beverages should be listed as well.

When the meal plan is complete, the HHA can make a shopping list. On another large sheet of paper, she can list categories, including produce, meats, canned goods, frozen foods, dairy, and other. She should leave space under each cat-

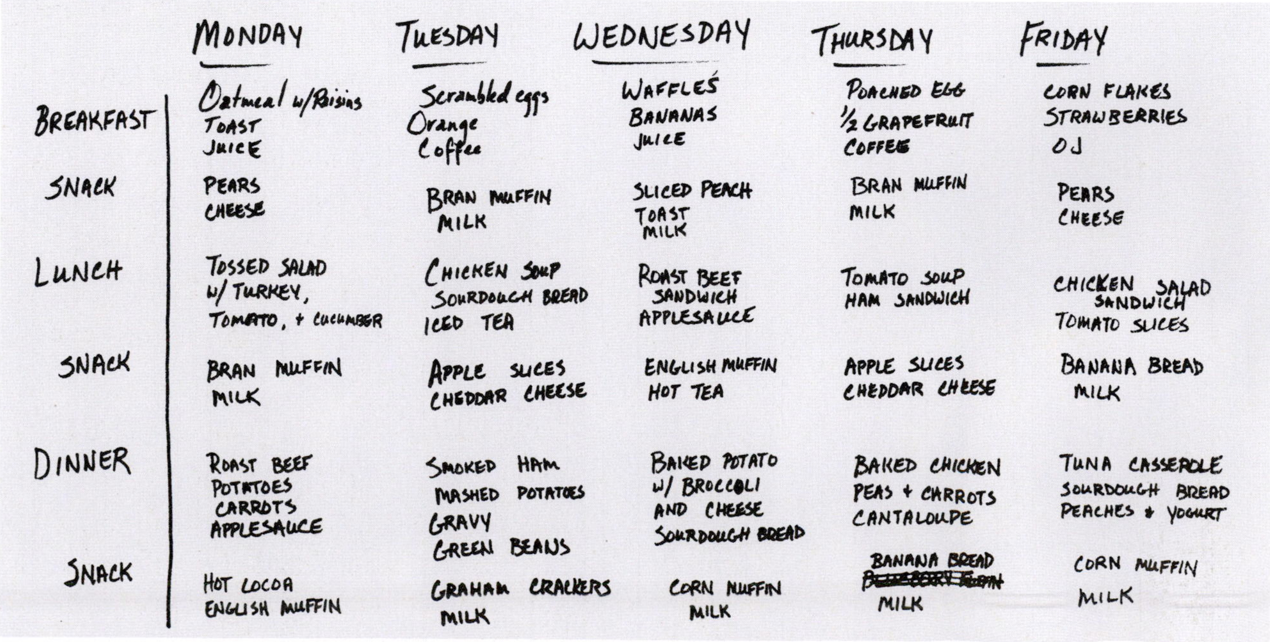

	MONDAY	TUESDAY	WEDNESDAY	THURSDAY	FRIDAY
BREAKFAST	Oatmeal w/Raisins Toast Juice	Scrambled eggs Orange Coffee	WAFFLES BANANAS JUICE	Poached Egg ½ Grapefruit Coffee	CORN FLAKES STRAWBERRIES OJ
SNACK	PEARS CHEESE	BRAN MUFFIN MILK	SLICED PEACH TOAST MILK	BRAN MUFFIN MILK	PEARS CHEESE
LUNCH	TOSSED SALAD w/ TURKEY, TOMATO, + CUCUMBER	CHICKEN SOUP SOURDOUGH BREAD ICED TEA	ROAST BEEF SANDWICH APPLESAUCE	TOMATO SOUP HAM SANDWICH	CHICKEN SALAD SANDWICH TOMATO SLICES
SNACK	BRAN MUFFIN MILK	APPLE SLICES CHEDDAR CHEESE	ENGLISH MUFFIN HOT TEA	APPLE SLICES CHEDDAR CHEESE	BANANA BREAD MILK
DINNER	ROAST BEEF POTATOES CARROTS APPLESAUCE	SMOKED HAM MASHED POTATOES GRAVY GREEN BEANS	BAKED POTATO w/ BROCCOLI AND CHEESE SOURDOUGH BREAD	BAKED CHICKEN PEAS + CARROTS CANTALOUPE	TUNA CASSEROLE SOURDOUGH BREAD PEACHES + YOGURT
SNACK	HOT COCOA ENGLISH MUFFIN	GRAHAM CRACKERS MILK	CORN MUFFIN MILK	BANANA BREAD ~~BLUEBERRY YOGURT~~ MILK	CORN MUFFIN MILK

Fig. 28-1. A meal plan helps a home health aide know what kinds and quantities of food to buy for a week.

egory to list the foods she needs to buy. Listing items by category saves time in the grocery store. The HHA can go through the plan meal by meal and write down all of the ingredients needed. Beverages should be included as well. The HHA should check the refrigerator, cabinets, and pantry for ingredients. Many needed ingredients may already be in the home. It is a good idea to keep a shopping list available so family members, clients, and caregivers can write down items they run out of during the week.

Nutritious Snacks

The client's dietary needs should be taken into account when planning snacks.

- Low-salt pretzels and low-sodium tomato juice
- Celery with peanut butter and milk
- Graham crackers and milk
- Rice cakes with peanut butter and milk
- Cereal and milk
- Yogurt
- Baked tortilla chips with salsa
- Carrot or celery sticks with hummus
- Crackers and cheese
- Gelatin with fruit
- Bran muffin and milk
- Raisins, dates, figs, prunes, or dried apricots
- Trail mix
- Smoothies made with yogurt, milk, and fruit blended together
- Fresh fruit
- Apple with peanut butter
- Apple with cheese

Meals that Make Good Leftovers

- Beef or vegetable stew
- Chili (meat or vegetable)
- Spaghetti with sauce
- Casseroles
- Red beans and rice
- Split pea soup
- Lentil soup

- Chicken soup
- Macaroni and cheese
- Lasagna (meat or vegetable)
- Meat loaf
- Pot roast

Guidelines: Shopping for Clients

G Use coupons. Check online for coupons or scan a newspaper if your client receives one. Print or clip coupons for items you have already planned to buy.

G Check store circulars for advertised specials. Compare foods by reading the unit price tags that are on the shelves in front of the products (Fig. 28-2). Store brands are usually cheaper than advertised brands.

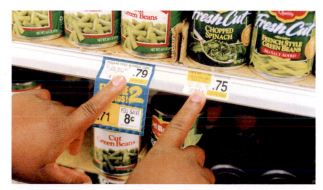

Fig. 28-2. *Compare foods by reading the unit price tags.*

G Buy fresh foods that are in season, when they are at peak flavor and inexpensive. You may also want to buy seasonal foods for canning, freezing, or preserving. Follow your client's preferences when buying in-season foods.

G Buy in quantity. Large amounts or larger sizes are usually more economical, but do not buy more than you can store.

G Shop from your list. Do not be tempted by items that are not on your list.

G Avoid processed, already-mixed, or ready-made foods. They are usually more expensive and less nutritious. When time allows, buy staples, or basic items.

G   Loaves of bread are generally a better buy than rolls or crackers. Day-old bread is usually sold at reduced prices. Buy whole-grain breads if the client agrees. Get different varieties from time to time.

G   Milk can be bought in many forms. Choose the type that the client prefers. Skim or one percent has lower fat content and is usually cheaper than whole milk. Evaporated milk is useful in cooking.

G   Buy a cheaper brand when appearance is not important. For example, store-brand mushroom pieces are fine to use in a casserole and cheaper than name-brand mushroom pieces.

G   Read labels to be sure you are getting the right product in the quantity you want. Read labels for ingredients that may be harmful to your client, such as excessive salt or sodium or sugar.

G   Estimate the cost per serving before buying. Divide the total cost by the number of servings to determine the cost per serving.

G   Consider the amount of waste in bones and fat when buying cheaper cuts of meat. Some cuts of less expensive meats yield only half of what leaner cuts yield per pound. For clients on low-fat/low-cholesterol diets, pick lean meats and take the skin off chicken and turkey parts. The skin holds much of the fat.

Inexpensive Meals

- Pasta dishes
- Baked stuffed potatoes
- Rice and beans
- Tuna casserole
- Chicken thighs or legs
- Hamburger casserole
- Pot roast
- Stews
- Lentil soup
- Split pea soup

When deciding what to buy, an HHA should keep these four factors in mind:

1. **Nutritional value**: Does this food contain essential nutrients, vitamins, and minerals? Is it unprocessed, without added salt or sugar?

2. **Quality**: Is this food fresh and in good condition? Fruits, vegetables, and meats should look fresh. Canned goods should not be dented, rusted, or bulging (bulging may be a sign of bacterial growth). Milk and dairy products should not have passed their expiration dates.

3. **Price**: Is this the most economical choice? If it costs more, is it worth it?

4. **Preference**: Will the client like this food? Can it be made into an appealing meal?

Environmentally-Friendly Care

Organic, Local, and Sustainably-Produced Foods

Planning healthy meals for clients is important. Proper nutrition is essential in improving health. More and more people are trying to include as much organic, local, and sustainably-produced food as possible in their diets, and this may be important to some clients.

Organic food is produced without using most conventional pesticides, synthetic ingredients, bioengineering, or ionizing radiation. Organic meat, poultry, eggs, and dairy products come from animals that are given no antibiotics or growth hormones. For foods to be labeled organic, they must meet certain legal standards.

The word *local* can have different meanings. Simply put, local foods are grown and produced as close to home as possible. Local foods are not necessarily organic, although they may be. One environmental benefit of buying food locally is that it is transported shorter distances, which may reduce the pollution associated with getting food to customers. Local foods may not require as much packaging or processing as foods that are shipped long distances, and that results in environmental benefits as well.

Although *sustainable* can also mean many different things, the main idea is that sustainably-produced foods cause minimal or no harm to the environment or to those involved in the work of producing the food.

The farming community is supported. Its workers are treated well, and the animals are treated humanely.

The HHA should buy and prepare the foods that each client wants. Organic, local, and sustainably-produced foods will almost always be more expensive than other options, and may not always be available. Choices should reflect the client's wishes. If unsure about exactly what the client wants, the HHA should talk to her supervisor.

2. List and define common health claims on food labels

Food packages often make claims about the health benefits of the food they contain. Food labels are a form of advertising designed to convince shoppers to buy a product. Although some regulations exist about what labels can claim, an HHA should read health claims carefully before making a decision to buy. Key claims in food label advertising include the following:

Low-fat, nonfat, fat-free, reduced fat, or light: If a product is labeled *low-fat* or *nonfat*, it usually does not contain much fat. However, it is still important to read the label to determine the fat content of the food.

Products labeled *reduced fat* or *light* contain less fat than other versions of the same product. For example, salad dressing labeled *reduced fat* should contain 25 percent less fat than regular salad dressing, but may still be high in fat. Salad dressing labeled *light* should contain 50 percent less fat than regular. Reading the label is the only way to determine fat content. Some foods that claim to have less fat may contain fat substitutes. In general, the best food and dollar value is found in products that do not contain these substitutes.

Cookies, cakes, and other treats labeled *fat-free* or *reduced fat* usually contain a lot of sugar and calories. All sweets should be used sparingly, as they provide little or no nutritional value. Extra calories, especially sugars, are quickly converted to fat by the body.

Low-sodium, very low-sodium, sodium-free, or no added salt (or no salt added): For clients who must reduce their sodium or salt intake, foods labeled *low-sodium, very low-sodium*, or *sodium-free* are important. *No added salt* or *no salt added* means that no salt was added during processing but these products may not be free of sodium. Most foods naturally contain some sodium. Foods that list salt or sodium as added ingredients should be avoided. In general, canned foods and prepared foods like soups and frozen dinners have a lot of added salt and should not be eaten regularly.

Cholesterol-free: Cholesterol-free foods may be helpful for clients who must restrict their cholesterol intake. However, the best way to limit cholesterol is to avoid foods containing animal fats, such as butter, cheese, whole milk, eggs, red meats, and organ meats.

Sugar-free or no added sugar: Clients who must restrict their weight or who have diabetes must be very careful about consuming sugar in any form. Sugar-free products can be helpful, but they may contain artificial sweeteners, such as saccharin or aspartame. These have no food value and should be used sparingly. Foods sweetened with fruit juice may still contain a lot of calories. People who have diabetes may need to avoid fruit-juice-sweetened products as well as sugar-sweetened ones.

Organic: Organic food differs from conventionally produced food in the way it is grown, handled, and processed (Fig. 28-3). Organic food is produced without using most conventional pesticides, fertilizers made with synthetic ingredients or sewage sludge, bioengineering, or ionizing radiation. Organic meat, poultry, eggs, and dairy products come from animals that are given no antibiotics or growth hormones. Before a product can be labeled organic by the USDA, a government-approved certifier inspects the farm where the food is grown to make sure all rules are being followed to meet USDA organic standards. Companies that handle or process organic food before it gets to the supermarket or restaurant must be certified, too.

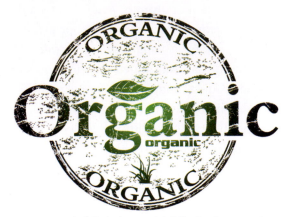

Fig. 28-3. *Foods labeled organic differ in the way they are grown, handled, and processed.*

Free range or free roaming: When poultry is labeled *free range* or *free roaming*, it means the chicken producing the eggs have access to the outside each day. However, the length of time of that access is not specified.

Natural, healthy, or good for you: These claims may have little or no meaning. In fact, due to consumers wanting clarification, in 2016 the U.S. Food & Drug Administration (FDA, fda.gov) asked the public for information and comment on questions related to the term *natural*. Buying whole, unprocessed grains, fresh fruits and vegetables, and lean meats, poultry, and fish is the best way to buy healthy, nutritious food. HHAs should not be swayed by the advertising on labels; they should check the facts.

3. Explain the information on the FDA-required Nutrition Facts label

The U.S. Food and Drug Administration (FDA) requires that all packaged foods contain a standardized nutrition label, called *Nutrition Facts*. This label contains information about the nutritional content of food (Fig. 28-4). Because the label is in the same format on all foods, it is easy to compare different products.

In 2016 major changes to the nutrition label became final. The changes make information easier to understand so that consumers can make informed decisions about what they eat. The Nutrition Facts label gives the following information:

Nutrition Facts	
12 servings per container	
Serving size	**1 cup (28g)**
Amount per serving	
Calories	**103**
	% Daily Value*
Total Fat 2g	3%
Saturated Fat 0g	1%
Trans Fat 0g	
Cholesterol 0g	0%
Sodium 186mg	8%
Total Carbohydrate 21g	7%
Dietary Fiber 3g	11%
Total Sugars 21g	
Includes 11g Added Sugars	25%
Protein 3g	
Vitamin D 2mcg	10%
Calcium 260mg	20%
Iron 8mg	45%
Potassium 235mg	6%

* The % Daily Value (DV) tells you how much a nutrient in a serving of food contributes to a daily diet. 2,000 calories a day is used for general nutrition advice.

Fig. 28-4. *The FDA-required Nutrition Facts label contains standard nutritional information that makes it easier to compare different products.*

Serving size and number of servings per container: In the updated label, serving sizes aim to reflect the amount people are actually eating, not what they should be eating. HHAs should check the size of the serving.

Calories per serving: The number of calories per serving tells how much food energy a serving contains. It does not explain how much nutritional value the food has. A candy bar is high in calories, providing quick energy, but has very few nutrients and lots of fat and sugar.

Total fat, cholesterol, sodium, total carbohydrate, and protein: The label provides information on total fat, including saturated fat and trans fat;

cholesterol; sodium; total carbohydrates, including dietary fiber and total sugars; and protein. In the updated version of the nutrition label, total sugars has a subcategory of added sugars to help consumers understand how much sugar has been added to a product. Studies have shown that excessive sugar may be linked to a variety of serious conditions and diseases.

Vitamins and minerals: The label lists the percentages of the recommended daily total for vitamin D, calcium, iron, and potassium. Manufacturers can voluntarily list amounts of other vitamins and minerals.

Percent daily values: The label tells a person what percent of the recommended daily total a serving contains. These recommended daily totals are based on a 2000-calorie diet, so someone who eats fewer than 2,000 calories per day should have less each day. Someone who eats more than 2,000 calories per day can have more.

4. List guidelines for safe food preparation

Foodborne illnesses affect up to 100 million people each year. Elderly people are at increased risk partly because they may not see, smell, or taste that food is spoiled. They also may not have the energy to prepare and store food safely. For people who have weakened immune systems because of AIDS or cancer, a foodborne illness can be deadly.

Guidelines: Safe Food Preparation

G   Wash hands frequently. Wash your hands thoroughly before beginning any food preparation. Wash your hands after touching non-food items, and after handling raw meat, poultry, or fish.

G   Keep your hair tied back or covered.

G   Wear clean clothes or a clean apron.

G   Wear gloves when you have a cut on your hands.

G   Avoid coughing or sneezing around food. If you cough or sneeze, wash your hands immediately.

G   Keep everything clean. Clean and disinfect countertops and other surfaces before, during (as necessary), and after food preparation.

G   Handle raw meat, poultry, fish, and eggs carefully. Use an antibacterial kitchen cleaner or a diluted bleach solution to clean any countertops on which meat juices or raw eggs were spilled. Wrap paper or packaging containing meat juices in plastic and discard immediately.

G   Once you have used a knife or cutting board to cut fresh meat, do not use it for anything else until it has been washed in hot, soapy water, rinsed in clear water, and allowed to air dry. Cutting boards made of plastic, glass, and nonporous acrylic can also be washed in the dishwasher. Use one cutting board for fresh produce and bread, and a separate cutting board for raw meat, poultry, and seafood (Fig. 28-5). This helps prevent contamination of food.

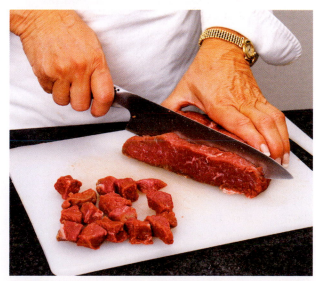

***Fig. 28-5.** Use a separate cutting board for raw meat, poultry, and seafood. After use, wash the cutting board in hot, soapy water, rinse in clear water, and allow it to air dry.*

G   Use hot, soapy water to wash utensils.

G   Use clean dishcloths, sponges, and towels. Change them frequently. Sponges should be washed in the dishwasher to disinfect them.

G   Defrost frozen foods in the refrigerator, not on the countertop. Do not remove meats or dairy products from the refrigerator until just before use.

G   Wash fruits and vegetables thoroughly in running water to remove pesticides and bacteria.

G   Cook meats, poultry, and fish thoroughly to kill any harmful microorganisms they may contain. Heat leftovers thoroughly. Never leave food out for over two hours. Put warm foods in the refrigerator before they are cool, so that bacteria does not have a chance to grow. Keep cold foods cold and hot foods hot. Use cooked meat, poultry, fish, and baked dishes within three to four days.

G   Do not use cracked eggs. Do not consume or serve raw eggs.

G   Never taste and stir with the same utensil.

5. Identify methods of food preparation

The following are basic methods of food preparation for preparing a variety of healthy meals:

Boiling: Food is cooked in boiling water until tender or done. This is the best method for cooking pasta, noodles, rice, and hard- or soft-boiled eggs (Fig. 28-6).

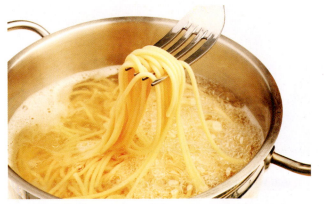

Fig. 28-6. Boiling works well for pasta and other grains.

Steaming: Steaming is a healthy way to prepare vegetables. A small amount of water is boiled in the bottom of a saucepan or pot, and food is set over it in a steamer basket or colander (Fig. 28-7). The pan is tightly covered to keep the steam in.

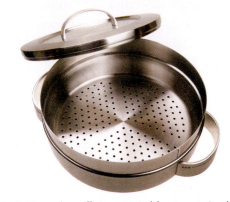

Fig. 28-7. Steaming allows vegetables to retain their vitamins and flavor and may be done in a steamer basket or colander.

Poaching: Fish or eggs may be cooked by poaching in barely boiling water or other liquids. Eggs are cracked and shells discarded before poaching. Fish may be poached in milk or broth, on top of the stove or in the oven in a baking dish (Fig. 28-8).

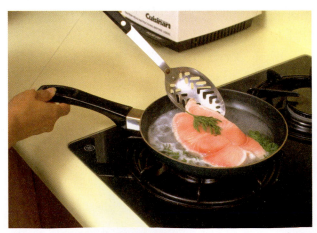

Fig. 28-8. Fish and eggs can both be poached.

Roasting: Used for meats, poultry, and some vegetables, roasting is a simple way to cook. Dry heat roasting means food is roasted in an open pan in the oven. Food may be tossed with oil and spices before roasting. Meats and poultry are **basted**, or coated with juices or other liquid, during roasting (Fig. 28-9).

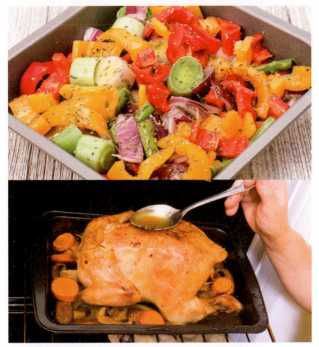

Fig. 28-9. *Vegetables, as well as meats and poultry, can be roasted. Meats roast well at high temperatures (450°F) but may need to be basted.*

Braising: Braising is a slow-cooking method that uses moist heat. Liquid such as broth, wine, or sauce is poured over and around meat or vegetables, and the pot is covered. The meat or vegetables are then slowly cooked at a temperature just below boiling. Braising is a good way to tenderize tough meats and vegetables, since the long cooking breaks down their fibers. Braising may be done in the oven or on the stove top.

Baking: Baking is used for many foods, including breads, poultry, fish, vegetables, and casseroles. Baking is done at moderate heat, 350°F to 400°F. Vegetables such as potatoes and winter squash bake very well (Fig. 28-10).

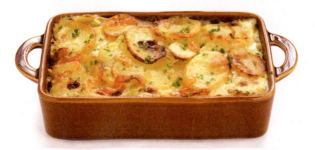

Fig. 28-10. *Potatoes are one type of vegetables that bake very well.*

Broiling: Used primarily for meats, broiling involves cooking food close to the source of heat at a high temperature for a short time (Fig. 28-11). Meat must be tender to be broiled successfully; inexpensive and lean cuts are often better cooked using moist heat. The broil setting on the oven can also be used to melt cheese or brown the top of a casserole. An HHA should leave the oven door ajar when broiling and never leave the kitchen; things can burn very fast.

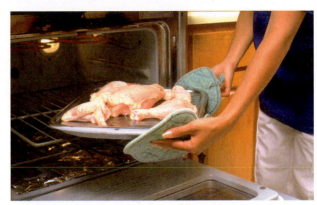

Fig. 28-11. *Broiling involves cooking at a very high temperature.*

Sautéing or stir-frying: These are quick cooking methods for vegetables and meats. A small amount of oil is used in a frying pan or wok over high heat (Fig. 28-12).

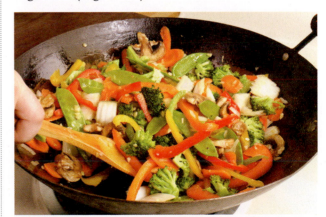

Fig. 28-12. *Stir-frying is quick and uses very little fat. Food must be stirred constantly to prevent it from sticking.*

Microwaving: Microwave ovens are safe to use for defrosting, reheating, and cooking. However, cold spots can occur in microwaved foods because of the irregular way the microwaves enter the oven and are absorbed by the food. If food does not cook evenly, bacteria may survive and cause foodborne illness. To minimize cold spots, food should be stirred and rotated once or twice during cooking. Arranging foods uniformly in a covered dish and turning large foods upside down during cooking can also help.

When defrosting food in the microwave, the store wrap should be removed first. Foam trays and plastic wraps may melt and cause chemicals to migrate into the food. The food should be placed in a microwave-safe bowl instead. Foods being reheated in the microwave should be steaming and hot to the touch. Covering foods and stirring them from the outside in will encourage safe, even heating.

To ensure that meat is properly cooked, an HHA should use a meat thermometer to verify that the food has reached a safe temperature. She should check in several places to be sure ground beef, pork, veal, and lamb is cooked to 160°F. Fresh beef, pork, veal, and lamb should be 145°F with a three-minute rest time. Ground or whole chicken and turkey should be 165°F. Visual signs of doneness include juices that run clear and meat that is no longer pink. Metal thermometers and other metal objects should not be placed in the microwave oven. Some clients cannot be near a microwave when it is in use.

Frying: Frying uses a lot of fat and is the least healthy way to cook. HHAs should avoid frying foods for clients (Fig. 28-13).

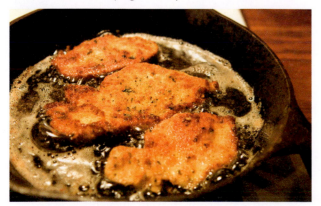

Fig. 28-13. Frying foods is one of the least healthy ways to cook and should be avoided.

Fresh, uncooked foods: Many fruits and vegetables have the most nutrients when eaten fresh, as in salads (Fig. 28-14). However, fresh fruits and vegetables may be difficult for some clients to chew or digest. Fruits and vegetables should be washed well to remove any chemicals or pesticides.

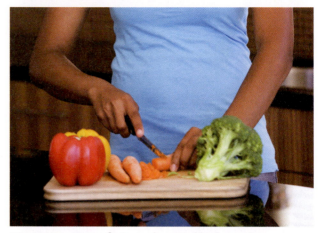

Fig. 28-14. Many fruits and vegetables have the most nutrients when eaten uncooked and fresh.

Preparing Mechanically Altered Diets

Information about special diets was introduced in Chapter 15. If a client has chewing or swallowing difficulties, weakness, paralysis, dental problems, or is recovering from surgery, the doctor may order a liquid, soft or mechanical soft, or pureed diet for a short time.

For soft, mechanical soft, or pureed diets, foods are prepared with blenders, food processors, meat grinders, or cutting utensils. Chopped foods are foods that have been cut up into very small pieces. When chopping food, use a sharp knife and a clean cutting board (separate boards for raw meat and for vegetables and other foods). Grinding breaks the foods up into even smaller pieces. Pureed foods are cooked and then ground very fine or strained. A little liquid is added to give them the consistency of baby food. Grinding and pureeing can be done in a blender, food processor, or meat grinder. However, fruits and vegetables can also be pureed by pushing them through a colander with the back of a spoon.

All equipment used must be kept very clean to help prevent infection and illness. The blender or food processor should be taken apart after every use. The pieces should be washed in hot, soapy water and rinsed thoroughly. The cutting board should be washed after each use. This is especially important after chopping raw meat, poultry, and fish. It can be washed with soap or in the dishwasher before using it again. Then the board can be air dried.

Changing the texture of food may make it lose its appeal. The HHA should season it according to the client's preferences to make it more appealing. He should talk about the food being served using positive words. Pureeing also causes nutrients to be lost, so vitamin supplements may be ordered. Constipation and dehydration are complications of a pureed diet. It is very important to follow directions exactly.

Preparing Nutritional Supplements

Illness and injury may call for nutritional supplements to be added into the client's diet. Certain medications also change the need for nutrients. For example, some medication prescribed for high blood pressure increases the need for potassium.

Nutritional supplements may come in a powdered form or liquid form. Powdered supplements need to be mixed with a liquid before being taken; the care plan will include instructions for how much liquid to add.

When preparing supplements, the supplement must be mixed thoroughly. The client should take it at the ordered time. Clients who are ill, tired, or in pain may not have much of an appetite. It may take a long time for him to drink a large glass of a thick liquid. The HHA should be patient and encouraging. If a client does not want to drink the supplement, the HHA should not insist that he do so. However, it should be reported to the supervisor.

6. Identify four methods of low-fat food preparation

1. **Cook lean**. Boiling, steaming, broiling, roasting, and braising are all methods of cooking that require little or no added fat. Broiling also allows fats in meat to drip out before food is consumed. This lowers the fat content even more.

2. **Drain fat**. When using ground meat, an HHA should brown it first. It should then be removed with a slotted spoon and drained on paper towels or put in a colander to remove excess fat.

3. **Plan lean**. Choosing foods with lower fat content to begin with will make low-fat cooking easier. Planning meals around grains will help cut the fat content. Low-fat meals based on grains include pasta dishes, rice and beans, baked or stuffed potatoes, and soups.

4. **Substitute or cut down**. Sometimes high-fat ingredients can be left out or replaced to lower the fat content of a recipe. An HHA can leave out cheese or reduce the amount of cheese used on sandwiches or to top casseroles. Plain nonfat regular or Greek yogurt can be substituted for mayonnaise or sour cream. Nonfat cottage cheese can also be used on a baked potato instead of sour cream.

Food Appearance, Texture, and Portion Size

The HHA should keep the color and texture of foods in mind when planning meals. For example, two types of green vegetables should not be served at the same meal. Rather than green beans and spinach, green beans and carrots may be a better option. Serving food that is similar in texture may make the meal less interesting. For example, mashed potatoes and mashed rutabagas are similar. A boiled or baked potato can be offered instead. To promote appetite, food should be arranged attractively on the plate and it should look appealing. Large portions should be avoided, unless the client normally eats larger amounts of food. Smaller portions should be given, but it is a good idea to have food available in case the client requests seconds. Small, frequent meals may be ordered for some clients. Chapter 15 contains more information about how to make mealtime appealing.

7. List four guidelines for safe food storage

1. **Buy cold food last; get it home fast**. After shopping, refrigerated foods should be put away first.

2. **Keep it safe; refrigerate**. The proper refrigerator temperature is between 36°F and 40°F. Freezer temperature should be 0°F. Refrigerated items that spoil easily should be kept in

the rear of the refrigerator, not the door. Jars and packages will state if food requires refrigeration (Fig. 28-15). Items should not be frozen again after they have been thawed.

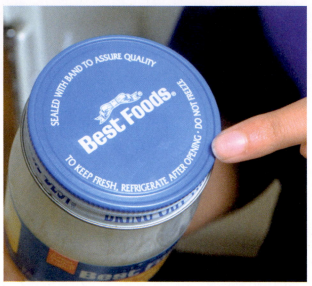

Fig. 28-15. *Refrigeration guidelines can be found on food labels.*

3. **Use small containers that seal tightly**. Foods cool more quickly when stored in smaller containers. They should be stored with enough room around them for air circulation. Foods should not be left out for more than two hours. They should be tightly covered. To prevent dry foods, such as cornmeal and flour, from becoming infested with insects, they should be stored in tightly-sealed or airtight containers. If an HHA finds items that are already infested, she should discard them and use a clean container to store a fresh supply. HHAs should check dry storage areas periodically for signs of insects and rodents.

4. **When in doubt, throw it out!** If an HHA is not sure whether food is spoiled, she must not take any chances. She should discard it. An HHA should check the expiration dates on foods, especially perishables, and check the refrigerator often for spoiled foods. Any expired foods should be discarded. Foods that have become moldy should be thrown away. Mold cannot just be scraped off.

Environmentally-Friendly Care

Composting

Clients may use scraps left over from food preparation, food that was not eaten, or expired food to make compost. **Compost** is a mixture of decaying food and garden waste that is used to improve and fertilize soil. Another benefit of composting is that it reduces the amount of waste sent to landfills. Only certain items can be composted. Fruits and vegetables (including rinds and cores), egg shells, coffee grounds and filters, tea bags, old bread and crackers (and other items made from flour), grains, many types of expired boxed foods, and spices can be composted. Meats, fish, dairy products, grease, and oils cannot be composted. If your client has a compost bin, the HHA should follow instructions about what to compost.

Chapter Review

1. When planning a meal for a client, what factors should the HHA take into account?

2. List ten examples of nutritious snacks.

3. What are two reasons that an HHA should buy fresh foods that are in season?

4. Why is more expensive meat sometimes a better deal?

5. Why are processed or ready-made foods not as desirable as food made from scratch?

6. What does it mean if a food is labeled organic?

7. On how many calories per day are the recommended daily totals based (as part of the Nutrition Facts label)?

8. What is the longest period of time that cooked food can safely be left unrefrigerated?

9. What needs to happen after an HHA has used a cutting board to cut fresh meat?

10. How can pesticides be removed from fresh fruits and vegetables?

11. How can a sponge be disinfected?

12. Briefly describe each of the following food preparation methods: boiling; steaming; poaching; roasting; braising; baking; broiling; sautéing; microwaving; and frying.

13. What equipment is used to prepare soft, mechanical soft, or pureed diets?

14. An HHA has browned ground beef to make soft tacos for her client. What should be done before adding the seasoning to make it lower in fat?

15. Give one example of a low-fat substitution in addition to those listed in the text.

16. When is it acceptable to refreeze an item?

17. What does the phrase "When in doubt, throw it out" mean?

18. If an HHA finds insects in the flour, what should he do?

Conversion Tables

Liquid Measures

1 gal=	4 qt=	8 pt=	16 cups=	128 fl oz
1/2 gal=	2 qt=	4 pt=	8 cups=	64 fl oz
1/4 gal=	1 qt=	2 pt=	4 cups=	32 fl oz
	1/2 qt=	1 pt=	2 cups=	16 fl oz
	1/4 qt=	1/2 pt=	1 cup=	8 fl oz

Dry Measures

1 cup=	8 fl oz=	16 tbsp=	48 tsp
3/4 cup=	6 fl oz=	12 tbsp=	36 tsp
2/3 cup=	5 1/3 fl oz=	10 2/3 tbsp=	32 tsp
1/2 cup=	4 fl oz=	8 tbsp=	24 tsp
1/3 cup=	2 2/3 fl oz=	5 1/3 tbsp=	16 tsp
1/4 cup=	2 fl oz=	4 tbsp=	12 tsp
1/8 cup=	1 fl oz=	2 tbsp=	6 tsp
		1 tbsp=	3 tsp

Emergency Substitutions

Emergency substitutions can sometimes be made, although it is best to use the ingredients called for in recipes.

Vegetables

Ingredient	Substitute
1 1/3 cups cut-up fresh tomatoes, simmered 10 minutes	1 cup canned tomatoes
1/2 lb fresh mushrooms	4-oz can mushrooms
Legumes	With the exception of lentils, dry beans can be used interchangeably to suit personal preference.

Herbs, Spices, Seasonings

Ingredient	Substitute
1 tbsp snipped fresh herbs	1 tsp same herb, dried, or 1/4 tsp powdered or ground
1 tsp dry mustard	2 tsp prepared mustard
1 tsp pumpkin pie spice	1/2 tsp cinnamon, 1/2 tsp ginger, 1/8 tsp ground allspice, 1/8 tsp nutmeg

Baking

Ingredient	Substitute
1 tsp baking powder	1/4 tsp baking soda plus 1/2 tsp cream of tartar
1 pkg active dry yeast	2 1/4 tsp dry yeast
1 cup oil	1/2 lb butter or margarine
1 cup brown sugar	1 cup granulated sugar

Thickeners

Ingredient	Substitute
1 tbsp cornstarch	2 tbsp flour, or 1 1/3 tbsp quick-cooking tapioca
1 tbsp flour	1/2 tbsp cornstarch, 2 tsp quick-cooking tapioca, or two egg yolks
1 tbsp tapioca	1 1/2 tbsp flour

29

The Clean, Safe, and Healthy Home Environment

1. Describe how housekeeping affects physical and psychological well-being

Providing a safe, clean, and orderly environment has always been an essential part of home health care. Illness and disability cause great stress. Clients feel better physically and psychologically and recover more quickly when their homes and families receive care and support. Infection and accidents are prevented. In addition, families who lack some knowledge about how to manage their homes can be taught valuable household management skills. These skills include sanitation, safety, personal hygiene, nutrition, meal planning, shopping, child care, food preparation, communication skills, and specific healthcare techniques. Home health aides can be role models for clients and their families by performing tasks efficiently and cheerfully.

2. List qualities needed to manage a home and describe general housekeeping guidelines

It takes efficiency, planning, knowledge, and skills to manage a household. An HHA needs to know how to use his time and energy well. Doing so allows him to focus on his primary responsibility—the personal care of the client.

The concept of person-centered care is important when caring for clients' homes, so sensitivity and respect are vital qualities as well. It is important that HHAs respect clients' customs, beliefs, and feelings. It may be helpful for a home health aide

to imagine how he would feel if a stranger were handling his personal items and possessions. It is not easy for a person to find himself unable to care for his own home, and it is important for home health workers to remember this and treat their clients with sensitivity and respect.

Sensitivity is also necessary when asking members of the household for help with housekeeping. Knowing when and how to appropriately ask for assistance is key. Some family members may be experiencing so much stress that they are unable to help at all.

An HHA's housekeeping assignments will vary. They may include simple cleaning and organizing of the client's room or general cleaning throughout the house. Some clients require management of all household functions, including finances. An HHA may be required to dust, straighten, vacuum, sweep, wash dishes, clean the bathroom and kitchen, and do laundry. The assignments will outline the specific duties to be performed (Fig. 29-1).

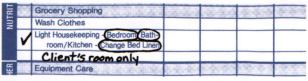

Fig. 29-1. An HHA's assignments will outline home maintenance tasks that he needs to perform.

Assignments may list specific days on which tasks should be performed, or the HHA may be allowed to make his own schedule. Flexibility is important and makes it easier to meet the client's and family's needs. If an HHA receives requests for services not listed in his assignments or if there are complaints about how tasks are done, he should contact his supervisor.

Most agencies require that aides perform light housekeeping. This usually involves dusting, straightening, vacuuming or sweeping floors and floor coverings, cleaning bathrooms and the kitchen, and disposing of trash. Light housekeeping does not involve moving heavy furniture, washing windows, taking down drapes, cleaning the attic or basement, or mowing the lawn.

Guidelines: Housekeeping

G Invite family participation. Depending on their abilities and availability, clients and family members may be asked to participate in housekeeping tasks.

G Invite family and client input when you determine the tasks that need to be done and the methods used.

G Use cleaning materials and methods that are acceptable to and approved by clients and their families. Any efforts you make toward improving the home environment should coincide with the client's choices, lifestyle, and values.

G Be organized when performing tasks. Write out detailed daily and weekly schedules. Seek feedback from your supervisor and the client and family.

G Build some flexibility into the schedule to allow for changes in the client's condition, needs, appointments, or social activities.

G Organize cleaning materials and equipment by placing them in one closet. Place cleaning materials in a pail, a carrying bin with a handle, a laundry basket, or a shopping bag (Fig. 29-2). Do not leave cleaning equipment around the home.

G Familiarize yourself with the cleaning materials and equipment. Read the labels and

instruction booklets. Ask the client, family members, or your supervisor how the equipment works if you are unfamiliar with it.

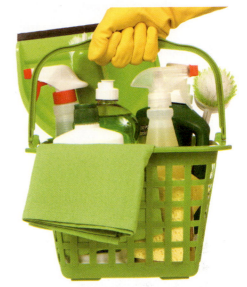

Fig. 29-2. *Keep cleaning materials and equipment organized.*

G Maintain a safe environment as well as a clean one. Do not wax floors if your client is unsteady. Mop up spills immediately.

G Use housekeeping procedures and methods that promote health. Many diseases may be transmitted through improper food handling, dishwashing, and handwashing, and unclean bathrooms and kitchens. Always wash from clean areas to dirty areas, so that you do not spread dirt into areas that have already been washed.

G Observe the home environment for signs of infestation by roaches, rats, mice, lice, and fleas. These insects and animals are common carriers of disease. Controlling them is vital to family health and cleanliness.

G Use proper body mechanics when performing activities to prevent injury. Housecleaning can require a great deal of bending, standing, stooping, and lifting. Watch your posture. Kneel instead of stooping for long periods.

G Clean up and straighten up after every activity. Clean spills as soon as they occur. Spills that have dried are difficult to remove later.

G   Carry paper and a small pencil to make note of items that must be purchased or replaced. Maintain a shopping list on a refrigerator door or other convenient location, and encourage family members to use the list.

G   Use your time wisely and efficiently. For example, prepare food while a load of wash is being done.

3. Describe cleaning products and equipment

Five basic types of home cleaning products are available:

1. All-purpose cleaning agents can be used for many purposes and on several types of surfaces. Surfaces include countertops, walls, floors, and baseboards.

2. Soaps and detergents are used for bathing, laundering, and dishwashing.

3. Abrasive cleansers are used mostly to scour hard-to-clean surfaces.

4. Specialty cleaners are used to clean special surfaces, such as glass, metal, or ovens.

5. Non-toxic, environmentally-safe cleaning products are made without toxic chemicals. They may be vegetable-based. Some of these products are even made at home with basic ingredients such as baking soda, vinegar, castile soap, and water (Fig. 29-3).

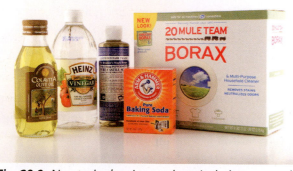

Fig. 29-3. *Non-toxic cleaning products include ones made with baking soda, vinegar, and castile soap, among other items.*

All cleaning products must be used properly. Many cleaning products are chemicals which can be irritating and can even cause burns. Some chemicals are poisonous when swallowed.

Guidelines: Using Household Cleaning Products

G   Read and follow the directions on the label of every product you use. Cleaning products can harm the materials you are trying to clean.

G   Wash your hands and don gloves before using cleaning products.

G   Do not mix cleaning products. This can cause a dangerous chemical reaction that may harm you or others. In particular, **never mix bleach or products containing bleach with ammonia. The fumes are toxic and can be fatal**.

G   Open windows when cleaning to provide fresh air. Some cleaning products have fumes that are unpleasant or even harmful if you are exposed to them for a long time.

G   Do not leave cleaning products on surfaces longer than the recommended time. Do not scrub too hard on soft surfaces.

G   Household bleach, diluted with four parts water, makes a strong disinfectant solution to clean bathroom surfaces. Diluted with nine parts water and stored in a labeled spray bottle, bleach makes a milder disinfectant to use on kitchen counters. Do not spill bleach or bleach solutions on carpets, clothing, or other surfaces that might be discolored.

Cleaning supplies generally include two types of tools:

1. Wet mops, pails, toilet brushes, and sponges are tools for softening and removing soil that has dried and hardened on washable surfaces.

2. A vacuum cleaner and attachments, carpet sweeper, dust mop, dust cloths, broom, and brush and dustpan are tools for removing dry dirt and dust.

Cleaning Solution Ideas

Several types of environmentally-safe, non-toxic cleaning solutions can be prepared from common household items.

- Baking soda can be used instead of scouring powder. Baking soda can also be diluted with warm water to make a solution that will eliminate odors when used to clean surfaces.

- White vinegar can be used to remove lime or other mineral deposits on sinks, toilets, or chrome fixtures. It cuts grease and removes mildew and odors. White vinegar diluted with water can be used instead of glass cleaner. Mix solution using one part white vinegar to three parts water (1:3). This solution can also be used to clean sealed wood and tile floors.

- Lemon juice, by itself or mixed with water or other ingredients, can be used to eliminate odors, clean and disinfect surfaces, and cut grease.

- Borax, or sodium borate, is a white powder that dissolves in water. Borax can be used to clean, eliminate odors, and disinfect. It is also used as an alternative insecticide. While borax is natural and is not an environmental toxin, it should not be swallowed, and it can cause skin irritation. Use care in handling borax; do not use it around food, and keep it out of reach of children and confused clients.

HHAs must be careful with equipment. Replacements can be expensive. HHAs should be familiar with how to use each piece of equipment and keep it clean and in its proper place. Brushes and bags of vacuum cleaners should be checked often.

4. Describe proper cleaning methods for living areas, kitchens, bathrooms, and storage areas

Not all housekeeping tasks must be performed daily. Some tasks may be done weekly. Others only need to be done once a month or seasonally. The special tasks can be spaced out. Each cleaning job should be done properly and as efficiently as possible. Housework can be made safer by eliminating unnecessary reaching, bending, and stooping. With a little experimentation, an HHA can find the most efficient way to do each job.

Cleaning can be done when a client is resting, sleeping, or doing another activity. Care of the client is the HHA's primary responsibility. However, he must not neglect housekeeping.

Guidelines: Straightening and Cleaning Living Areas

G Clear up clutter and put objects in their correct places.

G Pick up newspapers, magazines, and toys as needed.

G Empty wastebaskets and ashtrays daily.

G Make the beds each day.

G Keep essential and frequently-used items, such as eyeglasses, tissues, a wastebasket, phone, newspaper, magazines, laptop, tablet, and books, within reach. Organize them on an accessible table, magazine rack, or hanging organizer (Fig. 29-4).

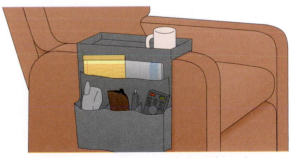

Fig. 29-4. A hanging organizer can help reduce clutter while keeping important items handy.

G Dust once a week or when necessary. If your client has allergies, you may need to dust daily.

G Vacuum floors and rugs once a week or more often if indicated. When vacuuming rugs, use long strokes and go over each area repeatedly. If the home does not have a vacuum, use a broom to sweep the floors and rugs. Take care not to raise too much dust.

G Floors covered with vinyl, ceramic tile, and linoleum may be washed. Some wood floors may not. Some floor coverings should be cleaned with water only. Check with the client or family before you begin. After removing loose dirt or crumbs with a vacuum or broom, wash floors with a cloth or mop dipped in warm, sudsy water. Dry the floor after you have washed it, or close off the area for the time it takes for the floor to dry (Fig. 29-5). Wet or waxed floors are slippery and are frequent causes of falls in the home.

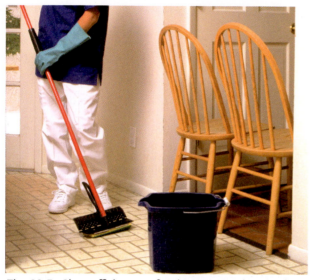

Fig. 29-5. Close off the area for the time it takes the floor to dry.

Handling food on contaminated surfaces, improper dishwashing, and contaminated food storage areas may transmit many diseases. Roaches, rats, and mice may cause disease and allergy by contaminating food with their saliva or through their droppings. Pest control is vital to health and cleanliness. An HHA should always report pest control problems to his supervisor.

Guidelines: Cleaning the Kitchen

G   Clean the kitchen after every use. Ask family members to do the same. Do not wait until the end of the day to clean up. Daily kitchen cleaning tasks include washing dishes, wiping surfaces, taking out garbage, and storing leftover food. Weekly tasks include cleaning the refrigerator and washing the floor. Cleaning cabinets, drawers, and other storage areas is usually done a few times a year.

G   Wash dishes in hot, soapy water using liquid dish detergent. Rinse them in hot water. When working with clients who have an infectious disease, use boiling water for rinsing and add a tablespoon of chlorine bleach to the soapy water. The combination of heat and chlorine will kill pathogens, or harmful microorganisms.

G   Wash glasses and cups first, then silverware, plates, and bowls. Pots and pans are washed last. Rinse with hot water and dry on a rack. Air drying dishes is more sanitary than drying with a dish towel.

G   If the house has a dishwasher, learn how to correctly load and start it. Dishwashers save time. They may also sterilize dishes because of the high temperature used in washing and drying. Scrape food from plates before placing them in the dishwasher. Empty cups and glasses. Do not place dishes, cups, and flatware too close together. This keeps them from being washed thoroughly. Place dishes and cups so that their eating or drinking surfaces are facing the water source. Use only a dishwasher detergent. Fill the well with the amount recommended on the label.

G   Do not wash the following items in the dishwasher: electrical appliances, certain plastic materials, wooden pieces or utensils, hand-painted or antique dishes, delicate china, crystal, cast iron, many pots and pans, and sharp or carbon steel knives.

G   Clean the outside of the stove, the trays, and burners with hot, sudsy water or an all-purpose cleaner, and rinse. Ovens should be cleaned according to manufacturer's recommendations. Be sure to follow the directions. Do not spray the light bulb inside the oven with cleanser, or it may break. Soak the broiler pan immediately after use.

G   The refrigerator should be completely cleaned once a week. However, you should wipe it out more frequently (Fig. 29-6). If the freezer is not a self-defrosting one, defrost it whenever necessary. One-half inch of frost usually means it should be defrosted. To defrost a freezer, turn the dial to the off position. Remove all food. Place foods in a cooler to keep them from thawing. Defrosting the freezer may take less time if you place pans of hot water in it. Do not use a knife to chip off the frost. This could damage the cooling unit.

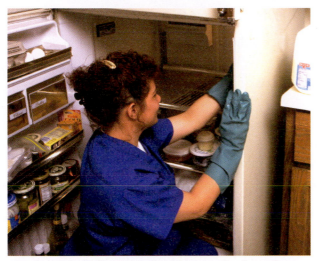

Fig. 29-6. The refrigerator should be totally cleaned once a week, but you should wipe it out more frequently.

G Mix two tablespoons of baking soda in one quart of warm water. Wipe the inside walls of the refrigerator and freezer. Baking soda will remove odors. Wash the shelves and trays with warm, soapy water.

G Clean countertops, tables, and the stove each time they are used. Clean cabinet and drawer fronts and the refrigerator once a week. If a cutting board or other surface has been used to cut fresh meat, scrub the surface thoroughly with hot, soapy water. Rinse well.

G An all-purpose cleaner or a vinegar or lemon juice solution may be needed to remove grease and cooked foods that have spilled or splashed on surfaces. Clean the sink with baking soda or a scouring powder or cream.

G Never place food on soiled work or storage areas or in unclean containers. Keep food covered. Close lids of cartons and cover food

storage containers to prevent contamination or infestation by insects and rodents. Place leftovers in covered containers and store them in the refrigerator immediately. Use them within two to three days.

G Vacuum, sweep, or dry mop the floor daily. Damp mop uncarpeted floors at least once a week, using hot water and a floor cleaner or vinegar solution. Rinse the floor if the label recommends it. Dry the floor or close off the area until the floor dries to prevent accidents.

G Dispose of garbage daily. To prevent odor and discourage insects and rodents, rinse out tin cans and bottles before placing them in the recycling bin or trash container. Follow the recycling procedures for your client's community. Periodically wash wastebaskets and trash cans with hot, soapy water.

G Store all cleaning materials away from food, food preparation utensils, and food preparation areas. Keep them out of reach of children and confused clients.

Environmentally-Friendly Care
Recycling

Recycling is the process of taking materials that would have been considered waste and turning them into new products. Recycling programs help reduce waste and the need for landfills. Recycling helps prevent pollution and saves energy, among many other benefits. Some clients will have recycling bins in their homes. Certain plastics, glass, steel, aluminum, and paper products are commonly placed in recycling bins. Other items, such as electronics and batteries, usually need to be recycled separately. The HHA should know which materials can be recycled and how to recycle in the client's community. Recyclable items may need to be rinsed and sorted into separate bins. If in doubt, the HHA should ask the client or the supervisor.

A clean, organized, and odor-free bathroom is an important part of improving a family's hygiene and safety. Because it is moist and warm, the bathroom is a reservoir for the growth of microorganisms, mold, and mildew.

Guidelines: Cleaning the Bathroom

G Involve the entire family in keeping the bathroom clean (Fig. 29-7). Remember to wash from clean areas to dirty areas.

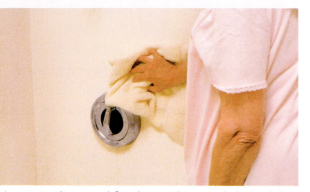

Fig. 29-7. Clients and family members can help by doing things like wiping out the shower after each use.

G Flush the toilet each time it is used.

G Clean toothbrushes and toothbrush holders.

G Scrub the tub and shower after use.

G Remove hair from drain strainers.

G Hang up all used towels to dry.

G Put away toiletries.

G Rinse the sink after brushing teeth, shaving, and washing.

G Place soiled towels in the laundry hamper after they are dry.

The bathroom is the location of many home accidents. All bathroom rugs should be nonskid, and puddles of water should be wiped up immediately. If a client has difficulty moving about in the bathroom safely and grab bars are not present, the HHA should report this to his supervisor.

Cleaning a bathroom

Equipment: approved disinfectant (a cleaning product that kills germs), scouring powder or baking soda, rags or disposable wipes, toilet brush, glass cleaner or white vinegar solution, paper towels, disposable or rubber gloves

1. Put on gloves.

2. Using the disinfectant and rag/wipe, wipe all surfaces and rinse as needed. Be sure to clean the sides, walls, and curtain or door of the shower or tub; the towel racks; holders for toilet paper, toothbrushes, and soap; and window sills.

3. Use a different rag/wipe to wipe the outside of the toilet bowl, seat, and lid. As a general cleaning rule, start with the cleanest surface first, then move to dirtier areas.

4. Use a different rag/wipe to clean the bathtub, shower stall, and sink. Use scouring powder or baking soda for tile and porcelain, and disinfectant or vinegar solution on other surfaces. Remember that scouring powder can scratch. Check with the client or a family member before using it. Be sure to scrub the sides, edges, and bottoms of all these areas. Clean faucets and scrub around their bases.

5. Scrub the inside of the toilet bowl with a toilet brush and scouring powder. Be sure to scrub under the rim. If you use a second, stronger toilet cleaner, flush the first cleaning product down the drain first to avoid possible chemical reactions. Wash the toilet brush with a disinfectant solution. Store it in a holder after letting it air dry.

6. Vacuum or dry mop the floor first, then wash if the floor is tile or linoleum. Use an all-purpose floor cleaner or vinegar solution in hot water. Wash the floor with a cloth or mop, taking special care to clean the areas at the base of the toilet and sink. Do not leave the floor wet. Dry it carefully to avoid accidents.

7. Clean the mirror and any glass or chrome surfaces using glass cleaner or vinegar solution and paper towels or clean rags.

8. Place dry, soiled rags in the laundry hamper or discard wipes. Empty the waste can into a garbage bag and dispose of the waste. Replace toilet paper and facial tissue when needed. Open the bathroom window for a short time, if possible, to air the room out.

Once a week, wash out waste can and laundry hamper. Launder the bath mats and rugs.

9. Store supplies.

10. Remove and discard gloves.

11. Wash your hands.

12. Document the cleaning.

Cleaning and organizing storage areas will contribute to the order and organization of the home.

Guidelines: Cleaning and Organizing Storage Areas

G Every item in the home should have a storage place that is convenient for use. That means storage places should be as close as possible to where they are used (Fig. 29-8). For example, bath towels should be stored in or near the bathroom. Frequently used pots and pans and cooking utensils should be near the stove. Less frequently used items, such as popcorn poppers, should be stored in the less accessible storage places.

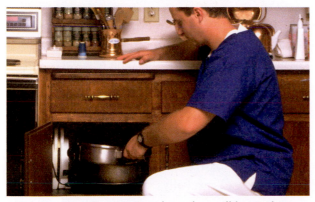

Fig. 29-8. *Store items near where they will be used.*

G Items that are frequently used should be easily seen and reached. Items that are used together should be stored near each other. Arrange food on shelves according to category to save time in searching for items. Dangerous materials such as cleaning products should be stored out of reach of children and confused adults.

G Some storage areas only need to be cleaned occasionally. Remove the stored items and any shelf or drawer liners. Wipe the shelves and drawers with a damp cloth and all-purpose cleaner. Replace the liners, or wipe them if they can be cleaned. Food storage areas and other storage areas that are used frequently should be cleaned more often.

G Do not change the client's or the family's storage arrangements without talking to them. If you think changes are needed, discuss your ideas with the family.

5. Describe how to prepare a cleaning schedule

Most housecleaning tasks should be done immediately, daily, weekly, monthly, or less often. The HHA will need to take into account the care plan, his assignments, how much help is needed, and how much time he has in a particular home to prepare a cleaning schedule. The HHA may not always follow the schedule exactly, but it will guide his work and help him get essential cleaning done. Establishing a schedule for cleaning can also help the family keep a housekeeping routine after home care has ended. A sample cleaning schedule follows. In this scenario, the client is unable to assist with household tasks. Her daughter comes in several times a week, but no family members live with the client.

Cleaning Schedule for Mrs. Hartman

Immediately: Wipe counters, wash dishes, store food, clean spills, put away supplies.

Daily: Straighten up: make bed, sort mail, remove clutter, empty trash, etc. Clean bathroom. (One hour)

Weekly: Wash kitchen floors, wipe refrigerator, scrub sink, vacuum other floors, dust all surfaces, scrub bathtub. (Two to three hours)

Monthly: Clean out refrigerator and freezer (defrost freezer if needed). (One hour)

Less often: Clean oven when needed. (One hour)

Cleaning schedules will be different for each client. The HHA should be flexible. Client care is the first priority, which means the schedule may need to be adapted after it is made.

6. List special housekeeping procedures to use when infection is present

Home health aides must follow Standard Precautions with every client. This is done because it is impossible to always know when infection is present (Chapter 5). However, when a client has a known infectious disease such as influenza, or one that weakens the immune system, such as cancer, the HHA should take these special precautions in housecleaning:

- Use disinfectant when cleaning countertops and surfaces in the kitchen and bathroom.

- Clean the client's bathroom daily. Have other family members use a different bathroom if possible.

- Use separate dishes and utensils for the infected client.

- Wash dishes and utensils in the dishwasher or wash dishes in hot, soapy water with bleach. Rinse in boiling water, and allow to air dry.

- Disinfect any surfaces that come into contact with body fluids, such as bedpans, urinals, and toilets.

- Frequently remove trash containing used tissues.

- Keep any specimens of urine, stool, or sputum in double bags and away from food or food preparation areas.

7. Explain how to do laundry and care for clothes

Hand or machine washing may be part of an HHA's assignments. Clean clothes, bed linens, and towels are important for hygiene and comfort.

Laundry Products and Equipment: Washing laundry requires laundry detergent, a washing machine or a basin for hand washing clothes, and a dryer or a clothesline and pins. The instructions for using washing machines are usually located on the inside of the machine lid.

In general, it is best to use all-purpose detergent. Some delicate fabrics, underwear, or stockings may require a special detergent. Some clients may prefer a non-detergent soap for use on baby clothes and diapers. Bleach, color brighteners, stain removers, and fabric softeners may also be used. An HHA should ask the client and family about their preferences for laundry products.

Pretreating: Pretreating means giving special treatment to items that have heavy soil, spots, and stains before washing them. Spots and stains should be treated immediately. The sooner they are treated, the easier they are to remove. Some oily stains harden with age and cannot be removed. Washing and ironing may set some stains, making them difficult or impossible to remove. It helps to identify the source of the stain and treat it according to a stain guide for the pretreating solution.

Bleach: Bleach is used with detergent. However, bleach cannot be used on all fabrics. The HHA should be familiar with the type of bleach and the fabric that is being washed. Two types of bleach are used in laundry: chlorine bleach and non-chlorine (called *oxygen* or *all-fabric*) bleach. Both types of bleach should be used with caution, and the instructions on the container should be read carefully.

Chlorine bleaches can come in liquid or powdered form. Liquid chlorine bleach is an excellent stain remover. It whitens clothing. However, it can be very damaging to fabric. Bleach should always be diluted in water. Water is added to the washing machine first, then the bleach is stirred in before the clothing is placed in the water. Liquid chlorine bleach must never be used on silk, spandex, wool, or any item that contains these fibers. Spraying or splashing liquid chlorine bleach can remove color or damage fabric, so it should be avoided. Powdered chlorine bleach is more gentle than liquid, but it can also damage clothing. Either type of chlorine bleach is also an excellent disinfectant. Non-chlorine bleach is used on washable fabrics, but it is most effective in hot water.

Water Temperature: The HHA should read the washing instructions for all materials and garments (Fig. 29-9). Warm water is the safest temperature for most garments. However, some must be washed in cold to prevent shrinking or colors from fading. Hot water is generally used for towels, bed linens, and white or colorfast cottons. Warm is usually used for permanent press, knit, synthetic, sheer, lace, acetate, fabric blends, rayons, and plastic. Cold water is used for brightly-colored fabrics or fabrics that are not colorfast.

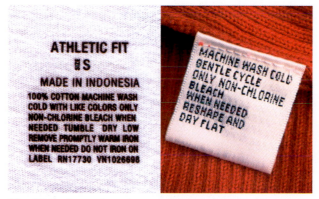

Fig. 29-9. A care tag gives washing and drying instructions. It can be found on most clothing.

Washing Action or Cycle: Cottons, linens, rayons, sturdy permanent press, knits, synthetics, blends, and most other items use the normal washer setting. The slow or gentle setting should be used for washable woolens, old quilts, curtains, and delicate or fragile items.

Drying Clothes: Settings on the dryer vary according to the model. The more delicate a fabric, the lower the drying temperature and the shorter the time in the dryer. Heavy items such as towels need higher temperature settings and a longer time in the dryer. The lint filter should be cleaned each time the dryer is used. If a cli-

ent does not have a clothes dryer, the HHA can hang clothes on a clothesline using clothespins.

Folding: Removing all clothes from the dryer immediately will reduce wrinkling. Clothes can then be folded neatly or placed on hangers. If clothes need to be ironed, they may be set aside; other clothes should be put away in drawers or in a closet.

Ironing: Special care is needed when ironing. Most care labels will indicate the best ironing temperature. If there is no tag, it is best to use the lowest temperature on the iron to avoid damaging the fabric. Pile fabrics like velvet and corduroy will keep their texture better if ironed on the wrong side over a towel. Dark fabrics, silks, acetates, rayons, linens, and some wools must be pressed on the wrong side to prevent them from becoming shiny. A pressing cloth can help protect the fabric.

Ironing fabrics lengthwise will prevent stretching. Collars, cuffs, and garment facings should be ironed first, followed by sleeves, then the front and back. As soon as clothes are ironed, they should be placed on hangers or folded. All hooks and buttons should be fastened and zippers closed. Clothes must be completely dry before they are put away.

Maintaining Clothing: An HHA may need to do basic mending or sewing occasionally. This is especially true if he is taking care of a family, an older person with impaired vision, or people who may not have the time or the ability to keep clothing and linens repaired. Some clients who can do their own mending may just need the HHA to thread the needle.

Doing the laundry

1. Sort clothes carefully. Make separate piles of whites, colors, and bright colors. Check clothing labels for special washing instructions. Do not wash anything labeled Dry Clean Only. If hand washing is recommended, do not wash in the machine.

2. As you sort laundry, check pockets and remove tissues, money, pens, and other items. Remove belts with buckles, trims, and non-washable ornaments. Close zippers, buttons, and other fasteners. Check garments for stains and areas of heavy soil. If appropriate, mend or repair any holes, snags, rips, tears, pulled seams, and weak spots in garments and other items.

3. Pretreat spots and stains before washing. A small amount of liquid detergent or dry detergent dissolved in water can be worked in with an old toothbrush (Fig. 29-10). Pretreat or soak clothing as soon as possible for best results. If you know something is stained, do not let it sit in the laundry hamper all week until you do the laundry.

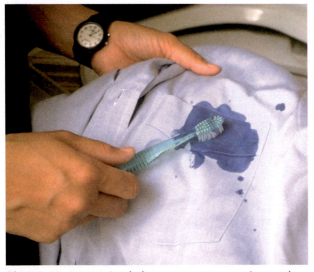

Fig. 29-10. Pretreating helps remove spots, stains, and areas that are heavily soiled.

4. Use the correct water temperature: hot for whites, warm for colors, cold for bright colors and delicate fabrics.

5. Use the appropriate laundry product(s). Follow the washing instructions on the container.

6. Follow written instructions or client or family instructions for using the washer. Use the correct washing cycle for the load you are laundering.

7. Dry clothes completely either in a dryer or on a clothesline. If using a dryer, follow the dry-ing instructions on clothing labels or the client's preferences. Some fabrics require cooler temperatures.

8. Hand wash items when necessary in cool or warm water, depending on the instructions. Use a mild detergent or special hand-washing liquid. Line dry or lay items flat on towels to preserve the shapes of the garments.

9. Fold or hang clean laundry and sort into categories. Store in drawers or closets.

8. List special laundry precautions to take when infection is present

When a client has a known infectious disease, the HHA must take these special precautions when handling laundry:

Guidelines: Handling Laundry for Infectious Clients

G   Keep client's laundry separate from other family members' laundry.

G   Handle dirty laundry as little as possible. Do not shake it. Sort it and put it into plastic bags in the client's room or bathroom. Take it immediately to the laundry area.

G   Wear gloves and hold laundry away from your clothes and body when you are handling it.

G   Use liquid bleach when fabrics allow.

G   Use agency-approved disinfectants in all loads.

G   Use hot water.

9. List guidelines for teaching housekeeping skills to clients' family members

In some assignments, an HHA will be asked to teach housekeeping skills to family members. This prepares them to take over housekeeping and care when home care is discontinued. By teaching household management skills, the HHA helps families meet their daily needs and become more self-reliant.

Guidelines: Teaching Family Members

G   Get to know the family before starting to teach them. Understand their needs or problems before beginning.

G   Be patient. Give people time to learn new skills. Praise their efforts.

G   Keep teaching sessions brief.

G   Break down tasks into simple steps. Explain each step and demonstrate it.

G   Answer all questions.

G   Assist the person as necessary. Do not do the task for him or her.

G   Remember that each person is an individual and will learn in different ways. Customize your teaching to allow for these differences.

Using Proper Body Mechanics in the Home

Body mechanics was discussed in detail in Chapters 6 and 10. The following additional tips should be used when working in a home:

- Bend the knees, not the back, when lifting things from the floor or when kneeling to pick up objects.

- Carry heavy objects close to the body and distribute the weight evenly. For example, when carrying a basket of clothes, the basket should be held directly in front of the body (Fig. 29-11). Do not twist at the waist.

- Stand close to the work area. When possible, the work area should be raised to a comfortable level so the back and neck are not bent. For example, the clothes basket can be placed on a chair before filling it (Fig. 29-12).

- Try not to lift heavy objects. If heavy objects such as furniture must be moved, pushing or rolling, using the entire body, is preferable.

- Avoid lifting heavy objects from the floor.

- Stand erect when doing tasks like washing dishes, with the knees slightly bent.

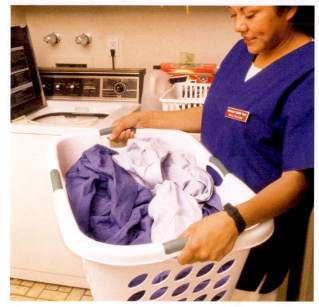

Fig. 29-11. Holding objects close to the body helps prevent back strain and injury.

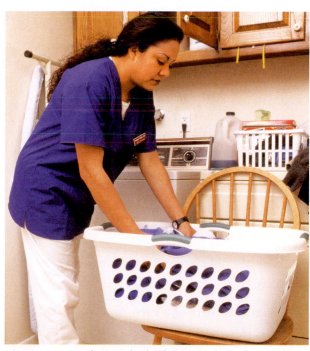

Fig. 29-12. By placing the basket on a chair close to her, this HHA avoids excessive bending and reaching.

10. Identify hazardous household materials

Any of the following household materials can have harmful effects:

- Household bleach

- Cleaning products

- Aerosol or spray cans

- Paint

- Chemicals such as turpentine or paint thinner

- Medicines, both prescription and over-the-counter

- Hair spray

- Nail polish remover

These products should be kept in separate cabinets with childproof latches or locks, or up out of the reach of children. If a client is confused, these cabinets should be marked with signs that indicate danger.

Chapter Review

1. What skills are important in household management?

2. What housekeeping assignments might an HHA be asked to do?

3. What are some housekeeping tasks an HHA should NOT be asked to perform?

4. List ten housekeeping guidelines.

5. Why is it important to read the directions for cleaning products?

6. Why should cleaning products never be mixed?

7. What two parts of a vacuum cleaner should an HHA check often?

8. How often should wastebaskets and ashtrays be emptied?

9. How should an HHA clean the floors if the home does not have a vacuum cleaner?

10. What should an HHA do when washing dishes for clients who have an infectious disease or cold?

11. How frequently should the refrigerator be cleaned?

12. In what time frame should leftover food be eaten?

13. What items should not be washed in the dishwasher?

14. Ideally, where should storage places be located?

15. Describe why it is helpful to make a cleaning schedule.

16. How frequently should an HHA clean the bathroom of a client who has an infectious disease?

17. What is pretreating?

18. What is the safest washing temperature for most garments?

19. How can an HHA reduce the amount of wrinkling after clothes have been dried in the dryer?

20. For a client with an infectious disease, what washing temperature should the HHA use?

21. List five guidelines to follow when teaching family members housekeeping skills.

22. Where should hazardous household materials be kept?

30

Managing Time, Energy, and Money in the Home

1. Explain ways to work more efficiently

Taking care of the client and other family members who need assistance and support is the home health aide's most important responsibility. For this to be accomplished, an orderly and clean environment must be maintained. To balance these responsibilities, HHAs must manage their time and energy efficiently. The following are guidelines to work as efficiently as possible:

Guidelines: Working Efficiently

G **Distribute tasks.** Look at the client care plan and your assignments. Note the assigned housekeeping tasks. Divide the tasks and schedule them for the week and the month. Make sure all your assignments can be completed in the time you have. Some tasks are best accomplished together. For example, it is most efficient to do all the laundry on one day. Then you are able to do larger loads and fold and iron all at once. Plan one morning or afternoon to do the laundry. For more efficiency, plan other tasks to do while loads are in the washer or dryer.

G **Prioritize tasks.** Prioritizing your tasks is an important time and energy management skill. Think about the jobs you want to complete throughout the day. Which ones must be done immediately? Which ones must be done at a certain time? Which activities are not absolutely essential and could be put off? Spend time on activities that are most important first.

G **Simplify tasks.** Take time to think about how you will go about doing a task. Try to eliminate a few steps but still get the same result. For example, when baking a cake, can you mix everything in one bowl? When you clean up, can you stack everything on a tray and take it all to the sink at one time?

G **Be realistic.** You may not be able to get everything done even if you plan carefully. Reassess your schedule during the day. Have you finished what you planned or are you behind? When tasks take longer than you expected, or unexpected tasks need to be done, be realistic about what you can do. Do not be afraid to change your plan. It is better to accomplish the highest-priority tasks and let others go unfinished than to do everything halfway. The key to success is to be flexible.

Here are ways to conserve time and energy:

G **Energize.** Use proper body mechanics. Take occasional breaks to restore your energy. Alternate longer tasks with shorter tasks, and high-energy tasks with low-energy ones. Take care of yourself—eat right, exercise, and get plenty of rest.

G **Organize.** At the beginning of the day, do a mental rundown of the tasks that must be done, and rearrange your schedule if necessary. Plan what must be done and do it. Store frequently used items in convenient places near the work area. Assemble your equipment and materials before you begin a task. Keep clutter under control, and work in good light. Think about how to organize activities and equipment to avoid unnecessary work. Make and use shopping lists.

G **Economize.** Save time and energy by doing a little extra ahead of time. Use trays, baskets, or carts to carry several things at once. Prepare often used food items ahead of time and freeze them. Cook in quantity and freeze meal-size portions. Cook more than one item in the oven at a time.

G **Minimize.** Look for ways to make tasks shorter and easier. Modify your workspace to make your work easier and more comfortable.

G **Specialize.** Use the right tool for each task. For example, a vegetable peeler is more efficient than a knife for peeling carrots. Take pride in what you are doing.

G Finally, be sure to thank family members who have picked up, cleaned up, or participated in household chores.

2. Describe how to follow an established work plan with the client and family

The client care plan and an HHA's assignments will explain the tasks that are required. The HHA can develop her own work plan. This will allow her to finish all of the assigned tasks as quickly and efficiently as possible. For each day or block of time spent in a home, the HHA can list all the tasks that need to be completed and then prioritize them. The most important should be marked *1*, the next most important *2*, and so on. Finally, the HHA can write out a schedule for the day, filling in the highest priority tasks first. If there are tasks that must be done at a certain time, those tasks must be put on the schedule at the appropriate time.

Tasks should be distributed so that the HHA is not trying to do all the house cleaning in one afternoon. She may then end up with no time to bathe or care for a client. Simplifying tasks whenever possible will allow the HHA to accomplish more.

Following an established work plan means more can be done in less time. It will also allow clients and families to know what to expect. The HHA may even want to discuss the plan with a client or family member as she is making it up or when it is finished (Fig. 30-1). Some people appreciate knowing what will be happening in their homes at any given time.

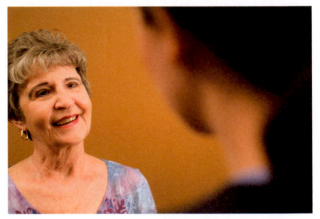

Fig. 30-1. *Prioritizing assignments will help an HHA to work more efficiently. The client should be included in the planning.*

3. Discuss ways to handle inappropriate requests

Occasionally, an HHA may be asked to do something that is not in the care plan or her assignments. Because each client's situation is unique, HHAs are not assigned the same tasks for every client. For example, the care plan may specify grocery shopping for Mrs. Singer, who lives alone and cannot drive. But if another client who lives with family members asks the HHA to run to the store, she has to say no if it is not in the care plan or her assignments.

Several things can help an HHA handle requests that she must refuse. First, she must explain that she is only allowed to do tasks assigned in the care plan. She can explain that nurses familiar with the client's condition give her assignments. It is helpful for the HHA to emphasize that she would like to help, but that she is limited to the tasks outlined in the care plan and her assignments. After explaining this to the client, she should contact her supervisor and discuss the request. The supervisor may add the task requested by the client to the HHA's assignments. It is possible it was left out by mistake. The HHA should document the client's request and the actions she took to address it.

Establishing a work schedule will also help an HHA handle inappropriate requests. If a client and family know what to expect, they may not be tempted to ask the HHA to do other tasks. Sharing a schedule of everything she must accomplish in a visit may help the client understand the HHA's job. If inappropriate requests continue, clients or family members should be referred to the supervisor.

4. List money-saving homemaking tips

The home health aide can use these tips to help save the client money:

Check store circulars for advertised specials. The HHA should plan menus around foods that are a good value; for example, raw foods are less expensive than prepared ones. Chapter 28 discusses more ways to plan economical meals.

Use coupons. The HHA can check online for coupons or scan the newspaper if a client receives one.

Shop from a list. The HHA should not be tempted by items that are not on the list, even if they are on sale.

Avoid convenience stores. Shopping at large supermarkets or discount stores usually guarantees the best prices.

Plan ahead. Restocking needed items before they run out will save money. Planning will also save

time and energy. For example, the HHA will not have to make a special trip when she discovers the client is out of laundry detergent.

5. List guidelines for handling a client's money

Different states and employers have different regulations and policies regarding healthcare employees handling clients' money. An HHA must find out from his employer whether he will be expected to handle clients' money. If he is not allowed to handle money, he should never agree to do so, even occasionally. He could get himself and his employer into serious trouble. If an HHA's state and his employer permit him to handle clients' money, there are several guidelines he must follow:

Guidelines: Handling a Client's Money

G   Never use a client's money for your own needs, even if you plan to pay it back. This is considered stealing. You could lose your job and/or be arrested.

G   Estimate the amount of money you will need before requesting it. If you are going to the grocery store, show the client your list and ask how much he is willing to spend on groceries, or how much is budgeted. You may need to take things off your list or calculate the total bill as you shop to stay within the budget allotted (Fig. 30-2).

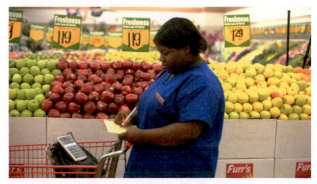

Fig. 30-2. Calculating items as you shop help you to stay within the client's budget.

G   Get a receipt for every purchase. This proves how much you spent and provides a record for the client and you.

G   Return receipts and change to the client or family member immediately. Do not wait until the end of the day or week to settle up. Do it right away while everything is fresh in your mind. Forgetting to return change could be viewed by the client or a family member as stealing.

G   Keep a record of money you have spent. Follow your agency's policies and procedures for documenting money issues. Write down how much you spent and where. Note any change returned to the client. The better record you have, the smaller the chance of any misunderstanding.

G   Keep a client's cash separate from yours. If you must use the client's cash, do not put it in your own wallet. Keep it in a separate, safe place. Do the same with change. This will prevent confusion.

G   Never offer money advice to clients. Do not refer clients to others regarding financial matters.

G   Remember, your clients' financial matters are private. Never discuss your clients' money matters with anyone.

Chapter Review

1. List three ways to work more efficiently.

2. What does it mean to prioritize tasks?

3. How should the HHA handle requests that are not in the care plan?

4. How might an HHA help a client and his family understand the HHA's job? How might this reduce inappropriate requests?

5. List five money-saving homemaking tips.

6. List six guidelines for handling a client's money.

7. Why is it important to get a receipt for anything purchased with a client's money?

8. When shopping for clients, how can using a calculator in the store be helpful?

31

Caring for Your Career and Yourself

The first 30 chapters of this book introduce readers to long-term care and home care settings. They cover the knowledge, skills, and qualities a person needs to work as a nursing assistant or home health aide. This final chapter is more personal. It has to do with finding and keeping a job. This chapter addresses the reader directly. It includes a step-by-step job-hunting guide and useful advice about building positive relationships with employers and coworkers. It also includes helpful tips for managing stress and staying healthy.

1. Discuss different types of careers in the healthcare field

There are many different types of careers in the healthcare field. Some of these are considered direct service. These are the positions that serve the resident, client, or patient directly. Nursing assistants, home health aides, patient care technicians, nurses, physician assistants, and doctors all provide direct service. Professionals in therapeutic services, such as occupational, speech, and physical therapists, also offer direct service.

Some specialized technicians, such as x-ray, lab, and ultrasound technicians, work in diagnostic services (Fig. 31-1), which are performed to determine a condition and/or its cause.

Medical social workers and substance abuse counselors are part of the psychology, counseling, and social work fields. Activities directors and assistants also work in health care. Admin-istrative and support staff, including directors or other executive staff, medical records personnel, receptionists, office managers, and billing staff are also part of the healthcare field.

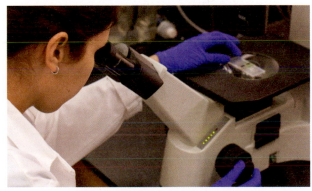

Fig. 31-1. *Lab technicians may conduct tests to help diagnose a condition.*

Career opportunities in health care also include the fields of dentistry, nutrition, and pharmacy. Complementary or alternative healthcare fields include chiropractic medicine and massage therapy (Fig. 31-2).

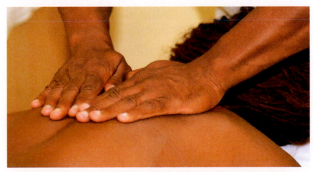

Fig. 31-2. *Massage therapists work on the body using pressure, which can help treat injuries and other problems, as well as promote circulation and relaxation.*

There are many opportunities for teachers within health care. Most of the career paths require classes before working in the field, as well as continuing education. Health educators and prevention professionals teach the general population or specific populations, such as people who have diabetes or pregnant women.

There are many opportunities available in the healthcare field, depending upon a person's interests, education, and abilities. The careers listed above are only a fraction of the jobs offered in health care. You are reading this textbook most likely because you want to become a nursing assistant and/or home health aide. Those positions may be the best fit for you or, at some point, you may want to try something different. Speak with your supervisor, instructor, or a career counselor if you want more information about other careers in the healthcare field. Review Chapters 1 and 2 for information on the different healthcare settings and educational requirements for care team members.

2. Explain how to find a job and how to write a résumé

You may soon be looking for a job. Nursing assistants may be able to work in long-term care facilities, in assisted living facilities, in hospitals, in the home, and in other settings. Home health aides usually look for jobs with home health agencies. To find a job, you must first find potential employers. Then you must contact them to find out about job opportunities. To locate potential employers, use the Internet, newspaper, or personal contacts. Try these resources:

- Check online, trying websites such as monster.com, indeed.com, and jobbankinfo.org (Fig. 31-3). You can also visit a search engine, such as google.com. Type *nursing assistant*, *nurse aide*, or *home health aide* and your city. See what employment opportunities are there. Check your local newspaper's website as well.

- Classified or employment sections of the newspaper list jobs currently available. Circle the positions for which you are qualified. Make a list of names, email addresses, and phone numbers to contact.

- Call the state or local Department of Social Services or Department of Aging. Many states hire or place nursing assistants or home health aides.

- Ask your instructor for potential employers. Some schools maintain a list of employers seeking nursing assistants or home health aides.

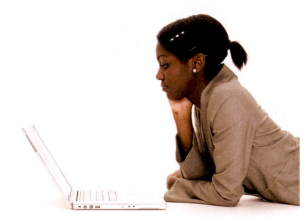

Fig. 31-3. *There are many online resources for finding a job.*

Once you have a list of potential employers, you need to contact them about job opportunities. Phoning or emailing first, unless they mention not to do so, is a good way to find out what opportunities are available. Ask how to apply for a job with each potential employer.

When making an appointment, ask what information to bring with you. Make sure you have this information with you when you go. Some of these documents include the following:

- Identification, including driver's license, social security card, birth certificate, passport, or other official form of identification.

- Proof of your legal status in this country and proof that you are legally able to work, even if you are a U.S. citizen. All employers must have files showing that all employees are le-

Caring for Your Career and Yourself

gally allowed to work in this country. Do not be offended by this request.

- High school diploma or equivalency, school transcripts, and diploma or certificate from your nursing assistant or home health aide training course. Take your instructor's name, phone number, and email address with you as well.

- References are people who can be called to recommend you as an employee. They include former employers and/or former teachers. Do not use relatives or friends as references. You can ask your references beforehand to write general letters for you, addressed "To Whom it May Concern," explaining how they know you and describing your skills, qualities, and habits. Take copies of these with you.

Some potential employers will ask you for a résumé. A **résumé** is a summary or listing of relevant job experience and education. When creating your résumé, include the following information:

- Your contact details: name, address, phone number, and email address

- Your educational experience, starting with the most current first (for example, nursing assistant training course, college degree, high school diploma, or G.E.D. courses)

- Your work experience, starting with the most current first (include name of company or organization, your title, dates worked, and a brief summary of duties)

- Any special skills, such as knowledge of computer software, typing skills, or speaking other languages

- Any memberships in professional organizations

- Volunteer work

State at the end of your résumé that references are available upon request. Try to keep your résumé brief (one page is best) and clear. Use nice white or cream-colored paper for printing your résumé.

The cover letter is a letter included with your résumé. It should be no longer than one page in length. This letter briefly states the position you are seeking and why you would be the best person for the job. Emphasize skills you have that would be a good match. Include the following in a cover letter:

- Date

- Your name, address, phone number, and email address

- Recipient's name, job title, and address

- Salutation (e.g., "Dear Ms. Orozco" or "Dear Human Resources Director")

- Introduction (position you are seeking)

- Body (skills/experience that fit job being offered)

- Closing and signature (e.g., "I look forward to hearing from you. Sincerely, Sarah Harris")

3. Demonstrate completing an effective job application

A job application may need to be completed (Fig. 31-4). Write down the general information you will need to complete the application. Take this information with you, along with your résumé, if you have one. This will save time and avoid mistakes. Include this information:

- Your address, phone number, and email address

- Your birth date

- Your social security number

- Name and address of the school or program where you were trained and the date you completed your training, as well as your certification number if you have one

- Names, titles, addresses, phone numbers, and email addresses of your previous employers, and the dates you worked there

- Salary information from your former jobs
- Reasons why you left each of your former jobs
- Names, addresses, phone numbers, and email addresses of your references

- Days and hours you are available to work
- A brief statement about why you are changing jobs or why you want to work as a nursing assistant or home health aide

Employment Application

Personal Information

Name: Sarah Harris   **Date:** 12 / 15 / 2019

Home Address:
1313 Iron Avenue SW

City, State, Zip:
Albuquerque, NM, 87102

Email Address: sarah@ hartmanonline.com

Home Phone: 505-555-1274   **Business Phone:** n/a

US Citizen? Yes   **If not, give visa number and expiration date:** n/a

Position Applying For

Title: Nursing Assistant   **Salary Desired:** $ 17.00/hr

Referred By: Ms. McClain, Instructor   **Date Available:** 12/15/2019

Education

High School (Name, City, State): Hobbs High School, Hobbs, NM

Graduation Date: May 2017

Technical or Undergraduate School: Hartman Medical Institute, Albuquerque, NM

Dates Attended: June - August 2017   **Degree Major:** Certified Nursing Assistant

References

Mr. Robert Castro, Instructor, Hartman Medical Institute, 505-291-1284

Ms. Scott, Health Occupations, Hobbs HS, 505-555-6255

Kate Crawford, Instructor, Hartman Medical Institute, 505-291-1294

Fig. 31-4. A sample job application.

Fill out the application carefully and neatly. Never lie on a job application. Before you write anything, read it all the way through once. If you are not sure what is being asked, find out before filling in that space. Fill in all of the blanks. You can write *N/A* (not applicable) if the question does not apply to you.

Your employer may require that a criminal background check be performed on new employees. If so, you may be asked to sign a form granting permission to do this. Do not take it personally; it is a law intended to protect patients, clients, and residents.

4. Demonstrate competence in job interview techniques

To make the best impression at a job interview, be professional and do the following:

- Shower or bathe and use deodorant.
- Brush your teeth.
- Wash your hands and clean and file your nails. Nails should be medium length or shorter. Do not wear artificial nails.
- Wear only simple makeup and jewelry or none at all.
- Your hair should be clean and out of your eyes. Wear it in a simple style (Fig. 31-5).

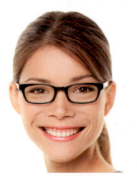

Fig. 31-5. *For job interviews, make sure your hair is clean and simply styled. Wear little or no makeup.*

- Shave or trim facial hair before the interview.
- Dress neatly and appropriately. Make sure clothing is clean, ironed, and has no holes in it. Do not wear jeans, shorts, or dresses or skirts shorter than knee-length. Do not wear

t-shirts or anything with a logo or writing on it. Make sure your shoes are clean and polished. Do not wear sneakers or flip-flops.

- Do not wear perfume or cologne. Many people dislike or are allergic to scents.
- Do not smoke beforehand because you will smell like smoke during the interview.
- Arrive 10 or 15 minutes early.
- Do not bring friends or children to the interview with you.
- Turn off your phone.
- Introduce yourself to the interviewer. Smile and offer to shake hands. Your handshake should be firm and confident (Fig. 31-6).

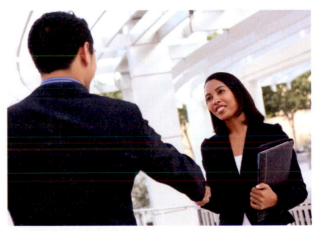

Fig. 31-6. *Smile and shake hands confidently when you arrive at a job interview.*

- Answer questions clearly and completely.
- Make eye contact to show you are sincere.
- Avoid using slang words or expressions.
- Never eat, drink, chew gum, or smoke in an interview.
- Sit up or stand up straight, and look happy to be there.
- Relax and be confident. You have worked hard to get this far. You understand the work and what is expected of you.

Be positive when answering questions. Emphasize what you enjoy or think you will enjoy about the job. Do not complain about any previous jobs you held. Make it clear that you are hard-working and willing to work with all kinds of clients.

The following are some questions you can expect to be asked:

- Why did you become a nursing assistant (or home health aide)?

- What do you like about working as an aide?

- What do you not like? (If this is your first job, you may be asked what you expect to like or dislike.)

- What are your best qualities? What are your weaknesses?

- Why did you leave your last job?

- What would your last supervisor tell me about you?

- Do you prefer to work with certain kinds of residents or clients?

Usually interviewers will ask if you have any questions. Have some prepared and written down so you do not forget things you really want to know. Questions you may want to ask include the following:

- What hours would I work? Is there any mandatory overtime I would need to work?

- What benefits does the job include? Is health insurance available? Would I get paid sick days or holidays?

- What is the average caseload for nursing assistants?

- What orientation or training is provided?

- How will I contact my supervisor when I need to do so?

- Are there any policies regarding ongoing education or advancement?

- How soon will you be making a decision about this position?

Later in the interview, you may want to ask about salary or wages if you have not already been given this information. Listen carefully to the answers to your questions. Take notes if needed. At the end of the interview, you will probably be told when you can expect to hear from the employer. Do not expect to be offered a job at the interview. When the interview is over, stand up and shake hands again. Say something like, "Thank you for taking the time to meet with me today. I look forward to hearing from you."

Send an email or a letter to the employer after the interview to say thank you and to express your continued interest in the job. If you have not heard anything from the employer within the time frame you discussed with your interviewer, call and politely ask whether the job has been filled.

5. Describe a standard job description

A job description is an agreement between the employer and the employee. When you start a new job, you will receive a job description. It states your responsibilities and the tasks you will be expected to perform. It also describes the skills required for the job, to whom you must report, and the salary range.

The job description provides protection for you and your employer. It protects you, the employee, from the facility or agency changing your duties without notifying you. It protects you from being fired based on something not related to your job description. The employer is protected if you were to ever claim you did not know certain duties were part of the job. The job description reduces misunderstandings and can be used to document what was agreed upon if misunderstandings or legal issues arise.

Tuberculosis Test and Hepatitis B Vaccine

Some employers are required to test employees for tuberculosis at least once per year. If so, you will get a notice when it is time to have a TB test. It is your responsibility to get the test.

As you learned in Chapter 5, hepatitis B (HBV) is a bloodborne disease that poses a serious threat to healthcare workers. Employers are required to provide free hepatitis B vaccines to all employees after hire to help protect against the spread of hepatitis B. This vaccine is given as a series of three or four shots.

6. Discuss how to manage and resolve conflict

Everyone experiences conflict at some point in his life. For example, families may argue at home, coworkers may disagree on the job, and so on. If conflict at work is not managed or resolved, it may affect a person's ability to function well. Productivity and the workplace environment may suffer. When conflict occurs, there is a proper time and place to address it. You may need to talk to your supervisor for help. In general, follow these guidelines for managing conflict:

Guidelines: Resolving Conflict

G Plan to discuss the issue at the right time. Do not start a conversation while you are helping residents or clients. Wait until the supervisor has decided on the right time and place. Privacy is important. Shut the door. Limit distractions, such as television and other conversations.

G Agree not to interrupt the person. Do not be rude or sarcastic, or name-call. Use active listening. Take turns speaking.

G Do not get emotional. Some situations may be very upsetting. However, you will be more effective in communicating and problem-solving if you can keep your emotions out of it.

G Check your body language to make sure it is not tense, unwelcoming, or threatening. Maintain eye contact and use a posture that says you are listening and interested. Lean forward slightly and do not slouch.

G Keep the focus on the issue at hand. When discussing conflict, state how you feel when a behavior occurs. Use "I" statements. First describe the actual behavior. Then use "feeling" words to describe how you feel. Let the person know how the problem is affecting you. For example, "When you are late to work, I feel upset because I end up doing your work along with my own."

G People involved in the conflict may need to come up with possible solutions. Think of ways that the conflict can be resolved. A solution may be chosen by a supervisor that does not satisfy everyone. In order to resolve conflict, you may have to compromise. Be prepared to do this.

7. Describe employee evaluations and discuss appropriate responses to feedback

From time to time you will receive evaluations from your employer. These evaluations contain ideas to help you improve your job performance, which is often referred to as *constructive feedback*. Constructive feedback involves giving opinions about a person's work and making helpful suggestions for change. The feedback may be positive or negative, but it is given in a non-aggressive way. Here are some ideas for handling feedback and using it to your benefit:

- Listen to the message that is being sent. Try not to become upset or angry, which may prevent you from truly understanding the message.

- Hostile criticism is not the same thing as constructive feedback. Hostile criticism is angry and negative. Examples are, "You are useless!" or "You are lazy and slow." You should not receive hostile criticism from your employer or supervisor. You may experience hostile criticism from residents, clients, family members, or others. The best response is to say something like, "I'm sorry you are so disappointed," and nothing more. Give the person a chance to calm down before trying to discuss their comments.

- Constructive feedback may come from your employer, supervisor, or other people. Constructive feedback is intended to help you improve. Examples are, "You really need to be more accurate in your charting," or "You are late too often. You'll have to make more of an effort to be on time." Listening to, accepting, and acting on constructive feedback can help you be more successful in your job. Pay attention to it.

- If you are not sure how to avoid a mistake you have made, always ask the person giving feedback for suggestions on improving your performance (Fig. 31-7).

- Apologize and move on. If you have made a mistake, apologize as needed (Fig. 31-8). This may be to your supervisor, a resident, or others. Learn what you can from the incident and put it behind you. Do not dwell on it or hold a grudge. Being able to respond professionally to feedback is important for success in any job.

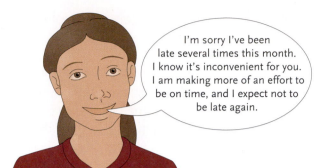

Fig. 31-8. Be willing to apologize if you have made a mistake.

Your evaluation will also cover overall knowledge, conflict resolution, and team effort. Flexibility, friendliness, trustworthiness, and customer service will also be considered. Evaluations are often the basis for salary increases. A positive evaluation can help you advance within the company. Being open to feedback and suggestions for improvement will help you be more successful.

8. Explain how to make job changes

If you decide to change jobs, be responsible. Always give your employer at least two weeks' written notice that you will be leaving. Otherwise, your facility may be understaffed. Both the residents or clients and other staff will suffer. In addition, future employers may talk with past supervisors. People who change jobs too often or who do not give notice before leaving are less likely to be hired.

9. Discuss certification and explain the state's registry

To satisfy the requirements set forth in the Omnibus Budget Reconciliation Act (OBRA), states must regulate nursing assistant training, evaluation, and certification. OBRA requires 75 hours as the minimum level of initial training and a 12-hour minimum for annual continuing education (called *in-services*). Many states' requirements exceed the minimum hours.

After completing an approved training program, nursing assistants (NAs) are given a competency

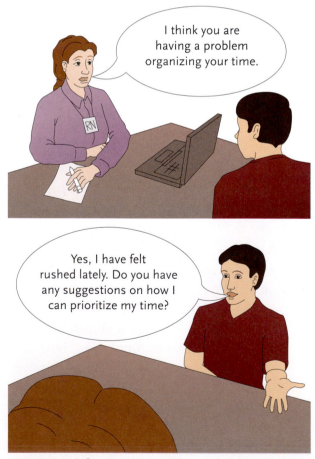

Fig. 31-7. Ask for suggestions when receiving constructive criticism.

evaluation (a certification exam or test) so that they can be certified to work in a state. This exam usually has both a written and skills evaluation. You must pass both parts in order to be certified to work as a nursing assistant.

OBRA also requires that each state keep a registry of nursing assistants. This registry is maintained by a state department, often by the state's Board of Nursing or Department of Health. The registry contains nursing assistants' training information, results of certification exams, and any findings of abuse, neglect, or theft by nursing assistants. Employers are able to access this list to verify that you have passed the certification exam, as well as to check if your certification is current. They are also able to see if you have been investigated for or found guilty of any abuse or neglect.

Nursing assistant registries are also a good source of information for nursing assistants. By contacting the department that oversees the registry, you can find out how you may be able to move your certification from one state to another state. This is called *reciprocity*.

Each state has different requirements for maintaining certification. Learn your state's requirements. Follow them exactly, or you will not be able to keep working. Once you are certified, you can lose your certification if you fail to follow your state's rules. Usually this occurs if you do not work in long-term care for a period of time or fail to get the required number of continuing education hours. You can also lose certification due to criminal activities, including abuse and neglect. For your state, make sure you know the following:

- How quickly after completing a training program you must take and pass the certification exam

- How many days per year you must work in long-term care to maintain your certification

- How many hours of continuing education you must take each year

Some states have a registry for home health aides like the one they maintain for nursing as-

sistants. Ask your employer how best to maintain your certification.

10. Describe continuing education

The federal government requires that nursing assistants and home health aides have a 12-hour minimum of annual continuing education. Many states may require more. In-service continuing education courses help you keep your knowledge and skills fresh. Classes may also provide you with more information about certain conditions, challenges you face in working with residents/clients, or regulation changes. You need to be up-to-date on the latest that is expected of you.

If you need more instruction in a particular area, speak to your supervisor. Perhaps she can arrange for an in-service continuing education class to be offered on that topic. Your employer may be responsible for offering continuing education courses. However, you are responsible for attending and completing them. Specifically, you must do the following:

- Sign up for the course or find out where it is offered.

- Attend all class sessions.

- Pay attention and complete all the class requirements.

- Make the most of your in-service programs. Participate (Fig. 31-9).

- Keep original copies of all certificates and records of your successful attendance so you can prove you took the class.

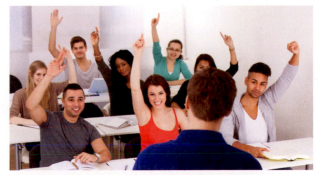

Fig. 31-9. *Pay attention and participate during continuing education courses.*

Caring for Your Career and Yourself

11. Define *stress* and *stressors*

Stress is the state of being frightened, excited, confused, in danger, or irritated. It is often thought that only bad things cause stress. However, positive situations cause stress, too. For example, getting married or having a new baby are usually positive situations. However, both can cause enormous stress because of the changes they bring to a person's life (Fig. 31-10).

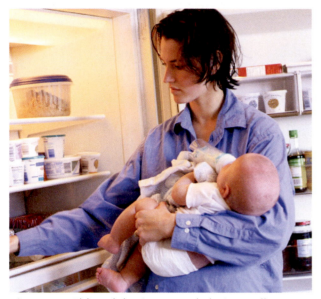

Fig. 31-10. *Although having a new baby is usually a happy time, it can also be a stressful one.*

You may be thrilled when you get your new job. But starting work may also cause you stress. You may be afraid of making mistakes, excited about earning money or helping people, or confused about your new duties. Learning how to recognize stress and what causes it is helpful. Then you can master a few simple techniques for relaxing and learn to manage stress. (Related to managing stress, defense mechanisms are unconscious behaviors used to cope with stress. Chapter 20 contains more information.)

A **stressor** is something that causes stress. Anything can be a stressor if it causes you stress. Some examples include the following:

* Divorce
* Marriage
* New baby
* Parenthood
* Children growing up
* Children leaving home
* Feeling unprepared for a task
* Starting a new job
* Problems at work
* New responsibilities at work
* Feeling unsupported at work (not enough guidance and resources)
* Losing a job
* Supervisors
* Coworkers
* Residents or clients
* Illness
* Finances

12. Explain ways to manage stress

Stress is not only an emotional response. It is also a physical response. When a person experiences stress, changes occur in the body. The endocrine system produces more of the hormone adrenaline. This can increase nervous system response, heart rate, respiratory rate, and blood pressure. This is why, in stressful situations, your heart beats fast, you breathe hard, and you may feel warm or perspire.

Each person has a different tolerance level for stress. In other words, what one person would find overwhelming might not bother another person. A person's tolerance for stress depends on his personality, life experiences, and physical health.

Guidelines: Managing Stress

To manage the stress in your life, develop healthy dietary, exercise, and lifestyle habits:

G Eat nutritious foods.

G Exercise regularly. You can exercise alone or with partners (Fig. 31-11).

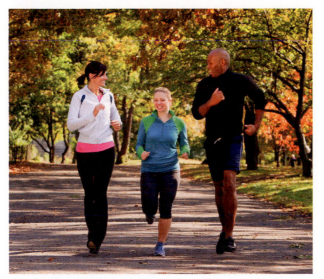

Fig. 31-11. Regular exercise is one healthy way to decrease stress.

G   Get enough sleep.

G   Drink only in moderation.

G   Do not smoke.

G   Find time at least a few times a week to do something relaxing, such as reading a book, watching a movie, sewing, or any of the following:

- Being in nature
- Doing something artistic (painting, drawing, writing, singing, etc.)
- Doing yoga
- Getting a massage
- Listening to music
- Meditating

Not managing stress can cause many problems. Some of these problems affect how well you do your job. Signs that you are not managing stress include the following:

- Showing anger or being abusive to residents/clients
- Arguing with your supervisor about assignments
- Having poor relationships with coworkers and residents/clients

- Complaining about your job and your responsibilities
- Feeling work-related burnout (burnout is a state of mental or physical exhaustion caused by prolonged stress)
- Feeling tired even when you are rested
- Having a difficult time focusing on residents/clients and procedures

Stress can seem overwhelming when you try to handle it yourself. Often just talking about stress can help you manage it better. Sometimes another person can offer helpful suggestions for managing stress. You may be able to think of new ways to handle stress by talking it through with another person. Get help from one or more of these resources when managing stress:

- Your supervisor or another member of the care team for work-related stress
- Your family
- Your friends
- A support group (Fig. 31-12)
- Your place of worship
- Your doctor
- A local mental health agency
- Any phone hotline that deals with related problems (check online)

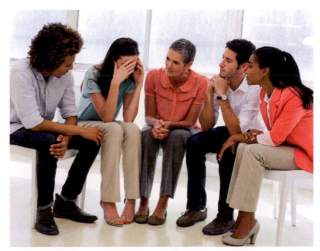

Fig. 31-12. Support groups can help people deal with different types of stress.

It is not appropriate to talk to your residents or clients or their family members about your personal or job-related stress.

Developing a plan for managing stress can be very helpful. The plan can include nice things you will do every day and things to do in stressful situations. When you think about a plan, first answer these questions:

- What are the sources of stress in my life?

- When do I most often feel stress?

- What effects of stress do I see in my life?

- What can I change to decrease the stress I feel?

- What do I have to learn to cope with because I cannot change it?

When you have answered these questions, you will have a clearer picture of the challenges you face. Then you can try to come up with strategies for managing stress.

13. Describe a relaxation technique

Sometimes a relaxation exercise can help you feel refreshed and relaxed in only a short time. Below is a simple relaxation exercise. Try it out. See if it helps you feel more relaxed.

The body scan. Close your eyes. Focus on your breathing and posture. Be sure you are comfortable. Starting at the balls of your feet, concentrate on your feet. Discover any tension hidden in the feet, and try to relax and release the tension. Continue very slowly. Take a breath between each body part. Move up from the feet, focusing on and relaxing the legs, knees, thighs, hips, stomach, back, shoulders, neck, jaw, eyes, forehead, and scalp. Take a few very deep breaths and open your eyes.

This exercise takes only about two minutes. If you find it helpful, try it the next time you need a break, at work or at home.

14. List ways to remind yourself of the importance of the work you have chosen to do

Look back over all you have learned in this program. Your work as a caregiver is very important. Every day may be different and challenging. In a hundred ways every week you will offer help that only a caring person like you can give.

Do not forget to value the work you have chosen to do. It is important. Your work can mean the difference between living with independence and dignity and living without. The difference you make is sometimes life versus death. Look in the face of each of your residents and clients. Know that you are doing important work. Look in a mirror when you get home and be proud of how you make your living (Fig. 31-13).

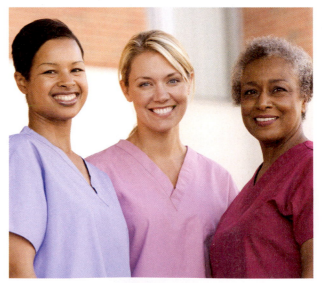

Fig. 31-13. *Being proud of the work you have chosen to do is important.*

Being able to reflect on how you spend your time is an important life skill. Learn ways to fully appreciate that what you do has great meaning. Few jobs have the challenges and rewards of working with people who are elderly, ill, or disabled. Congratulate yourself for choosing a path that includes helping others along the way.

Chapter Review

1. What are direct service positions?

2. List two resources that are helpful in identifying potential employers.

3. List three documents that a person should bring with him when applying for a job.

4. What should be done before writing anything on a job application?

5. List 10 ways to show potential employers professionalism during an interview.

6. How should a nursing assistant or home health aide follow up on a job interview?

7. What is contained in a job description?

8. List four guidelines to follow while working on resolving conflict.

9. What is constructive feedback?

10. Why might an employer not hire a person who has changed jobs often?

11. What information does a registry for certified nursing assistants include?

12. How many hours of continuing education does the federal government require that nursing assistants have each year?

13. What is stress? Give three examples of stressors you have experienced in the last year.

14. List five guidelines for managing stress.

15. What are five resources that are appropriate for an NA or HHA to use when trying to manage stress?

16. Before developing a stress management plan, what are four questions that a person should ask herself?

17. What do you think you will like best about being a nursing assistant or home health aide?

Abbreviations

abd	abdomen
ABR	absolute bedrest
ac, a.c.	before meals
ad lib	as desired
ADLs	activities of daily living
adm.	admission
AIDS	acquired immune deficiency syndrome
amb	ambulate, ambulatory
amt	amount
ap	apical
AROM	active range of motion
ASAP	as soon as possible
as tol	as tolerated
ax.	axillary (armpit)
BID, b.i.d.	two times a day
BM	bowel movement
BP, B/P	blood pressure
BPM	beats per minute
BR	bedrest
BRP	bathroom privileges
BSC	bedside commode
$\bar{c}$	with
C	Centigrade
CA	cancer
cath.	catheter
CBC	complete blood count

CBR	complete bedrest
CCU	cardiac care unit, cardiovascular care unit
CDC	Centers for Disease Control and Prevention
C. diff	*Clostridium difficile*
CHF	congestive heart failure
ck ✓	check
cl liq	clear liquid
CMS	Centers for Medicare and Medicaid Services
CNA	certified nursing assistant
CNS	central nervous system
c/o	complains of, in care of
COPD	chronic obstructive pulmonary disease
CPR	cardiopulmonary resuscitation
CS	Central Supply
CVA	cerebrovascular accident, stroke
CVP	central venous pressure
CXR	chest X-ray
DAT	diet as tolerated
DM	diabetes mellitus
DNR	do not resuscitate
DOA	dead on arrival
DOB	date of birth

DON	director of nursing
Dr., DR	doctor
drsg	dressing
DVT	deep vein thrombosis
Dx, dx	diagnosis
ECG, EKG	electrocardiogram
EMS	emergency medical services
ER	emergency room
exam	examination
F	Fahrenheit
FBS	fasting blood sugar
FF	force fluids
ft	foot
F/U, f/u	follow-up
FWB	full weight-bearing
FYI	for your information
geri chair	geriatric chair
GI	gastrointestinal
H_2O	water
h, hr, hr.	hour
H/A, HA	headache
HBV	hepatitis B virus
HHA	home health aide
HIPAA	Health Insurance Portability and Accountability Act
HIV	human immunodeficiency virus
HOB	head of bed
HS, hs	hours of sleep
ht	height
HTN	hypertension

hyper	above normal, too fast, rapid
hypo	low, less than normal
ICU	intensive care unit
inc	incontinent
I&O	intake and output
isol	isolation
IV, I.V.	intravenous (within a vein)
L, lt	left
lab	laboratory
lb.	pound
lg	large
LOC	level of consciousness
LPN	licensed practical nurse
LTC	long-term care
LTCF	long-term care facility
LVN	licensed vocational nurse
MD, M.D.	medical doctor
MDS	minimum data set
meds	medications
MI	myocardial infarction
min	minute
mL	milliliter
mm Hg	millimeters of mercury
mod	moderate
MRSA	methicillin-resistant *Staphylococcus aureus*

NA	nursing assistant
N/A	not applicable
N/C	no complaints, no call
NG, ng	nasogastric
NKA	no known allergies
NKDA	no known drug allergies
NPO	nothing by mouth
NVD	nausea, vomiting, and diarrhea
NWB	non-weight-bearing
OBRA	Omnibus Budget Reconciliation Act
OOB	out of bed
OR	operating room
OSHA	Occupational Safety and Health Administration
OT	occupational therapist/therapy
oz	ounce
$\bar{p}$	after
pc, p.c.	after meals
PCA	patient-controlled analgesia
PEG	percutaneous endoscopic gastrostomy
peri care	perineal care
per os	by mouth
PHI	protected health information
PNS	peripheral nervous system
PO	by mouth

post-op	after surgery
PPE	personal protective equipment
pre-op	before surgery
p.r.n., prn	when necessary
PROM	passive range of motion
PT	physical therapist/therapy
PVD	peripheral vascular disease
PWB	partial weight-bearing
$\bar{q}$	every
q2h	every two hours
q3h	every three hours
q4h	every four hours
qh, qhr	every hour
R	respirations, rectal
R, rt.	right
RBC	red blood cell/count
rehab	rehabilitation
res.	resident
resp.	respiration
RF	restrict fluids
R.I.C.E.	rest, ice, compression, elevation
RN	registered nurse
R/O	rule out
ROM	range of motion
RR	respiratory rate
$\bar{s}$	without
SDS	safety data sheet
SNF	skilled nursing facility

SOB	shortness of breath
SP	Standard Precautions
spec.	specimen
S&S, S/S	signs and symptoms
SSE	soapsuds enema
staph	*staphylococcus*
stat, STAT	immediately
std. prec.	Standard Precautions
STI	sexually transmitted infection
strep	*streptococcus*
T., temp	temperature
TB	tuberculosis
TIA	transient ischemic attack
t.i.d., tid	three times a day
TLC	tender loving care
TPR	temperature, pulse, and respiration
TWE	tap water enema
U/A, u/a	urinalysis
URI	upper respiratory infection
UTI	urinary tract infection
VRE	vancomycin resistant *enterococcus*
VS, vs	vital signs
WBC	white blood cell/ count
w/c, W/C	wheelchair
WNL	within normal limits
wt.	weight

Symbols

©	copyright
&	and
☣	biohazard
△	change, heat
°	degree
♀	female
♂	male
%	percent
☢	radiation

Appendix

Basic Math Skills

Nursing assistants need math skills when doing certain tasks, such as calculating intake and output. A basic math review is listed below:

Addition

```
      2,905                53,138
+       174          +      3,008
      3,079                56,146
```

Subtraction

```
     32,542               549,233
–     8,710          –     26,903
     23,832               522,330
```

Multiplication

```
      4,962                    79
x        13          x         41
     14,886                    79
+    49,620          +      3,160
     64,506                 3,239
```

Division

```
        34                     39
22 | 748             14 | 546
   – 660                  – 420
      88                    126
    – 88                  – 126
       0                      0
```

Converting Decimals, Fractions, and Percentages

Decimals, fractions, and percentages are different ways of showing the same value. For example, one-half can be written in the following ways:

As a decimal: 0.5
As a fraction: 1/2
As a percentage: 50%

Here are common values shown in decimal, fraction, and percentage forms:

Decimal	Fraction	Percentage
0.01	1/100	1%
0.1	1/10	10%
0.2	1/5	20%
0.25	1/4	25%
0.333	1/3	33.3%
0.5	1/2	50%
0.75	3/4	75%
1	1/1	100%

Follow these rules for converting decimals, fractions, and percentages:

To convert **from a decimal to a percentage**, you will multiply by 100 and add a percent sign (%).

.25 x 100 = 25%

To convert **from a percentage to a decimal**, you will divide by 100 and delete the percent sign (%).

80% ÷ 100 = 0.8

To convert **a fraction to a decimal**, you will divide the top number by the bottom number.

$$\frac{2}{3} = 2 \div 3 = 0.67$$

To convert a **decimal to a fraction**, write the decimal over the number 1.

Step 1 $\dfrac{0.5}{1}$

Then multiply top and bottom by 10 for every number after the decimal point (10 for 1 number, 100 for 2 numbers, and so on).

Step 2 $\dfrac{0.5}{1} \cdot \dfrac{\times 10}{\times 10} = \dfrac{5}{10}$

The resulting fraction is 5/10 (or 1/2 if you simplify the fraction).

To convert a **fraction to a percentage**, you will divide the top number by the bottom number. Then you multiply the result by 100, and add a percent sign (%).

Step 1 $\dfrac{3}{5} = 3 \div 5 = 0.6$

Step 2 $0.6 \times 100 = 60\%$

To convert a **percentage to a fraction**, first convert to a decimal by dividing by 100. Then use the steps for converting a decimal to a fraction.

Step 1 $15\% \div 100 = 0.15$

Step 2 $\dfrac{0.15}{1}$

Step 3 $\dfrac{0.15}{1} \times \dfrac{100}{100} = \dfrac{15}{100}$

The resulting fraction is 15/100 (or 3/20 if you simplify the fraction).

Other Useful Information

Multiplication Table

1	2	3	4	5	6	7	8	9	10	11	12
2	4	6	8	10	12	14	16	18	20	22	24
3	6	9	12	15	18	21	24	27	30	33	36
4	8	12	16	20	24	28	32	36	40	44	48
5	10	15	20	25	30	35	40	45	50	55	60
6	12	18	24	30	36	42	48	54	60	66	72
7	14	21	28	35	42	49	56	63	70	77	84
8	16	24	32	40	48	56	64	72	80	88	96
9	18	27	36	45	54	63	72	81	90	99	108
10	20	30	40	50	60	70	80	90	100	110	120
11	22	33	44	55	66	77	88	99	110	121	132
12	24	36	48	60	72	84	96	108	120	132	144

Conversions: Volume

1 ounce (oz) = 30 mL

¼ cup = 2 oz = 60 mL

½ cup = 4 oz = 120 mL

1 cup = 8 oz = 240 mL

1 liter (L) = 1000 mL

2 pints = 1 quart (qt) = 960 mL

2 quarts = ½ gallon (gal) = 2 liters (L)

4 quarts = 1 gallon (gal)

Conversions: Weight

1 kilogram (kg) = 2.2 pounds (lbs)

1 gram (g) = 1000 milligrams (mg)

1 pound (lb) = 16 ounces (oz)

Conversions: Length

1 inch (in) = 2.54 centimeters (cm) (or round off to 2.5)

12 inches = 1 foot (ft)

3 feet = 1 yard (yd)

10 millimeters (mm) = 1 centimeter (cm)

100 centimeters (cm) = 1 meter

Glossary

24-hour urine specimen: a urine specimen consisting of all urine voided by a person in a 24-hour period.

abdominal thrusts: a method of attempting to remove an object from the airway of someone who is choking.

abduction: moving a body part away from the midline of the body.

abrasion: an injury that rubs off the surface of the skin.

absorption: the transfer of nutrients from the intestines to the cells.

abuse: purposeful mistreatment that causes physical, mental, or emotional pain or injury to someone.

acquired immune deficiency syndrome (AIDS): the final stage of HIV infection, in which infections, tumors, and central nervous system symptoms appear due to a weakened immune system that is unable to fight infection.

active assisted range of motion (AAROM): exercises to put a joint through its full arc of motion that are performed by a person with some help from the affected person.

active neglect: the purposeful failure to provide needed care, resulting in harm to a person.

active range of motion (AROM): exercises to put a joint through its full arc of motion that are performed by the affected person alone, without help.

activities of daily living (ADLs): personal daily care tasks, such as bathing, dressing, caring for teeth and nails, eating, drinking, walking, transferring, and elimination.

acute care: 24-hour skilled care given in hospitals and ambulatory surgical centers for people who require short-term, immediate care for illnesses and injuries.

acute illness: an illness that has rapid onset, is usually short-term, and is treated immediately.

adaptive devices: special equipment that helps a person who is ill or disabled to perform activities of daily living; also called *assistive devices*.

additive: a substance added to another substance that changes its effect.

adduction: moving a body part toward the midline of the body.

adult day services: care for people who need some assistance or supervision during certain hours, but who do not live in the facility where care is given.

advance directives: legal documents that allow people to decide what medical care they wish to have if they are unable to make those decisions themselves.

affected side: a weakened side of the body due to a stroke or injury; also called *involved side*.

ageism: prejudice toward, stereotyping of, and/or discrimination against older persons or the elderly.

age-related macular degeneration (AMD): a condition in which the macula gradually deteriorates, causing vision loss and problems such as the inability to recognize faces, drive, read, and write.

agitated: the state of being excited, restless, or troubled.

agnostics: people who believe that they do not know or cannot know if God exists.

AIDS dementia complex: a group of symptoms including memory loss, poor coordination, paralysis, and confusion that occurs in the late stages of AIDS due to damage to the central nervous system.

alternative medicine: practices and treatments used instead of conventional healthcare methods.

Alzheimer's disease: a progressive, incurable disease that causes tangled nerve fibers and protein deposits to form in the brain, which eventually cause dementia.

ambulation: walking.

ambulatory: capable of walking.

amputation: the surgical removal of some or all of a body part, usually a hand, arm, leg, or foot.

anesthesia: the use of medication to block pain during surgery and other medical procedures.

angina pectoris: chest pain, pressure, or discomfort.

anorexia: an eating disorder in which a person does not eat or exercises excessively to lose weight.

antimicrobial: an agent that destroys, resists, or prevents the development of pathogens.

anxiety: uneasiness, worry, or fear, often about a situation or condition.

apathy: lack of interest in activities.

apical pulse: the pulse located on the left side of the chest, just below the nipple.

apnea: the absence of breathing.

arthritis: a general term that refers to inflammation of the joints, causing stiffness, pain, and decreased mobility.

artificial airway: any tube inserted into the respiratory tract to maintain or promote breathing.

aspiration: the inhalation of food, drink, or foreign material into the lungs.

assault: a threat to harm a person, resulting in the person feeling fearful that he or she will be harmed.

assisted living: residences for people who do not need 24-hour skilled care, but do require some help with daily care.

assistive devices: special equipment that helps a person who is ill or disabled to perform activities of daily living; also called *adaptive devices*.

asthma: a chronic inflammatory disease that causes difficulty breathing, coughing, and wheezing.

atheists: people who believe that there is no God.

atherosclerosis: a hardening and narrowing of the blood vessels.

atrophy: the wasting away, decreasing in size, and weakening of muscles from lack of use.

autoimmune illness: an illness in which the body's immune system attacks normal tissue in the body.

axillae: underarms.

baseline: an initial value that can be compared to future measurements.

basted: coated with juices or other liquid during roasting.

battery: the intentional touching of a person without his or her consent.

bed rest: stopping all activity and staying in bed in order to prevent labor from starting before a baby is ready to be born.

benign prostatic hypertrophy (BPH): a disorder that can occur in men as they age, in which the prostate becomes enlarged and causes problems with urination.

benign tumors: tumors that are considered noncancerous.

bias: prejudice.

biodegradable: capable of breaking down or being decomposed by bacterial or other living organisms.

bipolar disorder: a type of mood disorder that causes mood swings, changes in energy levels and the ability to function, periods of extreme activity, and periods of extreme depression.

bisexual, bi: a person whose physical, emotional, and/or romantic attraction may be for people of the same gender or different gender.

bloodborne pathogens: microorganisms found in human blood, body fluid, draining wounds, and mucous membranes that can cause infection and disease in humans.

Bloodborne Pathogens Standard: federal law that requires that healthcare facilities protect employees from bloodborne health hazards.

body mechanics: the way the parts of the body work together when a person moves.

bones: rigid connective tissues that make up the skeleton, protect organs, and allow the body to move.

bony prominences: areas of the body where the bone lies close to the skin.

brachial pulse: the pulse located inside the elbow, about one to one-and-a-half inches above the elbow.

bradypnea: slow breathing.

bronchiectasis: a condition in which the bronchial tubes are abnormally enlarged, causing chronic coughing, thick sputum, recurrent pneumonia, and weight loss.

bronchitis: an irritation and inflammation of the lining of the bronchi.

bulimia: an eating disorder in which a person eats huge amounts of foods or very fattening foods, and then eliminates the food by vomiting, using laxatives, or exercising excessively.

cancer: general term to describe a disease in which abnormal cells grow in an uncontrolled way.

cardiopulmonary resuscitation (CPR): medical procedures used when a person's heart or lungs have stopped working.

cataract: a condition in which cloudy spots develop in the lens of the eye, causing vision loss.

catastrophic reaction: reacting to something in an unreasonable, exaggerated way.

catheter: a thin tube inserted into the body to drain fluids or inject fluids.

causative agent: a pathogenic microorganism that causes disease.

C cane: a straight cane with a curved handle at the top.

cells: basic structural units of the body that divide, develop, and die, renewing tissues and organs.

Centers for Disease Control and Prevention (CDC): a federal government agency that issues guidelines to protect and improve the health of individuals and communities.

Centers for Medicare & Medicaid Services (CMS): a federal agency within the U.S. Department of Health and Human Services that is responsible for Medicare and Medicaid, among many other responsibilities.

central nervous system (CNS): the part of the nervous system that is composed of the brain and spinal cord.

cerebrovascular accident (CVA): a condition that occurs when blood supply to a part of the brain is blocked or a blood vessel leaks or ruptures within the brain; also called *stroke*.

Cesarean section (C-section): a surgical procedure in which a baby is delivered through an incision in the mother's abdomen.

chain of command: the line of authority within a facility or agency.

chain of infection: a way of describing how disease is transmitted from one human being to another.

chancres: open sores.

charting: documenting information and observations about residents.

chest tubes: hollow drainage tubes that are inserted into the chest to drain air, blood or other fluid, or pus that has collected inside the pleural cavity or space.

Cheyne-Stokes: alternating periods of slow, irregular breathing and rapid, shallow breathing, along with periods of not breathing.

chickenpox: a highly contagious viral illness that affects nearly all children.

child abuse: the physical, emotional, or sexual mistreatment of children.

child neglect: the purposeful or unintentional failure to provide for the needs of a child.

chlamydia: a type of sexually transmitted infection that is caused by organisms introduced into the mucous membranes of the reproductive tract; causes yellow or white discharge from the penis or vagina, burning during urination, swollen testes, painful intercourse, and abdominal and lower back pain.

chronic illness: a disease or condition that is long-term or long-lasting and requires management of symptoms.

chronic obstructive pulmonary disease (COPD): a chronic, progressive, and incurable lung disease that causes difficulty breathing, weakness, and a high risk for lung infections.

chronic renal failure (CRF): a condition that occurs when the kidneys cannot eliminate certain waste products from the body; also called *chronic kidney failure.*

circadian rhythm: the 24-hour day-night cycle.

circumcision: the removal of part of the foreskin of the penis.

cisgender: a person whose gender identity matches his or her birth sex (sex assigned at birth due to anatomy).

cite: in a long-term care facility, to find a problem through a survey.

claustrophobia: the fear of being in a confined space.

clean: in health care, a condition in which objects are not contaminated with pathogens.

clean-catch specimen: a urine specimen that does not include the first and last urine voided in the sample; also called *mid-stream specimen.*

clichés: phrases that are used over and over again and do not really mean anything.

closed bed: a bed completely made with the bedspread and blankets in place.

closed fracture: a broken bone that does not break the skin.

Clostridium difficile (C. diff, C. difficile): a bacterium that is spread by spores in feces that are difficult to kill; it causes symptoms such as diarrhea and nausea and can lead to serious inflammation of the colon (colitis).

cognition: the ability to think logically and clearly.

cognitive: related to thinking and learning.

cognitive behavioral therapy (CBT): a type of psychotherapy that is often used to treat anxiety disorders and depression and focuses on skills and solutions that a person can use to modify negative thinking and behavior patterns.

cognitive impairment: the loss of ability to think logically and clearly.

colorectal cancer: cancer of the gastrointestinal tract; also known as *colon cancer.*

colostomy: surgically-created opening through the abdomen into the large intestine to allow stool to be expelled.

combative: violent or hostile.

combustion: the process of burning.

coming out: a continual process of revealing one's sexual orientation or gender identity to others.

communication: the process of exchanging information with others by sending and receiving messages.

compassionate: being caring, concerned, considerate, empathetic, and understanding.

complementary medicine: treatments that are used in addition to the conventional treatments prescribed by a doctor.

complex carbohydrates: carbohydrates that are broken down by the body into simple sugars for energy; found in foods such as bread, cereal, potatoes, rice, pasta, vegetables, and fruits.

compost: a mixture of decaying food and garden waste that is used to improve and fertilize soil.

concentrated formula: a type of formula for infants that is sold in cans or bottles and must be mixed with tap or bottled water before using.

condom catheter: a type of urinary catheter that has an attachment on the end that fits onto the penis; also called *Texas catheter*.

confidentiality: the legal and ethical principle of keeping information private.

confusion: the inability to think logically and clearly.

congestive heart failure (CHF): a condition in which the heart muscle is damaged and is no longer able to pump effectively.

conscientious: guided by a sense of right and wrong; principled.

conscious: the state of being mentally alert and having awareness of surroundings, sensations, and thoughts.

constipation: the inability to eliminate stool, or the infrequent, difficult, and often painful elimination of a hard, dry stool.

constrict: to narrow.

contracture: the permanent and often painful shortening of a muscle or tendon, usually due to a lack of activity.

cross-dresser: typically a heterosexual man who sometimes wears clothing and other items associated with women.

cultural diversity: the different groups of people with varied backgrounds and experiences who live together in the world.

culture: a system of learned beliefs and behaviors that is practiced by a group of people and is often passed on from one generation to the next.

culture change: a term given to the process of transforming services for elders so that they are based on the values and practices of the person receiving care; core values include choice, dignity, respect, self-determination, and purposeful living.

cyanotic: skin that is blue or gray.

dandruff: an excessive shedding of dead skin cells from the scalp.

dangle: to sit up with the legs hanging over the side of the bed in order to regain balance and stabilize blood pressure.

defecation: the act of passing feces from the large intestine out of the body through the anus.

defense mechanisms: unconscious behaviors used to release tension or cope with stress.

degenerative: something that continually gets worse.

dehydration: a serious condition resulting from an inadequate amount of fluid in the body.

delegation: transferring responsibility to a person for a specific task.

delirium: a state of severe confusion that occurs suddenly and is usually temporary.

delusions: persistent false beliefs.

dementia: the serious loss of mental abilities, such as thinking, remembering, reasoning, and communicating.

dental floss: a special kind of string used to clean between teeth.

dentures: artificial teeth.

depression: a type of mood disorder that causes pain, fatigue, apathy, sadness, irritability, anxiety, sleeplessness, and loss of appetite, as well as other symptoms; also called *major depressive disorder*.

dermatitis: an inflammation of the skin causing swollen, reddened, irritated, and itchy skin.

developmental disabilities: disabilities that are present at birth or emerge during childhood that restrict physical and/or mental ability.

diabetes: a condition in which the pancreas produces too little insulin or does not properly use insulin.

diabetic ketoacidosis (DKA): a complication of diabetes that is caused by having too little insulin in the body.

diabetic retinopathy: a complication of diabetes caused by damage to the retina; causes spots, blurred vision, and difficulty seeing well at night and may lead to blindness.

diagnoses: medical conditions determined by a doctor.

dialysis: an artificial means of removing the body's waste products when the kidneys are no longer able to function properly.

diarrhea: the frequent elimination of liquid or semi-liquid feces.

diastole: phase when the heart relaxes or rests.

diastolic: the second measurement of blood pressure; phase when the heart relaxes or rests.

dietary restrictions: rules about what and when individuals can eat.

diet cards: cards that list the resident's name and information about special diets, allergies, likes and dislikes, and other dietary instructions.

digestion: the process of preparing food physically and chemically so that it can be absorbed into the cells.

dilate: to widen.

direct contact: a way of transmitting pathogens through touching the infected person or his secretions.

dirty: in health care, a condition in which objects have been contaminated with pathogens.

disinfection: a process that destroys most, but not all, pathogens; it reduces the pathogen count to a level that is considered not infectious.

disorientation: confusion about person, place, or time.

disposable: to be used only once and then discarded.

disposable razor: a type of razor that is discarded in a biohazard container after one use; requires the use of shaving cream or soap.

diuretics: medications that reduce fluid volume in the body.

doff: to remove.

domestic violence: physical, sexual, or emotional abuse by spouses, intimate partners, or family members.

don: to put on.

do-not-resuscitate (DNR): a medical order that instructs medical professionals not to perform cardiopulmonary resuscitation (CPR) in the event of cardiac or respiratory arrest.

dorsal recumbent: a body position in which a person is flat on her back with her knees flexed and her feet flat on the bed.

dorsiflexion: bending backward.

draw sheet: an extra sheet placed on top of the bottom sheet; used for moving residents.

durable power of attorney for health care: a signed, dated, and witnessed legal document that appoints someone else to make the medical decisions for a person in the event he or she becomes unable to do so.

dysphagia: difficulty swallowing.

dyspnea: difficulty breathing.

edema: swelling caused by excess fluid in body tissues.

edentulous: having no teeth.

electric razor: a type of razor that runs on electricity; does not require the use of soap or shaving cream.

elimination: the process of expelling wastes (made up of the waste products of food and fluids) that are not absorbed into the cells.

elope: in medicine, when a person with Alzheimer's disease wanders away from a protected area and does not return.

emesis: the act of vomiting, or ejecting stomach contents through the mouth and/or nose.

emotional lability: inappropriate or unprovoked emotional responses, including laughing, crying, and anger.

empathy: identifying with the feelings of others.

emphysema: a chronic disease of the lungs that usually results from chronic bronchitis and cigarette smoking.

epilepsy: a brain disorder that results from a disruption in normal electrical impulses in the brain, which causes repeated seizures.

episiotomy: an incision sometimes made in the perineal area during vaginal delivery that enlarges the vaginal opening for the baby's head.

epistaxis: a nosebleed.

ergonomics: the science of designing equipment, areas, and work tasks to make them safer and to suit the worker's abilities.

ethics: the knowledge of right and wrong.

eupnea: normal breathing.

expiration: the process of exhaling air out of the lungs.

exposure control plan: a plan designed to eliminate or reduce employee exposure to infectious material.

expressive aphasia: difficulty communicating thoughts through speech or writing.

extension: straightening a body part.

facilities: in medicine, places where health care is delivered or administered, including hospitals, long-term care facilities, and treatment centers.

fallacy: a false belief.

false imprisonment: the unlawful restraint of someone that affects the person's freedom of movement; includes both the threat of being physically restrained and actually being physically restrained.

farsightedness: the ability to see objects in the distance better than objects nearby; also called *hyperopia*.

fasting: not eating food or eating very little food.

fecal impaction: a hard stool that is stuck in the rectum and cannot be expelled.

fecal incontinence: the inability to control the bowels, leading to an involuntary passage of stool.

financial abuse: the improper or illegal use of a person's money, possessions, property, or other assets.

first aid: emergency care given immediately to an injured person by the first people to respond to an emergency.

flammable: easily ignited and capable of burning quickly.

flatulence: air in the intestine that is passed through the rectum, which can result in cramping or abdominal pain; also called *flatus* or *gas*.

flexion: bending a body part.

fluid balance: taking in and eliminating equal amounts of fluid.

fluid overload: a condition that occurs when the body cannot handle the amount of fluid consumed.

foot drop: a weakness of muscles in the feet and ankles that causes difficulty with the ability to flex the ankles and walk normally.

Fowler's: a semi-sitting body position, in which a person's head and shoulders are elevated 45 to 60 degrees.

fracture: a broken bone.

fracture pan: a bedpan that is flatter than a regular bedpan.

full weight-bearing (FWB): a doctor's order stating that a person has the ability to support full body weight (100%) on both legs.

functional grip cane: a cane that has a straight grip handle.

gait belt: a belt made of canvas or other heavy material that is used to help people who are weak, unsteady, or uncoordinated to walk.

gastroesophageal reflux disease (GERD): a chronic condition in which the liquid contents of the stomach back up into the esophagus.

gastrostomy: a surgically-created opening into the stomach in order to insert a tube.

gay: a person whose physical, emotional, and/or romantic attraction is for people of the same sex.

gender identity: a deeply felt sense of one's gender.

generalized anxiety disorder (GAD): an anxiety disorder that is characterized by chronic anxiety and worry, even when there is no cause for these feelings.

genital herpes: an incurable type of sexually transmitted infection that is caused by a virus; causes painful sores on the genitals.

genital HPV infection: a type of sexually transmitted infection caused by human papillomavirus; may cause genital warts and an abnormal pap test, and can lead to cervical cancer.

geriatrics: the study of health, wellness, and disease later in life.

gerontology: the study of the aging process in people from mid-life through old age.

gestational diabetes: a type of diabetes that appears in pregnant women who have never had diabetes before but who have high glucose levels during pregnancy.

glands: organs that produce and secrete chemicals called hormones.

glaucoma: a disease in which increased pressure inside the eye causes damage that often leads to vision loss and blindness.

glucose: natural sugar.

gonads: sex glands.

gonorrhea: a type of sexually transmitted infection caused by bacteria; signs include white, yellow, or green discharge from the penis, swollen testes, burning during urination, cloudy vaginal discharge, vaginal bleeding between periods, and rectal itching and soreness.

grief: deep distress or sorrow over a loss.

groin: the area from the pubis (area around the penis and scrotum) to the upper thighs.

grooming: practices to care for oneself, such as caring for fingernails and hair.

halitosis: bad breath.

hallucinations: false or distorted sensory perceptions.

hand hygiene: washing hands with either plain or antiseptic soap and water and using alcohol-based hand rubs.

hat: in health care, a plastic collection container that can be inserted into a toilet bowl to collect and measure urine or stool.

healthcare-associated infection (HAI): an infection acquired in a healthcare setting during the delivery of medical care.

health maintenance organizations (HMOs): a method of health insurance in which a person has to use a particular doctor or group of doctors except in case of emergency.

heartburn: a condition that results from a weakening of the sphincter muscle that joins the esophagus and the stomach and causes a burning sensation in the esophagus.

hemiparesis: weakness on one side of the body.

hemiplegia: paralysis on one side of the body.

hemorrhoids: enlarged veins in the rectum or outside the anus that can cause rectal itching, burning, pain, and bleeding.

hepatitis: inflammation of the liver caused by certain viruses and other factors, such as alcohol abuse, some medications, and trauma.

heterosexual: a person whose physical, emotional, and/or romantic attraction is for people of the opposite sex; also known as *straight*.

HIV (human immunodeficiency virus): the virus that attacks the body's immune system and gradually disables it; eventually can cause AIDS.

hoarding: collecting and putting things away in a guarded way.

holistic care: a type of care that involves caring for the whole person—the mind as well as the body.

home health agencies: businesses that arrange for health care and personal services to be provided in the home.

home health care: health care that is provided in a person's home.

homeostasis: the condition in which all of the body's systems are balanced and are working together to maintain internal stability.

hormones: chemical substances created by the body that control numerous body functions.

hospice care: holistic, compassionate care given to people who have approximately six months or less to live.

hygiene: practices that keep bodies clean and healthy.

hypertension: high blood pressure, regularly measuring 140/90 mm Hg or higher.

hyperthyroidism: a condition in which the thyroid produces too much thyroid hormone, causing body processes to speed up, resulting in rapid heartbeat, sweating, weight loss, and nervousness.

hypoglycemia: a complication of diabetes that can result from either too much insulin or too little food; also known as *insulin reaction*.

hypotension: low blood pressure, measuring 90/60 mm Hg or lower.

hypothyroidism: a condition in which the body lacks thyroid hormone, causing the body processes to slow down and resulting in fatigue, weight gain, constipation, and intolerance to cold.

ileostomy: a surgically-created opening into the end of the small intestine to allow stool to be expelled.

impairment: a loss of function or ability.

incident: an accident, problem, or unexpected event during the course of care that is not part of the normal routine in a healthcare facility.

incontinence: the inability to control the bladder or bowels.

indirect contact: a way of transmitting pathogens from touching an object contaminated by the infected person.

indwelling catheter: a type of urinary catheter that remains inside the bladder for a period of time; also called *Foley catheter*.

infection: the state resulting from pathogens invading the body and multiplying.

infection prevention: the set of methods practiced in healthcare facilities to prevent and control the spread of disease.

infectious: contagious.

inflammation: swelling.

informed consent: the process in which a person, with the help of a doctor, makes informed decisions about his or her health care.

input: the fluid a person consumes; also called *intake.*

insomnia: the inability to fall asleep or remain asleep.

inspiration: the process of inhaling air into the lungs.

insulin: a hormone that works to move glucose from the blood and into the cells for energy for the body.

insulin reaction: a complication of diabetes that can result from either too much insulin or too little food; also known as *hypoglycemia.*

intake: the fluid a person consumes; also called *input.*

integument: a natural protective covering.

intervention: a way to change an action or development.

intravenous therapy: the delivery of medication, nutrition, or fluids through a person's vein.

intubation: the passage of a plastic tube through the mouth, nose, or opening in the neck and into the trachea.

involuntary seclusion: the separation of a person from others against the person's will.

involved side: a weakened side of the body due to a stroke or injury; also called *affected side.*

irreversible: unable to be reversed or returned to the original state.

isolate: to keep something separate, or by itself.

jaundice: a condition in which the skin, whites of the eyes, and mucous membranes appear yellow.

joint: the place at which two bones meet.

Joint Commission: an independent, not-for-profit organization that evaluates and accredits healthcare organizations.

Kaposi's sarcoma: a rare form of skin cancer that appears as purple, red, or brown skin lesions.

karma: the belief that all past and present deeds affect one's future and future lives.

kidney stones: stones that form when urine crystallizes in the kidneys, which can block the kidneys and ureters, causing severe pain; also called *renal calculi.*

knee-chest: a body position in which the person is lying on her abdomen with her knees pulled towards the abdomen and her legs separated; arms are pulled up and flexed, and the head is turned to one side.

lactose intolerance: the inability to digest lactose, a type of sugar found in milk and other dairy products.

latent TB infection: a type of tuberculosis in which the person carries the disease but does not show symptoms and cannot infect others.

lateral: a body position in which a person is lying on either side.

laws: rules set by the government to help people live peacefully together and to ensure order and safety.

length of stay: the number of days a person stays in a healthcare facility.

lesbian: a woman whose physical, emotional, and/or romantic attraction is for other women.

leukemia: a form of cancer in which the body's white blood cells are unable to fight disease.

lever: something that moves an object by resting on a base of support.

LGBT: acronym for lesbian, gay, bisexual, and transgender.

LGBTQ: acronym for lesbian, gay, bisexual, transgender, and queer.

liability: a legal term that means someone can be held responsible for harming someone else.

lithotomy: a body position in which a person lies on her back with her hips at the edge of an exam table; legs are flexed, and feet are in padded stirrups.

living will: a document that outlines the medical care a person wants, or does not want, in case he becomes unable to make those decisions.

localized infection: an infection that is limited to a specific location in the body and has local symptoms.

logrolling: moving a person as a unit without disturbing the alignment of the body.

long-term care (LTC): care given in long-term care facilities for people who need 24-hour skilled care.

lung cancer: the growth of abnormal cells or tumors in the lungs.

lymph: a clear yellowish fluid that carries disease-fighting cells called lymphocytes.

major depressive disorder: a type of mood disorder that causes pain, fatigue, apathy, sadness, irritability, anxiety, sleeplessness, and loss of appetite, as well as other symptoms; also called *depression* or *clinical depression*.

malabsorption: the inability to absorb or digest a particular nutrient properly.

malignant tumors: tumors that are cancerous.

malnutrition: poor nutrition due to improper diet.

malpractice: injury to a person due to professional misconduct through negligence, carelessness, or lack of skill.

managed care: a system or strategy of managing health care in a way that controls costs.

mandated reporters: people who are legally required to report suspected or observed abuse or neglect because they have regular contact with vulnerable populations, such as the elderly in care facilities.

mastectomy: the surgical removal of all or part of the breast and sometimes other surrounding tissue.

masturbation: to touch or rub sexual organs in order to give oneself or another person sexual pleasure.

mechanical ventilation: the use of a machine to inflate and deflate the lungs when a person is unable to breathe on his own.

Medicaid: a medical assistance program for people who have a low income, as well as for people with disabilities.

medical asepsis: measures used to reduce and prevent the spread of pathogens.

Medicare: a federal health insurance program for people who are 65 or older, have certain disabilities or permanent kidney failure, or are ill and cannot work.

menopause: the end of menstruation (occurs when a woman has not had a menstrual period for 12 months).

mental health: the normal functioning of emotional and intellectual abilities.

mental illness: a disorder that affects a person's ability to function and often causes inappropriate behavior; confusion, disorientation, agitation, and anxiety are common symptoms.

metabolism: physical and chemical processes by which substances are broken down or transformed into energy or products for use by the body.

microbe: a living thing or organism that is so small that it can be seen only under a microscope; also called *microorganism*.

microorganism: a living thing or organism that is so small that it can be seen only under a microscope; also called *microbe*.

Minimum Data Set (MDS): a detailed form with guidelines for assessing residents in long-term care facilities.

mode of transmission: the method of describing how a pathogen travels.

modified diets: diets prescribed for people who have certain illnesses, conditions, or food allergies; also called *therapeutic* or *special diets.*

MRSA (methicillin-resistant *Staphylococcus aureus*): an antibiotic-resistant infection to methicillin.

mucous membranes: the membranes that line body cavities that open to the outside of the body, such as the linings of the mouth, nose, eyes, rectum, and genitals.

multidrug-resistant organisms (MDROs): microorganisms, mostly bacteria, that are resistant to one or more antimicrobial agents that are commonly used for treatment.

multidrug-resistant TB (MDR-TB): type of tuberculosis that is caused by an organism that is resistant to medication that is used to treat TB.

multiple sclerosis (MS): a progressive disease in which the myelin sheath breaks down over time; without this protective covering, nerves cannot conduct impulses to and from the brain in a normal way.

muscles: groups of tissues that provide movement of body parts, protection of organs, and creation of body heat.

muscular dystrophy (MD): a progressive, inherited disease that causes a gradual wasting away of muscle, weakness, and deformity.

myocardial infarction (MI): a condition that occurs when the heart muscle does not receive enough oxygen because blood flow to the heart is blocked; also called *heart attack.*

nasal cannula: an oxygen delivery device that consists of a piece of plastic tubing that fits around the face and two prongs that fit inside the nose.

nasogastric tube: a feeding tube that is inserted into the nose and goes to the stomach.

nearsightedness: the ability to see things near but not far; also called *myopia.*

neglect: the failure to provide needed care that results in physical, mental, or emotional harm to a person.

negligence: actions, or the failure to act or provide the proper care, that result in unintended injury to a person.

neonatal: pertaining to a newborn infant.

neonate: a newborn baby.

neonatologists: doctors who specialize in caring for newborn babies.

neuropathy: numbness, tingling, and pain in the feet and legs.

nitroglycerin: a medication that helps to relax the walls of the coronary arteries, allowing them to open and get more blood to the heart; comes in tablet, patch, or spray form.

non-intact skin: skin that is broken by abrasions, cuts, rashes, acne, pimples, lesions, surgical incisions, or boils.

nonspecific immunity: a type of immunity that protects the body from disease in general.

nonverbal communication: communication without using words.

non-weight-bearing (NWB): a doctor's order stating that a person is unable to touch the floor or support any body weight on one or both legs.

NPO: abbreviation for *nothing by mouth* from the Latin *nil per os*; medical order that means a person should not have anything to eat or drink.

nutrient: a necessary substance that provides energy, promotes growth and health, and helps regulate metabolism.

nutrition: how the body uses food to maintain health.

objective information: information based on what a person sees, hears, touches, or smells; also called *signs.*

obsessive-compulsive disorder (OCD): an anxiety disorder characterized by obsessive behavior or thoughts, which may cause the person to repeatedly perform a behavior or routine.

obstructed airway: a condition in which something is blocking the tube through which air enters the lungs.

occult: hidden; difficult to see or observe.

Occupational Safety and Health Administration (OSHA): a federal government agency that makes rules to protect workers from hazards on the job.

occupied bed: a bed made while a person is in the bed.

ombudsman: a legal advocate for residents in long-term care facilities who helps resolve disputes and settle conflicts.

Omnibus Budget Reconciliation Act (OBRA): a law passed by the federal government that includes minimum standards for nursing assistant training, staffing requirements, resident assessment instructions, and information on rights for residents.

onset: in medicine, the first appearance of the signs or symptoms of an illness.

open bed: a bed made with linen folded down to the foot of the bed.

open fracture: a broken bone that penetrates the skin; also known as *compound fracture*.

opportunistic infections: infections that invade the body when the immune system is weak and unable to defend itself.

opposition: touching the thumb to any other finger.

oral care: care of the mouth, teeth, and gums.

organs: structural units in the human body that perform specific functions.

orthopnea: shortness of breath when lying down that is relieved by sitting up.

orthosis: a device that helps support and align a limb and improve its functioning; also called *orthotic device*.

orthostatic hypotension: a sudden drop in blood pressure that occurs when a person sits or stands up.

orthotic device: a device that helps support and align a limb and improve its functioning; also called *orthosis*.

osteoarthritis: a common type of arthritis that usually affects the hips, knees, fingers, thumbs, and spine; also called *degenerative joint disease* or *degenerative arthritis*.

osteoporosis: a condition in which bones become porous and brittle, causing them to break easily.

ostomy: a surgically-created opening from an area inside the body to the outside.

outpatient care: care given to people who have had treatments, procedures, or surgeries and need short-term skilled care.

output: all fluid that is eliminated from the body; includes urine, feces, vomitus, perspiration, moisture that is exhaled in the air, and wound drainage.

oxygen concentrator: a box-like device that changes air in the room into air with more oxygen.

oxygen therapy: the administration of oxygen to increase the supply of oxygen to a person's lungs.

pacing: walking back and forth in the same area.

palliative care: care given to people who have serious diseases or who are dying that emphasizes relieving pain, controlling symptoms, and preventing side effects.

panic disorder: a disorder characterized by a person having regular panic attacks or living with constant anxiety about having another attack.

paralysis: the loss of ability to move all or part of the body, which often includes loss of feeling in the affected area.

paraplegia: the loss of function of the lower body and legs.

parenteral nutrition (PN): the intravenous infusion of nutrients administered directly into the bloodstream, bypassing the digestive system.

Parkinson's disease: a progressive, incurable disease that causes a section of the brain to degenerate; causes stiff muscles, stooped posture, shuffling gait, pill-rolling, and tremors.

partial bath: a bath given on days when a complete bed bath, tub bath, or shower is not done; includes washing the face, hands, underarms, and perineum.

partial weight-bearing (PWB): a doctor's order stating that a person is able to support some body weight on one or both legs.

passive neglect: the unintentional failure to provide needed care, resulting in physical, mental, or emotional harm to a person.

passive range of motion (PROM): exercises to put a joint through its full arc of motion that are performed by a caregiver, without the affected person's help.

pathogens: microorganisms that are capable of causing infection and disease.

payers: people or organizations paying for healthcare services.

pediculosis: an infestation of lice.

peptic ulcers: raw sores in the stomach that cause pain, belching, and vomiting.

percutaneous endoscopic gastrostomy (PEG) tube: a feeding tube that is placed into the stomach through the abdominal wall.

perineal care: care of the genital and anal area.

perineum: the genital and anal area.

peripheral nervous system (PNS): part of the nervous system made up of the nerves that extend throughout the body.

peripheral vascular disease (PVD): a disease in which the legs, feet, arms, or hands do not have enough blood circulation due to fatty deposits in the blood vessels that harden over time; causes cold legs, feet, arms, and hands, as well as pain, swelling, and ulcers of the legs and feet.

peristalsis: involuntary contractions that move food through the gastrointestinal system.

perseveration: the repetition of words, phrases, questions, or actions.

personal: relating to life outside one's job, such as family, friends, and home life.

personal protective equipment (PPE): equipment that helps protect employees from serious workplace injuries or illnesses resulting from contact with workplace hazards.

person-centered care: a type of care that places the emphasis on the person needing care and his or her individuality and capabilities.

phantom limb pain: pain in a limb (or extremity) that has been amputated.

phantom sensation: warmth, itching, or tingling from a body part that has been amputated.

phlegm: thick mucus from the respiratory passage.

Physican Orders for Life-Sustaining Treatment (POLST): a medical order that specifies the treatments a person wishes to receive, not what he wishes to avoid, when he is very ill; decisions are based on conversations between the patient and his healthcare providers.

phobia: an intense, irrational fear of or anxiety about an object, place, or situation.

physical abuse: any treatment, intentional or not, that causes harm to a person's body.

pneumonia: a bacterial, viral, or fungal infection that causes acute inflammation in lung tissue, causing fever, chills, cough, greenish sputum, chest pains, and rapid pulse.

policy: a course of action that should be taken every time a certain situation occurs.

portable commode: a chair with a toilet seat and a removable container underneath; also called *bedside commode*.

portal of entry: any body opening on an uninfected person that allows pathogens to enter.

portal of exit: any body opening on an infected person that allows pathogens to leave.

positioning: the act of helping people into positions that promote comfort and health.

postmortem care: care of the body after death.

postoperative: after surgery.

postpartum depression: a type of depression that occurs after giving birth.

posttraumatic stress disorder (PTSD): an anxiety disorder caused by experiencing or witnessing a traumatic experience.

posture: the way a person holds and positions his body.

powdered formula: a type of formula for infants that is sold in cans and is measured and mixed with tap or bottled water.

pre-diabetes: a condition that occurs when a person's blood glucose levels are above normal but not high enough for a diagnosis of type 2 diabetes.

preferred provider organizations (PPOs): a network of providers that contract to provide health services to a group of people.

prehypertension: a condition in which a person has a blood pressure measurement between 120/80 mm Hg and 139/89 mm Hg; indicates that although the person does not currently have hypertension, he is likely to have it in the future.

premature: the term for babies who are born before 37 weeks' gestation (more than three weeks before the due date).

preoperative: before surgery.

pressure injuries: injuries or wounds that result from skin deterioration and shearing; also called *pressure ulcers, pressure sores, bed sores,* or *decubitus ulcers.*

pressure points: areas of the body that bear much of the body weight.

procedure: a method or way of doing something.

professional: having to do with work or a job.

professionalism: the act of behaving properly when working.

progressive: something that continually gets worse or deteriorates.

pronation: turning downward.

prone: a body position in which a person is lying on his stomach, or front side of the body.

prosthesis: a device that replaces a body part that is missing or deformed because of an accident, injury, illness, or birth defect; used to improve a person's ability to function and/or to improve appearance.

protected health information (PHI): a person's private health information, which includes name, address, telephone number, social security number, email address, and medical record number.

providers: people or organizations that provide health care, including doctors, nurses, clinics, and agencies.

psychological abuse: emotional harm caused by threatening, scaring, humiliating, intimidating, isolating, or insulting a person, or by treating him or her as a child.

psychosocial needs: needs that involve social interaction, emotions, intellect, and spirituality.

psychotherapy: a method of treating mental illness that involves talking about one's problems with mental health professionals.

pulse oximeter: a noninvasive device that uses a light to determine the amount of oxygen in the blood.

puree: to blend or grind food into a thick paste of baby food consistency.

quad cane: a cane that has four rubber-tipped feet and a rectangular base.

quadriplegia: the loss of function in the legs, trunk, and arms.

queer: a term used by some people to describe sexual orientation that is not exclusively heterosexual and who may feel that terms such as lesbian and gay are too limiting.

radial pulse: the pulse located on the inside of the wrist, where the radial artery runs just beneath the skin.

range of motion (ROM): exercises that put a particular joint through its full arc of motion.

ready-to-use formula: a type of formula for infants that is sold in bottles and is ready to use.

receptive aphasia: difficulty understanding spoken or written words.

recycling: the process of taking materials that would have been considered waste and turning them into new products.

rehabilitation: care given by specialists to help restore or improve function after an illness or injury.

reincarnation: a belief that some part of a living being survives death to be reborn in a new body.

renovascular hypertension: a condition in which a blockage of arteries in the kidneys causes high blood pressure.

repetitive phrasing: repeating words, phrases, questions, or activites.

reproduce: to create new human life.

reservoir: a place where a pathogen lives and multiplies.

Residents' Rights: numerous rights identified in the OBRA law that relate to how residents must be treated while living in a facility; they provide an ethical code of conduct for healthcare workers.

resistant: a state in which drugs no longer work to kill specific bacteria.

respiration: the process of inhaling air into the lungs and exhaling air out of the lungs.

restorative care: care given after rehabilitation to maintain a person's function, improve his quality of life, and increase his independence.

restraint: a physical or chemical way to restrict voluntary movement or behavior.

restraint alternatives: measures used in place of a restraint or that reduce the need for a restraint.

restraint-free care: an environment in which restraints are not kept or used for any reason.

résumé: a summary or listing of relevant job experience and education.

rheumatoid arthritis: a type of arthritis in which joints become red, swollen, and very painful, resulting in restricted movement and possible deformities.

rigor mortis: the Latin term for the temporary condition after death in which the muscles in the body become stiff and rigid.

rotation: turning a joint.

routine urine specimen: a urine specimen that can be collected any time a person voids.

rummaging: going through drawers, closets, or personal items that belong to oneself or others.

safety razor: a type of razor that has a sharp blade with a special safety casing to help prevent cuts; requires the use of shaving cream or soap.

scabies: a contagious skin infection caused by a tiny mite burrowing into the skin, where it lays eggs; causes intense itching and a skin rash that may look like thin burrow tracks.

scalds: burns caused by hot liquids.

schizophrenia: a type of psychotic disorder that causes problems with thinking, communication, and the ability to manage emotions, make decisions, and understand reality.

scope of practice: defines the tasks that health-care providers are legally allowed to do as permitted by state or federal law.

sedative: an agent or drug that helps calm and soothe a person and may cause sleep.

sentinel event: an unexpected occurrence that results in grave physical or psychological injury or death.

sexual abuse: the forcing of a person to perform or participate in sexual acts against his or her will; includes unwanted touching, exposing oneself, and sharing pornographic material.

sexual harassment: any unwelcome sexual advance or behavior that creates an intimidating, hostile, or offensive working environment.

sexual orientation: a person's physical, emotional, and/or romantic attraction to another person.

sexually transmitted infections (STIs): infections caused by sexual contact with infected people; signs and symptoms are not always apparent.

sharps: needles or other sharp objects.

shearing: rubbing or friction that results from the skin moving one way and the bone underneath it remaining fixed or moving in the opposite direction.

shingles: a skin rash caused by the varicella-zoster virus (VZV) that causes pain, tingling, itching, and a rash of fluid-filled blisters.

shock: a condition that occurs when organs and tissues in the body do not receive an adequate blood supply.

shower chair: a sturdy chair designed to be placed in a bathtub or shower to help a person who is weak be able to bathe in the tub or shower, rather than in bed.

simple carbohydrates: carbohydrates that are found in foods such as sugars, sweets, syrups, and jellies and have little nutritional value.

Sims': a body position in which a person is lying on his left side with the upper knee flexed and raised toward the chest.

situation response: a temporary condition that has symptoms like those of mental illness; possible causes include a personal crisis, temporary physical changes in the brain, side effects from medications, interactions among medications, and severe changes in the environment.

sitz bath: a warm soak of the perineal area to clean perineal wounds and reduce inflammation and pain.

skilled care: medically necessary care given by a skilled nurse or therapist.

slide board: a wooden board that helps transfer people who are unable to bear weight on their legs; also called *transfer board*.

special diets: diets prescribed for people who have certain illnesses, conditions, or food allergies; also called *therapeutic* or *modified diets*.

specific immunity: a type of immunity that protects the body against a particular disease that is invading the body at a given time.

specimen: a sample that is used for analysis in order to try to make a diagnosis.

sphygmomanometer: a device that measures blood pressure.

spiritual: of, or relating to, the spirit or soul.

sputum: thick mucus coughed up from the lungs.

Standard Precautions: a method of infection prevention in which all blood, body fluids, non-intact skin, and mucous membranes are treated as if they were infected with an infectious disease.

sterilization: cleaning measure that destroys all microorganisms, including pathogens.

stethoscope: an instrument designed to listen to sounds within the body.

stoma: an artificial opening in the body.

straight catheter: a type of urinary catheter that is removed immediately after urine is drained.

stress: the state of being frightened, excited, confused, in danger, or irritated.

stressor: something that causes stress.

subacute care: care given in hospitals or in long-term care facilities for people who need less care than for an acute illness, but more care than for a chronic illness.

subjective information: information that a person cannot or did not observe, but is based on something reported to the person that may or may not be true; also called *symptoms*.

substance abuse: the repeated use of legal or illegal substances in a way that is harmful to oneself or others.

sudden infant death syndrome (SIDS): a condition in which babies stop breathing and die for no known reason while asleep.

suffocation: the stoppage of breathing from a lack of oxygen or an excess of carbon dioxide in the body that may result in unconsciousness or death.

sundowning: becoming restless and agitated in the late afternoon, evening, or night.

supination: turning upward.

supine: a body position in which a person lies flat on his back.

surgical asepsis: the state of being completely free of all microorganisms; also called *sterile technique*.

surgical bed: a bed made to accept a resident who is returning to bed on a stretcher.

susceptible host: an uninfected person who could become sick.

sympathy: sharing in the feelings and difficulties of others.

syncope: loss of consciousness; also called *fainting*.

syphilis: a type of sexually transmitted infection caused by bacteria; causes open sores on the penis or inside the vagina, as well as headache, fever, weight loss, and muscle aches.

systemic infection: an infection that travels through the bloodstream and is spread throughout the body, causing general symptoms.

systole: the phase where the heart is at work, contracting and pushing blood out of the left ventricle.

systolic: the first measurement of blood pressure; phase when the heart is at work, contracting and pushing the blood out of the left ventricle.

tachypnea: rapid breathing.

tactful: showing sensitivity and having a sense of what is appropriate when dealing with others.

TB disease: type of tuberculosis in which the person shows symptoms of the disease and can spread it to others.

telemetry: a cardiac monitoring device that sends information about the heart's rhythm and rate to a monitoring station.

terminal illness: a disease or condition that will eventually cause death.

therapeutic diets: diets prescribed for people who have certain illnesses, conditions, or food allergies; also called *special* or *modified diets*.

tissues: groups of cells that perform similar tasks.

tracheostomy: a surgically-created opening through the neck into the trachea.

transfer belt: a belt made of canvas or other heavy material that is used to help people who are weak, unsteady, or uncoordinated to transfer.

transgender: a person whose gender identity conflicts with his or her birth sex (sex assigned at birth due to anatomy).

transient ischemic attack (TIA): a warning sign of a CVA/stroke resulting from a temporary lack of oxygen in the brain; symptoms may last up to 24 hours.

transition: the process of changing genders, which can include legal procedures, medical measures, telling others, and using new pronouns.

transmission: passage or transfer.

Transmission-Based Precautions: a method of infection prevention used when caring for persons who are infected or may be infected with certain infectious diseases.

trauma: severe injury.

trigger: a situation that leads to agitation.

tuberculosis (TB): a highly contagious lung disease that causes fatigue, loss of appetite, slight fever, prolonged coughing, and shortness of breath.

tumor: a cluster of abnormally growing cells.

type 1 diabetes: a type of diabetes in which the pancreas does not produce any insulin; is usually diagnosed in children and young adults and will continue throughout a person's life.

type 2 diabetes: a common form of diabetes in which either the body does not produce enough insulin or the body fails to properly use insulin; typically develops after age 35 and is the milder form of diabetes.

ulceration: the process of eroding away.

ulcerative colitis: a chronic inflammatory disease of the large intestine that causes cramping, diarrhea, pain, rectal bleeding, loss of appetite, and weight loss.

umbilical cord: the cord that connects a baby to the placenta inside the mother's uterus.

unoccupied bed: a bed made while no person is in the bed.

upper respiratory infection (URI): a viral or bacterial infection of the nose, sinuses, and throat, causing nasal discharge, sore throat, fever, and fatigue.

ureterostomy: a surgically-created opening from a ureter to the abdomen for urine to be eliminated.

urinary catheter: a type of catheter that is used to drain urine from the bladder.

urinary incontinence: the inability to control the bladder, which leads to an involuntary loss of urine.

urinary tract infection (UTI): a bacterial infection of the urethra, bladder, ureter, or kidney that results in painful burning during urination and the frequent feeling of needing to urinate.

urination: the act of passing urine from the bladder through the urethra to the outside of the body; also known as *micturition* or *voiding*.

vaginitis: an inflammation of the vagina that may be caused by bacteria, protozoa, or a fungus.

validating: giving value to or approving.

vegans: vegetarians who do not eat any animal products, including milk, cheese, other dairy items, or eggs; vegans may also choose to not use or wear any animal products.

vegetarians: people who do not eat meat, fish, or poultry and may or may not eat eggs and dairy products.

verbal abuse: the use of spoken or written words, pictures, or gestures that threaten, embarrass, or insult a person.

verbal communication: communication involving the use of spoken or written words or sounds.

vital signs: measurements—temperature, pulse, respirations, blood pressure, pain level—that monitor the functioning of the vital organs of the body.

VRE (vancomycin-resistant *enterococus*): bacteria (*enterococci*) that have developed resistance to the antibiotic vancomycin.

walker: a type of walking aid with four rubber-tipped feet and/or wheels that provides stability when a person is unsteady or lacks balance.

wandering: walking aimlessly around the facility or facility grounds.

workplace violence: verbal, physical, or sexual abuse of staff by other staff members, residents, or visitors.

wound: a type of injury to the skin.

yarmulke: a small skullcap worn by Jewish men as a sign of their faith.

Index